Cannabis and Culture

World Anthropology

General Editor

SOL TAX

Patrons

CLAUDE LÉVI-STRAUSS
MARGARET MEAD
LAILA SHUKRY EL HAMAMSY
M. N. SRINIVAS

MOUTON PUBLISHERS · THE HAGUE · PARIS
DISTRIBUTED IN THE USA AND CANADA BY ALDINE, CHICAGO

Cannabis and Culture

Editor
VERA RUBIN

MOUTON PUBLISHERS · THE HAGUE · PARIS
DISTRIBUTED IN THE USA AND CANADA BY ALDINE, CHICAGO

Copyright © 1975 by Mouton & Co. All rights reserved.
No part of this publication may be reproduced,
stored in a retrieval system, or transmitted,
in any form or by any means, electronic, mechanical,
photocopying, recording or otherwise without the
written permission of Mouton Publishers, The Hague
Distributed in the United States of America and Canada
by Aldine Publishing Company, Chicago, Illinois
ISBN 90-279-7669-4 (Mouton)
0-202-01152-6 (Aldine)
Jacket photo: L'Institute pour la recherche
scientifique en Afrique centrale
Cover and jacket design by Jurriaan Schrofer
Indexes by John Jennings
Printed in the Netherlands

General Editor's Preface

This is probably the first exploration of any drug which brings together the range of knowledge required to understand the complexity of the substance and its multiple uses in a broad range of societies. The botany and pharmacology of cannabis, the history of its diffusion and use are examined and differential effects of its use in diverse social and cultural contexts are reported. The cases from many parts of the world which are the special virtue of this volume are especially significant in understanding sociocultural differences in reactions to this ancient and widespread substance. It was equally important that the papers should have been elicited for an international Congress, and discussed by scholars representing the major cultures of the world.

Like most comtemporary sciences, anthropology is a product of the European tradition. Some argue that it is a product of colonialism, with one small and self-interested part of the species dominating the study of the whole. If we are to understand the species, our science needs substantial input from scholars who represent a variety of the world's cultures. It was a deliberate purpose of the IXth International Congress of Anthropological and Ethnological Sciences to provide impetus in this direction. The *World Anthropology* volumes, therefore, offer a first glimpse of a human science in which members from all societies have played an active role. Each of the books is designed to be self-contained; each is an attempt to update its particular sector of scientific knowledge and is written by specialists from all parts of the world. Each volume should be read and reviewed individually as a separate volume on its own given subject. The set as a whole will indicate what changes are in store for anthropology as scholars from the developing countries join in studying the species of which we are all a part.

The IXth Congress was planned from the beginning not only to include as many of the scholars from every part of the world as possible, but also with a view toward the eventual publication of the papers in high-quality volumes, At previous Congresses scholars were invited to bring papers which were then read out loud. There were necessarily limited in length; many were only summarized; there was little time for discussion; and the sparse discussion could only be in one language. The IXth Congress was an experiment aimed at changing this. Papers were written with the intention of exchanging them before the Congress, particularly in extensive pre-Congress sessions; they were not intended to be read at the Congress, that time being devoted to discussions — discussions which were simultaneously and professionally translated into five languages. The method for eliciting the papers was structured to make as representative a sample as was allowable when scholarly creativity — hence self-selection — was critically important. Scholars were asked both to propose papers of their own and to suggest topics for sessions of the Congress which they might edit into volumes. All were then informed of the suggestions and encouraged to rethink their own papers and the topics. The process, therefore, was a continuous one of feedback and exchange and it has continued to be so even after the Congress. The some two thousand papers comprising *World Anthropology* certainly then offer a substantial sample of world anthropology. It has been said that anthropology is at a turning point; if this is so, these volumes will be the historical direction-markers.

As might have been foreseen in the first post-colonial generation, the large majority of the Congress papers (82 percent) are the work of scholars identified with the industrialized world which fathered our traditional discipline and the institution of the Congress itself: Eastern Europe (15 percent); Western Europe (16 percent); North America (47 percent); Japan, South Africa, Australia, and New Zealand (4 percent). Only 18 percent of the papers are from developing areas: Africa (4 percent); Asia-Oceania (9 percent); Latin America (5 percent). Aside from the substantial representation from the U.S.S.R. and the nations of Eastern Europe, a significant difference between this corpus of written material and that of other Congresses is the addition of the large proportion of contributions from Africa, Asia, and Latin America. "Only 18 percent" is two to four times as great a proportion as that of other Congresses; moreover, 18 percent of 2,000 papers is 360 papers, 10 times the number of "Third World" papers presented at previous Congresses. In fact, these 360 papers are more than the total of ALL papers published after the last International Congress of Anthropological and Ethnological Sciences which was held in the United States (Philadelphia, 1956). Even in the beautifully organized Tokyo Congress in 1968 less than a third as many members from developing nations, including those of Asia, participated.

The significance of the increase is not simply quantitative. The input of scholars from areas which have until recently been no more than subject matter for anthropology represents both feedback and also long awaited theoretical contributions from the perspectives of very different cultural, social, and historical traditions. Many who attended the IXth Congress were convinced that anthropology would not be the same in the future. The fact that the next Congress (India, 1978) will be our first in the "Third World" may be symbolic of the change. Meanwhile, sober consideration of the present set of books will show how much, and just where and how, our discipline is being revolutionized.

The conference on cannabis was held in conjunction with one on the use of alcohol, which resulted in a companion volume, *Cross-cultural approaches to the study of alcohol*, edited by M. W. Everett, J. O. Waddell, and D. B. Heath. In this series there are also many volumes directly related to these on mental health, religion, and medical and psychological anthropology; on food; on youth, urbanization, ethnicity and identity problems; and on the variety of cultures of the world as seen traditionally in a process of change.

Chicago, Illinois SOL TAX
July 15, 1975

Acknowledgments

The Conference was supported by a grant to the Smithsonian Institution from the Center for the Studies of Narcotic and Drug Abuse, National Institute of Mental Health. We wish to acknowledge the knowledgeable guidance of Miss Eleanor Carroll of the Center in developing the Conference program, and the able assistance of Mrs. Valerie Ashenfelter and Mr. William Douglass of the Center for the Study of Man (Smithsonian) in organizing the conference and travel arrangements. We also wish to express our appreciation to Mr. James Helsing, Office of Communications, National Institute of Mental Health, for his professional services and to Mrs. June Anderson and the Research Institute for the Study of Man staff for their invaluable support in the preparation of the manuscript for this volume. We are especially thankful to the participants, who made the Conference a pleasant as well as productive experience.

VERA RUBIN

Table of Contents

General Editor's Preface   v

Acknowledgments   IX

Introduction   1
   by *Vera Rubin*

PART ONE: ETHNOBOTANY AND DIFFUSION

Typification of *Cannabis sativa* L.   13
   by *William T. Stearn*

Cannabis: An Example of Taxonomic Neglect   21
   by *Richard Evans Schultes, William M. Klein, Timothy Plowman,* and *Tom E. Lockwood*

Early Diffusion and Folk Uses of Hemp   39
   by *Sula Benet*

The Origin and Use of Cannabis in Eastern Asia: Their Linguistic-Cultural Implications   51
   by *Hui-Lin Li*

Ethnobotanical Aspects of Cannabis in Southeast Asia   63
   by *Marie Alexandrine Martin*

Cannabis Smoking in 13th–14th Century Ethiopia: Chemical Evidence   77
   by *Nikolaas J. van der Merwe*

Dagga: The History and Ethnographic Setting of *Cannabis sativa* in Southern Africa   81
   by *Brian M. du Toit*

PART TWO: SOCIOCULTURAL ASPECTS OF THE TRADITIONAL COMPLEX

The Social Nexus of *Ganja* in Jamaica   119
    by *Lambros Comitas*

The Ritual Use of Cannabis in Mexico   133
    by *Roberto Williams-Garcia*

Cannabis and Cultural Groups in a Colombian *Municipio*   147
    by *William L. Partridge*

Patterns of Marihuana Use in Brazil   173
    by *Harry William Hutchinson*

Economic Significance of *Cannabis sativa* in the Moroccan Rif   185
    by *Roger Joseph*

Traditional Patterns of Hashish Use in Egypt   195
    by *Ahmad M. Khalifa*

The Traditional Role and Symbolism of Hashish among Moroccan Jews in Israel and the Effect of Acculturation   207
    by *Phyllis Palgi*

The Social and Cultural Context of Cannabis Use in Rwanda   217
    by *Helen Codere*

Réunion: Cannabis in a Pluricultural and Polyethnic Society   227
    by *Jean Benoist*

Social Aspects of the Use of Cannabis in India   235
    by *Khwaja A. Hasan*

Cannabis in Nepal: An Overview   247
    by *James Fisher*

The "*Ganja* Vision" in Jamaica   257
    by *Vera Rubin*

PART THREE: MEDICAL, PHARMACOLOGICAL AND ETHNOMETABOLIC STUDIES

Cannabis sativa L. (Marihuana): VI Variations in Marihuana Preparations and Usage — Chemical and Pharmacological Consequences   269
    by *Alvin B. Segelman, R. Duane Sofia*, and *Florence H. Segelman*

Social and Medical Aspects of the Use of Cannabis in Brazil   293
    by *Alvaro Rubim de Pinho*

Sociocultural and Epidemiological Aspects of Hashish Use in
Greece 303
by *C. Stefanis, C. Ballas,* and *D. Madianou*

Marihuana and Genetic Studies in Colombia: The Problem
in the City and in the Country 327
by *B. R. Elejalde*

Cannabis Usage in Pakistan: A Pilot Study of Long Term
Effects on Social Status and Physical Health 345
by *Munir A. Khan, Assad Abbas,* and *Knud Jensen*

The Significance of Marihuana in a Small Agricultural
Community in Jamaica 355
by *Joseph Schaeffer*

Chronic Cannabis Use in Costa Rica: A Description of Research
Objectives 389
by *W. E. Carter* and *W. J. Coggins*

PART FOUR: TRADITIONAL USAGE OF OTHER PSYCHOACTIVE PLANTS

Man, Culture and Hallucinogens: An Overview 401
by *Marlene Dobkin de Rios*

Peyote and Huichol Worldview: The Structure of a Mystic Vision 417
by *Barbara G. Myerhoff*

Magico-Religious Use of Tobacco among South American Indians 439
by *Johannes Wilbert*

Coca Chewing: A New Perspective 463
by *Roderick E. Burchard*

Cannabis or Alcohol: The Jamaican Experience 485
by *Michael H. Beaubrun*

PART FIVE: THE MODERN COMPLEX IN NORTH AMERICA

Cannabis Use in Canada 497
by *Melvyn Green* and *Ralph D. Miller*

Memories, Reflections and Myths: The American Marihuana
Commission 521
by *Louis Bozzetti* and *Jack Blaine*

Sociocultural Factors in Marihuana Use in the United States 531
by *William H. McGlothlin*

Intersections of Anthropology and Law in the Cannabis Area 549
  by *John Kaplan*

Cannabis Conference Participant-Observers 559

Biographical Notes 563

Index of Names 571

Index of Subjects 579

Plates between 266–267

Introduction

VERA RUBIN

Cannabis, the plant that produces hemp as well as hashish, is now known primarily as one of the leading psychoactive plants in world use, following only tobacco and alcohol in popularity. Probably one of the oldest plants known to man, cannabis was cultivated for fiber, food and medicine thousands of years before it became the "superstar" of the drug culture (Schultes 1973).

Public concern about the youth "drug culture," particularly in Western societies, has stimulated unprecedented support for research on various drugs, including cannabis. Most of the research on cannabis has dealt with botanical, biochemical and pharmacological aspects. Sociological surveys have also been undertaken, particularly in the work of various National Commissions, in an effort to determine the epidemiology of marihuana use. More recently, support has been made available for multidisciplinary studies of cannabis use and users in societies where there is long-term traditional use of the plant in various forms.

The papers in this volume were originally presented at a conference on Cross-Cultural Perspectives on Cannabis, convened in Chicago, August 1973, during the IXth International Congress of the International Union of Anthropological and Ethnological Sciences. It brings together much of the contemporary social science data and thought on many world areas where cannabis has been traditionally used as a multipurpose plant, about which there has previously been little or no scientific reporting. The volume also introduces new botanical classifications and presents data on clinical studies of cannabis users.

The Conference was attended by some sixty scientists, in the fields of anthropology, botany, genetics, pharmacology, psychiatry and sociology, involved in various aspects of research on the complexities of cannabis in relation to man and culture.

The major objectives of the Conference were to bring to light existing cross-cultural information on cannabis use in traditional areas and to locate social scientists familiar with cultural factors in cannabis use; to assemble information on ethnobotanical and ethnohistorical questions as well as on contemporary features of cannabis use; to review the work of National Commissions on marihuana and examine some of the legal issues; to provide comparative data on cultural and social class differences in use of and reactions to cannabis; and to compare the traditional uses of cannabis with the Amerindian uses of psychoactive plants such as tobacco and peyote.

While the exact place of origin of cannabis has not yet been determined, it is generally believed to have originated in central Asia and the oldest recorded references to its use are in the ancient literature of China, India and the Near East. Traditional folk use of cannabis undoubtedly has the greatest antiquity as well as the most extensive diffusion in these areas, and a number of the articles included in this volume present various aspects of cannabis use in this part of the world.

Hui-Lin Li, one of the contributors, maintains that the first documented medical uses of cannabis in China, in an herbal text of the second century A.D., chronicles oral traditions passed down from prehistoric times, based on archeological, botanical and linguistic evidence. The antiquity of cannabis as a cultivated species in China, Hui-Lin Li observes, is attested to by its multitudinal uses in ancient times and its important role in the practice of Shamanism. He posits that there was widespread ritual use by the Neolithic peoples of northeast Asia, and that the nomadic tribes carried the plant and its ritual uses to western Asia and to India, where it proliferated. As reported in the article by Khwaja Hasan, medical and sacred use in India is also known to have a long tradition, predating written records.

Sacred use of cannabis in Assyria, Babylon and Palestine has been recorded, and Herodotus described Scythian funeral rites involving purification with vapor from cannabis seeds. This was corroborated by the Soviet archaeologist, S. I. Rudenko. In her article in this volume, Sula Benet traces the derivation of the generic term *Cannabis* from the Hebrew term *kanebosm* that appears both in the Hebrew and Aramaic translations of the Old Testament. Hemp was used for sacred and secular purposes, for the ropes of Solomon's temple and the robes of the priests. Benet surmises that both Scythians and Semites diffused ritual use of the plant to southern and eastern Europe on their westward migrations from Asia Minor. According to the Old Testament, cannabis was among the merchandise carried by caravans on the trade routes of the ancient world. The Old Testament, like the medical and sacred writings of other ancient civilizations, is based on venerable oral traditions.

Determination of the origin of cannabis has recently become a matter for ethnobotanical reconsideration as well as for ethnohistorical reconstruction. The classification by Linnaeus, in 1753, of *Cannabis sativa* as a monotypic species, which has been generally accepted by Western botanists for almost two centuries, is critically examined in two of the articles in this volume. William Stearn, in his analysis of the botanical basis of the Linnaean classification, describes the problems of plant collection at the time and argues that these difficulties limited the possible recognition of other species. Developing this theme, and recognizing the need for investigating wild cannabis in its native habitat, Richard E. Schultes offers a completely revamped approach to cannabis taxonomy. Based on his own field studies and review of the work of Lamarck that has been generally rejected, and that of Soviet botanists, neglected because of linguistic barriers, Schultes proposes a polytypic classification. This article stands as the first major reexamination of the taxonomy of cannabis since Linnaeas and Lamarck and raises serious scientific questions which may well affect long established social and legal conventions.

Recent research interest in cannabis is part of an increased Western interest in the constituents and uses of folk medicinal plants, including psychoactive plants. Schultes has pointed out that only about twenty of the approximately sixty known plant species that have been used as "intoxicants" may be considered of major importance. And of these twenty species, "only a very few — the coca, the opium poppy, cannabis and tobacco — are numbered among the world's commercially important plants" (Schultes 1969:5). Of these four, cannabis is undoubtedly the most extraordinary with respect to the diverse range of purposes for which it has been used by man over the millennia — as food, for mercantile artifacts, for medication as well as an "intoxicant."

Variously known as *charas, dagga, hasish, ganja, kanebosm, kancha, kif, marijuana, mbange, la santa rosa, zamal* — among a myriad of terms — cannabis has had several streams of ethnobotanic diffusion, probably going back to the Neolithic. Two major cultural complexes appear to have encompassed use of the plant over time — a traditional folk stream which reveals remarkable continuity and a contemporary, more circumscribed configuration.

The folk stream is multidimensional and multifunctional, involving both sacred and secular use, and is usually based on small-scale cultivation: ancient use for cordage and clothing; and some use until recent times for home manufactures such as fiber skirts; use in the dietary for seasoning, soups, porridges, stews and sweets; extensive use in folk medicine, for man and beast; use as an energizer and invigorant; ritual use; and general use as a euphoriant and symbol of fellowship. Except for ritual purposes involving members of the priestly class, regular multipurpose use in the folk stream has been generally confined to the lower social classes: peasants, fishermen, rural and urban artisans and manual laborers. The sociocultural components of folk use were first described by the Royal Hemp Commission of 1893, sent to India to examine the alleged pathological effects of *ganja* uses. Given the antiquity and florescence of cannabis use in India and the thorough description in the *Report of the Indian Hemp Drugs Commission* (1969) which provides remarkable ethnographic coverage, it would not be inappropriate to adopt the Hindi term and refer to the folk stream as the "*ganja* complex."

The second stream of dispersion, or expansion, of cannabis use encompasses two major currents with different functions. The first is based on the use of hemp for commercial manufactures utilizing large-scale cultivation primarily as fiber for mercantile purposes mainly in Russia, Canada and the United States. Commercial production of hemp fiber predates the colonial period and was given further impetus with colonization and the rise of mercantile trade. The second current, going back only about a century to the formation of the Club des Hachichins in Paris, is linked mainly to the search for psychedelic experiences. Diffused in the mid-twentieth century to the United States and Canada and Western-oriented youth in traditional cultures, it generally is an upper- and middle-class social phenomenon, limited to the psychedelic function and may be called the "marihuana complex."

The two cultural complexes, then, differ in form, function, and social class composition. It is not possible, at this juncture, to reconstruct exactly the migratory routes of the plant and its uses, but the papers in this volume provide supportive evidence for the "two cultures" of cannabis which have emerged and some of the ethnohistorical background for the diffusion of traditional uses.

Whether through stimulus diffusion or independent experimentation, through the availability of wild species or the cultivation of introduced species, over a wide area of the Old World similar traditional uses and functions of cannabis may be traced. With few exceptions, there has been remarkable continuity in these patterns of use over the centuries, as may be seen in the articles on Asia, China and eastern Europe.

Diffusion on the African continent is examined by Brian du Toit in his article on the ethnohistory of cannabis smoking in southern and eastern Africa. He hypothesizes that cannabis and the pipes used were diffused by Arab traders during the first centuries A.D., and that once it had been introduced it spread to other parts of the continent. While other writers have suggested that cannabis use in Africa, south of the Sahara, is comparatively recent, du Toit's hypothesis is bolstered by Nikolaas van der Merwe's article on an archaeological find in Ethiopia of fourteenth century pipe bowls containing cannabis residue. The introduction of cannabis to Egypt is attributed to mystic devotees from Syria, arriving in the twelfth century, as noted in the article by Ahmad Khalifa.

Given the economic importance of hemp in the period of European expansion, somewhat more information exists on its introduction to the New World, although here, too, there is no precise ethnohistorical documentation and much of this has been reconstructed by anthropological and ethnobotanical research. Cannabis is one of the few psychoactive plants not indigenous to the Western Hemisphere, and was introduced to the New World colonies by the British, Spanish and Portuguese colonizers. Hemp was very important economically during the mercantile period, and the fibers, oil and seeds were of major value for a variety of essential manufactures. Hemp was introduced to the thirteen North American colonies during the seventeenth century and cultivation was vigorously encouraged.

Hemp, in fact, was an article of keen commercial competition among rival colonizing powers since Russia had the world monopoly and hemp manufactures were vital to the shipping industry and, consequently, to the plantation of the colonies. Spain, possibly following the lead of England, introduced hemp to its colonies for mercantile purposes. Introduction of cannabis to Brazil has been attributed to African slaves; however, W. H. Hutchinson proposes that Portuguese sailors may have been another source. Cannabis was used by the Portuguese Royal Court in both Lisbon and Rio de Janeiro. During the colonial period, slaves were permitted to plant *maconha* between the rows of sugar cane.

Hemp for commercial manufacture was also introduced to the West Indies at the end of the eighteenth century but never became an important source of fiber. Multipurpose use (other than for fiber) was introduced to Jamaica in the mid-nineteenth century by the indentured laborers from India, who may have brought with them a different species, *Cannabis indica*, and the essential cultural ingredients of the "*ganja* complex" that eventually spread to the black working class, rural and urban.

From behavioral as well as ethnohistorical considerations, comparison of the cannabis complexes affords an exceptionally interesting point of departure for the social sciences. In *ganja* complex areas, cannabis has been traditionally used by the folk — farmers, fishermen, artisans and manual workers — with elite usage generally confined to the priestly class (e.g., Brahmins in India, priests in the Near East). Upper-class attitudes toward cannabis users have generally been negative; in India, for example, the derogatory term "ganjeri" was used as an epithet, while in Colombia, as William Partridge points out, the poor are stigmatized as "marihuaneros" (whether or not they use marihuana). Nevertheless, traditional use has been extraordinarily well structured and regulated. *Ganja* is used to serve multiple functions, economic, energizing and medicinal, as well as recreational and psychoactive — it is sedative and stimulant, symbol of fellowship and network nucleus, sacred and secular. Reactions to *ganja* are conditioned by cultural expectations, i.e., according to the situational function which it is expected to serve.

The evidence now available concerning traditional use supports data gleaned from the Jamaica project, so far the most extensive multidisciplinary study of the effects of chronic cannabis use in the natural setting. Four papers from that project discuss different aspects of the Jamaican *ganja* complex. Lambros Comitas describes the social networks of cultivation and distribution and patterns of folk use. Vera Rubin discusses the standardized "vision" that sometimes occurs on initiation to *ganja* smoking and validates the role of smoker. Michael Beaubrun presents the medical and psychiatric findings and analyzes differences among alcohol and cannabis users and the effects of chronic consumption. *Ganja* may be a "benevolent alternative" to alcohol. Joseph Schaeffer reports on an intensive study of the acute effects of *ganja* on energy and productivity in a rural community, with data derived from videotaping, techniques for energy measurement and participant observation. Tentative conclusions indicate that while after smoking workers are less productive in certain tasks such as weeding, their productivity in other tasks such as sawing may not be affected and may be increased in tasks like cane loading. The workers' perception of increased energy and their motivation to work is enhanced by the use of *ganja*.

The studies from Morocco, Jamaica and Colombia indicate the economic importance of small-scale cannabis cultivation by peasants and farmers as a cash crop — another important aspect of the *ganja* complex. Cannabis cultivation, distribution and use are central to the development of intricate social networks, given the universal legal sanctions against all of these activities. Cannabis smokers are usually part of male-oriented peer groups, in work parties or recreational settings as reported in the

Introduction 7

papers on Colombia, South Africa, Southeast Asia, Nepal, Morocco, Jamaica and Pakistan. The lone user is a rarity seldom encountered. The "set and setting" determine both the stituational function of cannabis use and the psychocultural effects produced.

Furthermore, cultural screening devices have been developed to eliminate individuals who, for a variety of reasons, may "not have the head for it." This is a significant structural device in societies where the non-smoker is the deviant; it both avoids peer group ostracism and protects individuals who may be psychologically vulnerable to use of the plant. There are folk remedies to overcome any negative reactions that may occur.

An important source of research was brought to light, as a result of conference preparations by Madame Lucille Barash of the Le Dain Commission. The extensive botanical and pharmacological studies conducted in Czechoslovakia on the identification of plants with antibiotic properties have demonstrated the considerable antibiotic and analgesic properties of cannabis. After studying "the ancient herbaria, folk and primitive medicine," it was recognized that "these admirable properties of hemp have been utilized since ancient times" until the end of the nineteenth century when it was "forgotten and abandoned — without justification — in modern pharmacology" (Kabelik 1954:2). The medical conditions for which cannabis treatment is recommended by the Pharmaceutic Faculty of the Hygienic Institute of the Palacky University in Olomouc are among those still being treated by cannabis preparations in *ganja* complex societies.

These traditional uses are in sharp contrast to the contemporary cultural use of cannabis. The "marihuana complex," based primarily on exploitation of the mood-altering potential of the plant, has been the object of great public controversy, particularly in the United States. Apparently introduced to the United States by Mexican laborers about the turn of the century and taken up by black stevedores and jazz musicians, a furor about marihuana use — probably tinged with racist attitudes — was raised in the wake of the moral reform movements of the 1920s. Sensational, unfounded attacks in the following decade on its alleged criminal effects engendered the stereotype of marijuana as a "dangerous drug." Public concern was heightened during the 1960s as the social class character of the cannabis using population changed. Marijuana use spread to middle- and upper-class youth in the United States and was diffused to youth in other countries. The "alienation" and "amotivation" of youth were attributed to marijuana which was also held responsible for "escalation" to other drugs such as heroin and LSD. Scientific controversies sometimes still reflect the values engendered by the anti-marijuana campaigns of the recent past.

Several of the articles are concerned with various aspects of the contemporary middle-class use of marihuana in Colombia, Brazil, Egypt, Réunion, Canada and the United States. William H. McGlothlin examines the social class shift of users in the United States during the 1960s, from lower-class minority groups to youth of higher social classes. He argues that the symbolic role of marihuana in the counter-culture, rather than the pharmacological properties of the plant, was the most important factor in its widespread use. Consequently, he argues, the marihuana "epidemic" can be expected to decline, although a residual group of regular users will remain. Jack Blaine and Louis Bozzetti also indicate that marihuana use may be a "fad" expressing the rejection of social values that would recede in time.

Melvyn Green and Ralph D. Miller report that the "non-medical" use of cannabis in Canada, restricted to middle-class college students in the 1960s, was quickly diffused to older and younger persons of all class levels. In contrast to the reports from the United States, they indicate that cannabis use in Canada has been institutionalized as a *de facto* phenomenon and that its *de jure* legitimation for recreational purposes is a matter of time.

Modifications in the application of legal sanctions in Canada and the United States and recommendations for decriminalization reflect the decline of acrimonious, often violent, public attitudes directed at the counter-culture or minority groups as much as the "demon pot." Several of the papers from Latin America and other world areas indicate concern with the spread of the "marihuana complex" to new sectors of the population. This diffusion is frequently based on introduction by "nomadic" young North Americans or other channels of culture contact. Opinion in these areas tends to reflect the harsh moral and legal sanctions that accompanied the "marihuana epidemic" of the sixties in the United States, tending to link its use to "anti-social" behavior and to seek the etiology of various pathologies — chromosomal defects, spontaneous abortions, psychoses — in the alleged effects of marihuana smoking.

The ethnobotanical and ethnohistorical reports provide significant research leads that may afford a theoretical reconstruction of the different sociocultural frames of reference of cannabis use and its function. Data on the effects of cannabis use point up the problems of research comparability given different methodologies and points of departure. Research findings from clinical studies of cannabis smokers are presented for Brazil, Colombia and Pakistan. Alvaro de Pinho reports that in a study of 728 patients at the psychiatric hospital in Bahia marihuana was not a significant psychiatric factor. However, acute toxic psychoses occurred in some young people who were involved in youth movements and were known to have used marihuana. There was complete and rapid remission of the acute states. B. R. Elejalde reports that chromosomal studies of regular marihuana users in Colombia do not reveal any abnormalities. Munir Khan *et al.*, in a study of seventy male subjects in Pakistan who had consumed cannabis for at least twenty years, reported no findings of significant abnormalities, tolerance to, or dependence on cannabis and no evidence that it interfered with work abilities.

Possibly as an effect of the *Zeitgeist*, there is often as much scientific controversy about the reported effects of cannabis as there is public clamor about its alleged effects. One of the major problems in evaluating the alleged or attributed consequences of chronic cannabis use (e.g., "brain damage," psychoses, sterility, addiction to hard drugs) has been lack of specificity in defining research methodologies. This problem is confounded when there is inadequate or no data on the actual THC (the presently accepted major psychoactive element) content of the cannabis used, or on the duration and frequency of use; on the subject population, in terms of social class background and life histories, as well as medical histories, including use of other drugs and general medical status; and on the matching of smoker subjects and controls. As cannabis research becomes more sophisticated, the need for cross-disciplinary research on this complex subject also becomes more apparent. W. E. Carter and W. J. Coggins present a multidisciplinary research design for the study of the effects of chronic use of cannabis in Costa Rica.

Cultural factors in the use of other psychoactive plants are examined in several chapters. Johannes Wilbert discusses magico-religious use of tobacco among South American Indians. Tobacco, considered a sacred plant, is chewed to induce visions and trance in shamanistic rituals. The shift from sacred to secular use of tobacco is comparatively recent. Barbara Myerhoff presents the framework of ritual use of peyote among the Huichol, and Marlene Dobkin de Rios offers an overview of man's ritual and medicinal use of hallucinogens. Cultural belief systems and values contribute to the structuring of the subjective experience of visions.

The shift from sacred to secular use of tobacco points up the interdependence of cultural substitutions. In Colombia, for example, tobacco was used by African slaves and Spaniards to reduce fatigue and was allotted as part of the laborers' rations on *haciendas*. Tobacco was also used medicinally, for a variety of ailments. William Partridge believes that the medicinal use of cannabis may derive from that of tobacco, and

Sula Benet posits that the ready acceptance of tobacco in the Old World was based on familiarity with cannabis.

In both hemispheres, psychoactive plants have been used for a variety of purposes, secular as well as sacred, to serve a wide range of human needs. Different emphases on the use of such mind-altering substances become apparent in cross-cultural perspective as may be seen in the sacred and secular uses of tobacco and peyote, as well as in the two cannabis complexes. The collection of papers in this volume may also provide a new understanding of the cultural conditioning of human responses to psychoactive plants, regardless of their pharmacological content.

REFERENCES

INDIAN HEMP COMMISSION
   1969 *Report of the Indian Hemp Drugs Commission 1893–1894.* Silver Springs, Maryland: Thomas Jefferson Publishing Company.
SCHULTES, RICHARD EVANS
   1969 Plant kingdom and hallucinogens. *Bulletin on Narcotics* 21 (3):3–16.
   1973 Man and marijuana. *Natural History* 82:59–68, 78, 82.

PART ONE

Ethnobotany and Diffusion

Typification of Cannabis sativa *L.*

WILLIAM T. STEARN

ABSTRACT

The name *Cannabis sativa* L., published by Carl Linnaeus in 1753 in his *Species plantarum*, the internationally accepted basis for modern botanical nomenclature, is the first legitimate scientific name for the hemp grown in Europe where it had been extensively cultivated for many centuries previously. The cannabis material which Linnaeus had for study is fortunately represented by two good specimens in the Clifford Herbarium of the British Museum of Natural History. Although Linnaeus gave "India" as the country of origin of the species, he based his description on the hemp grown in northern Europe in 1737, which he knew in a living state and that had been described at length by Rabelais, in 1545, under the fictitious name "Pantagruelion."

The possibility that the genus *Cannabis* (Cannabaceae) comprises more than one species, as believed by Zhukovsky (1962) and other Russian botanists and as noted by Tutin *et al.* in *Flora Europaea* 1:67 (1964), or consists of one variable species divisible on fruit characters into several subspecies with differing chemical properties, has made it essential to examine the typification of the name *Cannabis sativa* so as to remove in advance any nomenclatural uncertainty which may otherwise come about if, for taxonomic reasons, the Linnaean epithet *sativa* has to be restricted to one member of the group.

The name *Cannabis sativa* L., having been published by Carl Linnaeus in his *Species plantarum* 2:1027 (1753), the internationally accepted starting point for modern botanical nomenclature, is the first legitimate scientific name for the hemp which was grown in Europe in the 18th Century. Here it had been extensively cultivated for many centuries, as is evident from both historical and palynological evidence (summarized by H. Godwin in 1967), being grown primarily for its tough fibres providing cordage and clothing but also for its oily seeds; fortunately, during the

For Plates, see pp. ii–iii, between pp. 266–267.

period of its maximum use in Europe, the narcotic properties of its resin were unknown there.

The flowers of hemp are either male (staminate) or female (pistillate). Normally an individual plant bears either male or female flowers but not both. Male and female individuals differ in appearance and longevity, the males having conspicuous loose few-leaved inflorescences and dying earlier than the females, which have compact more leafy inflorescences with much less conspicuous flowers.

Growers of hemp have probably always been familiar with the differences between male and female plants and have long distinguished them as such in a metaphorical manner completely opposed to their biological nature. According to Lefranc (1905), Antoine Rabelais, the father of François Rabelais (c. 1494–1553), grew much hemp on his property at Cinais, southwest of Chinon (Indre et Loire), and young Rabelais probably helped in its cultivation. Rabelais certainly knew everything known then about the character and cultivation of hemp; three chapters of his *Le tiers livre des Faictz et Dictz héroiques du noble Pantagruel* (1546) are devoted to *l'herbe nommée Pantagruelion*, which is simply hemp. Rabelais here duly mentioned its sexuality:

Et, comme en plusieurs plantes sont deux sexes, masle et femelle, ce que voyons es lauriers, palmes, chesnes, heouses, asphodele, mandragore, fougere, agaric, aristolochie, cypres, terebynthe, pouliot, peone, et aultres, aussi en ceste herbe y a masle qui ne porte fleur aulcune, mais abonde en semence, et femelle, qui foisonne en petits fleurs blanchastres, inutiles, et ne porte semence qui vaille, et comme est des aultres semblables, ha la feuille plus large, mains dure que le masle, et ne croist en pareille haulteur (Livre 3, chap. 49).

Sir Thomas Urquhart in his 1693 translation came closer to the original than he usually did, being swept along by his exuberant love of words which Rabelais would have appreciated, when he rendered this into English as follows:

And as in diverse plants and trees there are two sexes, male and female, which is perceptible in laurels, palms, cypresses, oaks, holmes [i.e. holmoaks], the daffodil [i.e. asphodel], mandrake, fern, the agaric [i.e. mushroom], birthwort, turpentine, pennyroyal, peony, rose of the mount and many other such like, even so in this herb there is a male which beareth no flower at all, yet it is very copious of and abundant in seed. There is likewise in it a female, which hath great store and plenty of whitish flowers, serviceable to little or no purposes, nor doth it carry in it seed of any worth at all, at least comparable to that of the male. It hath also a larger leaf and much softer than that of the male, nor doth it altogether grow to so great a height.

The seed-bearing hemp called "male" here is, of course, the female plant and the sterile hemp here called "female" is really the male.

Most pre-Linnaean botanical authors, except Ray and Morison, applied the terms *mas* (male) and *foemina* (female) in the same metaphorical way as Rabelais, without any concept of true sexuality in plants comparable to that of animals. Thus, of two kinds, usually distinct species, the more robust or more vigorous or more useful one, especially if having larger leaves or harder wood, was designated "male" and the inferior one "female." Hence, the names *Cannabis sativa* and *C. mas*, as used by D'Aléchamps, Dodoens and C. Bauhin, refer to female individuals of hemp; and the names *C. erratica*, *C. foemina* and *C. sterilis* refer to male individuals. The name *Cannabis sativa*, which Linnaeus used as a specific name covering both sexes, applied originally only to female individuals. This kind of usage died slowly. As late as 1884, Saint-Lager noted, in his erudite "Remarques historiques sur les mots 'plantes males' et 'plantes femelles'," that farmers in the Rhône basin were still calling pistillate plants of hemp "chanvre mâle" and staminate plants "chanvre femelle," because the pistillate plants remained green and robust after the weaker staminate plants had withered, their function as pollinators fulfilled.

In the same manner, C. Bauhin designated the useful female hop-bearing plant of *Humulus lupulus* as *Humulus mas* and the unproductive male as *H. foemina*.

The difference between male and female plants of hemp necessitates two periods of harvesting. Thus, Philip Miller in his *Gardeners dictionary*, 8th ed. (1768), recorded that in the east of England,

the first season for pulling the Hemp, is usually about the middle of August, when they begin to pull what they call the Fimble Hemp, which is the male plants.... These male plants begin to decay soon after they have shed their farina. The second pulling is soon after Michaelmas, when the seeds are ripe: this is usually called Karle Hemp, it is the female plants, which were left at the time the male were pulled.

The fruit is a small nut, i.e. it has a single seed tightly covered by the hardened wall of the ovary, and is enclosed within a sheathing hairy bract with abundant resin glands which presumably developed in the wild as a protection for the fruit against insects, like the glandular trichomes of other plants (cf. D. A. Levin 1973). The distinctions, which have been made between the taxa known as *C. sativa*, *C. indica* and *C. ruderalis*, relate to characteristics of the fruit; male plants seemingly provide no diagnostic features; hence for typification a pistillate specimen would be preferable to a staminate one on taxonomic as well as historic grounds.

Linnaeus's protologue in the *Species plantarum* 2:1027 (1753) is as follows:

1. CANNABIS *sativa*

Cannabis foliis digitatis. *Hort. cliff* 457.
    Hort. ups. 297. *Mat. med.* 457.
    Dalib. paris. 300. *Roy. lugdb.* 221.
Cannabis sativa. *Bauh. pin.* 320. ♀
Cannabis mas. *Dalech. hist.* 497. ♀
Cannabis erratica. *Bauh. pin.* 320. ♂
Cannabis femina. *Dalech. hist.* 497. ♂
Habitat in India.

Several matters in this protologue call for comment. In genera with several species, Linnaeus provided concise diagnostic phrase-names enabling the species thereby to be distinguished, e.g. *Hippophaë foliis lanceolatis* and *Hippophaë foliis ovatis* for *H. Rhamnoides* and *H. canadensis*. Such phrase-names were comparative; they contrasted specific features. In a genus with only one species, such as *Cannabis*, no such diagnostic phrase was required and would indeed have been illogical, since obviously the one and only species could not be contrasted with itself.

Typification of the generic name of such a monotypic genus is essentially the same as typification of the specific name; the nomenclatural type of the one must be the nomenclatural type of the other. Hence, the generic name *Cannabis* L. and the specific name *Cannabis sativa* L. must be permanently associated with the same element. The *Species plantarum* citations of literature begin with Linnaeus' own *Hortus Cliffortianus* (1738), where fuller synonymy will be found; the other citations likewise refer to plants cultivated in Europe. He used the terms *mas* and *femina* and the signs ♂ and ♀ for male and female plants in a purely biological sense and sorted his synonyms accordingly. Knowing hemp only as a cultivated plant in Europe, he evidently assumed that it must have been introduced from elsewhere, presumably Asia; he had earlier identified with this the male plant figured under the name "Kalengi-cansjava" in Rheede, *Hortus Malabaricus* 10:t. 60 (1690) and, with some doubt, the female plant figured there in t. 61 (1690); on this evidence, it would seem, he stated "Habitat in India." These Rheede illustrations were later cited by Lamarck under his *Cannabis indica* when he separated that as a species distinct from *C. sativa*.

Linaeus' account of *Cannabis sativa* in the *Species plantarum* (1753) is to be associated with the description of the genus *Cannabis* in his *Genera plantarum*, 5th ed., 453, no. 988 (1754), as stated in the *Internation-*

al Code of Botanical Nomenclature art. 13, note 3 (1972). This description is as follows:

988. CANNABIS*   *Tournef. 308*
        * Mas
CAL.   *Perianthuim* quinquepartitum: *foliolis* oblongis, acuminatoobtusis, concavis.
COR.   nulla.
STAM.   *Filamenta* quinque, capillaria, brevissima, *Antherae* oblongae, tetragonae.
        * Femina
CAL.   *Perianthium* monophyllum. oblongum, acuminatum, latere altero longitudinaliter dehiscens, persistens.
COR.   nulla.
PIST.   *Germen* minimum. *Styli* duo, subulati, longi. *Stigmata* acuta.
PER.   minimum. *Calyx* arcte clausus.
SEM.   *Nux* globoso-depressa, bivalvis.

The asterisk in the heading CANNABIS* here, as in the first edition, indicates that Linnaeus had based his account on living material, i.e. on plants cultivated in Sweden or Holland. This 1754 description comes, however, unchanged from the first edition of the *Genera plantarum* 304, no. 749 (1737) published at Leyden, when Linnaeus had charge of Cliffords' richly stocked garden at Hartekamp. That work, dealing with the genera, and his *Hortus Cliffortianus* (1738), dealing with the species, have the same close association as the 1754 *Genera plantarum* has with the 1753 *Species plantarum*. Thus, his principal reference under *Cannabis* in the 1753 *Species plantarum* is to the *Hortus Cliffortianus* 457, which, in turn, refers to the 1737 *Genera plantarum* no. 749.

In the *Hortus Cliffortianus*, Linnaeus provided a short diagnosis, *Cannabis foliis digitatis*, to distinguish the true hemp from a then imperfectly known plant diagnosed there as *Cannabis foliis pinnatis*, but named *Datisca cannabina* in the first edition of the *Species plantarum*. In short, Linnaeus' concept of *Cannabis sativa* in 1753 is identical with that of his *Cannabis foliis digitatis* of 1738. Just as John Ray had earlier distinguished functionally male individuals as *Cannabis sativa "mas s. sterilis"* and female individuals as *Cannabis sativa "foemina s. fertilis,"* so Linnaeus likewise distinguished male and female individuals, allocating pre-Linnaean synonyms to each. The material of *Cannabis* which Linnaeus had for study when preparing the *Genera plantarum* (1737) and *Hortus Cliffortianus* (1738) is fortunately represented in the Clifford Herbarium, Hortus siccus Cliffortianus, in the Department of Botany, British Museum (Natural History), London, by two good specimens, one (A) male (Plate 1.), the other (B) female (Plate 2.). Either is available for designation as lectotype. Since, however, the major characters for taxonomic division in *cannabis* come from fruiting material, *the Hortus siccus Cliffortianus fruiting specimen* (p. 457 *Cannabis no. 1, B*) of *Cannabis sativa* L. is here designated as the *lectotype*. This specimen represents *C. sativa* as currently commonly accepted. The fruit is about 5 mm. long, 3.5 mm. broad.

If Linnaeus had provided in 1753 a new diagnosis for *Cannabis sativa* or had modified in 1754 the generic description of *Cannabis* published in 1737 on the basis of later material — as he did for some other species and genera — then it would be judicious to select a lectotype from this material influencing his final concept of these. In fact, however, he did neither. Hence, as indicated above, the lectotype has to be taken from the earlier material on which his unchanged concepts were based. From this standpoint, the two specimens under *Cannabis* in his herbarium at the Linnaean Society of London have only a subsidiary relevance, because they in no way affected his publications. They are, however, of interest on account of their Linnaean association. Linnaean Herbarium specimen 1177.2, illustrated in Joyce & Curry, *The botany and chemistry of Cannabis* 22 (1970), is a pistillate plant, with fewer than the usual numbers of leaflets, which are narrowly lanceolate, long acuminate and sharply serrate. It has no epithet but is numbered "1" in Linnaeus' hand.

Linnaeus began to draft his *Species plantarum* long before he devised his method of consistent binominal nomenclature for species; even in 1748, he had not devised binomials for the whole vegetable kingdom; hence the most convenient method of arranging and designating his herbarium specimens was to number the species in each folder according to the numbered species entries in his manuscript *Species plantarum*. When, a few years after 1753, he began to prepare a second edition of the *Species plantarum*, with changed numbering of specific entries, he ceased to number his specimens but added instead the specific epithet introduced in that work. Thus, a numeral corresponding to an entry in the first edition of the *Species plantarum* is a valuable indication that Linnaeus possessed this specimen in 1753 or acquired it soon afterwards.

Hence, the numbered pistillate specimen with leaflets characteristic of European hemp, *Linn. Herb. 1177.2*, can be assumed to have been in his hands at this time if not much earlier. The other specimen, *Linn. Herb. 1177.1*, illustrated in Joyce & Curry, *Botany and chemistry of Cannabis* 21 (1970), is of very different aspect. It is a staminate plant with much shorter and broader almost obtuse more coarsely serrate leaflets. It has no number but is labelled "sativa" in Linnaeus' hand. Thus, this specimen, in no way typical of *Cannabis sativa* as commonly accepted, can safely be assumed to have come into Linnaeus' possession later than 1753.

The two *Hortus Cliffortianus* specimens belong to the old cultivated hemp stock of northern Europe. This is represented by another contemorary herbarium specimen in the British Museum (Natural History) which was grown in the Chelsea Physic Garden and presented in 1740 to the Royal Society of London under the number 908; for a discussion of the history and nomenclatural importance of these Chelsea specimens, see Stearn (1972). There are also specimens scattered through the herbaria assembled by Sir Hans Sloane (1660–1753) and now in the British Museum (Natural History): vol. 39, fol. 2 (c. 1660). vol. 83, fol. 161 (L. Plukenet, 1642–1706), vol. 85, fol. 62 (G. Bonnivert, fl. 1673–1703), vol. 91, fol. 47 (Plukenet), vol. 117, fol. 2 (A. Buddle, 1660–1715), vol. 167, fol. 393 (G. London, d. 1713), vol. 321, fol. 236 (H. Boerhaave, 1668–1738); see J. E. Dandy (1958).

SUMMARY

Although Linnaeus, when publishing the name *Cannabis sativa* in 1753, gave "India" as the country of origin of the species, he based his original description on the hemp grown in northern Europe in 1737, which he knew in a living state; this hemp belonged to the long-cultivated European stock which Rabelais had described at length in 1545 under the fictitious name "Pantagruelion." Linnaeus, like his predecessor Ray, correctly distinguished the staminate individuals as "male" and the pistillate and fruiting individuals as "female." Most pre-Linnaean authors, on the general masculine assumption that males were superior or more robust or more useful than females, metaphorically designated the relatively useless male individuals as "female" and the fruit-bearing female ones as "male." A female (pistillate) cultivated specimen in the Clifford Herbarium at the British Museum (Natural History), London, is taken as lectotype of the name *Cannabis sativa* L.

REFERENCES

DANDY, J. E., *editor*
   1958   *The Sloane herbarium.* London: Trustees of the British Museum.
GODWIN, H.
   1967   The ancient cultivation of hemp. *Antiquity* 41:42–50, 137–138.
   1967   Pollen-analytic evidence for the cultivation of *Cannabis* in England. *Rev. Palaeobot. & Palynol.* 4:71–80.

JOYCE, C. R. B., S. H. CURRY, *editors.*
  1970 *The botany and chemistry of Cannabis.* London: J. & A. Churchill.
LEFRANC, A.
  1905 Pantagruelion et Chenevreaux. *Rev. Études Rabelaissennes* 3:402–403.
LEVIN, D. A.
  1973 The role of trichomes in plant defense. *Quart. J. Biol.* 48:3–15.
SAINT-LAGER, J. B.
  1884 Remarques historiques sur les mots 'plantes males' et 'plantes femelles.' *Ann. Soc. Bot. Lyon* 11 (1883):1–48.
SCHULTES, R. E.
  1970 "Random thoughts and queries on the botany of *Cannabis*," in *The botany and chemistry of Cannabis.* Edited by C. R. B. Joyce and S. H. Curry, 11–38. London: J. &. A. Churchill.
STEARN, W. T.
  1970 "The *Cannabis* plant: botanical characteristics," in *The botany and chemistry of Cannabis.* Edited by C. R. B. Joyce and S. H. Curry, 1–10. London: J. &. A. Churchill.
  1972 Philip Miller and the plants from the Chelsea Physic Garden presented to the Royal Society of London, 1723–1796. *Bot. Soc. Edinburgh Trans.* 41:293–307.
ZHUKOVSKY, P. M.
  1962 *Cultivated plants and their wild relatives.* Translated by P. S. Hudson. Farnham Royal (Commonwealth Agricultural Bureau).

Cannabis: An Example of Taxonomic Neglect

RICHARD EVANS SCHULTES, WILLIAM M. KLEIN,
TIMOTHY PLOWMAN, and TOM E. LOCKWOOD

> The story of marijuana is not yet written.
> H. H. NOWLISS

ABSTRACT

Native apparently somewhere in central Asia, cannabis is at present one of the most widely disseminated cultivated plants. Cannabis as we know it has developed together with man as a multi-purpose economic plant; and, as a result of selection for desirable characteristics, it has become one of the most variable of cultivated plants. Due to the extraordinary plasticity and variability of cultivated cannabis, there can be no progress in unravelling the taxonomic complexities in the genus until the biology of the wild populations is investigated.

The genus has been and still is widely considered to be monotypic, especially by botanists who have not studied the classification of the genus in depth: we believe this results from lack of taxonomic investigations of wild cannabis in its native habitat or even of comparative studies of the range of variation in cultivated hemp. A polytypic concept of the genus is not new: in 1783 Lamarck recognized *Cannabis indica* as "very distinct" from the species which Linnaeus had named *Cannabis sativa*. In 1924, Russian botanists, who studied wild populations of cannabis, recognized a third species, *Cannabis ruderalis*. Their work has not been widely accepted, partly due to conservative attitudes to changing established beliefs in the monotypic nature of the genus. Several British and American taxonomists who have investigated the genus now favor the polytypic concept. There may be significant chemical differences in content of cannabinolic and other constituents among the species. The paper reviews the taxonomic history of the genus and presents data in support of the polytypic concept.

I. It is often true that we know less about the classification of our widely cultivated plants than we do about some of the rare wild species of limited or endemic distribution. The cultivation and dispersal of a domesticated plant tend to alter the organism in many ways, often so drastically that it may be difficult or even impossible to point to a wild species as its progenitor. Sometimes the plant is so dramatically changed that it becomes wholly dependent on man for its survival (Schwanitz 1966).

For Plates, see pp. iv–viii, between pp. 266–267.

The genus *Cannabis* provides an excellent example of an important group of useful plants the classification of which has long been clouded in uncertainty. One of man's oldest domesticates, dating back nearly to the beginnings of agriculture, cannabis as we now know it has developed together with man as a multi-purpose economic plant: the source of a fiber, a narcotic, a medicine, an oil, and an edible fruit (Camp 1936; Godwin 1967; Merlin 1972; Schultes 1970, 1973).

Native apparently somewhere in central Asia, where it occurs as a plant of open, disturbed habitats, such as riverbanks, bottomlands, and hillsides, hemp has spread to all parts of the world where conditions are suitable for its growth: in fact, it is at present one of the most widely disseminated cultivated plants (Davidian 1972; Quimby *et al.* 1973; Vavilov 1926; Zhukovsky 1964, 1971).

The effects of man's subconscious and later conscious selection for desirable characteristics combined with the effects of natural selection under the stress of new and sometimes inhospitable environments have acted significantly in morphologically and perhaps chemically altering the cannabis plant. As a result, today, possibly some 10,000 years after the beginnings of the man-hemp partnership, cannabis has become one of the most variable of cultivated plants.

It is precisely this variability and our lack of anything approaching a full understanding of its nature and extent that have created a most difficult problem for systematists who have attempted to delimit specific and subspecific boundaries in the genus.

Unlike some domesticated plants, cannabis is believed still to occur in wild populations in certain parts of Asia and to exhibit in these populations an appreciable amount of inherent natural variability (DeCandolle 1884; Vavilov 1926). Man took advantage of this variability as he domesticated cannabis by cultivating and artificially selecting for a number of useful traits, such as elongated bast fibres, large seeds with high oil content and copious production of narcotic resin. Under the pressures of selection for these characters, cannabis began to reveal characters and combinations of characters not found in wild or presumed wild populations, a phenomenon that has occurred in every plant domesticated by man.

Unlike many of man's other cultivated plants, however, hemp never became totally dependent on man. In many areas where hemp was cultivated, it readily escaped and became naturalized as an aggressive weed. Thus released from the pressures of artificial selection induced by cultivation, populations of naturalized cannabis underwent extensive adaptive radiation.

In this new role, cannabis invaded many disturbed habitats, especially habitats newly created by man, becoming established and spreading without man's direct intervention. Like many other weeds, hemp became one of man's camp followers along roadsides and in rubbish heaps and growing on the edges of fields (Anderson 1949; Camp 1936; Darwin 1868; Vavilov 1926). The changes invoked by the transition from domestication to naturalization included, at least in some cases, reversions to characteristics peculiar to wild hemp, as has been known to occur in other cultivated plants.

We thus perceive three "phases" of cannabis — the wild, the cultivated, the weedy. These "phases" are not necessarily three discrete states of existence. The last two "phases," occurring over vast areas of the world and under highly varied ecological conditions, have created the great array of phenotypic diversity which we witness today in cultivated and naturalized hemp. Cannabis in the wild state has probably adapted well to disturbed conditions. Its wild adaptive mode pre-adapted it in many cases to certain cultivated conditions and often made an easy transition back to the weedy state or "phase" (Davidian 1972; Schultes 1970, 1973; Vavilov 1926; Vavilov and Bukinich 1929).

As a result of the extraordinary plasticity and variability evident in present-day cultivated and weedy cannabis, there can be no hope of unravelling the complexities encountered in the genus through a study of cultivated types alone. No certain progress can be effected, until the biology of wild or presumably wild populations is carefully investigated — and it must constantly be borne in mind that there can be no *wild* hemp except in areas where it is native. The most critical studies on cultivated or weedy types of cannabis — in Europe, North America and South America, for example — can yield little new evidence toward an understanding of the species composition of the genus. There have been enough examples of cultivated plants, the classification of which has been clarified as a result of an investigation of wild ancestral types, of wild populations or of related wild species, to indicate the desirability and necessity of this approach in the case of cannabis.

II. Although the taxonomic literature on cannabis is complicated by a confusing plethora of specific and varietal names (most of which have never been properly published or described, according to the rules of botanical nomenclature), the genus has been and still is generally considered to be monotypic.

We are persuaded that this opinion is the result of an almost total lack of taxonomic investigation of wild cannabis as it occurs in its natural habitat or even of comprehensive and comparative studies of the range of variations found in cultivated hemp. Since botanists have not carried out such detailed and critical taxonomic studies, it has naturally been customary for authors of textbooks, check-lists, floras, manuals, botanical dictionaries, pharmaceutical publications, agricultural treatises and other generalized and summary-type publications to repeat the orthodox monotypic concept, thus establishing it even more firmly in the literature. This establishment of the monotypic concept is reflected in modern chemical publications and even in the drafting of laws in some of the countries that control the use of cannabis.

A polytypic concept of the genus is not new. It goes back 190 years to Lamarck's recognition of a collection from India as distinct from the species which Linnaeus thirty years earlier had named *Cannabis sativa*.

As an outcome of investigations carried out by Russian students of crop plant evolution in the 1920's and 1930's, the opinion that there are indeed several species of cannabis was, for the first time, offered on the basis of studies and experience in the field. They are the only taxonomists to have studied extensively wild populations of cannabis. Their work, however, has not been widely accepted. Failure to accept or at least to consider seriously their opinions has been the result of several factors: partly because their work was published in Russian journals of limited avaiilibity; partly because Western botanists were not able to visit the areas of presumed wild cannabis in Russian territory; and perhaps most significantly because of conservative unwillingness to contemplate change in the established belief in the monotypic nature of the genus.

We began to question the generally accepted view of *Cannabis* as a monotypic genus in 1969, when one of the writers (Schultes) was invited to address a symposium in London composed mainly of chemists and pharmacologists. He was asked to address himself to what is *not* known about the botany of cannabis. Although, in that lecture, essentially a review of the literature, he clung to the idea of the monotypic nature of the genus, his evaluation of the limited taxonomic studies raised serious doubt in his mind about the propriety of this viewpoint (Schultes 1970). Subsequent critical studies of the literature; examination of material from many areas preserved in several of the world's largest herbaria; preliminary fieldwork in Afghanistan; and a survey of the plantings of cannabis in Mississippi from seed imported from many localities around the world under the auspices of the National Institutes of Health — all have combined to convince us that *Cannabis* is not monotypic and that the Russian concept that there are several species may be acceptable.

It is not only the Russian sources (Komarov 1936; Vavilov 1926; Vavilov and Bukinich 1929; Zhukovsky 1964, 1971) that accept the polytypic concept of *Cannabis*. The British taxonomists who are editing *Flora Europaea* (Tutin *et al.* 1964) clearly indicate their belief that two species occur within the confines of the floristic area which they consider Europe. Although they have not published their opinions, several American taxonomists who have examined the evidence likewise favor the polytypic concept.

Other botanists who still maintain the monotypic nature of cannabis are receptive to the possibility that continued study may indicate more than one species. After a careful taxonomic evaluation of cannabis on a generic basis, for example, Miller (1970) suggested that only additional investigations could clarify the variability in characters on which several species have been set up. And Small (1972), who has carried out extensive cytological research on cannabis, has stated that... "there would not appear to be a basis for recognizing species or other taxonomic groupings in cannabis on the criterion of breeding isolation... [that] some of the numerous taxonomic entities that have been recognized... may be justified on the basis of morphological ground but, as no comprehensive morphological study of cannabis has yet been published, all recognized taxa in cannabis must be viewed with suspicion at present."

A complete clarification of the biology and systematics of *Cannabis* will, of course, require extensive field studies in those areas of Asia where the genus is presumably native or at least has not been subjected to intensive agricultural influence. Sufficient research has not been carried out to establish all of the general trends in the specific delimitation of the genus. Important aspects still remain unclear. Whether there are two or three — or possibly even more — species is still open to question, as is the correct nomenclature of the specific concepts involved.

But in the basic question of whether *Cannabis* be monotypic or polytypic we have little hesitation with the evidence available at this point in accepting the polytypic concept.

Central Asia and adjacent regions to the south and west comprise a vast area which includes a great diversity of geographical zones and ecological situations. It is here that cannabis is commonly believed to have originated, although it may be difficult to pinpoint any specific area of origin or to determine how great the geographical distribution of wild hemp was before the advent of man (DeCandolle 1884; Vavilov 1926; Zhukovsky 1964, 1971). In such a region, there could easily have arisen divergent populations sufficiently distinct both morphologically and ecologically, to be considered species, subspecies and varieties.

When man began to domesticate one or more of these species of cannabis and carry them from place to place, hybridization occurred between the wild species and the incipient cultigens.

Through continual introgressive hybridization with cultivated hemp, some of the original wild species of cannabis may have gradually become extinct. This process increased the variability in the gene pool of the cultivated plants and must have imparted to them some of the unique characters of the wild species. This belief is given credence by the fact that we find great morphological variations between populations of cultivated hemp in various parts of Eurasia in characters which have *not* been selected for by man, such as leaf size and shape and pigmentation of stem and fruit.

Studies in the reproductive biology of different strains of cultivated cannabis indicate that these plants are fully interfertile (Postma 1946; Small 1972). This does not mean, however, that sterility barriers may not exist within the genus, specifically in wild populations which have not yet been examined for this character. They may, indeed, show varying degrees of reproductive isolation.

Reproductive isolation can, of course, occur by means other than sterility barriers. It is well known that, in certain genera of plants, as in some animals, "acceptable" species exist where there are few or no sterility barriers present. The examples are many. These species have evolved with other types of isolating mechanisms, that are either mechanical, ethological or geographical.

The significant phenomenon in cannabis is that the combinations of morphological and anatomical (and possibly also chemical) characters have maintained their integrity, in spite of hybridization. The maintenance of these combinations of characters is a better indication of these reproductive barriers than that resulting from experimentation with cultivated strains of doubtful origin.

It is, furthermore, well recognized that species concepts must necessarily vary from one genus to another and from one family to another, dependent on the genetic peculiarities of the group under consideration. With the very different genetic backgrounds in different families, genera, etc., it is not at all surprising that the patterns of variation in these sundry groups may be quite different. There is not the equivalence of units amongst families of plants in the same sense of elements in chemistry. At one time, it was hoped that the species might be so rigorously defined that it would serve as the unit of evolution. Taxonomy has come a long way, however, since this belief, and taxonomists now hold that the population is the evolutionary unit, the biologically significant unit in plants.

Plants were not made to be catalogued and classified. They can never easily and with complete satisfaction be put into tight compartments. This simple and basic truth, usually not appreciated by non-scientists and sometimes overlooked by zealous taxonomists, should be borne in mind much more strongly for groups such as cannabis, where an historical perspective is imperative.

III. In view of the excessively confused taxonomic picture of cannabis that at present confounds botanical, chemical, legal and other considerations, a review of the specific history of the genus may be illuminating.

The history of *Cannabis* in modern taxonomic literature began in 1737, when Linnaeus established the genus *Cannabis*, basing it on pre-Linnaean concepts.

The name *Cannabis* (Greek Κάνναβις, Kannabis) is a very ancient classical vernacular name for hemp, with which the English word *hemp* itself, derived from the Anglo-Saxon *haenep* and the presumed Old Teutonic parental form *hanapiz*, are cognate; and, according to Laufer (1919), "is presumably a loan word pointing to Finno-Ugrian and Turkish," ancient languages of central Asia. Indeed, the principal difference between the Teutonic and the Graeco-Latin is due to the Gothonic consonant shift — Greek preserving the consonant *k* of an earlier Indo-European language which became *h* some five centuries or so B.C. in the primitive Teutonic languages. Thus, etymology accords with other evidence in indicating central Asia as the area whence plants of *Cannabis* spread outwards, mainly eastward, westward and to the south.

The binomial *Cannabis sativa* was published by Linnaeus in *Species Plantarum* in 1753, the internationally accepted starting point for modern botanical binomial nomenclature. *Cannabis sativa* hearkens back to pre-Linnaean literature.

Under *Cannabis sativa*, Linnaeus referred to several earlier synonyms: *Cannabis foliis digitatis*, used in his *Hortus Cliffortianus* of 1738; *C. sativa* and *C. erratica* of Bauhin in 1623; *C. mas* and *C. femina* of D'Aléchamps in 1587.

The Linnean Society of London preserves in the Linnean Herbarium two specimens of cannabis. One specimen, No. 1177.1[1] (Plate 1), is labelled "*sativa*" in Linnaeus' handwriting and respresents a staminate plant with much more abbreviated leaves than is usual for what we consider normal for *Cannabis sativa*. The other specimen, No. 1177.2 (Plate 2),

[1] Index number assigned to specimen in the Linnean Herbarium by the late M. Spencer Savage, Secretary of the Linnean Society of London.

without any specific epithet written on the sheet, represents a pistillate plant with the lanceolate leaflets that are commonly encountered in *Cannabis sativa*.

No locality data are found on these two collections, although, in *Species plantarum*, Linnaeus offers the information that the species has a "habitat in India." In his annotated copy of *Species plantarum*, preserved in the Linnean Society, Linnaeus had written in his own hand, as a note for any future edition, the word "Persia" as an additional habitat. It should, of course, be borne in mind that, in Europe in 1753, geographical delimitations were far from strict and that "habitat in India" and "Persia" represented extremely vague and wide areas, undoubtedly not corresponding precisely with today's India and Persia. Indeed, Linnaeus' "India" is often equivalent to modern China.

It is clear that these two specimens were not in Linnaeus' herbarium in 1753. He added them later. Linnaeus did not cite any specimens in his *Species plantarum*, nor did he offer any description of his *Cannabis sativa*. He based his recognition of *Cannabis sativa* on the kind of hemp commonly cultivated in northern European gardens at that period. Stearn has typified *Cannabis sativa* by choosing as lectotype a pistillate specimen from *Hortus Cliffortianus* and now preserved in the British Museum (Natural History). Until this typification was made, there might well have been doubt as to what Linnaeus actually meant by *Cannabis sativa*, regardless of the general use of this binomial for more than two centuries.

Although the two specimens in the Linnean Herbarium are of little taxonomic or nomenclatural significance, since neither one can be a type, there seems to be no reason to doubt that Linnaeus considered them to represent what he had already called *Cannabis sativa*. Consequently, it would be of interest if we could somehow ascertain the provenience of these two specimens. His annotation "habitat in India" does not constitute a guarantee that he had seen specimens that actually had come from Asia. Linnaeus was, of course, familiar with hemp as cultivated in northern Europe, including his native Sweden, and there is a strong probability that these two later specimens may have been locally collected.

Although very scanty, the two specimens in the Linnean Herbarium are of very different aspect. The pistillate specimen (1177.2) has leaves with fewer than the usual number of leaflets; the leaflets are long, linear-lanceolate, long-acuminate, with very sharply pointed but not coarse serrulation. The staminate specimen (1177.1) is very distinctive, with trifoliate leaves, the leaflets of which are short, elliptic to somewhat elliptic-lanceolate, apically almost blunt, with coarse, not markedly pointed serrulation.

Even though the type method in taxonomy was not employed in Linnaeus' time and although Linnaeus did not have these two specimens at hand in 1753, it is interesting and perhaps significant that the staminate specimen (1177.1), which does not resemble the concept that we now commonly recognize as *Cannabis sativa*, is actually the specimen upon which Linnaeus wrote "sativa." There is no indication of a specific epithet written on the other specimen (1177.2).

With the thousands of herbarium collections now available for study and years of attention to cultivated forms in many parts of the world, taxonomists should be able to examine these two specimens with much more perspicacity than Linnaeus himself was able to do. The question arises — even though this material is not critical to our taxonomic studies in the genus — Why are these two specimens so very unlike? Was the staminate specimen on which Linnaeus wrote "sativa" a branch from an abnormal plant? Or did perchance Linnaeus actually have at hand after 1753 representatives of two different species?

Although he did no basic taxonomic study on cannabis, Scopoli, in 1772, twenty years after Linnaeus' publication of *Cannabis sativa* and the name of the hop plants, *Humulus Lupulus*, reduced the genus *Humulus* to synonymy under *Cannabis*, calling the hop plant *Cannabis lupulus*. This point of view has never gained acceptance, although both genera, *Cannabis* and *Humulus*, are now almost unanimously considered to be closely allied and to be members of the same family, Cannabaceae.

Thirty years after Linnaeus' *Species plantarum*, in 1783, the French naturalist Lamarck described another species, *Cannabis indica*, in his *Encyclopédie méthodique*. This new species was based upon a specimen certainly of Asiatic origin. According to Lamarck, it was collected by a French naturalist, M. Pierre Sonnerat (1748(49)–1814) in India. Again, we are at a loss to indicate a definite area, partly because of vagueness of geographical terminology in that period and partly because, in the same paragraph, Lamarck reports that the plant grows in the "East Indies." He undoubtedly meant "eastern India," where Sonnerat did collect, for it is known that cannabis was introduced into what is now called "East Indies" much later. Sonnerat travelled between 1768 and 1771 in Madagascar, India, Ceylon, the Philippines, Indonesia and China; he spent some time collecting in Pondicherry and southern India.

Lamarck considerd his *Cannabis indica* to be a species "very distinct" from *C. sativa*. He reported it to be of a smaller stature, more profusely branched and provided with a much harder (woodier?), almost cylindrical stem. He further stated that the leaves are constantly alternate; the leaflets narrowly linear-lanceolate and very acuminate. The staminate plants have five or seven leaflets; whilst the pistillate plants are commonly threefoliolate, with the leaves near the summit being completely simple. The pistillate flowers he described as having a pubescent calyx and long parallel style. Because of its hard stem and thin cortex, the species, he maintained, was not capable of furnishing fibres similar to those provided by *Cannabis sativa*. The odor of Lamarck's species was, in his words, "strong and resembling somewhat that of tobacco." In a paragraph following the description of *Cannabis indica*, Lamarck pointed out that the principal virtue of this species lay in the strength of its narcotic properties.

At first glance, a photograph of the specimen on which Lamarck based the name *Cannabis indica* does not show a significant difference from Linnaeus' pistillate specimen No. 1177.2. But when one studies the photograph and the actual specimen (preserved in Paris) critically and against a background of experience with material of cannabis, the specimen appears to have been taken from a plant of much denser and more compact growth than the Linnaean specimen which gives the impression of having come from a rather laxly branched plant. We have also Lamarck's direct remark that the plant is "smaller" and "very much branched," which might well be interpreted to indicate a plant with branches more densely spaced than is the usual condition in what has long been called *Cannabis sativa*.

There were no further developments in cannabis taxonomy and nomenclature until 1792, when the French botanist Gilibert published *Cannabis foetens* in his *Exercitia phytologica*. This work, which is not consistently binomial, did not accept Linnaean names. After a very adequate description of what is obviously *Cannabis sativa* (as now typified), he commented mainly on differences in growth habits between the cannabis that he knew in France and that which he had found in Lithuania. There is no indication that he was attempting to differentiate *Cannabis foetens* from *C. sativa*. The name *Cannabis foetens* must, therefore, be considered a *nomen illegitimum*.

The next event in the nomenclatural history of cannabis was Sievers' casual enumeration in 1796 of "*Cannabis erratica*" (a binomial dating from pre-Linnaean times) in a list of plants encountered on a trip to Siberia. Since Sievers did not describe this binomial, it represents a *nomen nudum* without scientific status.

Half a century after Linnaeus' publication of *Cannabis sativa*, Stokes described *Cannabis macrosperma* in 1812 in his *A botanical materia medica*. While Stokes legitimately described the concept, no specimen is cited and no locality is given, although, by inference, Asia — and probably India — is indicated. There is little hope that we can now ascertain what

Stokes had at hand, but it is probable that he had an unusually large-seeded form of either *Cannabis sativa* or *C. indica*. He distinguished his *Cannabis macrosperma* from what he considered to be the *C. sativa* (with "nuts lenticular-globose") on the basis of its "oblong" achenes, indicating without explanation of his exact meaning, that the new species "is from *C. indica*."

In 1849, the name *Cannabis chinensis* appeared in a seed catalogue issued by the Montpellier Botanical Garden in France. This binomial is a *nomen nudum* referring probably to a form of cultivated hemp from China.

In Sturm's *Flora von Deutschland* of 1905, E. H. L. Krause published the description of a new species, *Cannabis generalis*, stating that its original home was Asia and, without distinguishing the two concepts, indicating that it represents a species present in the flora of Germany in addition to *C. sativa* and *C. indica*. No type specimen is cited. The description and illustration of *Cannabis generalis* indicate it to be one of the many European variants of the concept that has long gone under the name of *C. sativa*.

In 1908, Houghton and Hamilton published the binomial *Cannabis americana* to refer to "American grown hemp." The binomial is another *nomen nudum*, published without a description and with the clear indication that the authors believed it to be synonymous with *Cannabis sativa*. It need not enter any taxonomic consideration and is mentioned here only because — to the confusion of *Cannabis* nomenclature — it has been cited in later uncritical pharmacological literature.

Crévost published the binomial *Cannabis gigantea* in 1917 for a kind of hemp grown in Indochina. No description, no citation of specimen, no precise locality were given. The heading of his discussion of hemp in Indochina "*Cannabis sativa* (Lin.) et *Cannabis gigantea*" constitutes a clear indication that he considered the two concepts to be different species. Although referring possibly to a distinct kind of cannabis, the binomial cannot enter into any modern consideration of cannabis taxonomy.

The most recent taxonomic innovation in understanding the genus *Cannabis* is that of the Russian botanist Janischewsky who, in 1924, published a new species, *C. ruderalis*. This species is reputed to occur in the wild state in the Volga region, western Siberia, central Asia, and now to be widespread, probably in a weedy state, in northern and central Europe and Russia. According to its author, *Cannabis ruderalis* differs from *C. sativa* in a number of characteristics of a morphological nature (darker colored akene covered with a special coat representing the remains of the calyx and with a caruncle-like growth at the articulation of the akene) and of a biological nature (the akene falling easily and germinating the following spring).

IV. Preliminary examination of the wood anatomy of material which we collected in Afghanistan and which we believed to represent *Cannabis indica* (Plate 3) discloses differences from that of material of *C. sativa* grown in the United States. This research, being carried out by Dr. Loran C. Anderson of Kansas State University, is in its preliminary stages and will be the subject of a later paper.[2] The anatomical differences between these two species are very substantial, and Dr. Anderson feels that some comparable differences in other groups of plants might be given even generic status. In this connection, it should be noted that earlier anatomical investigations in Russia (Nassovov 1940) indicated important differences which seemed to point to three "types" of cannabis. It was also probably anatomical differences which were basic to Lamarck's statement in 1783 that one characteristic which distinguished *Cannabis indica* from *C. sativa* was its much harder, woodier stem.

The differences in growth habit are extraordinary. It is true that, in some localities, cultivated and escaped hemp may be of hybrid origin and/or, in strongly favorable habitats, may show some intergradation or ecotypical adaptation away from the norm.

These differences in growth habit we believe to be deeply significant. We have ascertained from our collections and studies in the extensive Mississippi plantation and elsewhere that the characters of growth habit seem to be genetically stable and are not obliterated by edaphic or environmental conditions. *Cannabis sativa* tends to be a tall — sometimes an extremely tall — very loosely branched plant, with the branches distant from one another; the habit of this species can perhaps best be described by the popular term *gangling*. What we consider to represent *Cannabis indica*, on the other hand, is usually a low, conical or pyramidal plant, normally three to four feet tall, very densely branched, with the branches extraordinarily close one to the other. Lamarck, in describing *Cannabis indica*, noted that it differed from *C. sativa* in its smaller stature and its more profuse branching. *Cannabis ruderalis* is reported to be very small, normally up to two feet in height, often only slightly branched or even unbranched at maturity.

---

[2] Anderson (1974) has found several anatomical differences in the wood morphology of *Cannabis sativa* and *C. indica* — differences of such magnitude that he believes that these two concepts must represent distinct species. Characters in the structure of wood are recognized by taxonomists to be extremely conservative.

We believe also that we can discern a general tendency in leaf variation, although, as in many plants, this character is far from being a conservative one. Furthermore, sufficient comparative studies have not been carried out for the full extent of the reliability of this character to be utilized. We would, however, indicate that the leaflets of *Cannabis sativa* appear, in the main, to be very narrowly linear-lanceolate, with fine and very sharp serrations. *Cannabis indica*, on the other hand, appears generally to have somewhat broader leaflets in relation to their length and to have somewhat coarser serrations that are not so sharp or which may be even somewhat obtuse. It is true that this character does not appear to be so striking in Lamarck's type specimen as it seems to be in the very ample herbarium material now at hand. The venation of the leaflets of *Cannabis indica* (Plate 4) likewise appears, as a general trend, to be much coarser than in *C. sativa*. In *Cannabis ruderalis*, the perceptible tendency seems to suggest leaflets which are very broad in relation to their length and which are much smaller (i.e., much shorter) than in either of the other two species. Since there is such extreme variation in leaf characters — at least, such *apparent* variation in view of the preliminary nature of our studies — we have preferred not to insert leaf characters into our key. The species can easily be distinguished, we feel, without recourse to characters which at present are not thoroughly investigated.

Furthermore, there may be — and we strongly suspect that there are — significant chemical differences, not only in the cannabinolic content but in other constituents, such as the essential oils, flavonoids and possibly several other classes of secondary compounds. Lamarck suggested as early as 1783 that the content of the intoxicating principal was higher in *Cannabis indica* than in *C. sativa*. In the intervening 200 years, during which the epithet *indica* has been used, there has usually been the inference that it is a more strongly intoxicating form of cannabis. Unfortunately, however, almost no chemical studies have been made in association with taxonomic studies nor on the basis of voucher specimens. Throughout the modern Russian literature there exists the inference, if not the outright claim, that the cannabinolic content of *Cannabis indica* is higher than that of *C. sativa* and *C. ruderalis*. Pertinent to species differentiation on a chemical basis may be the unexpected recent discovery, made independently by several workers (Doorenbos *et al.* 1971; Nordal and Braenden 1973; Turner and Hadley 1973; Turner *et al.* 1973), that chemical differences in cannabis appear to be based more on a genetic basis than on environmental or edaphic factors. If this be so, then it may add still another argument for specific differentiation in the genus.

Vavilov and Bukinich (1929), for example, after long field studies in

Afghanistan, maintained that cannabis comprised several species. In the *Flora of the U.S.S.R.* (1936), Komarov accepted the polytypic nature of the genus. Zhukovsky (1964, 1971) in his masterly *Cultivated plants and their wild relatives*, accepts three species of cannabis and indicates their morphological differences. In 1960, Soják asserted that *Cannabis ruderalis* (Plate 5) is spreading westward into Europe proper and described × *C. intersita* — a hybrid between *C. ruderalis* and *C. sativa* — on the basis of a Wallich collection in 1831. The *Flora Europaea* accepts a polytypic composition of cannabis, listing *C. sativa* and *C. ruderalis* — and this in a modern synthetic work which states that "all available evidence, morphological, geographical, ecological and cytological has been taken into consideration in delimiting species... [but which] are in all cases definable in morphological terms" (Tutin *et al*. 1964).

While we recognize our present incomplete knowledge of characters, we offer the following key to distinguish the several species discussed above:

1) Plants usually tall (five to 18 feet), laxly branched
   Akenes smooth, usually lacking marbled pattern on outer coat, firmly attached to stalk and without definite articulation   *C. sativa*
1A) Plants usually small (four feet or less), not laxly branched
    Akenes usually strongly marbled on outer coat, with definite abscission layer, dropping off at maturity
 2) Plants very densely branched, more or less conical, usually four feet tall or less. Abscission layer a simple articulation at base of akene
                                                                      C. indica
2A) Plants not branched or very sparsely so, usually one to two feet at maturity. Abscission layer forms a fleshy caruncle-like growth at base of akene   *C. ruderalis*

V. Acceptance of a polytypic composition of the genus *Cannabis* should not really lead to so much opposition as it seems to have caused in some botanical circles. As has been pointed out above, this opinion is nothing new and has been substantiated by critical work in wild populations.

But there have been greater changes in our concepts of cannabis. For many years, the family to which *Cannabis* belongs has been uncertain. Early taxonomists tended to put *Cannabis* in the Urticaceae, the Nettle Family. Then, botanists tended to allocate the genus to the Moraceae, the Fig Family. Now, almost all botanists are in agreement that *Cannabis* should be classified in a separate family, the Cannabaceae (sometimes incorrectly called the Cannabinaceae or Cannabidiaceae), which includes only two genera: *Cannabis* and the genus of the hop plant, *Humulus*. This change in outlook is much more drastic than the change from a monotypic to a polytypic concept of the specific composition of the genus — yet it has come about without the opposition which the proposal of several species instead of one extremely variable species has met in some circles. Furthermore, the change in understanding of the chemical makeup of the genus during the past few years — from four or five to more than twenty-nine cannabinolic structures — has been even more drastic.

VI. The principal fieldwork on cannabis was carried out more than forty-five years ago. We now have available more sophisticated and interdisciplinary techniques for arriving at taxonomic evaluation of generic, specific and subspecific classification of plants, especially of cultivated plants which have been manipulated and drastically altered through agricultural and horticultural practices extending over thousands of years.

The time is long overdue when a full study of cannabis taxonomy must be initiated. Cannabis has not received the taxonomic attention commensurate with its position as an ancient domesticate; as an important crop throughout most of man's history; as a genus with many interesting and varied uses; as the source of a narcotic, the use or abuse of which perplexes modern society; and as a plant which, through modern phytochemical investigations, holds promise for even greater significance to the material and cultural evolution of humankind.

VII. The genus *Cannabis* was described in 1737 by Linnaeus:

Cannabis Linnaeus Gen. Pl. (Ed. 1) (1737).

Since the beginning of modern botanical nomenclature in 1753, the following specific epithets have been proposed in cannabis.

Cannabis americana Houghton et Hamilton in Am. Journ. Pharm. 80 (1908) 17, *nomen nudum*.

Cannabis erratica Sievers ex Pallas Neue Nord. Beytr. 7 (1796) 174, *nomen nudum*.

Cannabis foetens Gilibert Exercit. Phytol. 2 (1792) 450, *nomen illegitimum*.

Cannabis generalis E. H. L. Krause in Sturm Fl. Deutschland, Ed. 2, 4 (1905) 199.

Cannabis gigantea Crévost in Bull. Econ. Indochine, n.s., 20 (1917) 613.

Cannabis indica Lamarck Encylc. 1 (1783) 695.

× *Cannabis intersita* Soják in Novit. Bot. Del Sem. Hort. Bot. Univ. Carol Praga (1960) 20.

Cannabis Lupulus Scopoli Pl. Carniol., Ed. 2, 2 (1772) 263.

Cannabis marcrosperma Stokes Bot. Mat. Med. 4 (1812) 539.

Cannabis pedemontana Camp in Journ. N. Y. Bot. Gard. 36 (1936) 114, *nomen nudum in synon.*

Cannabis ruderalis Janischewsky in Uchenye Zap. Gos. Saratov. Univ. 2, pt. 2 (1924) 14.

Cannabis sativa Linnaeus Sp. Pl. (1753) 1027.

REFERENCES

ANDERSON, E.
1949   *Introgressive hybridization.* New York: John Wiley & Sons.

ANDERSON, LORAN C.
1974   A study of systematic wood anatomy in cannabis. *Botanical Museum Leaflets,* Harvard University 23:29-48.

CAMP, W. H.
1936   The antiquity of hemp as an economic plant. *Journal of the New York Botanical Garden* 37:110-114.

DARWIN, C.
1868   *The variation of animals and plants under domestication* 2:201, 331. New York: Orange Judd & Company.

DAVIDIAN, G. G.
1972   Konoplia. *Bulletin of Applied Botany, Genetic Plant Breeding* (Technical Crops) 48 (3), Leningrad [in Russian].

De CANDOLLE, A. L. P. P.
1884   *Origin of cultivated plants.* London: Kegan Paul, Trench and Company.

DOORENBOS, N. J., *et al.*
1971   Cultivation, extraction and analysis of *Cannabis sativa* L. *Annals of the New York Academy of Sciences* 191:8-14.

GODWIN, H.
1967   The ancient cultivation of hemp. *Antiquity* 41:42-50.

HOUGHTON, E. M., H. C. HAMILTON
1908   A pharmacological study of *Cannabis americana (Cannabis sativa). American Journal of Pharmacology* 80:16-20.

HUTCHINSON, J.
1959   *The families of flowering plants 1 (Dicotyledons).* Ed. 2, 201. London: Oxford University Press.

KOMAROV, V. L., *editor*
1936   Flora of the USSR. *Israel Program for Scientific Translations.* Jerusalem. [Russian original: 5:383-384. Moscow-Leningrad: Academia Nauk SSSR.]

LAUFER, B.
1919   Sino-Iranica. Chinese contributions to the history of civilization in

ancient Iran.... *Field Museum of Natural History, Anthropology Series* 15:185–630.

MECHOULAM, R., *editor*
1937   *Marijuana.* New York: Academic Press.

MERLIN, M. D.
1972   *Man and marijuana.* Rutherford-Madison-Teaneck, New Jersey: Farleigh Dickinson University Press.

MILLER, N. G.
1970   The genera of the Cannabaceae in the southeastern United States. *Journal of the Arnold Arboretum* 51:185–203.

NASSOVOV, V. A.
1940   "Anatomical characteristics of geographical races of hemp," in *Vestnik Sotsialisticheskogo Rastenievostva* 4:107–120. Moscow: Institut Rastenievodstva. [in Russian].

NORDAL, A., O. BRAENDEN
1973   Variations in the cannabinoid content of Cannabis plants grown from the same batches of seeds under different ecological conditions. *Meddelelser Norsk Farmaceutisk Selskap* 35:8–15.

POSTMA, W. P.
1946   *Mitosis, meiosis en alloploidie bij Cannabis sativa en Spinacia oleracea.* Haarlem: H. D. Tjeenk & Zoon N.V.

QUIMBY, M. W., *et al.*
1973   Mississippi-grown marihuana — *Cannabis sativa.* Cultivation and observed morphological variation. *Economic Botany* 27:117–127.

SCHULTES, R. E.
1970   "Random thoughts and queries on the botany of Cannabis," in *The botany and chemistry of cannabis.* By C. R. B. Joyce and S. H. Curry. London: J. & A. Churchill.
1973   Man and marijuana. *Natural History* (August):59–63, 80, 82.

SCHWANITZ, F.
1966   *The origin of cultivated plants.* Cambridge, Mass.: Harvard University Press.

SMALL, E.
1972   Infertility and chromosomal uniformity in cannabis. *Canadian Journal of Botany* 50:1947–1949.

SOJÁK, J.
1960   In *Novitates Botanicae et Delectus Seminum Horti Botanici Universitatis Carolinae Pragensis*, 19–20.

STEARN, W. T.
1974   Typification of *Cannabis sativa* L. *Botanical Museum Leaflets*, Harvard University 23:325–336.

STOKES, J.
1812   *A botanical materia medica....* 4:539. London: J. Johnson and Company.

TURNER, C. E., K. HADLEY
1973   Constituents of *Cannabis sativa* L.II. Absence of cannibidol in an African variant. *Journal of Pharmaceutical Sciences* 62:251–255.

TURNER, C. E., K. HADLEY, P. S. FETTERMAN
1973   Constituents of *Cannabis sativa* L. VI. Propyl homologs in samples of

known geographical origin. *Journal of Pharmaceutical Sciences* 62: 1739–1741.

TUTIN, T. G. *et al., editors*
 1964 *Flora Europaea* 1. New York: Cambridge University Press.

VAVILOV, N. I.
 1926 Studies on the origin of cultivated plants. *Bulletin of Applied Botany* 16:1–248.

VAVILOV, N. I., D. D. BUKINICH
 1929 Agricultural Afghanistan. *Bulletin of Applied Botany 1, Genetic Plant Breeding, Supplement* 33:379–382.

ZHUKOVSKY, P. M.
 1964 *Cultivated plants and their wild relatives (systematics, geography, cytogenetics, ecology, origin)*. Ed. 2. Leningrad: Kolos Publishing House [in Russian]. Ed. 3. Revised and amended 1971. Leningrad: Kolos Publishing House [in Russian].

Early Diffusion and Folk Uses of Hemp

SULA BENET

ABSTRACT

Despite the growing volume of literature on the subject of hemp, the historical routes of its diffusion remain obscure and there is scant reference to its ubiquitous role in folk ritual, magic and medicine among European peasantry.

The term cannabis, itself, has been considered to be of Indo-European origin. The paper re-examines the origin of the term cannabis to demonstrate its derivation from Semitic languages. Both the word and its forms of use were borrowed by the nomadic Scythians from peoples of the Near East and diffused among the people with whom they came in contact. Ritual and other folk uses are described.

Hemp, one of the most versatile and important plants discovered by man and used for millennia, has been long neglected in scientific literature. Not until society's recent concern with drug addiction has the existing body of knowledge about hemp become so readily available. In the past, such information could be found in pharmacopoeia, in occasional historical references, or in ritual folkloristic material.

Although the body of literature concerning hemp has grown rapidly in the last decade, the exact origin of the plant has yet to be established; the historical routes of its diffusion remain obscure, and there is barely any reference to the role it played in the life of the European peasantry. The latter should be of special interest in view of the ubiquitous use of hemp in folk ritual, magic, and medicinal practices. A major reason for the obscurity as well as confusion that becloud the issue is that previously suggested theories of diffusion have been repeated and elaborated without critical examination of their historical sources. For example, the German scientists, Schrader, Hehn, and Bushan, as well as learned biblical commentaries and modern botanists, have claimed that ancient Palestine and Egypt did not know hemp and its uses (Dewey 1913; Moldenke 1952).

In this paper, I propose to reconsider the origin of the term *cannabis* to demonstrate that it is derived from Semitic languages and that both its name and forms of its use were borrowed by the Scythians from the peoples of the Near East. We will thus discover that the use of cannabis predates by at least 1000 years its first mention by Herodotus. Next, we will examine the diffusion of the plant to Europe and its continued use in peasant rituals, magic, and medical practices.

Western scholars have universally considered the term cannabis to be of Indo-European, specifically Scythian, origin. This widely-held opinion not only credited the Scythians with the name for hemp (which Linnaeus categorized as *Cannabis sativa*) but also with the initial introduction of the plant into Europe and Asia. There was barely any history of cannabis before the Greek historian Herodotus, in the fifth century B.C., observed that the Scythians used the plant to purge themselves after funerals by throwing hemp seeds on heated stones to create a thick vapor, inhaling the smoke and becoming intoxicated. "The Scythians howl with joy for the vapour bath" (Herodotus, IV: 142). To the Western world, Herodotus' account is the earliest source of knowledge of the ritual use of cannabis.

Tracing the history of hemp in terms of cultural contacts, the Old Testament must not be overlooked since it provides one of the oldest and most important written source materials. In the original Hebrew text of the Old Testament there are references to hemp, both as incense, which was an integral part of religious celebration, and as an intoxicant (Benet 1936). Cannabis as an incense was also used in the temples of Assyria and Babylon "because its aroma was pleasing to the Gods" (Meissner 1925 (II): 84).

Both in the original Hebrew text of the Old Testament and in the Aramaic translation, the word *kaneh* or *keneh* is used either alone or linked to the adjective *bosm* in Hebrew and *busma* in Aramaic, meaning aromatic. It is *cana* in Sanskrit, *qunnabu* in Assyrian, *kenab* in Persian, *kannab* in Arabic and *kanbun* in Chaldean. In Exodus 30:23, God directed Moses to make a holy oil composed of "myrrh, sweet cinnamon, kaneh bosm and kassia." In many ancient languages, including Hebrew, the root *kan* has a double meaning — both hemp and reed. In many translations of the Bible's original Hebrew, we find *kaneh bosm* variously and erroneously translated as "calamus"[1] and "aromatic reed," a vague term. The error occurred in the oldest Greek translation of the Hebrew Bible, Septuagint, in the third century B.C., where the terms *kaneh, kaneh bosm* were incorrectly translated as "calamus." And in the many translations

---

[1] Calamus, (*Calamus aromaticus*) is a fragrant marsh plant.

that followed, including Martin Luther's, the same error was repeated.[2]

Another piece of evidence regarding the use of the word *kaneh* in the sense of hemp rather than reed among the Hebrews is the religious requirement that the dead be buried in *kaneh* shirts. Centuries later, linen was substituted for hemp (Klein 1908).

In the course of time, the two words *kaneh* and *bosm* were fused into one, *kanabos* or *kannabus*, known to us from Mishna, the body of traditional Hebrew law. The word bears an unmistakable similarity to the Scythian "cannabis." Is it too far-fetched to assume that the Semitic word *kanbosm* and the Scythian word *cannabis* mean the same thing?

Since the history of cannabis has been tied to the history of the Scythians, it is of interest to establish their appearance in the Near East. Again, the Old Testament provides information testifying to their greater antiquity than has been previously assumed. The Scythians participated in both trade and wars alongside the ancient Semites for at least one millennium before Herodotus encountered them in the fifth century B.C. The reason for confusion and the relative obscurity of the role played by the Scythians in world history is explained by the fact that they were known to the Greeks as Scythians but to the Semites as Ashkenaz. Identification of the Scythian-Ashkenaz as a single people is convincingly made by Ellis H. Minns (1965) in his definitive work on Scythians and Greeks. The earliest reference to the Ashkenaz people appears in the Bible in Genesis 10:3, where Ashkenaz, their progenitor, is named as the son of Gomer, the great-grandson of Noah. The Ashkenaz of the Bible were both war-like and extremely mobile. In Jeremiah 51:27, we read that the kingdoms of Ararat (known later as Armenia), Minni (Medea), and Ashkenaz attacked Babylonia. In 612 B.C. Babylonians with the aid of the Medeans (Medes) and Scythians, coming from the Caucasus, dealt a deadly blow to Assyria (Durant 1954). Referring to the threat of war, Herodotus reports that Scythians attempted to invade Egypt by way of Palestine and that they withdrew only after the Pharaoh paid them to retreat.

There is evidence of the presence of the Scythians in Palestine. The city known as Beizan in modern times was originally called Bethshan and later renamed Scythopolis by the Greeks during the Hellenistic period, since many Scythians settled there during the great invasion of Palestine in the seventh century B.C.

---

[2] In Exodus 30:23 *kaneh bosm* is translated as "sweet calamus." In Isiah 43:24 *kaneh* is translated as "sweet cane," although the word "sweet" appears nowhere in the original. In Jeremiah 6:20 *kaneh* is translated as "sweet cane." In Ezekiel 27:19 *kaneh* is translated as "calamus." In Song of Songs 4:14 *kaneh* is translated "calamus."

The importance of the geographical position of Palestine cannot be overlooked when considering the trade routes through which caravans moved, laden with goods and precious "spices." Palestine was situated along the two most vital trade routes of the ancient world. One was between Egypt and Asia and the other ran west from Arabia to the coastal plain, from there branching off to Egypt to Syria. In the original Hebrew of the Bible (Ezekiel 27:19), in a description of Tyre, the royal city of the Phoenicians, famous in antiquity for its far-flung trade, it is noted that "Vedon and Yavan traded with yarn for thy wares; massive iron, cassia, and kaneh were among thy merchandise."[3] King Solomon, a contemporary and friend of King Hiram of Tyre (960 B.C.), ordered hemp cords among other materials for building his temples and throne (Salzberger 1912). Rostovtzeff (1932) describes the caravan trade between Babylonia, Egypt, Syria, and Asia Minor. Among the goods there was incense for the "delection of gods and men."

In addition to the caravan trade, the mobile, warlike Ashkenaz carried their raids to the Caucasus in the north and westward to Europe, taking with them their knowledge of the use of hemp as well as their dependence on its intoxicating qualities. So mobile were the Scythians that there is a good probability that as they spilled across much of Europe and Asia, they were the ones to introduce the natives to the ritual use of the plant and the narcotic pleasures to be derived from it. The Scythians apparently did not use hemp for manufactures such as weaving and rope-making. Yet, despite the plentiful quantity of wild hemp, the Scythians cultivated the plant in order to increase the amount available for their use. Apparently their need for it was great indeed.

Since hemp was originally used in rituals, it may be assumed that the Scythians spread their custom among the people with whom they came into contact. The Siberian tribes of Pazaryk in the Altai region (discovered by the Soviet archaeologist, S. Rudenko) left burial mounds in which bronze vessels containing burnt hemp seeds to produce incense vapors were found. Rudenko believes that these objects were used for funeral purification ceremonies similar to those practised by the Scythians (Emboden 1972:223).

Another custom connected with the dead in parts of Eastern Europe is the throwing of a handful of seeds into the fire as an offering to the dead during the harvesting of hemp — similar to the custom of the Scythians and of the Pazaryk tribes, two-and-a-half thousand years ago. There is no doubt that some of the practices, such as funeral customs,

---

[3] The markets of Tyre were frequented by the Jews. Biblical quotation from *The Holy Scriptures*, the Jewish Publication Society of America.

were introduced by the Scythians during their victorious advance into southeast Russia, including the Caucasus, where they remained for centuries.

Hemp never lost its connection with the cult of the dead. Even today in Poland and Lithuania, and in former times also in Russia, on Christmas Eve when it is believed that the dead visit their families, a soup made of hemp seeds, called *semieniatka*, is served for the dead souls to savor. In Latvia and the Ukraine, a dish made of hemp was prepared for Three Kings Day.

Since the plant was associated with religious ritual and the power of healing, magical practices were connected with its cultivation. In Europe, peasants generally believed that planting hemp should take place on the days of saints who were known to be tall in order to encourage the plant's growth. In Germany, long steps are taken while sowing the seed which is thrown high into the air. In Baden the planting is done during the "high" hours, between 11:00 a.m. and noon. Cakes baked to stimulate hemp growth are known as *hanfeier*.

Following the planting, magical means are applied to make the hemp grow tall and straight. The custom of dancing or jumping to promote the growth of the plant is known throughout Europe. In Poland, married women dance "the hemp dance" on Shrove Tuesday, leaping high into the air. The hemp dance ('for hemp's sake') is also danced at weddings by the young bride with the *raiko*, the master of ceremonies (Kolberg 1899). In the wedding rituals of the Southern Slavs, hemp is a symbol of wealth and a talisman for happiness. When the bride enters her new home after the wedding ceremony, she strokes the four walls of her new home with a bunch of hemp. She is herself sprinkled with hemp seeds to bring good luck. In Estonia, the young bride visits her neigbors in the company of older women asking for gifts of hemp. She is thus "showered" with hemp.

The odor of European hemp is stimulating enough to produce euphoria and a desire for sociability and gaiety and harvesting of hemp has always been accompanied by social festivities, dancing, and sometimes even erotic playfulness.

Women play a leading role in the festivities. In Poland, initiation ceremonies are held during the harvest. Young brides are admitted into the circle of older married women on payment of a token fee. Since the Catholic Church never deemed it necessary to interfere with these festivals, it must have regarded them as harmless and perhaps even socially benevolent. In Eastern Europe hemp is evidently not considered addictive and no case of solitary use among the peasants has been reported: it is always used in a context of group participation. In many countries, hemp gathering is an occasion for socializing. The Swiss call it *stelg* (Hager 1919). Young men come to the gathering wearing carnival masks and offer gifts to the girls.

Hemp gathering rituals also reveal the sacred character of the plant. In certain areas of Poland, at midnight, a chalk ring is drawn around the plant which is then sprinkled with holy water. The person collecting the plant hopes that part of the flower will fall into his boots and bring him good fortune. The flower of a hemp plant gathered on St. John's Eve in the Ukraine is thought to counteract witchcraft and protect farm animals from the evil eye.

Although it is believed that witches can use the plant to inflict harm, they are not likely to do so in fact, and hemp is often used against persons suspected of witchcraft. In Poland, it is used for divination, especially in connection with marriage. The eve of St. Andrews (November 30th) is considered a most propitious time for divination about future husbands. Certain magical spells, using hemp, are believed to advance the date of marriage, perhaps even signal the very day it will occur. Girls in the Ukraine carry hemp seeds in their belts, they jump on a heap and call out:

Andrei, Andrei,
I plant the hemp seed on you.
Will god let me know
With whom I will sleep?

The girls then remove their shirts and fill their mouths with water to sprinkle on the seed to keep the birds from eating them. Then they run around the house naked three times.

The sacred character of hemp in biblical times is evident from Exodus 30:22–33, where Moses was instructed by God to anoint the meeting tent and all its furnishings with specially prepared oil, containing hemp. Anointing set sacred things apart from the secular. The anointment of sacred objects was an ancient tradition in Israel: holy oil was not to be used for secular purposes.

And thou shalt speak unto the children of Israel, saying, "This shall be a holy anointing oil unto me, throughout your generations." (King James Version, Exodus 30:31).

Above all, the anointing oil was used for the installation rites of all Hebrew kings and priests. Dr. R. Patai (1947) expresses the opinion that the use of sacred oil is based on the belief in its nourishing, conserving and healing powers. Dr. Patai discusses the spread of this custom from the ancient Near East to most of Africa where we find the ritual of anointing among other parallels in the rites of installation of kings.

Almost all ancient peoples considered narcotic and medicinal plants sacred and incorporated them into their religious or magical beliefs and practices. In Africa, there were a number of cults and sects of hemp worship. Pogge and Wissman, during their explorations of 1881, visited the Bashilenge, living on the northern borders of the Lundu, between Sankrua and Balua. They found large plots of land around the villages used for the cultivation of hemp. Originally there were small clubs of hemp smokers, bound by ties of friendship, but these eventually led to the formation of a religious cult. The Bashilenge called themselves *Bena-Riamba* — "the sons of hemp," and their land *Lubuku*, meaning friendship. They greeted each other with the expression "*moio*," meaning both "hemp" and "life."

Each tribesman was required to participate in the cult of *Riamba* and show his devotion by smoking as frequently as possible. They attributed universal magical powers to hemp, which was thought to combat all kinds of evil and they took it when they went to war and when they travelled. There were initiation rites for new members which usually took place before a war or long journey. The hemp pipe assumed a symbolic meaning for the Bashilenge somewhat analogous to the significance which the peace pipe had for American Indians. No holiday, no trade agreement, no peace treaty was transacted without it (Wissman *et al.* 1888). In the middle Sahara region, the Senusi sect also cultivated hemp on a large scale for use in religious ceremonies (*Ibid.*).

USE OF CANNABIS IN FOLK MEDICINE

Hemp, both because of its psychoactive properties and its mystical significance, became a popular and widely-utilized plant in the folk medicine of Europe and Asia. Since ancient times its soothing, tranquilizing action has been known. The Atharvaveda (1400 B.C.) mentions hemp as a medicinal and magical plant. In the Zend-Avesta, hemp occupies the first place in a list of 10,000 medicinal plants given to a doctor Thrita. According to Dioscorides (100 A.D.), the resin of fresh hemp is an excellent treatment for earaches (Dioscorides 1902). In an old Germanic catalogue of medicinal plants, hemp is listed as a tranquilizer (Hofler n.d.). An edition of Diocletian also mentions the use of cannabis as a medicament (Bretschneider 1881). Medieval Arab doctors considerd hemp a sacred medicine which they called *schâhdânach*, *schâdâbach* or *kannab* (Dragendorff 1898). Syrenius wrote in 1613 that ointment made from hemp resin is the most effective remedy for burns (Syrenius 1613) and that diseased joints could be straightened with the roots of hemp boiled in water.

In Russia and Eastern Europe hemp was widely used in folk medicine, and references can also be found to its use in Western Europe. In Germany for example, sprigs of hemp were placed over the stomach and ankles to prevent convulsions and difficult childbirth, and in Switzerland hemp was also used to treat convulsions. In Poland, Russia and Lithuania, hemp was used to alleviate toothache by inhaling the vapor from hemp seeds thrown on hot stones (Biegeleisen 1929). Szyman of Lowic (16th century) gives the following prescription: "For worms in the teeth, boil hemp seeds in a new pot and add heated stones. When this vapor is inhaled the worms will fall out." This method is varied somewhat in Ukranian folk medicine, the fumes of cooked hemp porridge are believed to intoxicate the worms and cause them to fall out. In Czechoslovakia and Moravia, as in Poland, hemp was considered an effective treatment for fevers. In Poland, a mixture of hemp flowers, wax and olive oil was used to dress wounds. Oil from crushed hemp seeds is used as a treatment for jaundice and rheumatism in Russia. In Serbia, hemp is considered an aphrodisiac (Tschirch 1911). Hemp is also thought to increase a man's strength. In the Ukraine there is a legend of a dragon who lived in Kiev, oppressing the people and demanding tribute. The dragon was killed and the city liberated by a man wearing a hemp shirt.

Hemp is also used to treat animals. A cat that eats *mukhomor*, a poison mushroom, is kept in a hemp field to eat the plant until it "comes to its senses." And if chickens are given hemp seeds on Christmas Eve, they will lay all year round.

In central Asia, for cure or pleasure, hemp is eaten, chewed, smoked, rubbed over the body, inhaled and made into numerous elaborate concoctions. Since the Soviet Union leads a determined fight against the use of hashish, the subject is taboo, and the literature on *nasha*, as hemp is called in central Asia, is virtually nonexistent. Prof. Antzyferov (1934) wrote a short but most interesting report on the use of hashish in central Asia. Hemp has also been used for the cure of chronic alcoholics in central Asia quite succesfully, according to Dr. Antzyferov.

At the time of his report, Prof. Antzyferov was the head of the State Hospital at Tashkent where he collected among his patients and their relatives and friends numerous recipes for *nasha*. All of his informants believed that a great deal of fat taken in food counteracts any harmful effect of *nasha*. Some recipes are family secrets, others are well known and used for centuries by the general public, native and European settlers alike.

A mixture of lamb's fat with *nasha* is recommended for brides to use on their wedding night to reduce the pain of defloration. The same mixture works well for headache when rubbed into the skin; it may also be eaten spread on bread.

A candy called *guc-kand,* popular among women for a "happy mood," is made of hemp boiled in water, put through a sieve with added sugar, saffron and several egg whites. The ingredients are mashed and formed into small balls and then dried in the sun. The candy is given to boys before circumcision to reduce pain and to children to keep them from crying. An ointment made by mixing hashish with tobacco is used by some women to shrink the vagina and prevent fluor alvus.

There is also "the happy porridge" made of the following ingredients: (1) almond butter mixed with *nasha,* (2) dried rose leaves, (3) root of Anacyclius pyrethrum, (4) carnation petals, (5) crocus, (6) muscut nut, (7) cardamon, (8) honey, and (9) sugar. This mixture is the most expensive of all hashish preparations. It is eagerly sought by men who consider it the strongest aphrodisiac.

The use of hemp in Europe and Asia is, of course, much older than archaeological, historical or linguistic evidence would indicate. Early man roaming around in search of edible plants must have easily discovered the seeds and powerful odor of the ripened tips of the weeds.

There is considerable difference of opinion concerning the place of origin of the plant and its diffusion, specifically, its appearance in Eastern Europe, but it is generally understood that it should be searched where it grows in the wild.[4] The Russian botanist, N. Vavilov (1926) considers the region where the greatest number of varieties of a particular plant grow is the center of its evolutionary differentiation and variation. The common mid-European hemp is known as "Russian" or "German" hemp. This variety is spread over most of Europe except for the southern part. Hemp belongs to the group of plants which are self-planting and self-fertilizing. Yanishevski observed that it draws to its fatty tissue a bug, *Pirrhocoris apterus* L., which clings to the base of the hemp seeds. The *Pirrhocoris* and birds contribute to the dissemination of hemp seeds. De Candolle (1883), seeing the wild plant in the Black Sea and Aralian regions, concluded that this was the place of origin. We now know that hemp is also indigenous to the Russian plains, the Caucasus, Transcaucasia, the Crimea and the Urals, in fact, the whole area from China to the Balkan Peninsula (Vavilov 1926).

We must, therefore, conclude that there was not one but probably several origin sites and that whenever man discovered hemp he used it for

---

[4] Editor's note: see article by Schultes in this volume.

food and probably as a stimulant. However, the ritual use of hemp as well as the name, cannabis, in my opinion originated in the Ancient Near East. From there in the middle of the second millennium B.C. through trade contacts, migrations and wars, the ritual uses of the plant were carried to Egypt and Africa, westward to Europe, and eastward to central Asia. Whether India received the plant from China or central Asia is not clear.

Hemp, as used originally in religious rituals, temple activities, and tribal rites, involves groups of people rather than the solitary individual. The pleasurable psychoactive effects of hemp were then, as now, communal experiences.

I believe that the acceptance of tobacco in Europe was undoubtedly enhanced by European familiarity with smoking hemp. Tobacco was, in many ways a counterpart to hemp, all the familiar features were there. Brought to Spain from the New World as a medicinal plant, it came to be regarded as a cure-all; the Amerindian ritual use of tobacco may also have been known, and eventually also its psychoactive qualities. Even the use of pipes for smoking tobacco in the Near East was adopted from the water-pipes used for smoking hemp. Like hemp, tobacco is chewed, sniffed and smoked.

Perhaps the spread of tobacco was so rapid and overwhelming in the Old World, because a receptive ground had been laid by the traditional folk uses of hemp.

REFERENCES

ANTZYFEROV, L. V.
    1934   Hashish in Central Asia. *Journal of Socialist Health Care in Uzbekstan.* Tashkent [in Russian].

BENET, SULA (BENETOWA)
    1936   Le chanvre dans les croyances et les coutumes populaires. *Comtes Rendus de Séances de la Société des Sciences et des Lettres de Varsovie* XXVII.

BIEGELEISEN, H.
    1929   *Lecznictwo ludu Polskiego* [Polish folk medicine]. Crakow.

BRETSCHNEIDER
    1881   Gotanicon sinicum. *Journal of Northern China, Branch of the Royal Asia Society* I:569.

DE CANDOLLE, ALPHONSE LOUIS P. P.
    1883   *Origine des plantes cultivées.* Paris: G. Bailliere.

DEWEY, L. H.
    1913   Hemp. *Yearbook of the Department of Agriculture.* 289.

DIOSCORIDES, ANAZARBEUS PEDACIUS
　1902　*Arzneimittellehre* [Pharmacology]. Translated by J. Berendes. Vol. III. Stuttgart: F. Enke.
DRAGENDORFF, GEORG
　1898　*Die Heilpflanzen der verschiedenen Völker und Zeiten* [The medical plants of various peoples and times]. Stuttgart: F. Enke.
DURANT, W.
　1954　*Our oriental heritage.* Vol. I. New York: Simon and Schuster.
EMBODEN, WILLIAM A. JR.
　1972　"Ritual use of Cannabis sativa L," in *Flesh of the Gods: the ritual use of hallucinogens.* Edited by Peter T. Furst. New York: Praeger Publishers. 223.
HAGER, K.
　1919　Flachs und Hanfund ihre verarbeitung im Bundner Oberland. *Yahrbuch des Schweizer Alpenclub* 147.
HOFLER
　n.d.　Altgermanische Heilkunde [Old-Germanic medicine]. *Neubuerger-Pogel's Handbuch* I: 466.
KLEIN, SIEGFRIED
　1908　*Tod und Begrabnis in Palistina.* Berlin: H. Itzkowski.
KOLBERG, O.
　1899　*Mazowsze Lud.* Towarzystwo Ludoznawcze V: 206.
MEISSNER, B.
　1925　*Babylonien und Assyrian.* II: 84. Heidelberg: von W. Foy.
MINNS, ELLIS H.
　1965　*Scythians and Greeks.* Vol. I. New York: Biblo and Tannen.
MOLDENKE, H., A. MOLDENKE
　1952　*Plants of the Bible.* Waltham, Massachusetts: Cronica Botanica Co.
PATAI, R.
　1947　Hebrew installation rites. *Hebrew Union College Annual* XX.
ROSTOVTZEFF, M.
　1932　*Caravan cities.* London: Oxford.
SALZBERGER, G.
　1912　*Salomons Tempelbau und Thron* [The building of Solomon's temple and throne]. Berlin: Mayer and Muller.
SYRENIUS, SZ.
　1613　"Zielnik [Medicinal plants]," in *Typographia Basilii Skalski.* Krakow: [in Polish].
TSCHIRCH, A.
　1912　*Handbuch der Pharmakognosie* [Pharmaceutical handbook]. II. Leipzig: Verlag von chr. Herm. Tauchnitz.
VAVILOV, N.
　1926　Tzentry proiskhozhdenia kulturnksh rastenii [Centers of origin of domesticated plants]. *Trudy no Prile Bot. I. Sel.* XVI: 109 [in Russian].
WISSMANN, H., et al.
　1888　*Im innern Afrikas* [In inner Africa]. Leipzig: F. A. Brockhaus.

The Origin and Use of Cannabis in Eastern Asia: Their Linguistic-Cultural Implications

HUI-LIN LI

ABSTRACT

Archeological evidence has shown that cannabis was used as a fiber plant in northeastern Asia in neolithic times — about 6,000 years ago. The Chinese character for hemp, *ma*, dates to about 3,000 years ago and was derived from an ideogram depicting the plant's fiber producing character. In early writings separate characters were assigned to male and female hemp plants, its seeds, fruits, etc. This differentiation indicates the antiquity of its cultivation as it points to an enduring and varied relationship of man to the plant.

The cannabis plant had multitudinal uses in ancient times in China, another fact attesting to its antiquity as a cultivated species. Besides its importance as a plant fiber, cannabis was an important food plant, being listed as one of the five major "grains."

The medicinal properties of the plant were first recorded in the classical herbal *Pen Ts'ao Ching*, first compiled in the second century A. D. but undoubtedly based on traditions passed down from prehistoric times. The stupefying nature of cannabis and its hallucinogenic effect were clearly described. The drug was used as a cure for various diseases and as an effective pain killer. Later pharmacopoeias repeated or confirmed these properties but indicated that the plant was rarely used, and then only by necromancers for its hallucinogenic effect.

The original character *ma* in later usage assumed two additional connotations. One connotation meant numerous or chaotic, derived from the nature of the plants' fibers. The second connotation was one of numbness or senselessness, apparently derived from the stupefying effect of the fruits and leaves. *Ma* was used in these ways as a radical for many other characters.

It is suggested that the drug use of the plant was widely known to the neolithic peoples of northeastern Asia and that it played an important part in the practice of shamanism — widespread in that northern area. The great mobility of these nomadic tribes apparently carried the plant to western Asia and from there into India, where its use proliferated. While cannabis use and shamanism in general were on the upswing in these other Asian locales, its hallucinogenic practices slowly declined in China from the age of Confucius onwards. Only in sporadic small areas did the shamanistic traditions continue.

The discontinuation of cannabis in China as a "drug" apparently had its reasons. The Chinese were not averse to taking drugs to alter states of consciousness. "Wu shih," a mineral drug, was used in the third century by certain of the intelligentsia. In more recent times tobacco has been accepted with the same enthusiasm it has met in other parts of the world. Opium, first introduced from western Asia in about the 8th century as a drug, gradually became adopted as a narcotic. In the nineteenth century, under pressure from foreign powers, its use became common throughout China. The adoption of the introduced opium, a euphorica, and the non-adoption of the indigenous cannabis, a phantastica, is explained herein with its cultural implications.

Cannabis sativa is one of man's oldest cultivated plants. Botanically it is distinct from all other plants and readily recognized. Yet among individual plants it is extremely variable. It now grows spontaneously in great abundance and ubiquity. While most botanists consider the plant monotypic, some regard it as consisting of more than one species and a number of varieties, and so propose several different systems of classification. The systematics of this plant still awaits classification by further botanical studies.

Cannabis is generally believed to be an Asiatic plant. There is no concerted agreement among botanists as to where the plant originally grew wild and where its cultivation first began. Estimates range within the wide span of temperate Asia from the Caucasus Mountains and the Caspian Sea through western and central Asia to eastern Asia. There is no easy way to distinguish between wild and spontaneous or adventitious, and semi-cultivated or cultivated plants. And so much remains to be done in determining the geographical origin of the plant.

These difficulties in classification and origin arise from the long and close association of cannabis with man. Man has caused its extreme variations and wide dispersion. It will no longer suffice to study the plant itself alone. The influence of man must be considered side by side with the botanical fact in order to unveil the complex nature of this plant.

Historically, the oldest records in existence seem to place the origin of cultivation in northeastern Asia, a portion of which falls in present northern China where the early Chinese civilization began. Cannabis has left a continuous record of its presence in this area from Neolithic times down to the present and its uses were closely integrated with the life and culture of the people throughout all periods.

As a cultivated plant, cannabis had multitudinous uses in ancient times in China, another fact attesting to its antiquity as a cultivated species. Besides its importance as a fiber plant, it was also an important food plant, one of the major "grains" of the ancients. And it was an important medicinal plant.

The earliest or primary use of the plant was probably for its fibers. It was the only fiber plant (hemp) known to ancient peoples in northern and northeastern China, and eastern Siberia. In China its use was so extensive and important that from the earliest times the phrase, "land of mulberry and hemp," was used as a synonym for cultivated fields. Mulberry trees were planted for their leaves used to feed silkworms. These, in turn, produced the unique product, silk, that made China famous in other lands. Silk fabrics were used by the wealthy while hemp cloth was the textile of the masses.

Textile fibers are next to cereal grains in social and cultural importance to early man. From the standpoint of textile fibers, three centers can be recognized in the ancient Old World; the linen culture in the Mediterranean region, the cotton culture in India, and the hemp culture in eastern Asia. Each of these seems to have developed independently and their uses were unknown to each other for quite a long time.[1]

Evidence of the use of hemp fibers has been found in Neolithic records in northern China. This evidence appears as paintings of or impressions of ropes and woven cloth on pottery, as well as stone or pottery instruments of weaving: spinning-whorls and bone needles. Andersson[2] first discovered the Neolithic culture in Honan province. It has become known as the Yang-shao culture and is characterized by painting pottery; Andersson believed that these traces pertained to hemp. Relics of this culture are now dated by the carbon-14 method as around 5,200 to 6,200 years ago.[3] Many subsequent excavations have revealed that this culture extended along the Yellow River Valley to northeastern China. The presence of hemp has been supported by the findings of several other workers. Hemp was also found in discoveries of later Neolithic cultures such as the Lung-shan culture of about 3,200 to 4,200 years ago. Archeological records have shown that hemp was continuously present in northern China from Neolothic times through all historic time down to the present.[4]

The ancient use of hemp as a fiber is substantiated by written records. Ancient literature indicates that hemp fibers were used since time immemorial for making ropes and fishing nets. Knots were tied in ropes as a

---

[1] Berthold Laufer, in his work *Sino-Iranica*, 1919, makes a point of great culture-historical interest about the "fundamental diversity between East-Asiatic and Mediterranean civilizations, — there hemp, and here flax, as material for clothing" (p. 293). In a footnote he says that he hopes to demonstrate in a subsequent study that hemp had been cultivated by the Indo-Chinese nations, especially the Chinese and Tibetans, in a prehistoric age. However, no such paper seems to have been actually published.
[2] Andersson, J. G., An early Chinese culture. *Bulletin of the Geological Survey of China* 1923 5 (1):26.
[3] An Chih-min, On the problem of dating in the Neolithic culture of our country. *K'ao-ku* 1972, 6:35–44.
[4] A more detailed account of the archeology and history of hemp in China will be given in a separate paper.

means of record keeping before written language. Fishing is believed to have preceded the domestication of animals.

The great cultural importance attached to hemp as a textile fiber is clearly indicated by the practice, since Confucian times, of wearing hemp fabric clothes while mourning the death of a parent or parents. The practice was prescribed in the *Li Chi* (Book of Rites) of the second century B.C. and was meticulously followed through all ages down to recent times. The great emphasis on filial piety in Chinese culture indicates the significance of such a long tradition.

A further distinctly important contribution of hemp fiber to Chinese culture, as well as to the culture of mankind as a whole, is the role it played in the invention of paper. Paper originated in China in the late Han dynasty. According to the dynastic history *Hou-Han shu*, the Marquis Ts'ai Lun used old fish nets, ragged cloth, hemp fibers, and tree bark in making paper and presented his new invention to the throne in 105 A.D. Fish nets and cloth were also made of hemp fibers. Ts'ai Lun probably perfected a technique that had been in use for some time. The oldest existing paper made of hemp was recently discovered in a grave in Shensi province that dates before the reign of Emperor Wu (104–87 B.C.) of the Early Han dynasty.[5]

There is also linguistic evidence for original and primary use of cannabis as a fiber plant. The character *ma*, in the ancient *chuan* script, was derived from ideographic components representing fibers hanging on a rack and placed under a roofed shack. Having evolved from the ancient to the later styles, it remains the character for hemp (Fig. 1). When other fiber plants from the warmer regions of the south, as well as introduced plants from foreign countries became known, the character *ma* developed into a generic name for fiber, and hemp itself was known as *ta-ma* (great *ma*), or sometimes as *Han-ma* (Chinese *ma*), or *hou-ma* (fire-*ma*).

At a very early period the Chinese recognized the cannabis plant as dioecious. While the name *ma* was applied to the plant in general, the male and female plants were accorded distinct names. The male plant, called *i* or *hsi*, yields the superior fiber. The female plant, known as *tsà* or *chü*, yields edible seeds and inferior fibers from the stem. Furthermore, the male flower clusters were called *p'o*, the fruiting clusters *fên* or *pên*, and the seeds *ma-jên* (Fig. 2). This ancient differentiation reflects the antiquity of the cultivation of the plant in the same way that it points to an enduring and varied relationship between man and plant.

This differentitation also suggests that the use of cannabis as a food

---

[5] Pan Chi-hsin, [The earliest plant-fiber paper in the world.] *Wen-wu* 1964. 11:48–49.

The Origin and Use of Cannabis in Eastern Asia

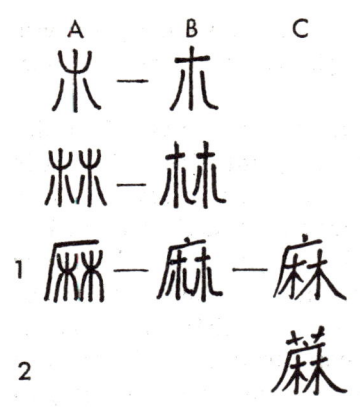

```
      A     B     C
1   朮 — 木
    林 — 林
    㡛 — 麻 — 麻
2              蔴
```

Figure 1. Evolvement of the character *ma* or hemp (line 1.) Column A, archiac *chuan* script, B, plain *chieh* script, C, cursive *hsing* script. Line 2 represents the vulgar word for *ma* with the added "grass" radical

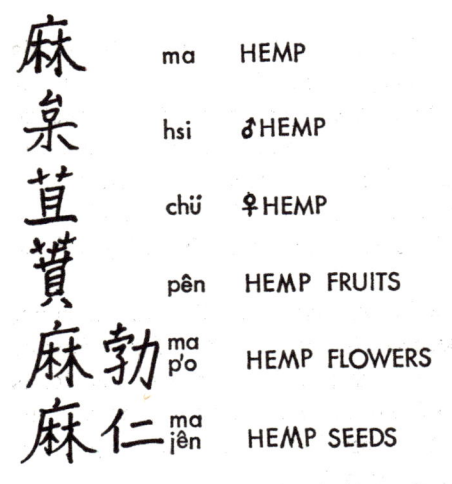

麻	ma	HEMP
枲	hsi	♂HEMP
苴	chü	♀HEMP
蕡	pên	HEMP FRUITS
麻勃	ma p'o	HEMP FLOWERS
麻仁	ma jên	HEMP SEEDS

Figure 2. Different names for the hemp plant and its parts

plant had a very early beginning. Hemp seeds were considered, along with millet, rice, barley and the soybean, as one of the major grains of ancient China. Its use as a fiber as well as a grain was mentioned in such classical literature as the *Shi Ching* (Book of Odes), and *Li Chi* (Book of Rites), both of about the first and second centuries B.C. or earlier. Detailed instructions on the cultivation of hemp as both a fiber and a grain crop were given in the most ancient works on agriculture in existence.

The use of oil from hemp seeds was a later development since it involved the more complicated process of extraction. As grains, the seeds were used until at least the 6th century A.D. In later times the grain was completely forgotten, due apparently to its replacement by other, superior, cereal grains.

As ancient man used hemp seeds for food, it was quite natural for him to also discover the medicinal properties of the plant. The edible seeds are enclosed in fruit-coverings which contain a toxic resinous substance. In the earliest medical literature this differentiation was clearly noted.

Definitive records of the medicinal and physiological effect of cannabis are found in the earliest pharmacopoeia in existence. The famous *Pên-ts'ao Ching*, attributed to the legendary Emperor Shên-nung of about 2,000 B.C., was compiled in the first or second centuries A.D., but was undoubtedly based on traditions passed down from earlier — even prehistoric — times. It states that "ma-fên (the fruits of hemp)... if taken in excess will produce hallucinations (literally "seeing devils"). If taken over a long term, it makes one communicate with spirits and lightens one's body."[6]

The famous physician Hua T'o (110-207 A.D.) lived at about this time. The dynastic history, *Hou-Han shu*, records that Hua T'o used *ma-fei-san* (hemp boiling compound), to be taken with wine, to anesthetize his patients during surgical operations on abdominal organs. After the operation magical balm was applied, and the patient recovered in due time. Wu Pu, a disciple of Hua T'o, wrote an herbal in 200 A.D. in which he made a clear distinction between the toxic hemp fruits (*ma-fên*) and the non-poisonous seeds or kernels.

Worthy of note is the work of the famous physician, T'ao Hung-ching, of the 5th century A.D. In his *Ming-i pieh-lu*, he noted the difference between the non-poisonous seeds (*ma-tze*) and the poisonous fruits (*ma-fên*). Of the latter he said, "Ma-fên is not much used in prescriptions [now a days]. Necromancers use it in combination with ginseng to set forward time in order to reveal future events."

In addition to the above statement about the temporal distortion caused by cannabis, there is a similar passage in the later work *Chêng-lei pên-ts'ao* by T'ang Shên-wei of the 10th century A.D. He stated that "Ma-fên has a spicy taste; it is toxic; it is used for waste diseases and injuries; it clears blood and cools temperature; it relieves fluxes; it undoes rheumatism; it discharges pus. If taken in excess it produces hallunications and a staggering gait. If taken over a long term, it causes one to communicate with spirits and lightens one's body."

[6] Passages of most of these older works were quoted or cited by Li Shih-chên in his *Pên-ts'ao kang-mu*, *Materia Medica*, 1590; Bretschneider, E.V., *Botanicon sinicum*, pt. 3, 1895, translates many of these entries into English.

That the stupefying effect of the hemp plant was commonly known from extremely early times is also indicated linguistically. The character *ma* very early assumed two connotations. One meaning was, "numerous or chaotic," derived from the nature of the plant's fibers. The second connotation was one of numbness or senselessness, apparently derived from the properties of the fruits and leaves which were used as infusions for medicinal purposes.

As a radical, *ma* combines with many other radicals to form such characters as *mo*, demon (combining *ma* with "devil"), *mo*, grind (combining *ma* with "stone"), *mi*, waste (combining *ma* with "negative"), *mo*, rub (combining *ma* with "hand"), *mi*, porridge (combining *ma* with "rice") (Fig. 3). As a character it combines with other characters to form such bisyllabic words as *ma-tsui*, narcotic (*ma* and "drunkenness"); *ma-mu*, numb (*ma* and "wood"); and *ma-p'i*, paralysis (*ma* and "rheumatism") (Fig. 4).

It should be mentioned that in ancient China, as in most early cultures, medicine had its origin in magic. Medicine men were practicing magicians. The evidence quoted above suggests that the medicinal use of the hemp plant was widely known to the Neolithic peoples of northeastern Asia and shamanism was especially widespread in this northern area and also in China, and cannabis played an important part in its rituals. The great mobility of the nomadic tribes north of China apparently assisted the movement of the plant to western Asia and from there to India, where its use as a drug intensified. While shamanism, and the use of cannabis in particular, were on the upswing in these other Asiatic locales, hallucinogenic practices slowly declined in China beginning with the Age of Confucius. Only in scattered small areas did shamanistic traditions continue in China during later ages.

The discontinuation of the use of cannabis as a drug in China was due to certain traceable causes. The Chinese were not adverse to taking drugs in order to alter states of consciousness. Wine was taken from very early times, though in general it was never used excessively. An exception was during the earliest historic dynasty when the Yin-Shang people of the 18-12th centuries B.C. were known to imbibe wine in great quantities. They created many kinds of elaborate bronze wine vessels which are among the greatest artistic achievements of ancient peoples. During the 3rd century the *Wu-shih san* (5 minerals compound), a prescription containing cinnabar (mercuric sulfide), was widely used in China by certain groups. As a drug, it produced certain physiological effects and some mental stimulation. Since it was expensive, its use was confined to the wealthy upper class, especially the intelligentsia. During this period of great poli-

麻 醉 narcotic

麻 木 numb

麻 痺 paralysis

麻 亂 tangle

麻 煩 troublesome

Figure 3. *Ma* as a component radical with the connotation of "numbness" in the 3 characters above and of "numerous" in the 2 lower ones

麻 + 鬼 = 魔
    devil   demon

麻 + 石 = 磨
    stone   grind

麻 + 非 = 靡
    negative waste

麻 + 手 = 摩
    hand   rub

麻 + 米 = 糜
    rice   porridge

Figure 4. *Ma* as a character in several bisyllabic words

tical disorder, the intelligentsia, seeking escape from oppressive circumstances, resorted first to excessive drinking and later to the use of this drug. Its high toxicity apparently led to the subsequent decline of its use. But even in the T'ang dynasty (618-906), this or similar drugs containing mercury and sulfur were used as elixirs of longevity.

In more recent times tobacco has been adopted with the same enthusiasm it has met in other parts of the world. Opium was first introduced, perhaps by the southern sea route, as a medicine from western Asia. From the time of its introduction in the 8th century A.D., it was gradually adopted as a narcotic. Its adoption was undoubtedly aided in the beginning by the use of tobacco as an accompaniment. In the 19th century, under military pressure from foreign powers, its import and use became common throughout China.

The adoption of the introduced substance opium, in contrast to the lack of general use of the indigenous cannabis, can be explained on a cultural basis. Opium is an *Euphorica*, a sedative of mental activity. Cannabis, on the other hand, is a *Phantastica*, an hallucinogenic drug that causes mental exhilaration and nervous excitation. It distorts the sense of time and space. Overuse may cause rapid movements and under certain situations stimulate uncontrollable violence and criminal inclinations.

These effects were duly noted by Chinese physicians at least from the second century A.D. or earlier. They were in every respect inconsistent with the philosophy and traditions of Chinese life. The discontinuation of the use of cannabis by the Chinese can perhaps simply be referred to its unsuitability to the Chinese temperament and traditions.

From ancient times Chinese culture was characterized by two basic streams of thought, closely interwoven and permeating the life of its people at all levels of education. The dominant stream was Confucianism, or more correctly *Ju-chia*, which had its beginning long before Confucius, although it was greatly developed by him. Confucianism is more a moral system or philosophy of life than a religion, though it has been, for many people, a substitute for the latter.

The teachings of the Confucian School set up a body of ethical doctrines emphasizing the principle that the Universe is regulated by a Natural Order which is moral in essence. Man, the superior being, is a moral entity who can refrain from wrong doing through education and through the observance of the doctrines of uprightness and moderation (the doctrine of the Mean). Education involves such outward means of development as studying classical teachings, rules of propriety and ceremony, as well as an inward means of self-improvement through the recognition of one's own nature as a moral being and by constant watchfulness over one's self in solitude. Goodness consists of such fundamental virtues as *Jên* (benevolence), *I* (righteousness), *Li* (propriety), *Chih* (intelligence), and *Hsin* (faithfulness). Having achieved a state of knowledge of this self-discipline, the learned scholar has the responsibility of setting himself up as an example for the masses. Furthermore, the practical virtues of filial piety, reverence for ancestors, and respect for elders are emphasized.

The other stream of ancient thought, a more passive and fundamental one, is Taoism. Taoism actually encompasses two quite distinct movements. The Taoist school of philosophy, as expounded by ancient philosophers, emphasized the doctrine of nonaction. *Tao* has the meaning of a road or way. It signified the course of nature, and the harmony between nature and man. The teachings of these Taoist philosophers were adopted by priest-magicians and passed down from generation to generation, developing gradually into a religion, or pseudo-religion, in the later Han dynasty. This religion involved a multiplicity of gods and idols. The priests offered divination and magic as a means to inward power, restored youth, superhuman abilities and immortality. To most Taoist followers, who simultaneously followed Confucianism and Buddhism, the Taoist religion was essentially a sanction of the ethics of simplicity, patience, contentment and harmony.

At about the time that Taoism had developed into a religion and, therefore, was more capable of satisfying deeper instincts within human nature, Buddhism was introduced into China from India. While Buddhism had a more complete theology and, in the beginning, underwent years of rivalry with Taoism and Confucianism, all eventually settled down in peaceful coexistence, borrowing and lending ideas and methods. Buddhism in many ways became highly sinicized. Ch'an (Zen) Buddhism, or the Meditation School, became the dominant school of Buddhist thought in China. It professed the doctrine of self-improvement, which, while difficult, offered man a means whereby he could use his innate resources to overcome obstacles. This doctrine closely approaches Confucianism. In the last analysis Ch'an is more a moral philosophy than a religion. It is also interesting to note that meditative Buddhism developed mainly among the Chinese rather than among the peoples of India. On the other hand, the neo-Confucian School, which became the main stream of thought in the thousand years since the Sung dynasty, has been considerably affected by Buddhism and Taoism.[7]

---

[7] The literature of Chinese culture is too extensive for citation here. As representative of relevant subject matter, see the work of Hsü, F. L. K., *Under the ancestors' shadow: Chinese culture and personality*, 1949 New York and London.

Chinese culture is characterized by its uniformity and continuity. In spite of the vicissitudes of war, invasion and natural disaster, the culture is remarkable in its continuous, unbroken history. An historical orientation permeates every level of Chinese society, and is manifested in everyday life in the strong family system, ancestor worship and filial piety. Geographically, the uniformity of basic philosophy at all levels of culture is remarkable, defying wide distances, climatic variations and linguistic differences.

We cannot fail to ascribe this uniformity and continuity in part to the unique written Chinese language. Its monosyllabic characters can be traced back continuously for thousands of years to the early ideograms from which they were derived. The oldest documents can thus be read or deciphered. Even though there are numerous spoken dialects in China, the same non-phonetic, ideographic written language can be used and understood in every part of the vast country.

Despite the risk of oversimplification, we can conclude that Chinese culture, in conditioning the reflexes of the Chinese mind, is characterized by a dislike of metaphysics and its commonsense view of morality. The traditional Chinese philosophy of life is centered on humanism; it thus emphasizes in particular interpersonal relations. Compounded by its universally adopted doctrine of the Mean and its strong social system based on the family, these cultural influences seem to provide sufficient background for the universal failure to adopt a drug which causes hallucination and fantasy.[8]

If we consider first the question of the Chinese family, which is the primary socializing agency, the difference between the effects of cannabis and opium can be readily seen. The fantasy, unreality and sometimes violence caused by cannabis would disrupt family life, a life which follows the doctrine of moderation and frowns on extremes and excess. On the other hand, the sedative effect of opium is more compatible, especially in view of the large size of families where several generations live together. It could be used communally, often in surroundings containing other amenities. In a way it incidentally served to preserve the large extended family system, thus reinforcing the teachings of filial piety and ancestor

[8] The conformity of an individual in Chinese society is regulated by a culturally instilled sense of shame. The Confucian personality is a shame-oriented personality (Eberhard, W., *Guilt and sin*. 1967, Los Angeles and San Francisco). The Western personality tends to be more guilt-oriented. The adoption of opium and the non-adoption of cannabis reflect a behavioral response to traditional Chinese society. The opium user was more likely to remain pacific and sedated, and thus not challenge social norms. Cannabis, with its stimulating of erratic effects, was likely to induce acts that might bring shame upon the user or his family.

reverence. In reality, it was not uncommon to find the use of opium by the younger generation encouraged by their elders who were eager to keep the family and its fortune intact.

That there is a cultural background associated with the non-use of cannabis can be illustrated vividly by a situation in the remote hinterlands. To the northwest in the Sinkiang province (often known to the West as Chinese Turkestan), the Han Chinese, mostly immigrants, live side by side with the native tribes, the Uigurs being the majority. A travel record of 1919[9] showed that during the first quarter of the 20th century, the Chinese were outnumbered 5 to 1. Large quantities of cannabis were grown there at that time for export to Kashmir and India. It was also smoked locally by the young and old of the Uigurs and other native tribes, whose languages are different from that of Han Chinese. These non-Han people had adopted the Moslem religion. Before that, in the 13-14th centuries and earlier, they were largely shamanistic. In contrast to these tribal peoples, the Han Chinese minority were observed to entirely refrain from the use of cannabis.

[9] Hsieh Ping, *Hsin-chiang yu-chi*. Account of travel in Sinkiang, 1919, Shanghai.

Ethnobotanical Aspects of Cannabis in Southeast Asia

MARIE ALEXANDRINE MARTIN

ABSTRACT

Cannabis indica, originating in central Asia, was probably introduced into Southeast Asia about the sixteenth century. The vernacular name used throughout Southeast Asia is derived from the Sanskrit *ganja*. Cultivation of the plant is on a family basis, several roots planted around the house. *Ganja* is openly sold in the markets. The female plants are smoked, together with tobacco. The occasional cases of intoxication are remedied by decoctions of native plants. *Ganja* leaves and stalks are used extensively in the cuisine, to provide both an euphoric quality and agreeable flavor. Recognized as an analgesic, cannabis is used to combat, among other conditions, cholera, malaria, dysentery, anorexia, and loss of memory; it relieves asthma and calms the nerves; suppresses polyps, coughing, dizziness and convulsions; facilitates digestion and childbirth; it stimulates lactation, purifies the blood and clears the bile, regulates the function of the heart, liver and lungs; eliminates intestinal parasites, decongests the organism and is a treatment for paralysis. Cannabis is considered a source of social well-being, to be shared with friends and is also used to ease difficult work tasks.

Data are presented principally from Cambodia with some observations about Thailand, Laos and Vietnam. There are marked similarities in the use of cannabis in these countries.

Cannabis, better known by the name of Indian hemp, hashish or marihuana, is famous throughout the world for its psychoactive properties. Its chemical components are well-known and will be referred to here only in relation to certain uses of the plant. Psychopathological reactions have also been examined by numerous writers and are still subject to active research. I shall limit myself here to noting the different uses of cannabis and attitudes regarding the plant. It is therefore from an ethnological rather than a pharmacodynamic perspective that this study is presented.

The field of study is based essentially on Cambodia. Some observations

I wish to acknowledge the assitance of Mlle Uraisi Varasarin and M. Pierre Marie Gagneux in carrying out this study.

For Plates, see p. ix, between pp. 266–267.

were also made in Thailand, Laos, and Vietnam; and we shall see that, within this area, there are great similarities among the different countries.

ORIGIN AND INTRODUCTION OF CANNABIS

While it is known with certainty that hemp grows wild in central Asia, it is less clear when it was introduced into the above mentioned countries: Was it in the thirteenth or fourteenth century, by the Arabian conquerors; or by the Spanish and Portuguese who set up commercial activities in the region in the sixteenth century? For the inhabitants, it would be the Indians who brought in the plant. In Vietnam, one of the names of the species is *gai âṅdô*, or Indian grass-cloth plant, and as we shall see the Sanskrit name is widespread throughout the peninsula.

Vocabulary

In these four countries of Southeast Asia the vernacular name is directly derivable from the Sanskrit *guñja*:

> Thailand: *kancha:* or *kanhcha:*; there would also be *kanhcha:*(thai), *kanhcha:thĕt* (foreign), and *kanhcha:cin* (Chinese). In the absence of plant samples, I cannot say what these different names correspond to botanically.
> Cambodia: *kânhcha:*.
> Laos: *kan xa*.
> Vietnam: *cân xa* or *gai âṅdô*.

These names seem to be quite old, except in Vietnam where *cân xa* has become popular since the massive introduction of drugs in the last few years. Previously, the term *gai âṅdô* or *dai áṅdô* were used. Names given to the seed and the kernel, which were frequently used in medicine, underwent some Chinese influence as well: *dai ma tử* or *dai ma hôt* (seed); *dai ma nhân* (kernel); *dai* or *gai* (Vietnamese name designating the grass-cloth plant); *ma*, a term encountered in several Chinese plant names, e.g., *ta ma* (cannabis), *tchou ma* (Boehmeria), and *pi ma* (Ricinus); *tử* (Chinese word to denote seed); *hôt* (Vietnamese word to denote seed); and *nhân* (Vietnamese word to denote the kernel).

The inhabitants also recognize male and female plants. In Cambodia, this distinction crosscuts scientific reality, perhaps because the normal criterion for differentiation of the male plants from the female ones is, at least for the peasants of this country, the size of the leaves. It will be noted that, in the case of cannabis, the male, slender plants have smaller leaves than the females, whose leaves are more developed, which conforms to the data derived from empirical analysis. We, therefore, have male cannabis (botanical) *kanhcha*: (*chmọ:l*) and female cannabis (botanical) *kanhcha*: (*nhi:*).

We are led to make a similar comment for Laos, where yet another division within the female group was pointed out to me: male cannabis (botanical) *kan xa*: (*phu:*), also called *kan xa*: *dɔk* (flower), probably because its flowers are grouped together in a broad panicle visible from a distance, the more discrete female inflorescence being composed of single flowers with axillae of foliacious bracts often requiring closer examination before being recognized; and female cannabis (botanical) *kan xa:mè* including *hua nok khao* (owl head), and *kali*.

This last dichotomy seems to rest on superficial characteristics, the extremity of the leafy stem thus being the significant trait determining the assignment of a particular name. We might be tempted, by analogy with *hua nok khao*, to translate *kali* as "elephant," a word which is part of the current *lao mais* vocabulary. It is not obvious what this resemblance corresponds to in reality; the word *kali* occurs also in Cambodia and Thailand. In Thailand, it denotes inflorescences; and in Cambodia, *kali* denotes seed, which explains why the use is limited to female flowers. To my knowledge, it is used exclusively for cannabis. The term appears in no Khmer or Sanskrit dictionaries, therefore, it is not possible to give a translation or etymology for it.[1]

In Laos, it is by the common term *dɔk* that the flowers of the hemp plant are named. There is no special vocabulary for the other parts used:

	leaf	stem
Cambodia	slɤk	daəm
Thailand	bai	tôň
Laos	bai	tôň
Vietnam	la	thân

It should be noted that we are not talking here of the resin, for the natives smoke the raw plant simply chopped up. This material does not have any special name; whether the entire plant is chopped up ready to smoke, mixed with tobacco, or put into the pipe, it is always *kânhcha*. In Vietnam, the preparation with a resinous base that has been recently introduced

---

[1] *Kali* is a word of Hindi origin, meaning "bud" (personal communication with Dr. Vera Rubin). Linguistics, therefore, argues in favor of introduction of hemp through India, either directly by the Indians, or indirectly by the Spanish and Portuguese explorers in the sixteenth century.

(*cân xa:*) is smoked mostly by foreigners. It is since this period that more severe controls over growing and using intoxicating plants have appeared in this country.

GROWING AND SELLING

Commercial growing of hemp is not legally authorized in Cambodia. Under the French Protectorate, Customs and Excises controlled the entire territory of French Indochina. After independence, King Suramarinth, under the edict of *kram* No. 10 NS of May 30, 1955, halted all growing of cannabis. The Bureau of Narcotics created last year in Phnom Penh (by *kret* No. 481.72 PRK of July 14, 1972) emphasized the repression of opium traffic and updated complementary clauses relative to hemp. These plants have apparently never been intensively cultivated; and neither the poppy nor "grass" seems to have been smoked regularly by the inhabitants. While the former does not exist anywhere in Cambodia, on the other hand, there can frequently be found small plots of cannabis around houses (see Plate 1); the largest garden we observed contained about seventy plants. Although the species require rich and humid soil, it grows quite often in sandy dry soil with only water and chicken or cattle manure required from time to time. Female *kânhcha: nhi:* plants yield a small number of seeds which are left to soak in water for three days before being planted in open ground. The best time for sowing the seeds is during the rainy season (hemp is harvested during the dry season), but cultivation can be started at any time during the year provided that the amount of water indispensable to growth is provided. When the inflorescence develops after four or five months, it is called *laəng kali: haəy* (*laəng*, the verb "to climb," also used to translate the completion of an action; *haəy*, particle marking the past). However, along the river and closer to Vietnam, cultivation of these plants is of greater importance.

Nearly all the harvest is bought from the grower, at 3000 *riels* per kilo for female plants, by an intermediary who resells them, either on the open market at ten *riels* per package of seven or eight tops from flowering female plants, or to restaurateurs or individual buyers (male or female plants). In Laos, a package of smoking hemp (ten flowering stems) costs ninety *kips*[2], or twenty kips for the same amount of stems without flowers, both male and female, for making soup. Retail sale of the plant is absolutely free in Cambodia and Laos, as may be seen in Plate

[2] Officially, in April 1973, 26 *riels* = 1 *franc* at the same rate, 45 *riels* = 1 *franc*; 600 *kips* = 1 U.S. dollar, at the same rate, 840 *kips* = 1 U.S. dollar.

2. In Thailand, since the formation of the new government in December 1971, cannabis has not appeared openly and its use in popular medicine has been regulated: it must always be used together with other plants in medical preparations and may not be the sole ingredient of any medication.

Cultivation is hardly more widespread in Laos than in Cambodia, nor is it in Thailand, except perhaps in the north and in a few central regions. In Vietnam, it is important in Chaudec, a Cambodian border region. At any rate, cultivation here does not achieve the significance of the opium fields of Laos; hemp may formerly have been cultivated on a larger scale locally. Thirteen kilometers downstream from Vientiane, on the banks of the Mekong, is the village of Ban Het Kansa, or the village of the hemp-covered sand bank; there is no longer any trace of this plant, which must have been cultivated here some time in the past (Taillard 1971).

The male and the female plants have different destinations which we will now consider.

USES

Psychoactive

Unlike the *kif* of Arab countries and the marihuana of others, which are preparations with resinous bases derived from the stem or the flowers of the plant, hemp in Southeast Asia is smoked with no prior treatment at all. It is essentially the flowering female plant that is used; the bracts are known to produce the desired state of euphoria, because of the cannabinol they contain. However, the entire plant is used, after being dried in the sun — the stem, the leaves, and the inflorescence. The plant is cut into small pieces, and tobacco is added to it; more rarely, it is smoked alone. Cigarettes of the mixture are made wrapped in the same way as ordinary cigarettes; for example, paper, leaf of maize (*slɤk po:t*) leaves of the *Combretum quadrangulare* (*slɤk sângkaê*), parts of banana leaves (*slɤk ce:c*); more frequently, the mixture is placed in the bowl of a water pipe made of bamboo (*ru sey*). It should be noted that the chopping block on which the plant is cut is a slab of Cambodian *strychnos* wood (*slaêng*) (*phya:mu: lêk* in Thailand), as it is thought that bits of this wood added to the hemp constitute a cough remedy, and that a pleasant taste is derived from the *strychnos* (*khlɤm*). Another practice in Cambodia consists of cooking down the hemp and sprinkling the tobacco with the juice from the boiled plant.

The Khmers smoke only the female plants, because it is said that cigarettes made from the male plant cause an eye disease, or rheum (*a:c phnêk*). Moreover, the female plants are more effective in that they contain more resin.

In Laos, several qualities of hemp are distinguished: first quality: harvested in the winter when covered with dew (the strongest variety); second quality: harvested at other times; and third quality: comprised of the plants that were not gathered at the proper time and whose development may be incomplete, with the euphoric power thus reduced. This particular point concerning the qualities cannot be more precisely stated at this time.

In certain regions of Laos, the dried leaves of the *kan xa: hua nek khao* are used for their euphoric quality. In Cambodia, the *kânhcha:nhi:* are sometimes smoked without the flowers; the effects produced by the flowers are less strong, and we shall see later that they are used in cooking.

Substitutes

When there is a lack of cannabis, there is recourse to other plants. In Thailand in particular, *lêw*, an indeterminate species, would be a good replacement. Leaves are also smoked of the *Mitragyna speciosa*, a bush growing profusely in Chieng Mai, but this yields secondary reactions which will be noted later. For medication, in the absence of *kancha*, the entire *Grangea darerasparana* (composite) plant is used, or the *phya:muti*. Users are reluctant to employ the root of the *Mitragyna* for they say it makes breathing difficult. According to Burkill (1966), the effects of *Mitragyna speciosa* are worse than those ascribed to hemp and are more like those caused by opium. It seems that the narcotic power of this species was known in ancient Siam; its use then spread to Malaysia.

In Cambodia, no substitutes are noted. In the absence of *kânhcha*, people smoke a quality of tobacco called "strong" (thnam khlang); but this is only a short-term solution, and it is rare that hemp is unavailable for long periods of time. In medications, it may be replaced, but not necessarily, by the *Cananga latifolia* (*chkaê sraêng*), which also produces a reaction (*chuəl*), but not a serious one.

Frequency of Use

In Cambodia, it is essentially the males who smoke *kânhcha*. Their first attempts generally occur when they are around fifteen years old; more rarely, young Cambodian girls use the pipe, although they are not authorized to do this before the age of eighteen. This practice is common, however, among the women of certain northeastern tribes (at least, this is what I have observed in a Bu nong village). On the whole, there are few Khmers who become intoxicated by the plant, for they do not smoke regularly, taking only a few puffs from time to time when the opportunity presents itself. However, some have assumed the habit, especially among strangers, of lighting their pipes several times a day. It is in this way that one often meets former members of the French army who can no longer do without the "benefits" of cannabis. For these few people, we can consider the plant is used to provide intoxication, or at least habitude (five or ten pipes three times a day). When there is some deficiency in the drug, reactions are immediate — anorexia, extreme nervousness, irritability, aggression. Return to daily use rapidly dissipates these symptoms.

In Thailand, if the user wishes to nullify the effects, he goes to the medicine man to get the root of the *ra:k ya: nang dêng (Anacardiacée?)* used to cure all sorts of intoxication. Two types of cures are possible:

Intoxication is temporary, due to occasional use; the root is rubbed on a stone until the plant is completely pulverized and a bit of rice water is added. The small glass of boiled root and rice water obtained is then drunk all at once.

Intoxication is due to prolonged use; the remedy must be taken each time there is a desire to smoke and until hemp can be completely relinquished. For this purpose, the medication may consist of a tea made of the root, taken in limitless quantities.

In Cambodia, smokers prefer to consume large quantities of sugar or sweet meats for which they seem to feel a great need, or even acidic foods. During the cure period, one showers frequently.

Besides the fact that these daily doses do not seem — at least in the first twenty years of life — to lead to "depravity," it sometimes happens that the accidental ingestion of a large quantity of hemp all at once can result in serious problems. The ones observed were the following: repeated loss of consciousness, except in these moments of weakness, however, complete lucidity; excessive nervousness; increased hilarity or anxiety, depending upon the subject; accentuation of the dominant individual character trait; increased heart rate, pupil dilation, and pains in the chest. Pupil dilation persisted for several days, the chest difficulties and nervousness disappeared only after ten to twelve days.

The noxious effects of cannabis are sometimes exploited for criminal purposes. It has been pointed out to me, in one of the countries I visited, that the suppression of an individual was easily resolved by increasing the dosage of hemp in a medicinal preparation. These preparations are quite numerous, as will be seen below.

Medicinal Uses

Besides the restrictions in Thailand, already noted, there is no regulation of the use of hemp in popular medicine. Everywhere it is considered to be of analgesic value, comparable to the opium derivatives. Moreover, it can be added to any relaxant to reinforce its action. Cooked leaves, which have been dried in the sun, are used in quantities of several grams per bowl of water. This decoction helps especially to combat migraines and stiffness; taken before sleep and before meals, it relaxes the nerves. Other plants may eventually be added. This beneficial medical action is recognized both by the peasants and by the official pharmacopoeia of these countries. This is not the case, however, for all the remedies to be enumerated, since popular medicine sometimes includes magical elements. At any rate, it is interesting to note the significance attached by the peasants to a plant which seems never to have been widespread in the region.

In Cambodia, the entire male or female plant is used for the cure of numerous maladies. By the entire plant, is meant all of the vegetative and reproductive organs; often, however, the female flowers are only added in small amounts to give the sick person a feeling of well-being. A glass of the decoction, taken before the two principal meals of the day, restores the appetite; treatment generally lasts for only a day, but may be continued longer if necessary. The identical result is achieved by smoking a mixture of male and female plants.

Cigarettes made of hemp and the stem of the *Cananga latifolia* (Hook f. and Thoms.) Finet and Gagnep (*chkaê sraêng*) smoked daily will make polyps of the nose disappear (*ruѩh do:ng*).

The fragrant bark of the *têpiru*, a myrtle which grows among the giants of the dense Cambodian forests, and that of the *sâmbɔ lvêng*, a species of *Cinnamomum*, when boiled with hemp yield a beverage which facilitates digestion (*rumliəy mho:p* — "to dissolve food"); a glass is taken before each meal. According to the Cambodians, this medication has a stronger effect than injections, which are however considered the most effective remedy in western pharmacopoeia.

After delivery of a baby, cannabis is extensively used: the infusion made from the tops (*cong*) of both male and female plants — about ten per liter of water — brings a feeling of well-being (*sruəl khluən*) to the mother. It is preferable to limit consumption to one small glassful before each meal, for fear of intoxication. The female flowers are used just as much as are the male: young mothers who do not have enough milk to nurse their babies twice daily take a concoction made of hemp, the stems of a bush, *Cinnamomum* sp. (*sâmbɔ lvêng*), and different tropical creepers:

Tetracera Loureiri Craib (*dâng kwən*), *Walsura villosa* Wall. ex. Hiern (*sdok sdao*), *Illigera* sp. (*vɔ: kro:c*); the alcoholic extract of hemp and the bark of several trees: *Aegle marmelos* (L.) Correa, *Mitragyma* sp. (khtom), *Cinnamomum* sp. (*sambə lvêng*), *Walsura villosa*, ? Myrtle (*têpiru*) combats postpartum stiffness (*chu: khluən, chu: ch'ɤng*).

Cambodians attribute all sorts of complications (təəh) that may occur after the baby's birth to non-observance of nutritional taboos during pregnancy. As a remedy, the mother must take — among other preparations, three times a day until she is well — an alcoholic extract (or decoction) prepared from the following plants: hemp, bark of the *Mitragyna* sp., the *Aegle marmelos* (*preah phnəv*), the *Annona squamosa* L. (*tiəp khmae*), the Psidium *Guajava* L. (*trâbaêc*), and the *Antidesma Ghaesembilla* Gaertn (*dângkiəp khdam*).

Individuals affected by malaria use hemp as a cure: one kilogram of male and female plants inhaled (*câmha:y*) twice a day until the end of the crisis. The same amount of hemp and of water, in a preparation taken in 2cc. doses before each meal, sometimes replaces the inhalation method, but is not as effective.

Cigarettes or pipes filled with hemp and tobacco are used not only to produce a state of narcosis, but are also used to reduce biliousness (*thla: tuik prâma:t*).

While these remedies are being taken, the patient is not subject to nutritional taboos, contrary to what is often the case.

In Thailand, numerous curative virtues are attributed to cannabis. It is used in medications to eliminate dizzy spells (*lom*). Sandalwood (*can thĕt*) and hemp have a beneficial effect on the functioning of the heart, the liver, and the lungs; this is taken in the form of tea. Used alone, cannabis is a remedy for cholera. In such cases, water from the pipe that has been smoked is also drunk.

To suppress convulsions, hemp is ground up in honey with many other plants such as ? *Ferula* sp. (*ma hă: hĭng*), *Garcinia Hanburyi* Hook f. (*rong thong*), wild *Dioscorea* (*klɔy*), fruit from the *Terminalia chebula* Retz (*sà mɔ̆ thai*) and the *Terminalia belerica* Roxb. (*sà mɔ̆ phĭ phĕk*), wild Piper (*sa khàn*), *Piper retrofractum* Vahl (*di: phli:*), an araceous plant (*ka dàt thâng sŏng*); *Eugenia aromaticus* H. Bn (*ka:n phlu:*), leaves from the *Vitex trifolia* L. f. (*khon thi sɔ̆:*), leaves from the *Caesalpinia* sp. (*swà:t*), *Abroma augusta* L. (*thiam dam*), *Lawsonia inermis* Roxb. (*thian khă:w*), *Cinnamomum* sp. (*òp chəy*), *Piper nigrum* L. (*prĭk thai*), unripened fruit from the *Aegle marmelos* (*matum*), and heart of the *Aegiceras corniculatum* Blanc. (*samĕ*).

Another preparation consists of an alcoholic extract from hemp and various ground-up plants such as: *Artemisia vulgaris* L. (*kòt cù la: lampha:*), the fruit and flower of the *? Myristica* (*can*), *Piper nigrum*, *Piper chaba* Hunter, *Zingiber officinale* L., wild *Piper*, *Cinnamomum* (woodland) (*sà mŭn la wéng*), *Cinnamomum* sp. (*òp chəy*), *?Salacia flavescems* Kruz (*Khŏp chà nang tháng sŏng*), a chemical product (arsenic?) (*sǎ:nnŭ:*). This medication cures hemorrhoids and polyps of the throat, intestines, and the sex organs.

To counteract dysentery, the fruit and flower of the *can* (*? Myristica*) are dried in a pan with the bark of *Eugenia aromaticus*, and tubers from *?Curcuma zedoaria* and the *phlai*. These plant materials constitute the number one, indispensable, element of the preparation. The second element, or the *krâ sǎ:y*, is the water derived from mashing the hemp and the *diń kinh* (indeterminate); its significance is secondary. The plants that are soaked vary according to the first element. Both elements are mixed if there is no second element, the products of the first are taken alone, soaked in pure water.

Cannabis is frequently used to stimulate the appetite of sick people and make them sleep. In cigarettes, mixed with tobacco, it relieves asthma. Its use to counteract diarrhea and dysentery is equally common. During difficult periods of childbirth, preparations made with hemp facilitate contractions.

Despite its multiple uses, hemp must be taken wisely, especially to avoid the heavy doses that might induce tetanus.

In Vietnam, our information is scarce. Outside of its use as an analgesic the plant is used as a vermifuge to eliminate *taenia*. Traditional medicine, on the other hand, which has been largely inspired by Chinese medicine, makes great use of cannabis. It is generally the seeds — and preferably the kernels — that are used. The preparation (*sac thuoc*) is used to combat loss of memory and mental confusion; aging; ailments due to "unhealthy breezes" that engender psoriasis, with dark spots; decongest the organism; eliminate blood wastes; cure dysmenorrhea; and produce a feeling of well-being after childbirth. In obstetrics, if the presentation of the child is awkward, twenty-one kernels boiled in water have the power of replacing him in the normal position.

Paralysis due to *phong* (allergy, rheumatism, anaphylaxia) is treated by roasting the kernels, and mashing them in baby's urine; the juice is then extracted and a small glassful drunk three times a day. The pulverized kernels, mixed with cooking water from rice, arrest the fall of hair.

In Laos, medicinal uses of hemp seem few, perhaps because of all the opium derivatives available to the inhabitants. However, it is used to cure stomach ailments (*ciep thong*) and *béng thong* or *nhung thong*, the swollen stomach (of cattle as well as people); the sick person drinks a preparation from the male and female leaves. Sorcerers also use hemp to treat an individual affected by a *phi, phi kha,* or *phi khom;* if the *phi* responsible for the malady smokes, an offering is made of several leaves of kan xa: to restore the health of the patient.

Alimentary Uses

Hemp soup is common throughout Southeast Asia. *Sngao* in Cambodia, especially *sngao mɔən,* flavored with male or female leaves of *kânhcha:* that have been roasted. These are also added to other soups, *sâmlâ kâko:, Kɛ:ng phe:t* from Thailand with ground-up *kancha:* flowers added; Chinese soup sold throughout the region incorporates hemp — the male or female stems in Laos — in order to induce clients to return; this was eventually replaced by green tea.

In Cambodia, the leaves are used in diverse ways: fresh, they are condiments (*kruəng*) for curry or vegetables (*bânlâê*) to accompany vermicelli soup (*num bânhcɔk*); they are eaten as vegetables (*ânlwək*) in the form of fritters with fish paste (*prâhok*).

It is not only the intoxicating power of hemp but the pleasant flavor it imparts to food that makes it good to use in cooking.

Textile Uses

The fibers in the stem of cannabis seem to be scarcely used today, except perhaps by montagnard tribes people. The plains inhabitants are not acquainted with this use, which is completely unknown in Khmer country and no samples harvested in Cambodia can be found in the herbarium of the National Museum of Natural History, in Paris. There are speciemens from Tonkin and Laos, whose labels show they were used as "textile plants." Crévost and Lemarié (1919–1921) speak of a variety (?) cultivated at the beginning of this century on the high plateaus of Laos and the Tonkin area; skirts worn by the *meo* and *nhung* ethnic groups were then made of hemp. According to the authors, the *meo,* from China, would have imported textile hemp north of the Annamese chain in the seventeenth century.

At the beginning of the French Protectorate, attempts at cultivation were made more extensively in the south; faced with the mediocre results obtained — plant growth reduced to 0m60 instead of several meters — production of hemp was halted beyond a southern limit, north of Indochina. Today, grass-cloth plants and jute are the primary textile plants in Southeast Asia.

REACTIONS AND ATTITUDES OF THE PEOPLE OF SOUTHEAST ASIA REGARDING CANNABIS

Traditionally, cannabis has not been prohibited in Southeast Asia. In Cambodia, it is not considered a dangerous product, as opposed to opium, which leads to depravity. For the Khmer people, smoking hemp is an added pleasure to give oneself, and it is agreeable to smoke with friends. Aside from intoxicated individuals we have mentioned, solitary pipe smokers are rare; it is a group pleasure. After the evening meal (5:00 or 6:00 o'clock), the head of the house lays out a straw mat and invites others to accompany him in his search for euphoria. It is not a question of forgetting one's troubles or escaping from heavy obligations; smoking is to avoid being sad, to experience a feeling of well-being (*sruəl khluən*). It is the same for enjoying the soup, which, moreover, acquires a pleasant taste. Those who use cannabis speak of its effects: "you are in a drunken mood (*srâvwəng*) as with morphine, you are happy, laughing, eating well, you have strength, and can remain in the water for several hours. For military people, consumption of *kânhcha:* gives resistance to combat."

As a result of these latter properties — giving strength, allowing one to remain in the water for several hours — hemp is often used to accomplish difficult tasks. Those who smoke daily tend to increase their dosage before going to work in the forest or to harvest jute. Others smoke several pipes before the two principal meals of the day; throughout the time the job takes, their endurance is thus increased. Certainly, it may happen that an individual who wishes to prolong the feeling of strength and well-being experienced on these occasions gradually turns to regular use of hemp. On the whole, this trend is not frequent. Let us note further that this particular use of *kancha:* is far from being general and that it is exclusively a male activity, more kinds of jobs being performed only by men. This was also pointed out to me as the case in Laos. In Cambodia, hemp is also a way of combating cold during the cold season.

Being in possession of *kânhcha:* does not constitute an offense; the normal reaction is rather to laugh and wish pleasure to the person who has it. The medicine men of Cambodia (*kru: thnam*) no longer share the distrust of hemp of some of their colleagues in neighboring countries. This is doubtless because they are accustomed to using it and are well acquainted with the proper amounts to prescribe. Hence, people seldom talk anymore of untoward reactions which occur following excessive doses.

In Thailand, users describe what they feel in the following way: "after having used hemp, you want to eat sweets or drink a lot of water; you have red eyes and heavy eyelids; you see everything in a good light and feel very gay. This state doesn't last long if you eat while smoking."

Generally, in Southeast Asia, distrust regarding hemp appears among individuals having cultural and social attitudes patterned after those of the West. As for the peasants, they experiment with everything that belongs to their universe, often have complete knowledge of all the elements that compose it, and how to use them in moderation. There is thus nothing surprising in the fact that they consider cannabis to be a plant that is socially beneficial.

This is an example of application of knowledge regulated by folk understanding.

REFERENCES

BURKILL, ISAAC HENRY
    1966 *A dictionary of the economic product of the Malay peninsula*. Two volumes. Kuala Lumpur, Malaysia: Ministry of Agriculture and Co-operatives.

CRÉVOST, C., C. LEMARIÉ
    1919–1921 Catalogue des produits de l'Indochine. *Bulletin Économique Indochine*, p. 116. Saigon.

TAILLARD, C.
    1971 *Les berges de la Nam Ngun et du Mékong*. Commissariat Général au Plan. Vientiane, Laos.

Cannabis Smoking in 13th–14th Century Ethiopia: Chemical Evidence

NIKOLAAS J. VAN DER MERWE

ABSTRACT

Two ceramic smoking-pipe bowls, excavated in Lalibela Cave, Begemeder Province, Ethiopia, were radiocarbon dated to 1320 ± 80 A.D. A modified thin-layer chromatographic technique, applied to the pipe residues, yields positive tests for cannabis-derived compounds. Long-lived cannabinoids, produced by the heat of smoking from short-lived psychoactive ingredients in cannabis, makes identification possible.

The origins and spread of *Cannabis sativa* are obscure, although the plant has achieved worldwide distribution, and is commonly known under such names as *bhang, ganja, dagga, hemp, marijuana*, etc. The psychoactive properties especially of its tropical varieties are well-known as they have apparently been since the 3rd millennium B.C. The plant is mentioned in a 2737 B.C. pharmacological treatise attributed to the Chinese emperor Shen-Nung (Merlin 1972). Another possible reference occurs in Vedic texts from India around 2000-1400 B.C., while Herodotus gives a clear description of the Scythian practice of throwing hemp seeds on hot rocks in a confined space. By 950 A.D. the use of cannabis was well-established in Arabia; Marco Polo's account of the alleged hashish-related assassin's cult of Hasan-ibn-al-Sabbah (11th century) is also well-known, if not necessarily accurate. We now have chemical evidence that the plant was smoked in Ethiopia in the 13th–14th century A.D.

According to Vavilov's phytogeographic postulates, the site of species formation of *Cannabis sativa* was in central or Southeast Asia; the plant was probably domesticated in the same region. The cultigen is of the same species, while a more strongly psychoactive form has been named *Cannabis indica;* the latter may or may not be a separate species.[1] Since the same psychoactive compounds are involved in both cases, the differen-

---

[1] Editor's note: see paper by Schultes in this volume.

ces can be ignored here. The main psychoactive constituent is tetrahydrocannabinol (THC); this, along with cannabinol and cannabidiol, is the substance commonly tested for in the chemical identification of cannabis (Turk et al. 1969). They occur naturally only in the cannabis plant (THC has been produced synthetically). All three compounds degrade at least partially when burned (as in smoking), and also deteriorate rapidly with time. These attributes provide difficulties when testing for evidence of cannabis use in residues from ancient smoking pipes.

Two ceramic pipe bowls, excavated by J. C. Dombrowski (1971) at the site of Lalibela Cave in the Begemeder Province of Ethiopia (near Lake Tana), were tested for the presence of cannabinolic compounds. The pipes came from level 2 of the cave, with an associated radiocarbon date of 1320 ± 80 A.D. (Y-2433); calibration on the bristlecone pine curve produces no significant change in age. This date is clearly earlier than the introduction of tobacco to Africa from the New World, following Columbus' journey. Archaeological remains from Lalibela level 2 differ but little from the present-day material culture of the region, and the workmen at the site were able to identify the pipe bowls and their mechanical operation. Both bowls formed part of waterpipes; an aperture at the bottom of the bowl allows for the attachment of a vertical stem, which presumably descended into a water container. Pipe B2 was well preserved, contained a "pipe-cake" as thick as 1 mm in places, and was identified as an Awraja's pipe or the pipe of a "big man." Pipe A2 was broken and contained only a small amount of residue.

A standard thin-layer chromatographic technique, used in hospital and police testing for the presence of cannabis, was used in the experiment.[2] A small sample (less than 100 mg) of the unknown (plant material or pipe residue) is soaked in petroleum ether, with appropriate stirring to break up caked materials. (Ether can also be poured directly through a pipe if no obvious residue is present.) Cannabinolic compounds dissolve in about 10 minutes. The ether solution is then poured off, evaporated in a stream of hot air, and the residue is reconstituted with a few drops of chloroform. Using a capillary tube, a drop of the solution is "spotted" about 3 cm from the lower edge of a 20×20 cm glass plate, coated with a 250 micron layer of silica gel G. Spots from different samples are spaced about 2 cm apart, the same distance from the edge. The plate is then placed upright in a container with about 1.5 cm of benzene in the bottom,

[2] We thank Wilson Memorial Hospital of Johnson City, N. Y. for the use of their Toxicology Laboratory; hospital toxicologist, S. James, for his patient instruction and supervision; and archaeologists J. C. Dombrowski (University of Ghana) and J. Atherton (Portland State College, Oregon) for providing pipes for testing.

the container tightly covered, and left for 30 minutes. During this time the benzene rises about 15 cm in the silica gel. As it passes the sample spots, cannabinolic compounds separate and travel upwards on the plate for a distance proportional to their affinity for benzene. The distance travelled, relative to the total height reached by the benzene, provides the R_f value of a given compound. When the plate is removed from the benzene container and sprayed with a solution of fast blue B salt (naphthanil diazo dye, K & K laboratories), cannabinolic compounds appear as orange-red spots. In testing fresh samples of *Cannabis sativa*, a major spot (THC) developed at an R_f value of 0.53, with lesser spots at 0.62 (cannabinol) and 0.45 (cannabidiol).

Residue samples from the two Ethiopian pipes (A2 and B2) were compared on the same plate with a 60% THC resin extract and positively identified samples of *Cannabis sativa*. The standards produced the customary spots in each case, while A2 and B2 did not. Two faint spots, representing unidentified cannabinoids, developed from A2 and B2 at R_f values of 0.69 and 0.84; these spots were absent in the standards. In a second experiment, a 60% THC resin standard and several modern pipes which had previously tested positively for cannabinolic compounds were used for comparative purposes. The THC standard and the modern pipes exhibited the familiar spot for THC, cannabinol, and cannabidiol, while pipes A2 and B2 did not; the modern pipes exhibited faint spots at R_f values of 0.69 and 0.84, as did pipe B2 (from which sufficient residue had been available). In a third experiment, no spots could be developed from A2 and B2 (probably due to insufficient sample material), but modern pipe samples once again developed faint spots at 0.69 and 0.84. Lack of sample material prevented further testing of A2 and B2.

A third pipe, excavated by J. Atherton from a pre-tobacco context in Liberia, yielded no results in three attempts. The pipe lacked visible residue, and ether was poured through it in an attempt to obtain sample material.

We conclude that THC, cannabinol, and cannabidiol have relatively short lifetimes and cannot be identified in ancient samples. (A figure of 50 years is often mentioned, but remains untested.) When subjected to the heat of smoking, however, one or more of these compounds degrade to form two unidentified cannabinoids, with R_f values of 0.69 and 0.84, and lifetimes in excess of 500 years. The presence of these cannabinoids in a pipe positively identifies its use for the smoking of *Cannabis sativa* or one of its relatives or extracts. The evidence is difficult to detect, with success probably dependent on sample size (not determined) and on the strength of the material smoked (highly variable).

Archaeologically, we conclude that some variety of *Cannabis sativa* was smoked around Lake Tana in the 13th–14th century, in much the same way as it is today. This is evident for pipe B2 (two positive tests), somewhat less so for A2 (one positive test). How and when the plant, and knowledge of its psychoactive properties, reached this area is unknown; an Arabic source seems probable.[3] In view of these results it may be necessary to review archaeological interpretations relating to smoking pipes in early African contexts. A prime example could be the chronological system based on pipe designs which has been established in West Africa, where the exclusive use of tobacco has been assumed.

REFERENCES

DOMBROWSKI, J. C.
   1971   "Excavations in Ethiopia: Lalibela and Natchabiet Caves, Begemeder Province." Boston: Boston University Ph. D. Thesis.

MERLIN, M. D.
   1972   *Man and marijuana*. Teaneck, New Jersey: Fairleigh Dickinson University Press.

TURK, R. F., *et al.*
   1969   Method for extraction and chromatographic isolation, purification and identification of tetrahydrocannabinol and other compounds from marihuana. *Journal of Forensic Sciences* 14:385–391.

---

[3] Editor's note: see paper by du Toit in this volume.

Dagga: The History and Ethnographic Setting of Cannabis sativa *in Southern Africa*

BRIAN M. DU TOIT

ABSTRACT

Cannabis sativa has been used throughout southern and eastern Africa for centuries, yet we know little about its origin, diffusion, and patterns of use. This paper deals with the likely migratory routes and diffusion patterns of cannabis in Africa. It traces the historic presence of the herb among various African peoples, recording their patterns of use and the paraphernalia associated with cannabis smoking. Terminologically, we are able to construct three geographical complexes in Africa: a southern area where cannabis is referred to as *dagga*, an east-central area where we find variations of the term *bangi*, and a western area where variations on *diamba* are used. Cannabis was not present in West Africa prior to World War II.

The methods of smoking the herb among the African peoples of southern and east-central Africa have been changing. Throughout this region the old water-pipe has almost completely disappeared, and today the young people are employing either various forms of the chilam pipe, which is bought from Indians, or the cigarette.

INTRODUCTION

Historical

The herb we are discussing probably originated in the semi-desert regions south and east of the Caspian Sea and gradually spread to the Himalayas and throughout central Asia. While it is known to have been used by man

---

This paper is being written while I am involved in a full-time research project, funded by the Center for Studies of Narcotics and Drug Abuse, National Institute of Mental Health. While there are distinct and immediate advantages to being in the field while writing, the library and research facilities are sometimes not completely satisfactory.

A word of very sincere appreciation is due the staff of the Killie Campbell Africana Library in Durban, South Africa, and in particular to Monica Sauer and Jeanette Langner who were always more than ready to assist in searching for items, obtaining photocopies, or tapping the resources of inter-library loan facilities.

as early as 6000 years ago, it may in fact constitute one of the earliest plants cultivated for material use rather than food. The herb most likely supplied man with fiber from its stem for many centuries before the oil from its stem and the medicinal value of its resin were discovered.

The early uses and diffusion of hemp in Europe, Asia, and the Middle East and its botany have been extensively described in the literature (Emboden 1972; Schultes 1970; Rosenthal 1971; Grinspoon 1969).

In Egypt cannabis has been grown for almost a thousand years. While the domesticated variety was used for the production of rope, the wild variety (transplanted to gardens) was specifically recommended for use as a drug. "In certain parts of the Delta of the Nile, the major crop sown was hashish, and the daily consumption of hashish in Cairo was quite considerable" (Rosenthal 1971:132). Despite the fact that the use of hashish was adjudged a crime in Muslim society and was thus punishable by religious law and judicial authorities, it was very commonly used. Part of the geographical spread of cannabis is due to its association with Muslim migrant communities.

We also know that it spread down the east of Africa with Arab traders. The terms *Bangalah* and *Bhang* were names for Bengal and the word *bhang*, used for the herb, could thus have spread into east Africa centuries ago to refer to its Indian origin. The spread of its use was compounded with more recent Arab trading from Saudi Arabia, and it was almost certainly used in the southern part of the continent in pre-Portugese times, i.e. before A.D. 1500.

Likely Migratory Route

One of the potentially most hazardous pastimes is to postulate "origins" and "migration routes" for plants which are well-nigh universally distributed. In the case of cannabis, we are entering such a problem area. Few, if any, archaeological site reports mention pollen counts or seed distribution; neither have I come across descriptions of early occupied sites in southern Africa in which the pipe is mentioned. For later material in this regard Walton (1953) has summarized the evidence. We are thus forced to the use of analogy and assumption.

Plant distribution can be brought about by winds, currents, and similar natural forces. It can also follow animal activity and migration by becoming attached to their feet or hooves, or by being eaten by birds (Darwin 1900; Polunin 1964).

We know that the herb was present in Persia and India, and from there reached Arab settlements in the northern and northeastern borders of the

African continent. The fairly early trade contacts with Zanzibar should thus be accepted as a likely migratory route.

The literature contains a number of suggestions on the spread of cannabis into southern Africa:

1. Watt (1961:9) has suggested that "the plant may have been introduced by the early travellers circumventing the Cape from the east." Almost all our historical documentation and linguistic evidence, however, suggest a date long before this.

2. Theodore James (1970:575), basing his argument on a single case of terminological agreement [namely Hindi and Shangaan (Thonga)] states that: "the plant was first carried to the coast of Mozambique ... by the Portuguese militant traders returning from India." This sets the date even later, and certainly does not recognize documents regarding early use.

3. Morley and Bensusan (1971:409) point out that the plant is not indigenous to southern Africa: "It appears most likely that it was brought by Arab traders to the Mozambique coast from India. From there it was carried southwards by the migrating Hottentots and Bantu." In general, this position is supported by Goodwin (1939:456). While recognizing an earlier date of introduction of cannabis, this hypothesis is rather vague as to "Hottentots and Bantu."

4. Walton (1953:85) refers to his own survey of archaeological reports which mention pipes found in early Bantu settelements, and also to Dos Santos' description of cannabis cultivation by the Eastern Shona in the sixteenth century. He then suggests that cannabis "was introduced into southern Africa by the very first waves of Bantu invaders from the north." The use of the herb would then have spread from Bantu to Hottentot and Bushmen. Walton's suggestion comes closest to the way in which the material will be reconstructed here.

The early contact between Indonesia and Madagascar may suggest the latter as a stepping stone. Copland (1822:327) points out that a "plant resembling hemp" was used, but I would doubt that this could be cannabis for this *ahetsmanga*, as it was called, had a green pod with about twelve seeds. Subsequent authors report the presence of hemp for its fiber (Shaw 1885) or for smoking (Ellis 1838; Sibree 1870 and 1880). Cannabis here is identified as *rongona* or *rongony*. Its use was illegal by this time in the Portuguese colonies in Africa. I would discount a migratory route via Madagascar on linguistic evidence, and because the Arab link to the

African mainland is much better documented. Berthold Laufer (1930) points out that hemp was smoked in Madagascar by the middle of the seventeenth century. He suggests that the term *ahetsmanga* is, in fact, based on *ahets* (herbs) and *mangha* derived from *bhang*. One possibility for the introduction of cannabis into Africa is the trade route through Ethiopia. It is well accepted that the Amhara people very early on came from southern Arabia (Simoons 1970). There was also a well-established trade route from Ethiopia to the Great Lakes — a route employed by the Turks (Greenway 1944–1945).

The most likely migratory route of the herb, however, is down the east coast of Africa. In his discussion of the introduction of tobacco into Africa, Laufer states that "hemp was introduced into East Africa from India through the medium of the Arabs, as has well been demonstrated by Count de Ficalho ..." (1930:13), but does not amplify. Although I have been unable to locate a copy of the source, I would agree with this statement regarding the origin and distribution of hemp. Trade links between Arabia (and possibly Turkey, India, and Persia) and the East African coast, existed during the first centuries A.D. According to classical sources an Arabian settlement existed at Rhapta, and gradually spread southwards, with permanent Muslim settlements on Zanzibar and Pemba, and at Kilwa no later than the twelfth century.

This is also the period during which the use of hemp spread westward to Egypt (Rosenthal 1971) and, according to our suggestion here, down the East African coast. During this period Bantu-speaking peoples were resident on the east coast and groups were migrating southward. The Arab traders had also expanded the gold trade with Sofala (Chittick 1965) and permanent Arab settlements on the African coast were being established. Much of the trade with the interior was by way of the rivers, but these frequently rendered travel impossible during the rainy season, thus necessitating extended periods in the interior. It is quite conceivable, as McMartin has suggested, that "this led to the eventual establishment of inland settlements by the Arabs where they would spend one or two years away from the coast" (1970:16). When the Portuguese made their way up the Zambezi in 1531 to establish a trading post, a small Arab community already existed at Sena, almost 100 miles from the coast. Livingstone (1857;1865) during his early explorations, repeatedly commented on the presence of Arabs and Arab cultural influences.

Even without the actual Arab presence in the interior, trading did exist. As far back as the second and third centuries A.D. "imports" were reaching the interior via the Zambezi valley, and Iron Age Africans were cultivating cereals and keeping cattle (Fagan 1969). We also know from early pottery traditions that the people in central Africa were soon producing pipes (Fagan 1963) and by the time that hemp was introduced would have been able to construct crude hubble-bubble pipes. Once it had been introduced into central Africa the avenues existed for its spread further west — either by an extensive series of trade routes into the Congo basin (Vansina 1962) or, more likely, by Swahili-speaking traders coming to the Great Lake region.

Further to the south we have documentation that around 1835 "the Matabele had considerable traffic with the Amasili/Masarwa off the edge of the Kalahari, exchanging iron, *dagga* [sic], spears, hoes and knives for ostrich-eggshell beads, ivory, feathers, horns and skins" (Sutherland-Harris 1970:253–254; Dornan 1925:122–123). The same kind of trade into the Kalahari region from the peoples in South West Africa also existed, as did various trade links among the local populations who cultivated and used cannabis (see others mentioned below; Vedder 1938). The migratory route proposed above has been outlined in general terms in Map 1.

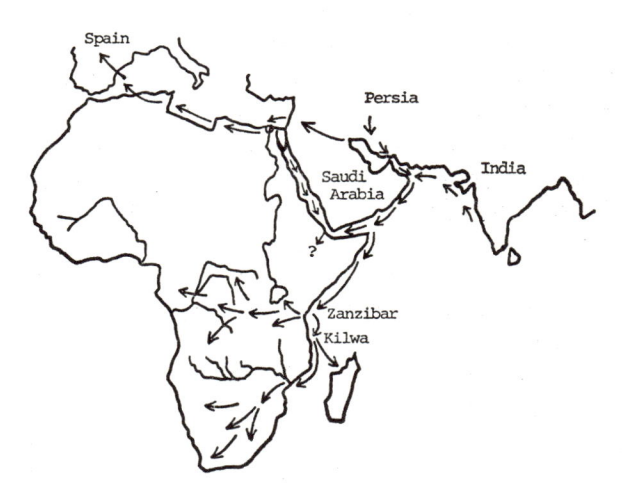

Map 1. Sketchmap representing the distribution of *Cannabis sativa*

Linguistic evidence for this spread must at this stage be based simply on the terms by which hemp is known. The Thonga who use cannabis live in the general vicinity of the Zambezi River mouth. In a complicated saliva contest (see later for a similar game among the Zulu) they distinguish between *matjafula* (ordinary white saliva) and *ntjutju* (black saliva produced by hemp). The Thonga (Junod 1962) refer to hemp as *mbange*, and the Rhodesian Shona use *mbanji*, while the Hindu term is *bangi* or *bhang*. The Venda who live just south of the Limpopo Divide, southwest of the Thonga, refer to hemp as *mbanzhe*. Among the Sotho it may be called *matokwane, lebake,* or *patse*. The Swazi-Zulu complex refers to it as *ntsangu,* while the Hottentot use the term *daXab,* which refers also to tobacco, and so gave rise to the common reference to *dagga*. The Lamba, in the current Zambia, speak of *uluwangula* (Doke 1931) while the people around the Great Lakes, and immediately to the south of Lake Victoria, refer to it as *bhangi* (Kollmann 1899). When the famous explorer Speke made his way from the coast to the Great Lakes he also found Arab communities and the use of cannabis. Among the Swahili around the coast the use of *banghi* was common as it still is.

Crossing into the general area now known as Zaire, and also northern Angola, we find the term *riamba* or *chamba* as the standard referent. Map 2 outlines this linguistic material.

Looking at the historical and linguistic evidence, we have two possible explanations regarding the introduction of cannabis into southern Africa:

1. If we accept *dagga*, or the traditional names from which it was derived, as the oldest and original referent, we would be on safe ground, provided we adhere only to that material. *Dagga* is the term used furthest south. This would force us to postulate that the Hottentot herders were grazing their stock along the east coast during the twelfth and thirteenth centuries, and were first contacted by the Arabs. Here again, we could assume: (a) that this contact occurred prior to the spread of the word *bhang* from India and that the water-pipe (of Persian origin) came by way of the early Arab settlers. Hemp was introduced simply as a form of *duXan* or tobacco (*vide* the discussion below regarding the etymology of the term *dagga*). As the herders migrated southward, and were replaced on the coast by Bantu speakers, the latter took over the same practice. (b) Since this would now be after the twelfth or thirteenth centuries, the Arabs would have already been using the terms *bhang* or *bangi* which came with the new spread of the herb from India, the Bantu then took over the referent *bangi* and its derivatives which are today recorded. While this hypothesis might explain the geographical distribution of the terminology, there is no evidence for Hottentot-Arab contacts and little evidence for the latter smoking anything before tobacco was introduced to them (Rosenthal 1970).

2. The more likely hypothesis is that Bantu-speaking negroids along the east coast, from Lamu to the Zambezi, had contact with Arabs who smoked *bangi,* a practice which they had brought from India. As the Bantu adopted the custom of smoking cannabis, they also adopted the water-pipe and referrents which underwent linguistic adaptation. The

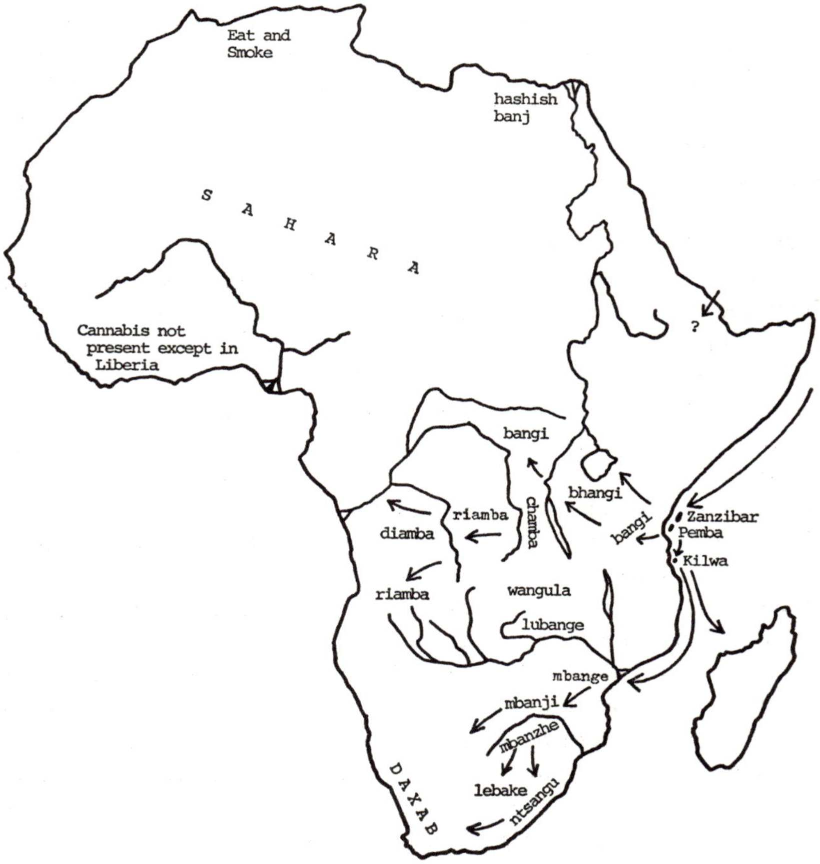

Map 2. Sketchmap showing terms by which *Cannabis sativa* is known

Sotho terms are linguistically the most distant and also the most distant geographically — measured in terms of degrees of contact with the original people who introduced the practice and the term. This hypothesis suggests that when the Hottentot herders were introduced to smoking hemp, they saw it in much the same way as they looked on other kinds of tobacco (including *Leonotis leonurus*) which were used for snuff or perhaps smoked. Thus they called it *daXab*, but qualified that it actually was "green" tobacco.

I would suggest that the same factors influenced the westward spread of cannabis. It was carried by traders, both Swahili and Arab, and traded from the east coast to the Great Lake region. Due to local frames of reference or cultural equivalents among the Luba or other people who first accepted the practice, we find the reference to *riamba*. Further research is underway regarding the origin and meanings of the latter term.

As far as can be ascertained, cannabis has been growing in southern Africa for the past four or five centuries, While it was originally an imported plant, most likely carried southward by early migrants, it has long since become naturalized, and grows with much vigor in the warmer regions.

It should be recognized that the botanical specimens present in this region today have been influenced by cross-breeding with plants grown from seed imported from Europe and also from South America.[1]

It should also be recognized that in southern Africa there are at least two cultural traditions which blended folk knowledge and uses of cannabis. At the beginning of the seventeenth century in the southern part of the continent, there were indigenous cultural traditions of use among the "Bushmen," "Hottentot" and Bantu-speaking peoples of negroid extraction. Into this setting came European settlers who had had contact with the East Indies and in time, introduced their own folk beliefs concerning the use of cannabis. Most of these beliefs seem to have been medicinal. In the process, due to errors in identifying plant species, they included a number of other plants in the general folk nomenclature. While the term "dagga" (spelled in a number of ways) was accepted to refer to *Cannabis sativa* L., we find numerous cases where the term "dagga" also refers to various species of *Leonotis*. In almost every case, however, it is used with a qualifier, such as *Wilde dagga*, *Klip dagga*, *Rooi dagga* (wild *dagga*, stone *dagga*, red *dagga*), and so forth. These various plants formed an integral part of the folk medicines of both African indigenes and white Boer settlers.

Etymology of the Term "Dagga"

The earliest use of this referrent of which I am aware occurs in the diary of Jan van Riebeeck, the first governor of the new Dutch Settlement at the Cape of Good Hope. The date was 1658, and it was spelled "daccha." It is almost certain that in this and subsequent references we are not dealing with *Cannabis sativa* but with *Leonotis leonurus*. Van Riebeeck describes *daccha* as "een droogh cruyt dat de Hottentoos eeten ende droncken van worden" (a dry powder which the Hottentots eat and which makes

---

[1] Whether this has greatly affected the growth cycle, size or foliage of the local *indica* variety is not known.

them drunk). Watt and Breyer-Brandwijk (1932), discussing the medicinal and poisonous plants of southern Africa, point out that *Leonotis leonurus R. Br.*, also referred to as *Rooi dagga, Wilde dagga*, or *Klip dagga*, was in early times smoked by the Hottentots instead of tobacco. They also quote early authors to the effect that white colonists employed the plant and that "the preparation produces narcotic effects if used incautiously" (*Ibid.:* 156) and that "Laidler records that in olden times the Namas formed the powdered leaf into cakes which were chewed evidently for the intoxicating effect" (*Ibid.*: 157). Many of the same properties are ascribed to *Leonotis leonurus R. Br.*, also referred to as *Knoppies dagga* or *Klipdagga*.

While it is impossible to confuse the adult plant of *Cannabis sativa* and adult specimens of the *Leonotis* groups with their bright red flowers, it is likely that the common use and related effects of these two plants lead to the common term. This classificatory error also underlies suggestions that cannabis products were eaten or drunk. The *Leonotis* leaves were smoked, usually after being mixed with tobacco.

One of the most complete linguistic analyses of the term "dagga" has been made by Nienaber (1963) who suggests two possible origins for this term: following Lichtenstein (1928) it is possible that the Dutch term *tabak* (tobacco), which frequently appears as *twak*, was corrupted to *twaga*, later *toaga*, and finally *dagga*. This seems an unlikely origin. A more plausible theory is that the Hottentot term *daXa-b* or *baXa-b*, which among other things refers to tobacco, is the root noun. When referring specifically to *dagga* one finds the qualifier *!am* (green) being added to the root, and the result is *!amaXa-b* namely, "green tobacco" or *dagga*.

Lichtenstein (1928) and Nienaber (1963) doubt that *dagga* is an original Hottentot word. Meinhof suggested that *dagga* is a derivative of the Arabic word *duXan* or "tobacco" (cited in Nienaber 1963:243), which came in with the early Hottentot migrants. We should immediately point out that no other language group in South Africa used this term.

Early European observers in South Africa had problems in phonetically recording the terms they heard among indigenous peoples. In time a variety of spellings for this Hottentot word appeared. Thus we find *daccha* (1658), *dacha* (1660), *dackae* (1663), *dagha* (1686), *daggha* (1695), *dagga* (1708), *tagga* (1725), *dacka* (1775) and *daga* (1779) (*vide* Nienaber 1963 and Raven-Hart 1971). It should be repeated that not all these writers in fact referred to *Cannabis sativa*, or to the *smoking* of the herb.

AN ETHNOGRAPHY OF CANNABIS

An Ethnohistorical Outline

As far as we know today the first people to occupy the southern part of Africa were hunters and gatherers and perhaps also herders. These groups who were occupying the Cape when the Portuguese first rounded the southern tip of Africa are known as the "Bushmen" and "Hottentot," terms that have created a great deal of confusion.

There was a tendency to lump together all yellow-skinned, hunting and gathering peoples whose language was characterized by "clicks." These peoples were called "Bushmen" after the early reference of *Bosjesmans* assigned by the Dutch settlers to the little people who would appear as if from nowhere from behind a shrub or bush. They were differentiated from the taller, yellow-skinned people, who also employed "clicks" in their language, but were cattle and sheep herders and were called "Hottentot." The literature in time contained descriptions of yellow-skinned people who employed various "clicks" in their language, and could be differentiated on the following bases: culturally, by the fact of herding versus hunting and gathering; linguistically, or physically, by stature and a few other minor traits.

Among themselves these early settlers had differentiated between the "Khoikoin" or "men of men" as the herders referred to themselves, and the "San" as they referred to all yellow-skinned hunters and gatherers. It has become accepted — partly due to a derogatory note attached to the term "Hottentot" — to refer to all these peoples as the Khoisan. There is a growing insistence that physical descriptions or names be based on physical criteria only, while linguistic classification should be based on linguistic criteria.[2]

In addition to the Khoisan groups there were also a few groups of negro hunters who were marked by an extremely simple material culture. Some of these spoke a Khoikhoi language (Nama) and they are together referred to as the "Dama," "Damara" or "Bergdama."

The first people to be contacted by the Portuguese who rounded the Cape in 1487 were yellow-skinned herders. They were not settled villagers but seemed to migrate with available grazing and water supplies and built temporary camps. According to Jan van Riebeeck, the first Dutch Commander at the Cape, they met small groups of Khoikhoi who subsis-

---

[2] One of the persons who has made this insistence on the clearest linguistic grounds is Westphal (1963; 1971), who is rewriting the linguistic prehistory of southern Africa.

ted on hunting, fishing and collecting along the seashore. These people became known as the Strandloopers (literally, "Beach Walkers").

From the north at about this time came a number of negroid groups who were village dwellers and iron workers. We know that Iron Age people crossed the Zambezi River somewhere between A.D. 100 and A.D. 300 (Inskeep 1969), but most of these groups seem to have remained in the central plateau region. It is believed that the ancestors of the present Bantu-speaking negroids migrated into this region after the sixth century and by A.D. 1000 were widely spread throughout the present Rhodesia, Transvaal and Orange Free State. This information is based on well-defined pottery traditions, mining undertakings and carbon-14 dates of remains found in early Iron Age settlements. Two important facts are known, namely, that by 1552 "Kaffirs" occupied the coastal plains on the east coast (according to a diary by the survivors from the wreck of the *Sao Joao*) and "a ship from Sofala was expected annually at Lourenço Marques to buy ivory" (Wilson 1969:78). We find shortly after this that the Nguni peoples, comprised of the Zulu and Swazi in the north and the Xhosa, Tembu, Fingo and smaller groups in the south, occupied the region between the coastal plains and the foothills into the interior. The coast itself was sparsely populated. These mutually intelligible Nguni groups spread from the Lebombo mountains and Khosi Bay region in the north to the Sundays River in the south.

Quite extensive interaction accompanied by cultural, linguistic and genetic exchanges occurred between the local hunters and gatherers and the herders as well as between the latter and Iron Age negroid settlers. Since Nguni may have been in the foothills of the Drakenberg from as early as A.D. 1300 (Wilson 1959), this exchange and interchange was well advanced at the time of the first written record. This does not suggest that the Nguni people adopted the use of cannabis from the yellow-skinned herders when they settled in the south, but merely that a degree of interchange, especially regarding the methods of use, did occur. Cannabis may have been introduced to the herders by these latecomers.

Early Records of Use Among the Herders

It will be recalled that the first observers confused various preparations which were eaten or drunk (these were not cannabis), preparations which were smoked in various mixtures (which included cannabis), and products which were smelled and inhaled (which might have included cannabis but were usually restricted to roots such as the *gannabossie*, i.e., the *Ganna* shrub).

Six years after arriving at the Cape, Jan van Riebeeck reports on the "daccha" which the herders ate in the form of a dry powder. Dapper in 1668, touched on the same subject when he referred to the fact that the Khoikhoi were wealthy herders and did not practice agriculture at all except for a "zekeren krachtigen wortel, dien zy dacha noemen, en eeten om dronken te worden" ("certain potent root, which they call dacha, and which they eat to get drunk") (Dapper 1933:40). He also refers to the effects on persons who have *eaten* this root. It is almost certain that we are here dealing with *Leonotis leonurus*. Its leaves were also frequently smoked alone or mixed with tobacco. Dapper mentions particularly the Heusequas as being involved in cultivating the plant.

Writing two years later, John Ogilby states that "these Heusequas onely maintain themselves with planting (for the rest of the Hottentots neither sowe nor plant) of a powerful Root, which they call Dacha: sometimes eating it, otherwhiles mingling it with water to drink: either of which ways taken, causeth Ebriety" (1670:583).

Almost identical statements are found in Bogaert published in Amsterdam in 1711 (*vide* Raven-Hart 1971), and in Johan Schreyer published in Saalfeld in 1679 (*Ibid.*). The latter speaks of this dried herb which they *chew* and which then produces the same results already mentioned. Wilhelm Ten Rhyne, who was a physician of the Dutch East India Company in 1686 wrote *A short account of the Cape of Good Hope and of the Hottentots who inhabit that region*. He obviously did not have ideal rapport with his Khoikhoi informants, for he stated that one could not always get all the information one wanted from these people, "For in the first place the Hottentots lie, and, in the second, they are determined to keep their secret remedies to themselves. They cure colic quickly by a certain aromatic root. They employ also a certain species of Datura, as I think, called dacha. This they bray carefully, and after braying, make it into balls and eat it, as many Mahommedans do with Amsion or opium. It makes them monstruous drunk" (1933:153). Also Schrijver, writing in 1689, states that the Khoikhoi bartered for *Dagha* "which is used by them as the Indians use opium amphion" (1931:234). In a lengthy letter written in 1695, de Grevenbroek explains that the Khoikhoi "set very great store by the plant Daggha, as they call it, the roots of which they make into little cakes not exceeding in size the silver coin known in the vernacular as a rix dollar: and these they chew, as the Indians do opium and the Egyptians oetum. It puts them to sleep, but never maddens them" (1933:263).

In almost all cases thus far we may in fact be dealing with *Leonotis leonurus* and other shrubs and not with *Cannabis sativa*, though all references are to *dagga*. We know that this *dagga* was grown domestically, for Mentzel, writing in 1785, explains that white settlers who employed Khoikhoi paid them with "a few head of cattle, a little tobacco, dagga, some knives, glass beads..." (1944:85). Latrobe (1969), in fact, was so incensed at this use of *dacha*, "a species of wild hemp (cicuta)," that he proposed the first penal code against its use and distribution — a penalty fully as severe as that which exists today.

In addition to the use of *dagga* at this time, we also find reference to the use by the Khoikhoi and the San, of *kanna*, a root which was greatly valued as it was burned and the smoke inhaled (Kolb 1968).[3] In addition, it seems that the leaves of *ganna* bush were "also dried and powdered, and used both for chewing and smoking. When mixed with dacha it was very intoxicating" (Stow 1905:53): Lichtenstein (1928:154) identifies it as *Salsola sphylla* and *Salicornia fruticosa* and as being used by indigenous peoples and white settlers. We are told that *kanna, canna* or *ganna* could be identified as "several species of Salsola" which were chewed in much the same way "as the natives of India use betel or areca" (Schapera and Farrington 1933:264–265). It was thus another of a group of stimulants used by the Khoisan peoples.

While so many of the early writers used the term *dagga* without clearly identifying it, I would suggest that they might have been observing the use of *Cannabis sativa* along with other herbs and roots, including different species of *Leonotis* and *Salsola*. This is suggested by the trade routes and migration patterns and by documentation from other writers who were the contemporaries of our earlier observers. Thus Le Vaillant (1796:71) while speaking of the Gonaqua, a Khoikhoi group whom he visited, explains: "They smoke the leaves of a plant which they name dagha, and not daka, as some authors have written. This plant is not indigenous: It is the hemp of Europe."

In much the same way, John Barrow (1801:18) stated that the Khoikhoi cultivated hemp, "not, however, for the purpose of being manufactured into cordage or cloth, but merely for the sake of the leaflets, flowers, and young seeds which are used by the slaves and Hottentots as a succedaneum for tobacco." An almost identical statement is found in Anderson's (1967:79) description of his travels into southwest Africa. The Damara whom he visited in the 1850's, cultivated hemp for the young "leaves and seeds." It seems that the Damara were the main *dagga*

---

[3] Arbousset and Daumas, speaking of the Free State Bushmen whom they met on their visit to a settlement, state: "The old mama took from her neck a bit of some narcotic root, lit it at the fire; and bringing it near her nose, snuffed in the smoke" (1846: 251). This seems to have been a common practice, for Stow (1905) also describes it.

cultivators in the region. In addition to small gardens of melon, pumpkins and *dagga*, they also planted tobacco and in this respect "they far surpass the Ovaherero and the Namaqua" (Stow 1905:259). We are told that they "did a regular trade with the Ovambo tribes, from whom they got cows, goats, iron and copper in exchange for dagga, for dagga was at that time the Bergdamas' money with which they could buy anything" (Vedder 1938:175). The author in the latter case identified *dagga* as a "kind of intoxicating hemp" (*Ibid.*: 53). This position is confirmed by Jenny (1966), referring to another early missionary, Hugo Hahn. William Burchell, speaking of a "mixed Hottentot" settlement he visited in 1811, also refers to the cultivation of "dakka" in a garden that was "irrigated by a trench which conducted water from a spring not far off" (1967, II:7). The practice of cultivating *dagga* seems to have been concentrated among the Nama (and the Nama-speaking negroid Bergdama) and the Hancumqua.

We are not too sure about the cultivation of *dagga* among the Khoikhoi. Van Riebeeck suggested that the Hancumquas were the actual cultivators while Stow (1905:243) also speaks of the Hancumquas and Chainouquas (sub-groups of the same tribe) as subsisting by the breeding of cattle and the "cultivation of the plant *dagga*." Schrijver also named the Ganumqua (note H equals G), Namkunqua and the Ganaqua as the people who cultivated the *dagga* and traded it to other groups, including the hunters or San.

Trade and Use by Hunters

While the Khoikhoi were herders and practiced a minimum of garden cultivation, the San were hunters and gatherers. Their hunting sites are distributed over most of southern Africa and the now famous "Bushmen Paintings" adorn the ledges and domes of countless caves and mountain shelters. From numerous early sources we learn of trading relations between the hunters and other groups in southern Africa and even suggestions that the hunters might have been the earliest smokers. The noted writer George Stow states that "the hunters were addicted to smoking, and used these pipes generations before they came in contact with the stronger races" (1905:53). In exchange for tobacco and *dagga* they supplied feathers, game, and other products collected in the hunt (Dornan 1925). While Dornan refers to *dagga* as *Leonotis leonurus* we now have sufficient reason to accept the evidence of Schapera who states that "as narcotics, the Bushmen use chiefly tobacco and dagga [*Cannabis sativa*]" (1960:101).

The hunters used the water-pipe, one of the older forms of use, which may have diffused from Persia via the Arabic region.

The hunting and gathering San people did not settle down easily and did not take to being employed by the newly arrived white settlers. Describing a missionary garden in a Khoikhoi settlement, Burchell refers to "the common hemp" which is raised there and "given as presents to the Bushmen" (1967, I:366). Gutsche quotes a number of cases in which white settlers gave *dagga* to Bushmen (1968) in an attempt to create friendly relations. In other cases "the whites who seldom use the dacha themselves [should] cultivate it for their servants. But it is, I believe, an inducement to retain the wild Bushmen in their service..." (Gutsche 1968: 46). This was also the practice further into the interior where farmers cultivated *dagga* to keep the herders and the hunters, in their service; the latter became sheep herders *par excellence* (Fritsch 1868).

The Kalahari hunters of recent times also used *dagga* (Tobias 1961) as do a number of hunting groups today.[4] Among these groups are the Bugakwe people who live north of the Dkavango Swamps. They also use the same kind of composite water-pipe common in the past (Heinz 1972, personal communication): this form of smoking is described by Theal (1910).

The question will remain whether the smoking of *dagga* was introduced relatively late by the arrival of the negroid migrants or whether it had been present among hunters and herders prior to the arrival of the negroid cultivators. One thing can be accepted without doubt: smoking long preceded the arrival of whites in southern Africa. It is thus difficult to understand on what basis Raven-Hart states that the indigenous wild *dagga* was chewed, since "the idea of smoking anything came in with the Dutch" (1971:507).

Later Arrivals: The Agriculturalists

The Bantu-speaking negroids spread their gardens and pastures over most of the eastern and northern parts of southern Africa. Documents which are readily available recount early meetings first on the eastern frontier and later further north and east.

As white settlers and explorers moved eastward they met the Xhosa, Fingo and other southern Nguni people, and both tobacco and *dagga* were valued (Alberti 1968) and smoking was practiced by men and women

---

[4] Silberbauer (1965) produces a photograph of a young Bushmen woman smoking a typical short-stem pipe, but does not indicate whether these people use *dagga* or only tobacco.

(as is still the case). Andrew Smith (1939:312) who gained a very thorough knowledge of the people, states that "Dakka has from time immemorial been known to the Caffers. They are very partial to smoaking it. Those that can procure both tobacco and dakka snuff the former and smoak the latter. They smoak it through water." The smoking of *dagga* among the Baralong and Bathlapin, both sub-groups of the Tswana, is also mentioned by Andrew Smith, and hemp smoking by the Bechuana, another Tswana group, is mentioned by Conder (1887). Baines (1964:213) gives a full description of the water-pipe and presents a drawing of an African smoking "dakka" (1864).

Related to neighboring Tswana we find the Sotho who occupy the present Lesotho. One of the early missionaries described and diagrammed the pipe they used for smoking. He states that "tobacco has long been in use among the natives, and must have come to them from the Portuguese of Mozambique but, in a song consecrated to the praise of this favorite plant, they confess that the use of dagga (a kind of hemp, of which the Arabs make Hagschisch), is much more ancient" (Casalis 1965:141). Much the same position was taken by Nienaber (1963) who states that the Hottentot smoked long before tobacco was introduced. We are told that there was a time when the Sotho did not know tobacco "but they used to smoke hemp" (Ellenberger and Macgregor 1912:9).

The Zulu occupy most of Natal, and, as Nguni, are related to the Xhosa in the south and the Swazi in the north. John Bird raises an interesting problem; he writes that "dakka, the dried leaf of the wild hemp, is indigenous to the country" (1888, I:306). Later in the same volume we read of "sangu which is only European hemp, and raised for smoking." This is a problem, because in most of the subsequent references and also in current usage, *intsangu* is synonymous with *dagga* which is used to refer to cannabis. It would seem that we are back to the mistaken identity of *dagga* as "wild hemp." (See also Gardiner 1836:106, who suggests that the Zulu made a snuff of dagga leaves.)

Writing even before Bird, the Reverend Grout who spent half his lifetime among the Zulu, speaks of smoking the pipe in which the bowl is filled "with the leaves and seed of the insangu" (1970:110). This "filthy and baneful" practice, as the Reverend Tylor describes it, "has a narcotic even intoxicating effect, similar to that of Indian hemp" (1891:122–123). The latter author is reminiscent of Latrobe who almost a century earlier in the Cape, suggested that smokers of hemp should be denied church membership (*Ibid.*).

In a traditional Zulu community it was common for men to smoke *intsangu*, even daily, and it seems that the effects reported were as varied as the individual personalities. Some turned to extraordinary hilarity, others to moroseness. It was especially at times of war that men would smoke the herb and, as saliva collected in the mouth, it would be passed through "a hollow stem of tambootie grass and so made to trace a labyrinth (*tshuma sogexe*) on a smooth floor" (Samuelson n.d.: 81).[5] The young warriors smoked *dagga* before an attack and were then capable of accomplishing almost any feat. Bryant states that "the hemp [*intsangu, Cannabis sativa*] the Zulus smoked was home grown in every kraal..." and the best quality leaves were terminologically differentiated from the poorer kind (1949:222–223). In all cases the traditional form of the pipe was used. The Zulu did not smoke tobacco as a rule but ground it into snuff. That is why they have only a single term for tobacco and snuff.

The Swazi also used the *dagga* pipe as well as the method by which a hole is made in the ground and the smoke sucked through a mouth-piece. The herb seems to have been associated here primarily with diviners who used a pipe. Following a puff of smoke each would fill his mouth with water to cool down the hot smoke (O'Neil 1921). It was also used as a stimulant by young warriors, as among the Zulu, and by the praise singer who must intone the praises of the king or some prominent person. "It is contended by natives that the drug stimulates the brain. If a man is faced with an extraordinary knotty problem he will smoke his *shawulo* [pipe] and concentrate on the problem and the solution will present itself to him without trouble" (Marwick 1940:80).

The water-pipe was found among all of these people. Slight variations obviously occurred as with the Venda, who, however, did not use *dagga* very extensively (Stayt 1931). An identical description for the pipe as it was used by the Matabele is given by Decle (1898).

The Neighbors to the North

Since it has been suggested that cannabis was introduced into Africa from the northeast, and not from the south, it would be fruitful to follow briefly the patterns of its distribution and use.

Dagga is a weed which can only grow well under cultivation in Rhodesia. The distribution of the plant in or through this ecosystem must thus

---

[5] Braatvedt (1949:134) gives a very good description of this game. The level ground in front of the smokers represented the battlefield and the saliva bubbles they blew through the hollow reed represented the respective armies. Due to the *insangu* influence, the saliva formed bubbles which would not break for a considerable time. As the smokers took turns with the hollow reed their respective armies tried to encircle one another. This was the pastime, and a very exciting one, for the old men.

have accompanied people. For normal growth it needs "a rich soil, fairly good rainfall and personal attention" (Editor 1958:500). In Mashonaland it is known as *mbanji* and is said to be a stimulus both sexually and in terms of increasing working efficiency. It is interesting to note how varied the effects or contradictory the information is from one author to the next.

Having arrived at the great falls which he named after Queen Victoria, David Livingstone observed cannabis smoking among the Makololo, a Sotho offshoot. It is of interest that they call it *matokwane*. He describes its use as follows:

We had ample opportunity for observing the effects of this matokwame smoking on our men. It makes them feel very strong in body, but it produces exactly the opposite effect upon the mind. Two of our finest young men became inveterate smokers, and partially idiotic. The performances of a group of matokwane smokers are somewhat grotesque; they are provided with a calabash of pure water, a split bamboo, five feet long, and the great pipe, which has a large calabash or kudu's horn chamber to contain the water, through which the smoke is drawn Narghille fashion, on its way to the mouth. Each smoker takes a few whiffs, the last being an extra long one, and hands the pipe to his neighbour. He seems to swallow the fumes; for, striving against the convulsive action of the muscles of chest and throat, he takes a mouthful of water from the calabash, waits a few seconds, and then pours water and smoke from his mouth down the groove of the bamboo. The smoke causes violent coughing in all, and in some a species of frenzy which passes away in a rapid stream of unmeaning words, or short sentences, as, "the green grass grows," "the fat cattle thrive," "the fish swim" (1865:286–287.)

It was also used to impart self-confidence; Livingstone states that when the soldiers of the chief Sebitwane came in sight of their enemies, they "sat down and smoked it, in order that they might make an effective onslaught" (1857:540). Whatever hallucinogenic and stimulating properties may be present in cannabis, and whatever psychoactive material in THC, it was long since recognized in daily living by southern African people.

In the region of the present Malawi, Johnston (1897) observed it being planted and smoked as did Livingstone (1865). Hughes states that in the Malawi-Zambia area cannabis is smoked and it is known here as *bange*. This he recognizes as "a term introduced by the Arabs, the same word as the Indian *Bhang*" (1933:70). Turning further to the interior, we find that among the Ila-speaking peoples cannabis was extensively grown and "smoked in a kind of narghile." It is of interest that the native word for hemp is *lubange* (Smith and Dale 1920:152).

Tracing another route northward, i.e., along the western part of the continent, we find cannabis being smoked in Angola where the usual horned water-pipe was used (Schachtzabel 1923) and where its use "by a slave is considered a crime" by the Portuguese (Livingstone 1857:541; Monteiro 1968:257). Across the Angola highlands one descends into the present Zaire, where hemp-smoking was said to be "the curse of the Batetela in Kasai province" (Hilton-Simpson 1911:256).

One of the most interesting areas to look at is the Congo drainage area and its border districts. Harry Johnston summarizes the picture by stating that "hemp as a narcotic is not much used in the Congo basin except in the southern, south-western, and south-central parts, and the western Mubangi. This practice has nearly died out in the kingdom of Kongo, though it was prevalent once. Of late years hemp-smoking has developed in a rather sensational fashion among the excitable Bashilange..." (1908:607–608). The latter, a sub-group of the larger Luba people, occupy the area around the confluence of the Lulua and the Kasai. It seems that Swahili traders from Zanzibar (Keane 1920:114) introduced cannabis into the region after the 1850's and the original *bhang* was here referred to as *rhiamba*. During the civil strife in the early 1870's a secret society calling itself *Bena-Riamba* was formed.[6]

In time there was concern about the increasing use of the herb and secret societies were formed to counter its use. A quarter of a century later Wissman pointed out that "among the younger generation it is already beginning to decrease" (1891:308). It is interesting that, in the same region, we should find the Badjok, a southern Bantu people, who "denied ever smoking hemp, but a great quantity of it grew near Mayila's hut — probably as an ornament" (Torday 1925:271).

Cannabis was also smoked in the northern part of Zaire (Dorman 1905:88) and had spread into the former French Congo. Cureau states that people smoke tobacco moderately, but "the same cannot be said for Indian hemp, the habit of indulging in which is making frightful progress" [sic] using what was then recognized as a "peculiar pipe for smoking it" (1915:229, 238).

Looking to the east we learn that cannabis use was "in 1883 greatly on the increase" among the Nyamwezi in the current Tanzania (Wissman 1891:308). Half a century later Raymond stated that the use of hemp had become so widespread that the word *njemu* (hemp) was also used to refer to a "senseless person." They had a different term to refer to insanity

---

[6] Early writers translated this as "Sons" of hemp, but Johnston points out that we should recognize *bena* (meaning "brothers") not *bana* (meaning "children"). He suggests the use of an initial D rather than R (1908:608) to read *Bena-Diamba*, but due to the widespread use of *Riamba* we will retain it here.

1938:74). North of this region, the area frequently referred to as East Africa, we find the term *chamba* which is smoked in the absence of food or drink when they are tired, but which they admit "catches their legs" (Werner 1906:179). The linguistic connection between *diamba* and *chamba* is obvious.

Roscoe states emphatically that the "Basoga are addicted to smoking Indian hemp, and this makes them stupid and often stubborn" (1921: 249). The Baganda, however, did not take to the new smoking habit (Roscoe 1911). Since cannabis was introduced among the Bagishu, probably by some Arab traveller, it has spread from family to family. We find here an interesting belief in the potential harm cannabis smoking may have on a developing fetus. Purvis states that "a man will even forbid his wife to smoke it on account of some evil effect it is said to have upon her or her child, should she be about to become a mother" (1909:336–337). Children were free to use it, however, for individual freedom of decision and choice was highly developed in Masaba.

We have not yet mentioned the non-negroid peoples in this part of Africa. Until fairly recently, there has been speculation about links between the hunters and herders in southern Africa and the Hadza and Sandawe in Tanzania. It has been suggested that since the San and these northern groups had a hunting and gathering economy, they must be related. Others suggested that since the languages of the Khoikhoi and San in the south and Hadza and Sandawe in the north were marked by "clicks" these people had to be related. Westphal (1963 and 1971) argues that "clicks" cannot be any criterion of linguistic affinity. The debate will continue. We do know that the Sandawe grow tobacco and "a plant with the same effect as the 'dagga' of South Africa" (Bagshawe 1924–1925: 226). They also use the water-pipe which seems to be associated with cannabis throughout the continent irrespective of region, socioeconomic level or linguistic group membership.

Referring to the Pygmies, the other major non-negroid peoples of the region, Torday (1925:240) notes that the smoking of cannabis "is practised to some extent among the Bangongo (a group living in the present Zaire), who say that they have learned it from the Pygmies, who were addicted to it since times immemorial...."

The author immediately allows for the more plausible explanation — that of Arab introduction — but continues by stating that "should it be proven that the Pygmies are responsible for its propagation, hemp would have to be considered as the oldest narcotic known to the Africans" (*Ibid.*: 240).

Regarding the Efe (one of the Pygmy groups) Schebesta explains that they believe that smoking the *bangi* would give them the "power to kill elephants" (1933:229). The same variety of water-pipe they used was found among the Bambuti, made from either calabash or of clay (Schebesta 1952:167). The reasons given for the migration of the pygmies to the vicinity of Atoli and Arambi are that in this part of the forest there are plentiful growths of banana and *bangi* (Schebesta 1936:248). A photograph in this latter volume is described as Schebesta giving a plate of soup to a pygmy, but he seems to be holding a water-pipe (*Ibid.*: 192).

The most interesting fact about southern and eastern Africa is that we have found amazing uniformity in several respects: the water-pipe, with clay bowl, gourd, or horn; only smoking of cannabis; and a pattern of names (a) derivatives of the Arabic word *duXan*, or of the Khoikhoi *daXab*, in the south; (b) derivatives of the Indian term *bang* in the southeast and central regions; and (c) derivatives of the Swahili trader's term *riamba* in the Congo drainage region.

But what about West Africa? If the herb entered Africa from Egypt one would certainly expect its diffusion along caravan routes across the Sahara. If, on the other hand, the main routes were Arab traders' down the east coast, we may well ask how long it would take cannabis to spread across the continent from east to west, given the fact that the major population movements were southward and considering the fact of ecological changes. If we can believe specialists who have published to date, cannabis either was not introduced to West Africa or was not accepted due to various factors. Asuni states that "Cannabis sativa is not indigenous to Nigeria, and evidence indicates that it was introduced to the country and most likely to other parts of West Africa during and after the second World War by soldiers returning from the Middle East and the Far East, and North Africa, and also by sailors" (1964:18). Furthermore, there is no traditional name for it though a number of local terms have since emerged. By 1965 Nigeria supplied for local consumption and "illicit traffic between neighbouring countries and in international illicit traffic" (Tella *et al.* 1967:40). It is then not strange to find the herb used primarily by "marginal" Africans, by young migrant workers, and by "organized political thugs" or "recently evolved secret societies with criminal aims, such as Odozi Obodo and the Leopard-men Society of Nigeria" (Lambo 1965:3, 6). In contrast to some of the cases in East Africa where cannabis is well-accepted and used by males and females alike, we find that it is "almost entirely confined to the male sex" in this region (Boroffka 1966:378).

Moving further west to Ghana the picture remains almost identical. The first illegal cultivation of cannabis in Ghana was reported by police in 1960 where the herb is called *Wee*, which Sagoe sees as "a corruption of 'weed,' by seaman" (1966:8). The only way of using cannabis is by smoking it in a rolled cigarette. We can thus see it as a recent introduction without the normal accompanying paraphernalia.

Types and Methods of Smoking[7]

As all evidence suggests, there is an association of hemp smoking and some kind of water-pipe, or at least the use of water in the mouth. The order in which these pipe types are discussed here may not follow an evolutionary sequence, but suggest some historical association with the Persian origins of the hubble-bubble.

Type I: Gourd Water Containers

Calabash, a variety of gourd, is used as a water container: the neck is cut off or a hole is made in its side to apply to the mouth of the smoker. Another hole is made in the body of the gourd, into which the pipe bowl is placed, either directly or attached to a connecting reed. The smoker inhales through the aperture, thus drawing the smoke through the water. This kind of water-pipe is found throughout the northern, northeastern and northwestern parts of the region under discussion. It is found also among the San hunters of Angola, the Kung and Heikum of the Kalahari region and peoples all along the Zambezi. These people "use a plain, narrow, oval gourd, narrower at the top end, where is inserted a reed which goes right down to the bottom of the gourd and has a bowl fixed at its top. The smoker inhales through a square hole cut in the side of the gourd" (Shaw 1938:282).

Type II: Horn Water Containers

In the area marked by large antelope and long-horned cattle the gourd is replaced by a hollow horn. The pipe stem now enters the horn at an angle, the horn is half-filled with water and the smoke is inhaled through the open end of the horn, usually that of an ox or one of the larger antelope species, e.g., the Kudu (*Strepsiceros strepsiceros*). Once again the clay bowl is attached to the horn by a hollow wooden tube or reed and the

---

[7] While smoking leads to certain uniformities, we find a wide variety of "pipe" forms and diverse ways of inhaling the smoke. The classificatory categories to be employed in this section have been used by a number of authors, notably Miss M. Shaw of the South African Museum in Cape Town, and James Walton.

gum or wax may be applied to seal the junction of the reed and the horn; the mouth is applied to the large open end of the horn and the smoke is drawn through the water. Should the open end of the horn be too large, it is placed in such a way that half the opening presses against the cheek and the other half is covered by the mouth. There are various ways of inserting the reed stem into the horn, either at an angle as was done by Zulu, Sotho, Tswana and the Transkeian Nguni, or vertically as was done by the Cape San hunters. The Swazi, Thonga, and Venda used a longer reed stem but instead of cutting an aperture in the side of the horn, the long reed was placed down into the horn through the large open end. Stayt explains that the Venda hemp smoker "inhales by placing both hands over the opening and around the reed and drawing through the aperture made by slightly parting the hands. The smoke passes through the water at the bottom of the horn. It is taken in huge breaths, and exhaled with great coughing and spluttering" (1931:50–51). Among the Herero, and some of the San and Khoikhoi living in the Cape region the reed was absent as the bowl was placed directly on the horn.

A logical development was to block the open end of the horn by a piece of wood or horn, or to cover it with skin as the Cape San and Khoikhoi did. Schachtzabel (1923:88) illustrates another variation from Angola in which the large open end of the horn is completely closed and a small opening made in the top of the horn.

A simpler form of this type was the use of a short piece of the shin bone of some animal. Shaw (1938:285) mentions it as "possibly the earliest tobacco pipe," and variations on it are found among the San (Schapera 1960:101–102) and the Bambuti (Schebesta 1952:167) for hemp smoking.

Type III: Sandstone and Earthenware Water Containers

Some of the Transkeian Nguni and the Tswana, Sotho and Matabele developed a water container consisting of a hollow rectangular block. "Two holes were made, one to hold the pipe bowl and the other for the insertion of the reed mouthpiece" (Walton 1953:91). The water-vessel may be molded by hand, constructed and baked in the form of a block: "In one ingenious example half an actual brick has been used, and passages bored, one right through the centre and corked at each end, in which water is placed, and two others joining from the top, one for the bowl and the other for the mouthpiece" (Shaw 1938:282–283). Pipes with water containers of the same type are illustrated in Baard (1967:231–232).

Type IV: Ground and Wet Sand Pipes

These variations on the portable water container are apparent responses "when portable pipes are lacking, or when hemp smoking has to be practiced surreptitiously" (Balfour 1922:65). The pipe is made in the ground, i.e. formed below the surface, or may be built up on the ground surface.

Campbell, writing in 1822, explained how the Batapin (in present Botswana) "dug a hole in the ground the shape of a basin, in which they formed with their finger, a round passage, down one side and up the other, in the shape of an inverted bow, this they arched over with clay, and filled their tobacco (or rather wild hemp) with a lighted cylinder at one end, and putting their mouths close to the other they sucked out the smoke" (1822:281).

This variation was also found in the eastern Zambezi river region as well as among the Ngoni, a Zulu offshoot who migrated into the present Malawi. An interesting description by Moszcik which first appeared in the *Internationale Archiv für Ethnographie* in 1910 is given by Balfour (1922:66):

Two pits, about 8 cm deep are excavated in the ground, the bottoms of which are united by a groove of about a span's length, formed by removing the earth between the pits. Some moistened straws or rushes are laid along the groove, their ends projecting from both pits. The earth is then replaced in the groove and firmly pressed down and after a short time, the straws are withdrawn, a duct being thus formed. A hollow tube is stuck into one of the pits to act as mouthpiece and prevent particles of earth entering the smoker's mouth. Hemp is then placed in the bowl and kindled. A little water is poured into the duct and the native lies flat or kneels down and inhales the smoke through the water.

This method was also common among the Tswana and Matabele while the Heichware (a San group) as well as the Gonaqua (a Khoi group) carried a pipe stick with them and could thus prepare a small hollow in wet sand when available (Shaw 1938).

A brief statement should be made concerning the clay and stone bowls of pipes. Archaeological evidence points to the early presence of stone or earthenware pipe bowls in Rhodesia and Transvaal. Shaw states: "Presuming, as we may, that dagga came into the country before tobacco, *we may take the water pipe to be the earliest form of pipe in the country....* These pipe bowls have been found over a large area from Zimbabwe to the Natal Coast" (1938:281) [italics mine].

Balfour confirms the presence of cannabis among "some unconsumed remains" in the bowl of a pipe (1922:66). The types of and designs on these pipe bowls are extremely varied and complex. Walton (1953) has made an initial typological classification of *dagga* pipe bowls, arriving at seven basic types. He also pays attention to the design on these bowls, while Baard (1967), with less success, attempted to look more closely at the design patterns. Walton concludes: "Eventually dagga pipe bowls should prove a valuable supplement to pottery and beads as a diagnostic cultural feature" (1953:112).

Large-scale agriculture in southern Africa until very recently was based on grazing animals and the cultivation of cereal and fruit crops. Most of the work was done by hired labor, usually African or Coloureds.[8] It was customary for the white farmers to give their laborers a daily "tot" of wine or brandy, or a daily ration of rolled tobacco or *dagga*. The "tot-system" still exists in the western Cape, but the practice of rewarding workers with a handful of *dagga* was outlawed during the early part of the present century as *dagga* smoking became illegal.

What had been an institutionalized and even ritualized use, was thus legally prohibited. The old Xhosa or Zulu with his horn-pipe, taking his daily smoke is now encountered only in ethnographies.[9] And so the custom was forced underground, resulting in new kinds of ground pipes or in cigar-type preparations.

Type V: Modern Adaptations

Modern variations on nearly all these types of pipes have appeared, showing great initiative and ways in which elements are substituted.

The Illustrated London News of September 30, 1911 explains how the ground pipe was adapted by employing a glass bottle of which the neck and the bottom had been broken away. Baard (1967:223) describes a pipe found at a building contractor's site in Bloemfontein, made of cement and glass tubing in much the same way as those described above.

Variations on the horn and bone pipes have also been recorded and Schapera states that "nowadays the most prevalent form of pipe is an empty cartridge case" (1960:101).

In modern times, there are a number of interesting innovations; two specimens taken in a police raid in a slum area in Cape Town are described by Shaw: "One is made of a pickle jar and the other of a coconut shell...."

---

[8] The racial classification "Coloured" includes Cape "Coloured" (Mestizo), Cape Malay, Chinese and other Asiatics and Griqua. After the Population Registration Act of 1950 the latter was classified as "Native."
[9] We should remember that "accustomed smokers used *dagga* in moderation and in somewhat formal fashion; intemperance was frowned upon then, and probably, among the rural Bantu, it is even now" (James 1970:576).

In another specimen "the water vessel consists of a round enamel basin about sixteen inches in diameter, built up on top with clay into a cone, in the centre of which is a large depression for the dagga..." (1938:285). A reed stem was used. Such substitutions may go back many years if we correctly interpret Baines' description of a Fingoe hemp pipe, made of bullock's horn that had a clay or stone bowl attached to it by a tube; "a can of water and a wooden tube bound with strips of raw hide" formed part of the apparatus (1964:213). The smoker here would take a puff at the pipe and quickly add a draught of water before expelling both.

We find two basic forms of use under modern urban conditions: some people, mostly older men, still use the pipe but with a clay bowl purchased at the Indian Market in Durban. Most young people, males and females, use a cigar form and dispense with all the elaborate paraphernalia of the water-pipe.

The different patterns of use are due partly to urban living conditions and partly to the danger of police interruption. As the pipe was replaced so, too, was the calm relaxed atmosphere of use. Stott (1959:20) points out that *dagga* was commonly smoked by older men who came home from a hard day's work: "They have a smoke after their meal and then sleep off the effects before morning."

STATUS OF RECENT RESEARCH

While *Cannabis sativa* L. is mentioned in various botanical studies the first complete discussion with ethnographic references appears in Watt and Breyer-Brandwijk (1932), and the first full-fledged study of *dagga* plants was published in 1936 by Watt and Breyer-Brandwijk. Study of chemical and pharmaceutical properties of the plant has been going on at universities and at the South African Institute of Medical Research.

Speight (1932), along with a great number of writers, suggested that "ill-health and insanity" are the inevitable results of continued *dagga* use, while Steyn (1934) quoted an earlier allegation that cakes prepared from the seed of *Cannabis sativa* have been suspected of causing poisoning in stock.

In 1935 the South African Medical Congress requested that "the Minister of the Interior arrange for a controlled investigation into the possible relationship of dagga-smoking with acute psychotic conditions and with the ultimate production of a state of mental degeneration in addicts." Non-white inmates at the Pretoria Mental Hosptial were selected as research subjects. The results of the investigation were published by the Medical Staff in February, 1938. While participation in the project was voluntary, three classes of patients were included: the "confirmed addict" [sic]; the regular smoker; the patient who had never smoked *dagga*.[10] The Medical Staff conclusion states that "the facts observed appear to indicate that *dagga*, as an intoxicant, produces symptoms very similar to those produced by alcohol.... Many natives apparently use *dagga* as the European uses alcohol, i.e., as a so-called "stimulant." It is difficult to determine whether the moral degeneration, which often exists in an addict, is the cause or the result of his addiction" (1938:87-88).

Little attention was paid to *dagga* in the ensuing period until the recent interest in marihuana in the United States hit the headlines, and the South African Government proposed its new drug law.

In 1923 the government of the then Union of South Africa proposed to the League of Nations Advisory Committee on traffic in Opium and Dangerous Drugs that "the whole or any portion of the plants C. Indica and C. Sativa" should be treated as habit-forming drugs and included in the international convention.

Under the provisions of the Medical, Dental and Pharmacy Act No. 13 of 1928 (as spelled out in Articles 61-70), it became illegal to grow, use, sell or supply in any form products denoted as "habit-forming drugs." Under this heading *dagga* was included. Article 69 states: "No person shall smoke, or use, or shall import, manufacture, sell or supply, or possess for purpose of sale or supply to any other person, any pipe, receptacle or appliance for smoking opium, Indian hemp or dagga or intsangu, or save and except in the circumstances contemplated in sections sixty-two, sixty-four...."

The latter section made provision for licenses to be issued for the cultivation and export of *dagga*. Since the law came into effect in 1928 only one license was issued for the cultivation of *dagga* and one license for the export of the herb. These licenses were not renewed. The reason for the non-renewal is quite likely that the foreign market for legally importing *dagga* had evaporated.

Under the provisions of Act 42 of 1937 which followed, a farmer was subject to prosecution should he cultivate or permit *dagga* to grow on his land. Figures in the Government Report of 1952 on *dagga* trade and

---

[10] The subjects mostly used the regular pipe method of smoking in which they would take a mouthful, inhale the fumes, and then spit out the water. Dosage varied from 30 grains of *dagga* taken by "confirmed addicts" to 10 grains used by beginners. "These experiments, carried on over a period of approximately six months, did not show the development of a tolerance to *dagga* in the latter case" (Medical Staff 1938: 85).

"abuse" indicate that the African and Coloured groups, who comprised about 76 percent of the total population, represented 96 percent of all *dagga*-associated prosecutions.

The general public has thought of *dagga* use as a problem identified with African or other political minority groups. A number of writers have pointed out that it was increasingly associated with the "poor-White" and James warned that "it has become permissive among the White Elite male youth of this country" (1970:581). It was thus with somewhat of a shock that conservative white South Africans read a report on drug-taking among the national servicemen at Voortrekkerhoogte — the South African West Point. Levin, who conducted the study on 188 drug-dependent white males, made a number of rather startling statements:

It was found that cannabis usage was by far the most common; all 188 drug users used cannabis. In fact, except for sniffing agents and cough syrups, it was apparently used as the initial product in all the cases. It was found that 76.3 percent of all regular cannabis users proceeded to take other drugs regularly..." and that "the longer one uses cannabis the severer the addiction becomes "(1972: 1691–1692).

Levin concluded that "without cannabis there was no progression toward other drugs, including the so-called 'hard drugs'" (1972:1693). Does this imply that the other 23.8% in time will become hard drug users and that all drug users started with cannabis?

Since Levin acknowledged that multiple drug use was the rule (*Ibid.*: 1691), he is evidently reporting on the users of amphetemines, barbiturates, LSD, opium, cocaine, cough syrups, glue, alcohol, weight-reduction agents, and/or *Datura stramonium*, alone or in combination, with cannabis. A recent review of the South African medical literature indicates the lack of carefully controlled studies of users versus non-users.[11] The study of cannabis and its effects alone is lacking in sweeping studies of "drug-taking."

In this light it is of interest that Shapiro twenty years ago, as editor of the *South African Medical Journal*, pointed out that "a careful study of the social effects and psychological actions of dagga is long overdue" (1951:286).

A number of academicians are conducting research on the psychological effects of *dagga* use, and the National Institute of Personnel Research

---

[11] James reviews the available information concerning *dagga* and concludes that "there are very few recorded firsthand clinical observations and assessments in our medical literature presented as case histories, and none in South African medical literature, which is surprising for a country with such a long experience with the drug" (1970:578).

is working on the neuropsychological effects and developing appropriate tests. The critical fact is that research should not be culture-bound, nor be limited by language barriers between the various peoples of South Africa.

In 1972, the Secretary of Social Welfare and Pensions sent a memorandum to universities seriously urging research of all kinds (mentioning social sciences by name), on drugs, drug users, and the effects of drug use, including *dagga*.

A Sociocultural Study of Cannabis in Africa[12]

In September 1972, a research project was initiated in the province of Natal. While focusing on the Zulu population, it is by no means restricted to them; it is hoped that in time the research might be extended cross-culturally to other ethnolinguistic groups and cross-nationally to other geographical regions so that it more closely approximates a study of *Cannabis in Africa*.

The study will investigate a number of basic questions.[13] The first of these is to establish the type of persons who uses *dagga*. We believe it is possible to ascertain a profile of the "typical *dagga* user," but whether this alone is of predictive value is open to question. The social survey will cover urban and rural residents and gather data on residential and demographic questions, income categories and economic implications of use, social ties and interaction sets as well as descriptions of living routines and life-style. Our research is also aimed at elucidating rural-urban patterns, age groups, differences and patterns which involve uni-ethnic versus multi-ethnic groups of users: production sources of *dagga*, distribution patterns and networks, and associated stimulant and drug use. The study will also include biographical interviews with long-term users.

---

[12] (As Principal Investigator I would like to express my sincere appreciation to the National Institute of Mental Health in Washington D. C. for funds provided under grant RO1-DA-00387.)

[13] The attempt to find references to *dagga* in current social science research reports is a matter of utter frustration. I have searched in vain through anthropological monographs and urban studies on southern Africa. Phillips, in his classic study of the Bantu in the City has a single reference to "dagga smoking" (1938:104-105), while numerous others hardly mention the subject or make the usual easy exit by linking "drinking and smoking dagga," or "young tsotsis smoking dagga" (*Tsotsis* are young urban gang members).

CONCLUSION

This paper brings together for the first time most of the published historical and ethnographic material available to date which deals with cannabis in southern and eastern Africa. However, this background information and the hypothesis regarding origin, dates and distribution of cannabis, represent only the beginning of our study. As this is being written our research returns are starting to come in. The final analysis and reports will follow the completion of this research project and our return to university facilities.

REFERENCES

ALBERTI, LUDWIG
    1968   *Account of the tribal life and customs of the Xhosa in 1807*. Translated by William Fehr. Cape Town: A. A. Balkema.

ANDERSON, CHARLES JOHN
    1967   *Lake Ngami or explorations and discovery during four years of wanderings in the wilds of South Western Africa*. First published 1856. Reprinted in Cape Town: C. Struik Pty. Ltd.

ARBOUSSET, T., F. DUMAS
    1846   *Narrative of an exploratory tour to the north-east of the Colony of the Cape of Good Hope*. Cape Town: Saul Soloman and Co.

ASUNI, T.
    1964   Socio-psychiatric problems of cannabis in Nigeria. *Bulletin on Narcotics* 16:17–28.

BAARD, E.
    1967   Dagga stone pipes in the collection of the National Museum. *Researches of the Nationale Museum* 2:216–233.

BAGSHAWE, F. J.
    1924–1925   The peoples of the happy valley. *Journal of the Royal African Society* 24:226–227.

BAINES, THOMAS
    1964   *Journal of residence in Africa 1842–1853*, Vol. 2. Edited by R. F. Kennedy. Cape Town: The Van Riebeeck Society.

BALFOUR, HENRY
    1922   Earth smoking pipes from South Africa and Central Asia. *Man* 22:65–67.

BARROW, JOHN
    1801   *An account of travels into the interior of southern Africa in the years 1797 and 1798*. London: A. Strahan.

BIRD, JOHN
    1888   *The annals of Natal 1495–1845*, Vol. 1. Pietermaritzburg: Leonard Bayly & Co.

BOROFFKA, A.
    1966   Mental illness and Indian hemp in Lagos. *East African Medical Journal* 43:377–384.

BRAATVEDT, H. P.
1949 *Roaming Zululand with a native commissioner.* Pietermaritzburg: Shuter and Shooter.
BRYANT, A. T.
1949 *The Zulu people as they were before the White man came.* Pietermaritzburg: Shuter and Shooter.
BURCHELL, WILLIAM
1967 *Travels in the interior of southern Africa,* Vol. I and II (1824). Cape Town: C. Struik Africana Publishers.
CAMPBELL, J.
1822 *Travels in South Africa undertaken at the request of the London Missionary Society.* London: Francis Westley.
CASALIS, E.
1861 *The Basutos or twenty-three years in South Africa.* Reprinted 1965. Cape Town: C. Struik Pty. Ltd.
CHITTICK, NEVILLE
1965 The 'Shirazi' colonization of East Africa. *Journal of African History* 6:263–273.
CONDER, C. R.
1887 The present condition of the native tribes of Bechuanaland. *Journal of the Anthropological Institute* 16.
COPLAND, SAMUEL
1822 *A history of the island of Madagascar.* London: Burton and Smith.
CUREAU, A. L.
1915 *Savage man in central Africa: a study of primitive races in the French Congo.* Translated by E. Andrews. London: T. Fisher Unwin.
DAPPER, O.
1933 "Kaffrarie, of lant der Hottentots," in *The early Cape Hottentots.* Translated and edited by I. Schapera and B. Farrington. Cape Town: The Van Riebeeck Society.
DARWIN, CHARLES
1900 *The origin of the species.* First ed. 1859. London: John Murray.
DECLE, L.
1898 *Three years in savage Africa.* London: Methuen and Co.
DE GREVENBROEK, J. G.
1933 "An elegant and accurate account of the African race living round the Cape of Good Hope commonly called Hottentots," in *The early Cape Hottentots.* Translated and edited by I. Schapera and B. Farrington. Cape Town: The Van Riebeeck Society.
DOKE, CLEMENT
1931 *The Lambas of Northern Rhodesia.* London: George G. Harris & Co.
DORMAN, M. R. P.
1905 *A journal of a tour in the Congo Free State.* London: Kegan Paul.
DORNAN, S. S.
1925 *Pygmies and Bushmen of the Kalahari.* London: Seeley, Service & Co. Ltd.
DU TOIT, BRIAN M.
1958 Dagga (*Cannabis sativa*) smoking in Southern Rhodesia. *The Central African Journal of Medicine* 4:500–501.

ELLENBERGER, D. F., J. C. MAC GREGOR
  1912   *History of the Basuto, ancient and modern.* London: Caxton Publishing Co. Ltd.
ELLIS, WILLIAM
  1838   *History of Madagascar,* Vol. I. London: Fisher, Son & Co.
EMBODEN, WILLIAM A., JR.
  1972   "Ritual use of Cannabis sativa L.: a historical-ethnographic survey," in *Flesh of the Gods; ritual use of hallucinogens.* Edited by Peter T. Furst. New York: Praeger.
FAGAN, BRIAN M.
  1969   Early trade and raw materials in south central Africa. *Journal of African History* 10:1–13.
FRITSCH, GUSTAV
  1868   *Drie Jahre in Süd-Afrika.* Breslau: Ferdinand Hirt.
GARDINER, ALLEN F.
  1836   *Narrative of a journey to the Zoolu country in South Africa undertaken in 1835.* London: William Crofts.
GOODWIN, A. J. H..
  1939   The origin of certain African food plants. *South African Journal of Science* 36:445-463.
GREENWAY, P. J.
  1944–1945   The origin of some east African plants. *East African Agricultural Journal* 10:250–255.
GRINSPOON, LESTER
  1969   Marihuana. *Scientific American* 221:17–25.
GROUT, LEWIS
  1861   *Zululand: or life among the Zulu-Kafirs of Natal and Zululand, South Africa.* New impression 1970. London: African Publication Society.
GUTSCHE, THELMA
  1968   *The microcosm.* Cape Town: Howard Timmins.
HEINZ, H. J.
  1972   Personal communication.
HILTON-SIMPSON, M. W.
  1911   *Land and peoples of the Kasai.* London: Constable & Company Ltd.
HUGHES, J. E.
  1933   *Eighteen years on Lake Bangweulu.* London: The Field House.
INSKEEP, R. R.
  1969   "The archaeological background," in *The Oxford history of South Africa,* Vol. I. Edited by Monica Wilson and Leonard Thompson. Oxford: The Clarendon Press.
JAMES, THEODORE
  1970a   Dagga: a review of fact and fancy. *South African Medical Journal* 44: 575–580.
  1970b   Dagga and driving. *South African Medical Journal* 44:580–581.
JENNY, HANS
  1966   *Südwestafrika: land zwischen den extremen.* Berlin: W. Kohlahammer Verlag.
JOHNSTON, HARRY H.
  1897   *British central Africa.* London: Methuen & Co.

1908 *George Grenfell and the Congo*, Vol. 2. London: Hutchinson & Co.
JUNOD, HENRI A.
1962 *The life of a south African tribe*. First Edition 1912. New York: University Books Inc.
KEANE, A.
1920 *Man, past and present*. Cambridge: The University Press.
KOLB, PETER
1968 *The present state of the Cape of Good Hope*, Vol. I. First edition 1731. Edited by W. Peter Carstens. London: Johnson Reprint Corporation.
KOLLMANN, PAUL
1899 *The Victoria Nyanza*. London: Swan Sonnenschein & Co.
LAMBO, T. A.
1965 Medical and social problems of drug addiction in West Africa. *Bulletin on Narcotics* 17:3–13.
LATROBE, C. I.
1969 *Journal of a visit to South Africa in 1815 and 1816*. Reprint. Cape Town: C. Struik Pty. Ltd.
LAUFER, BERTHOLD
1930 "The introduction of tobacco into Africa," in *Tobacco and its use in Africa*. Edited by Berthold Laufer, W. D. Hambly, and R. Linton. Anthropology Leaflet 29. Chicago: Field Museum of Natural History.
LE VAILLANT, M.
1796 *Travels into the interior parts of Africa by the way of the Cape of Good Hope; in the years 1780–1985*, Vol. II. 2nd edition. London: Robinson.
LEVIN, AUBREY
1972 The pattern of drug-taking among drug-dependent South African national servicemen. *South African Medical Journal* 46:1690–1694.
LICHTENSTEIN, HENRY
1928 *Travels in Southern Africa in the years 1803, 1804, 1805, and 1806*, Vol. I. First published 1812. Translated by Anne Plumtre. Cape Town: The Van Riebeeck Society.
LIVINGSTONE, DAVID
1857 *Missionary travels and researches in South Africa*. London: John Murray.
LIVINGSTONE, DAVID, CHARLES LIVINGSTONE
1865 *Narrative of an expedition to the Zambesi and its tributaries*. London: John Murray.
MARWICK, BRIAN
1940 *The Swazi*. Cambridge: The University Press.
MC MARTIN, A.
1970 The introduction of surgarcane to Africa and its early dispersal. *The South African Sugar Year Book 1969–1970*, Durban.
MEDICAL STAFF
1938 Mental symptoms associated with the smoking of dagga. *South African Medical Journal* 12:85–88.
MENTZEL, O. F.
1944 *A geographical and topological description of the Cape of Good Hope 1785*. Translated and edited by G. V. Marais and J. Hoge. Cape Town: The Van Riebeeck Society.

MONTEIRO, JOACHIM
- 1875 *Angola and the River Congo*, Vol. 2. Reprinted 1968. London: Frank Cass and Co.

MORLEY, J. E., A. D. BENSUSAN
- 1971 Dagga: tribal uses and customs. *Medical Proceedings* 17:409–412.

NIENABER, G. S.
- 1963 *Hottentots*. Pretoria: J. L. van Schaik Ltd.

OGILBY, JOHN
- 1670 *Africa: being an accurate description of the regions.* London: Tho. Johnson.

O'NEIL, OWEN ROWE
- 1921 *Adventures in Swaziland.* London: George Allen and Unwin Ltd.

PHILLIPS, RAY E.
- 1938 *The Bantu in the city.* Lovedale, South Africa: Lovedale Press.

POLUNIN, NICHOLAS
- 1964 *Introduction to plant geography.* London: Longmans.

PURVIS, J. P.
- 1909 *Through Uganda to Mt. Elgon.* London: Fisher Unwin.

RAVEN-HART, R.
- 1971 *Cape Good Hope 1652–1702. The first fifty years of Dutch colonization as seen by callers*, Vol. I. Cape Town: A. A. Balkema.

RAYMOND, W. D.
- 1938 Native Materia medica. *Tanganyika Notes and Records* 5: 73–75.

ROSCOE, JOHN
- 1911 *The Baganda.* Reprinted 1965. London: Frank Cass & Co.
- 1921 *Twenty-five years in East Africa.* Cambridge: The University Press.

ROSENTHAL, FRANZ
- 1971 *The herb.* Leiden: E. J. Brill.

SAGOE, E. C.
- 1966 Narcotics control in Ghana. *Bulletin on Narcotics* 18:5–13.

SAMUELSON, L. H.
- n.d. *Some Zulu customs.* London: Church Printing Company.

SCHACHTZABEL, ALFRED
- 1923 *Im Hochland von Angola.* Dresden: Verlag Deutsch Buchwerksätten.

SCHAPERA, I.
- 1960 *The Khoisan peoples of South Africa.* London: Routledge and Kegan Paul (Ltd.).

SCHAPERA, I., B. FARRINGTON, editors
- 1933 *The early Cape Hottentots.* Cape Town: The Van Riebeeck Society.

SCHEBESTA, PAUL
- 1933 *Among Congo Pygmies.* Translated by Gerald Green. London: Hutchinson & Co.
- 1936 *Revisiting my Pygmy hosts.* Translated by Gerald Green. London: Hutchinson & Co.
- 1952 *Les Pygmées du Congo Belge.* Brussel: Memoires, Institut Royal Colonial Belge.

SCHRIJVER, ISAQ.
1931 "The diary of an island expedition made in the Cape Province in the year 1689," in *Journals of Expeditions of Olaf Bergh (1682-1683) and Isaq. Schrijver (1689)*. Translated and edited by E. E. Mossop. Cape Town: The Van Riebeeck Society.

SCHULTES, R. E.
1970 "Random thoughts and queries on the botany of cannabis," in *The botany and chemistry of cannabis*. Edited by C. R. B. Joyce and S. H. Curry. London: J. & A. Churchill.

SHAPIRO, H. A.
1951 Editorial: dagga. *South African Medical Journal* 25:284-286.

SHAW, GEORGE
1885 *Madagascar and France*. London: Willian Clowes & Sons.

SHAW, M.
1938 Native pipes and smoking in South Africa. *Annals of the South African Museum* 24:277-302.

SIBREE, JAMES
1870 *Madagascar and its people*. London: W. Clowes & Sons.
1880 *The great African island*. London: Trübner & Co.

SILBERBAUER, GEORGE B.
1965 *Report to the government of Bechuanaland on the Bushman survey*. Gaberones: Government Printer.

SIMOONS, FREDERICK J.
1970 "Some questions on the economic prehistory of Ethiopia," in *Papers in African prehistory*. Edited by J. D. Fage and R. A. Oliver. Cambridge: University Press.

SMITH, ANDREW
1939 *The diary of Dr. Andrew Smith (1834-1836)*, Vol. I. Edited by Percival Kerby. Cape Town: The Van Riebeeck Society.

SMITH, EDWIN, ANDREW M. DALE
1920 *The Ila-speaking peoples of Northern Rhodesia*, Vol. I. London: Macmillan.

SPEIGHT, W. L.
1932 Dagga. *The Pharmaceutical Journal and Pharmacist* 128:372.

STAYT, HUGH A.
1931 *The Bavenda*. London: Oxford University Press for the International Institute of African Languages and Cultures.

STEYN, DOUW G.
1934 *The toxicology of plants in South Africa*. London: William Clowes & Sons.

STOTT, H. H.
1959 A pilot health study of the Zulu community of Botha's Hill, Natal. South Africa. *WHO/PHA/33*.

STOW, GEORGE
1905 *The native races of South Africa*. London: Swan Sonnenschein & Co.

SUTHERLAND-HARRIS, NICOLA
1970 "Trade and the Rozwi Mambo," in *Pre-colonial African trade*. Edited by Richard Gray and David Birmingham. London: Oxford University Press.

TELLA, A., et al.
1967 Indian hemp smoking. *Journal of Social Health in Nigeria* 40–50.
TEN RHYNE, WILHELM
1933 "A short account of the Cape of Good Hope and of the Hottentots who inhabit the region," in *The early Cape Hottentots*. Translated and edited by I. Schapera and B. Farrington. Cape Town: The Van Riebeeck Society.
THEAL, GEORGE
1910 *Ethnography and condition of South Africa before A.D. 1505*. London: George Allen and Unwin Ltd.
TOBIAS, PHILLIP V.
1961 Physique of a desert folk. *Natural History* 70:16–24.
TORDAY, E.
1925 *On the trail of the Bushongo*. London: Seeley, Service & Co Ltd..
TYLOR, JOSIAH
1891 *Forty years among the Zulus*. Boston: Congregational Sunday School and Publishing Society.
VANSINA, J.
1962 Long-distance trade-routes in Central Africa. *Journal of African History* 3:375–390.
VEDDER, HEINRICH
1938 *South West Africa in early times*. London: Humphrey Milford.
WALTON, JAMES
1953 The dagga pipes of Southern Africa. *Researches of the National Museum* 1:85–113.
WATT, J. M.
1961 Dagga in South Africa. *Bulletin on Narcotics* 13:9–14.
WATT, J. M., M. G. BREYER-BRANDWIJK
1932 *The medicinal and poisonous plants of Southern Africa*. Edinburgh: E. and S. Livingstone.
1936 The forensic and sociological aspects of the dagga problem in South Africa. *South African Medical Journal* 10:573–579.
WERNER, A.
1906 *The natives of British Central Africa*. London: Archibald Constable & Co. Ltd.
WESTPHAL, E. O. J.
1963 The linguistic prehistory of southern Africa: Bush, Kwadi, Hottentot and Bantu linguistic relationships. *Africa* 33:237–264.
1971 "The click languages of southern and eastern Africa," in *Current trends in linguistics: linguistics in sub-Saharan Africa*. Edited by Jack Berry and Joseph H. Greenberg. The Hague: Mouton Publishers.
WILSON, MONICA
1959 "The early history of the Transkei and Ciskei," *African Studies* 18.
1969 "The Nguni people," in *The Oxford history of South Africa*, Vol. I. Edited by Monica Wilson and Leonard Thompson. Oxford: The Clarendon Press.
WISSMAN, H.
1891 *My second journey through equatorial Africa*. London: Chatto and Windus.

PART TWO

Sociocultural Aspects of the Traditional Complex

The Social Nexus of Ganja *in Jamaica*

LAMBROS COMITAS

ABSTRACT

The contemporary complex of behavior and values associated with cannabis use among the working-class population of Jamaica is considered as an institution. Preceding the main discussion, brief summaries of the East Indian paternity of the complex as well as the extent of current cannabis use are presented. Substantive sections are organized around three principal themes: patterns of activities related to cannabis (cultivation, distribution, and consumption); social groupings of cannabis users (as related to specific activities and to age factors); beliefs and values underlying the cannabis institution (variations related to different modes of consumption, cannabis as energizer, and "the motivational syndrome"). A final section considers cannabis use as a social class marker; cannabis and social mobility; and stereotypes and misconceptions about cannabis reportedly held by the socially superordinate sections of Jamaican society.

Although not native to Jamaica, cannabis has become a plant of major social and economic significance in that West Indian nation. Its illegal but widespread proliferation, the extent and variety of uses to which it has been put by the folk, and the legal and political problems it has raised make cannabis, or *ganja*, a social phenomenon of vital interest.

The nature of *ganja*-related behavior and beliefs in Jamaica lends itself

This paper summarizes part of the anthropological material collected by the Jamaica Marihuana project of the Research Institute for the Study of Man in collaboration with the University of the West Indies. This research was funded under Contract No. HSM-42-70-97, with the Center for Studies of Narcotic and Drug Abuse, National Institute of Mental Health. The full report of this anthropological and medical project (Rubin and Comitas 1972) is entitled *Effects of chronic smoking of cannabis in Jamaica*. While responsibility for interpretations and conclusions presented in this paper rest solely with the author, grateful acknowledgement is made for the considerable contribution of Melanie C. Dreher, member of the RISM anthropological team, now on the faculty of the School of Nursing, University of Massachusetts. The bulk of community-level cases and examples cited was collected and initially analyzed by Mrs. Dreher during the first phase of the project.

easily to a form of institutional description and analysis. S. F. Nadel, the noted British anthropologist, has defined institutions as "standardized modes of co-activity" (1951:108) with charters of values, distinctive forms of social grouping and personal relationships, set cycles of activities, material apparatuses, and purposive character. The Jamaican *ganja* complex, as it presently exists, fits well within this definition, exhibiting as it does a series of definable and repetitive activities, characteristic social groupings, and a coalescing corpus of beliefs and values. Also, by pursuing an institutional approach, it is possible to attain an efficient ordering and presentation of the materials which follow.

The roots of the Jamaican *ganja* complex can be traced to the Indian sub-continent. During the latter part of the 19th century, its prototypical forms were carried to the island by East Indian indentured laborers recruited to replace the emancipated slaves in the cane fields. Present day techniques and types of *ganja* use, critical parts of the *ganja* lexicon, as well as much of the justificatory ideology lend strong support to a claim of a direct India to Jamaica diffusion. The great majority of *ganja* users in contemporary Jamaica, however, are not East Indians, who form only a small minority of the population, but Black laboring people, both rural and urban, descendants of the African slaves forcibly brought to the New World in the 17th and 18th centuries. Although the exact process is not known, it appears that *ganja* and associated behaviors were relatively quickly incorporated and reworked into the cultural inventory of the Black lower section of Jamaican society and, despite sixty years of stringent sanctions against its cultivation, distribution, and consumption, it, as a complex, has thrived and proliferated throughout the country. At this point in time, the Indian paternity of the complex has, for all intents and purposes, been forgotten. In fact, some culturally militant Black users now claim Africa as the original source of Jamaican *ganja*, and cite Biblical references to the existence of "the herb," or marihuana, on King Solomon's tomb.

Putting questions of derivation aside, it is clear from *prima facie* evidence that *ganja* use in Jamaica is extraordinarily widespread. Although national statistics on these illegal practices are non-existent, estimates of the number of users range from one-third to two-thirds of the "lower class." A somewhat more precise estimation can be made based on the work of the Research Institute for the Study of Man anthropological team. For example, a survey of *ganja* smoking in one of the seven study communities indicated that of all males over the age of 15, fully 50% were smokers (half of these being classified as heavy smokers); 7.3% were former smokers: only 20% were non-smokers; and 22.3% were unclassifiable due either to conflicting information or reluctance to provide information by respondents. If we were to include only half the unclassifiables (11.1%) to the smoker group, a conservative procedure, we would generate a figure for adult smokers of over 60%. If we were to add the 7.3% former smokers, then over 68% of the adult males in the community at the time of the study were either current smokers or had smoked *ganja* in the past. After comparing these data with those derived more generally from the other six study localities, we believe that 68% does not seriously misrepresent the extent of male smoking in the rural parts and, in fact, supports the higher ranges of earlier, somewhat more impressionistic estimates.

Male *ganja* smokers, however, make up only part of the *ganja* using population. Women, in lesser numbers, also smoke. A larger pool of individuals, including women and children, adult smokers and adamant non-smokers, drink *ganja* teas and tonics for medicinal or prophylactic purposes. Many utilize preparations from the plant as external salves and a relatively small number will make occasional use of *ganja* in food. Given the extent of non-smoking uses, one could estimate with confidence that some 65 to 75% of the lower section of the rural population, men, women, and children, inhale, ingest or use *ganja* in some form and to some degree — undoubtedly one of the highest rates of marihuana use for any non-deviant population in the Western world.

What are the institutionalized characteristics of the *ganja* complex? What are its constituent activities, its social groupings, its rules, ideas and values? We shall deal with each in order.

PATTERNS OF ACTIVITIES

Ganja activities can be divided for analytic purposes into three distinctive categories — cultivation, distribution, and consumption.

Cultivation: Jamaica does not import *ganja*. In fact, in recent years, it has developed an illegal export trade with North America and the United Kingdom. In most regions of the island, two crops a year can be harvested, the growing cycles generally running from April to August and from June to November. The physical conditions for growing *ganja* are good, individual land ownership, particularly in the hilly interior, is high, and unattended bush lands are available for cultivation. In essence, all the potential grower requires is access to relatively isolated land removed from regular traffic. In Jamaica, this is not difficult to find. In one quite typical farming community, at least 25% of all households are known to include members who cultivate *ganja*, almost always on land away from the settlement. And given the secrecy attached to this cultivation, there can be little doubt that this figure underestimates the total number of *ganja* growers. Of 39 known cultivators, 56% grow only for personal or household use; 31% cultivate for sale as well. Only five growers (13%) cultivate primarily for commercial purposes. Significantly, members of this latter group do not smoke *ganja* and are of higher social standing in the community.

In the main, however, the cultivation of *ganja* is a poor man's enterprise which fits well with the agricultural patterns of mixed cropping common to the Jamaican folk. Not unexpectedly, then, the amount of *ganja* grown by any given individual is relatively small. In our typical community, for example, the largest "planter" will cultivate some 200 "roots" or plants, the next four in importance might cultivate 100 on the average, and the rest of the cultivators who sell some of their crop for profit may put in anywhere from 30 to 100 roots. Those who grow for their own use generally plant about ten, and sometimes less, per growing season. For the great majority of growers, *ganja* is an agricultural side line, which may bring some much needed income, but which does not seriously impinge on established patterns of economic and social life.

The very physical conditions which permit the cultivation of *ganja* may well become impediments to successful harvesting. Since remote and not easily guarded land must be utilized, the cultivator is at constant risk of theft from outsiders, competitors, and adolescent boys. Statistically, praedial larceny of legal crops is one of the most common crimes in Jamaica. *Ganja* is certainly no exception to the rule. But the victimized *ganja* grower, even if he knows the thief, has little direct recourse to the law. As a consequence, he is left to his own and group resources to protect his crop. Although violence against suspected depredators has been reported as have allegations of police protection, these means do not appear to be as important in controlling indiscriminate theft as more subtle and informal methods. The principal mechanisms of control are, in fact, firmly rooted in the cultural patterns and social alignments of the folk as broadly illustrated in the following cases:

Mr. A, a *ganja* cultivator, discovered that Mr. B, another *ganja* cultivator, had been stealing his 'herbs.' Recognizing the futility of directly confronting Mr. B, he went to people closely associated with the culprit and told them that he knew B was stealing his *ganja*, that he planned to put poisonous seeds that looked like *ganja* seeds into a few of his plants; and that this poison would bring instant death to the consumer. All this was imparted with an air of great secrecy and with the plea that his plan not be told to B. Predictably, Mr. B's friends warned him of the "plot" and the depredations of Mr. A's *ganja* fields ceased.

If such a tactic fails, the *ganja* cultivator has recourse to other alternatives. For example, the Pastor of the Pentecostal Church in our typical community is also the local "science man," or practitioner of magic. In this dual capacity, he keeps well informed of local events and has intimate and current knowledge of village relationships and alignments. With such information and skillful use of his position, he has amassed sufficient power so as to be able to manipulate effectively a given situation for the advantage of his client, as in this case:

> Mr. C discovered that a large quantity of *ganja* that he had cut and left for curing was stolen. After making discreet inquiries, he determined who the thief was. Unable to go to the police, he turned to the Pastor with his problem. The Pastor, while not promising that he could guarantee the return of the stolen *ganja*, instructed Mr. C as to the steps that should be taken to punish the thief. Following these instructions, Mr. C posted a parchment on a pear tree near the place where the *ganja* had been stolen. On the parchment, inscribed with doveblood, was a biblical psalm decorated with magical symbols. A few days after the posting, the wife of the thief came to Mr. C with the half-cured *ganja*, begged for forgiveness, and asked him to remove the curse. Mr. C, gratified with the results, assumed that the thief had seen the parchment and recognized its significance. In reality, the wife of the thief was a member of the Pastor's congregation, and he had called her in, lectured her strongly on the evils of theft, and told her to return the *ganja* before serious misfortune befell her and her husband.

In the somewhat unlikely event of arrest for illegal cultivation, again the local system of relationships may come into play. It would not be unusual for an apprehended grower to turn for advice, influence, and even financial assistance to powerful "science men" who often count police and civil servants among their clientele. Other local power brokers may also be petitioned for help.

Distribution: The distribution of *ganja* can best be characterized as a small, albeit illegal, individual business activity engaged in by a relatively large number of occasional and part-time vendors. In the abstract, and given the patterns of occupational multiplicity found in rural Jamaica (Comitas 1973:157–173), *ganja* selling can be viewed as another supplementary economic enterprise available to the poor. In the seven communities studied, no evidence was found of any centralized, hierarchically organized distribution net that operated on either the local, regional, or island-wide basis.

In our illustrative community, sixteen men out of a total of 178, or nearly 9%, sell *ganja* in some quantity to others in the community. This figure does not include the five "commercial" producers who grow locally and sell in Kingston, the capital city. Of these sixteen, twelve are also *ganja* growers. Eight of this latter group sell *ganja* in small quantities to friends and acquaintances until their stock is depleted, when they become buyers for their own use; the remaining four cultivators also sell their crop during the season but buy additional stock in the capital as the need arises. Four vendors are not cultivators and buy their entire *ganja* supply in Kingston. None of the sixteen vendors are full-time specialists; all combine selling with agricultural or other work, even though dealing in *ganja* may, for some, bring in a major portion of their income.

In general, the life style of *ganja* vendors adheres closely to that of the majority of the population. Almost all can be classified as belonging to the upper levels of the working class or lowest social sections. Nearly all rely on general cultivation of their own land for their primary source of livelihood. With an occasional exception, all have stable marital unions; all have children and established households. None are active in community level organizations. Significantly, these vendors are not known frequenters of rum shops; they appear quiet and law abiding, except for their activities in selling *ganja;* and they voice the same attitudes and make the same protests against criminality and violence as do the more affluent and respected members of the community. In all visible respects, the personality and demeanor of vendors tends to be pleasant and friendly, and they are thought of as "nice guys," jocular, inoffensive, and not given to quarrels or anger.

Consumption: There are four major methods of *ganja* use: smoking; drinking as medicinal teas and tonics; applying externally as plaster and ointments; and cooking food. *Ganja* is smoked in spliffs, or *ganja* cigarettes about four inches in length containing variable amounts of marihuana and tobacco, or in the *chillum*, the Jamaican equivalent of the "hookah" or Middle Eastern water pipe. Spliff smoking, however, is far more popular in Jamaica than smoking the *chillum*. It is more convenient, and safer than pipe smoking which generally requires the gathering of several smokers, the apparatus itself, and substantially greater security precautions. Individual consumption levels vary considerably. For example, in the sample of 30 smokers intensively examined in the clinical phase of the Research Institute for the Study of Man study, the consumption range was from one to twenty-four spliffs a day, the average number consumed per day being seven.

Of all methods of *ganja* consumption, tea drinking, which is widely reputed to have therapeutic and prophylactic properties for specific or general complaints, is the most prevalent, and is used across socioeconomic lines. It is particularly recommended for infants and children who may well consume, in this form, a substantial part of the *ganja* used in rural Jamaica. Tonics blended from rum and/or wine poured on *ganja*, bottled, and allowed to set, are also used for therapeutic and prophylactic purposes. *Ganja* poultices and compresses are utilized for the relief of pains and for open wounds. Topical *ganja* preparations for neonates are not unusual.

Consumption of *ganja* with food has been noted and reported. The occasional use of marihuana in soups or with assorted greens or with cooked bananas is not unknown but this method of ingestion appears to be limited.

SOCIAL GROUPINGS

The proliferation of *ganja* use in Jamaica has generated distinctive social groupings and alignments in all areas of *ganja* activity — with one significant exception. *Ganja*, in the main, is cultivated individually without assistance rather than as a group activity. Such a pattern, induced by the severe legal sanctions against *ganja* cultivation, runs counter to traditional small farming practices among Jamaicans who, in order to avoid or decrease outlays for necessary farm labor as well as to solidify social ties within the community, have developed patterns of ongoing work partnerships and other forms of labor exchange for legal cultivation. Throughout most of Jamaica, *ganja* partnerships are non-existent, thereby avoiding the recriminations that would almost inevitably follow if a jointly worked *ganja* field is raided by the police, plundered by others, or neglected by one of the partners. For the somewhat precarious venture of *ganja* cultivation, the grower assumes full responsibility and expects all the profit. In so doing, he minimizes the social risks of rupturing harmonious work relationships in ordinary cultivation as well as legal risks. There appear to be few exceptions to this rule.

In *ganja* distribution, however, patterns of social clustering are clearly discernible. As already indicated, Jamaican communities tend to have substantial numbers of occasional or part-time vendors. Each vendor of this type establishes his own network of clients, usually from ten to twenty trusted individuals. These networks are relatively contained, with entry generally based on the personal knowledge of the client by the vendor. But these networks are also flexible, occasionally adding potential clients vouched for by older members. Nevertheless, much *ganja* buying on the island is indirect — an ultimate consumer requesting some trusted person to purchase *ganja* for him. This friend, in turn, may ask another, so that *ganja* often passes through an amorphous screen of middlemen who may receive little or no cash reward. Given this pattern, the consumer may well end up having purchased *ganja* from a nearby neighbor without either knowing. Consequently, while vendors sell directly only to those few they can trust, they may indirectly supply a much larger number. Individual amounts of *ganja* sold are generally small. The most common quantity purchased, variously called a "stick," "bump," or "head," with weight ranging from two to six grams, is sufficient at the very least for one spliff.

Larger-scale distributors may service anywhere from 50 to 100 smoker-clients. Their operations, unlike the small vendors, are usually localized in what are commonly referred to as "herb camps" and "herb yards." Often the major vendor in the community will operate a "herb camp" in the immediate vicinity of his house. In addition to *ganja*, he may offer beer, ale, or stout for sale. He provides a recreational atmosphere with dominoes, a record player, and occasionally even a television set for his customers. Less important dealers run "herb yards," places where a user can come to smoke. No other facilities are provided and a user-client may either purchase limited quantities of *ganja* from the vendor, or bring his own.[1]

The nature of social groups directly involved with *ganja* consumption is heavily influenced by age factors. Social patterning changes as individuals move from one significant period of their life to another. For the average rural user, at least four such periods are discernible.

During the first period, infancy-childhood, infants and young children are introduced to *ganja* through the ingestion of *ganja* teas. Even though these brews are consumed in a familial setting, an aura of secretiveness often surrounds this ordinary practice; words denoting *ganja* are not commonly used to identify the tea served, and since its taste is almost always obscured by milk and sugar, the young drinker may well be unaware of the basic ingredient. Significantly, tea drinking is the only method of *ganja* use and childhood is the only period of life in which the social use of *ganja* is not peer related but intergenerational, with adults prescribing and providing *ganja* for minors in their care.

Adolescence characterizes and influences the form of social grouping in the second phase. While young boys are warned about the evils of smoking *ganja*, such occasional admonitions, sometimes modified by cautions not to get caught, appear to have minimal impact particularly in households where fathers or surrogate fathers are regular smokers. While parental example undoubtedly serves as a role model, there is substantial evidence indicating that the initial experience with *ganja* smoking is in the

---

[1] For the distinction between "herb camp" and "herb yard," I am grateful to Claudia Rogers, member of the Research Institute for the Study of Man anthropological team, now in the Department of Anthropology, University of Miami.

company of friends of similar or slightly older age. In contemporary Jamaica, boys may begin smoking during pubescence, with the more precocious starting as early as ten years of age.

During the first years after introduction, smoking is more often a sporadic rather than a systematic and regular activity. Not until boys begin to earn their living is it economically feasible for them to indulge habitually. Adolescent smokers typically interact in relatively large and amorphous peer groups, sometimes dominated by a *ganja* vendor of roughly equal age. Since boys, as a rule, do not purchase *ganja* from adult vendors in their communities for fear of exposure, they rely on young distributors who are also friends and confidantes. Participation in these youthful groups varies in relation to the individual's ability to buy as well as his commitment to *ganja:* some young boys are essentially only curious bystanders; others may smoke an occasional spliff; still others, particularly the oldest, are confirmed and steady smokers. This adolescent phase may best be characterized as experimentation in *ganja* smoking.

The third period is that of adulthood. In their twenties, young men begin to establish their own households, choose mates, acquire children, and settle into their adult occupational routines. As their life style changes, so do their *ganja*-related alignments. For one, regular *ganja* users may begin to cultivate their own supply in order to save money and to decrease dependence on vendors. More significantly, groups diminish in size and stability in membership as choice of smoking companions is deliberately limited to work mates and trusted neighbors. Finally, smoking *ganja* is no longer the central preoccupation of these small networks, as it is for the younger age grades, but rather a natural part of the daily round, an almost unnoticed routine at work parties, lunch breaks, evening visits, and the like. These more tightly knit groups are also more egalitarian than adolescent ones, with no discernible hierarchical structure. Typically, each man supplies his own *ganja* and smokes his own spliffs or, on occasion, members take turns supplying all the *ganja* needed for an evening.

Old age is the fourth and last period. Compared to younger age groups, there is a smaller percentage of regular *ganja* smokers over the age of sixty and a corresponding breakdown of smoking groups. Explanations for this vary: some villagers claim that the brains of old people become weak and "dem kyáan take ganja"; some old people say that as they become older and closer to death they become more Christian, feel guilty about *ganja* smoking, and give it up. It is possible, however, that other factors are operative. For one, the incidence of *ganja* use was considerably less when these men were in their formative and young adult years so that there should be proportionately fewer confirmed smokers among the older males. Second, older males who are smokers tend to lose their customary settings and incentives for smoking as they lose their smoking companions through illness or death. Finally, there are physical and economic factors: many old men are simply incapable of working their own fields, so that their incomes are markedly reduced and their supply of *ganja* is limited.

BELIEFS AND VALUES

What are the principal beliefs and values which give life to the *ganja* complex in Jamaica? Most importantly, users firmly believe in the efficacy of the substance. Nevertheless, a sharp distinction is made between the effects of tea drinking and those of smoking. The folk explanation is that teas and tonics are absorbed into the blood stream, strengthen the blood, and enable it to ward off disease, whereas *ganja* when smoked goes directly from the lungs to the brains where it may have sometimes unpredictable consequences. Whatever the objective truth, beliefs about the differential effects of *ganja* drinking and smoking are reinforced and perpetuated by differences in the general attitudes of those who only take *ganja* as tea, primarily members of the higher social levels and aspirants for higher status, as compared to those who smoke as well as drink *ganja*, members of the lowest social level.

Ganja, primarily in the form of teas and tonics, is widely believed to have medicinal properties, both prophylactic and therapeutic. It keeps the user in good health, prevents constipation, colds, gonorrhea and a host of other ills. It is held that it is particularly good for children, preventing disease in general and marasmus in particular. With *ganja* tea, the youth grow stronger and smarter. For the mass of users, *ganja* is valued as a cure for a wide assortment of complaints from arthritis to stomach ailments.

There are strong beliefs related to physiological, psychobiological and psychodispositional effects of *ganja* — beliefs related to sleep, appetite, sex, reflection, relaxation, and the like. Descriptions of these effects, however, are typically qualified by mention of necessary, prior conditions. For example, if a user is in the mood to go to bed, *ganja* will make him sleepy. More importantly, however, there is little evidence indicating that *ganja* is systematically consumed by adults specifically for the purpose of inducing these states.

There is one important exception to this rule — *ganja* is regularly taken to increase work capacity. Almost universally, users maintain that *ganja* enhances their ability to work, that is, to perform manual labor, and they regularly consume *ganja* with this objective. In this regard, *ganja* is believed to take effect in two ways. One is the cumulative benefit that comes with "building" one's blood and strength with regular dosages of *ganja*. The other is that *ganja* has the immediate effect of producing a burst of energy sufficient for completing laborious tasks. If there is difficult land to clear, it is claimed, a farmer-user will sit down, smoke a spliff, and a few minutes later he is able to face and then complete the task. Almost unanimously, informants categorically stated that *ganja*, either in teas or smoked, made them work harder, faster, and longer. For energy-related purposes, *ganja* can be and is taken in the morning, during breaks in the work routine, or immediately before particularly onerous labor.

Putting objective assessments of these claims aside, the belief that *ganja* acts as a work stimulant, and the observable behavior that this induces, casts considerable doubt on the universality of what has been described in the literature as "the amotivational syndrome," or "a loss of desire to work, to compete, to face challenges — interests and major concerns of the individual become centered around marihuana and drug use becomes compulsive" (Smith 1968:37–41). In Jamaica, and we would suspect in other marihuana-using agricultural countries, cannabis, at least on the ideational level, might well be central to a "motivational syndrome." *Ganja*, in the rural reaches of Jamaica, is a substance that apparently permits the individual to face, start, and carry through the most difficult and distasteful manual labor. Following from this, it could be argued that in certain types of non-industrial economies based on small-scale agriculture faced with difficult ecological conditions and complex land tenure systems, marihuana use may well have positive social value.

Ganja carries other values of considerable sociological significance. On one level, smoking the substance is considered adventurous by the adolescent boy: by participating in an illegal practice, even though it is widespread among his elders, the young smoker believes he is demonstrating courage, defiance, and, most importantly, manhood. In subtle ways, the smoking of *ganja* is considered by the young almost as a *rite de passage*, an audacious act signifying transition from adolescence to maturity. On another level, particularly for males from the lowest socioeconomic rung of the society, smoking symbolizes camaraderie, equality, and belonging; it is a sign of friendship and trustworthiness. Confidence can be placed in a man who joins in a smoke; those who will not have, potentially, "somet'ing over you." In such a milieu, adult males who do not smoke *ganja*, with the exception of avowed "Christians," can almost be considered deviant — often "loners" and withdrawn; these non-users are rarely included in male gatherings and are even sometimes thought of as simple-minded or deranged. Well based on customary behavior, *ganja* smoking has developed into a social activity limited only to age, work, and status peers. Therefore, among the rural poor, to smoke is to conform; not to smoke may mean social marginality — the reverse of the situation found on the higher social levels.

In the preceding sections, the case for a working-class Jamaican *ganja* institution has been sketched. Whether proven or not, it is nevertheless true that for a large part of the population the *ganja* complex or institution is of considerable consequence with well demarcated social parameters and culturally bounded behavior and effects. However, it is a complex that is legally condemned and publicly denounced by the socially more important sections of Jamaican society. Consequently, an individual's position regarding *ganja* is typically linked to his social status and to his aspirations for upward mobility in the society. In the Jamaican context, *ganja* usage and particularly *ganja* smoking implies participation with others in an illegal activity uniformly judged to be "lower class" and, therefore, "bad" by those with or hopeful of higher status. Public use of *ganja* by such individuals would leave them socially vulnerable and would affect their chances for maintaining or obtaining higher status and the benefits derived from such positions. These individuals, as a consequence, predictably avoid as well as denounce *ganja* and *ganja* smoking as they do other forms of clearly "lower-class" behavior such as common law marriage, bastardy, or reliance on the magical practices of *obeah*.

Not suprisingly, differences in class or sectional *ganja* attitudes are strongly correlated with differences in the prevalence and frequency of *ganja* use between the major social groupings. The social factor is vital to the understanding of cannabis in Jamaica. Most revealing in this regard are the *ganja* patterns of the mobile or socially aspiring individuals of the working or lowest social stratum. To rise in status in a sharply stratified society such as Jamaica is no mean accomplishment. At a minimum, it requires the shedding of obvious "lower class" markers. *Ganja* use is one such marker and from observation appears one of the easiest to divest. In our typical community, the mobiles present a dramatically different smoking profile from that of their more socially static peers in the working class. Despite the fact that many were known to be committed *ganja* smokers in the past, most mobiles are now non-smokers; none are heavy smokers; very few are regular or even intermittent smokers.

The upper elements of Jamaican society hold *ganja* responsible for increases in delinquency and criminality. Such views are continually reinforced by a stream of newspaper reports vividly describing assaults, robberies, and murders allegedly perpetrated by individuals under the influence of *ganja*. Little, if any, objective and substantiated evidence exists, however, which can support these charges. On the contrary, our research indicates that compared with non-smokers of similar stations in Jamaican life, smokers are similar in every major dimension — certainly no less hard-working and no less socially capable. The overwhelming majority of even the heaviest smokers are law-abiding citizens, except with regard to cannabis, with no criminal involvement with police or court. Nevertheless, the stereotypes held and promulgated by the upper elements persist and flourish in Jamaica.

The Jamaican *ganja* laws which date back to 1913 appear, in historical retrospect, to have been based on class and racial factors rather than on objective medical and social evidence (Rubin and Comitas 1972:43–90). In any case, they are so viewed by the *ganja*-using population who see this legislation and its enforcement as arbitrary, directed against the laboring masses, and utilized by those in control for purposes far beyond the intent of the letter of the law. Some users hold the relatively benign opinion that "government" simply does not understand that *ganja* causes no harm and does not lead to violence. Most, however, cling to conspiratorial views: "government" is antagonistic to poor people having anything good and will take *ganja* away; or, legalizing *ganja* would adversely affect the "big men" who make "plenty profits" from the plant; or, medical doctors are against *ganja* because users do not get sick; or, more generally, *ganja* laws make the vulnerable people of Jamaica more vulnerable.

Granting the biases and distortions in these convictions, they should not and cannot be summarily dismissed. From one perspective, they reflect more general feelings of societal abuse harbored by many in the laboring population. From another, they underscore the social danger of institutional and institutionalized misunderstanding in a sharply stratified society.

REFERENCES

COMITAS, LAMBROS
    1973 "Occupational multiplicity in rural Jamaica," in *Work and family life: West Indian perspectives*. Edited by Lambros Comitas and David Lowenthal. Garden City, New York: Anchor Press/Doubleday.

NADEL, S. F.
    1951 *The foundation of social anthropology*. London: Cohen & West.

RUBIN, VERA, LAMBROS COMITAS
　1972　*Effects of chronic smoking of cannabis in Jamaica.* Report by the Research Institute for the Study of Man to the Center for Studies of Narcotic and Drug Abuse, National Institute of Mental Health, Contract No. HSM-42-70-97.

SMITH, D. E.
　1968　Acute and chronic toxicity of marijuana. *Journal of Psychedelic Drugs* 2:37–41.

The Ritual Use of Cannabis in Mexico

ROBERTO WILLIAMS-GARCIA

ABSTRACT

Members of an Indian tribal group living in small communities, near the Gulf of Mexico, use marihuana, which they call *la santa rosa*, in their religious ceremonies. *La santa rosa* is considered a sacred plant, as revealed in a myth of divine origin. Chewed in small quantities, the major observed psychomotor effect is extensive verbalization. The devotees say that the herb makes them speak. By contrast, several cases are presented of secular use of marihuana among urban mestizos.

The plant always rests on the altar of the divine. Only a knowing eye can perceive the contents of the bundles of paper placed on the altar table. *La santa rosa*, the sacred rose, rests there alongside small bells, whistles, incense pots, and a tray of artifacts and fragments of crystal and obsidian which are called *antiquas*, "ancient things." These antiquities are the gods who live in the mythical Hill of Gold. On that table set on the earthen floor, there are usually also paper figures and images of the Catholic saints cult resting against the wall. On the table there is also always cannabis, which the villagers and the diviners call *la santa rosa*. Branches with dry leaves suggest a recently celebrated ritual.

La santa rosa is an object of daily care and attention: it is given offerings of water and refreshments, and is perfumed with incense. If a priest, male or female, has to leave the village, the sacred rose is entrusted to a colleague who is provided with money for the daily offerings, served every morning and every afternoon. The offering is necessary the *curandera* explains, because the sacred rose is a companion of the ancient things, before which the deputy intercedes if a question arises during the absence of the priest. The sacred rose is consumed by the men and women connected with the altar. Male and female priests have the same status in the relationship with the supernatural. In cases where the wife of the male priest has her own ritual activities, she is not his collaborator, but a companion at the same level of activity. It is also consumed by guests who are invited by the priests to care for the plant and participate in the ceremonies in which it is consumed. The caretakers are called the *padrinos* and *madrinas*, the godparents, of *la santa rosa*. During the ceremonies, cult music is played and the players also consume the holy plant. Everyone connected with the cult eats the plant. It is not considered prudent for anyone to take it alone, since one may become intoxicated, dizzy, or experience temporary anxiety.

On special occasions one consumes the sacred rose: the festival of the favored harvest celebrated by a diviner and his followers, or when an aspirant to the profession of priest fulfills his vows. There are other motives for celebrating the ceremonies. The vow is signalled by a *gatanit*, "cat-like," shout which specifies a fiesta. In the case of the consecration of a priest, the cry signifies acceptance of the vows because the ritual has a religious character for the individual; and community values confer great prestige to the priestly occupation. To achieve this status one is required to have had revelatory dreams or have manifested exceptional interests. During the fulfillment of the vows, it is indispensable for the aspirant to eat the sacred rose.

One priest, Pedro Agustin, told me of the effects of his first experience with the sacred herb. He ate it late one afternoon, and remained sleeping. At dawn he was awakened by the noise of rockets which he believed to be the effect of the sacred rose. He sat in a chair before the altar and remained there with a fixed gaze. In a moment, he felt that someone ordered him to speak; someone urged him to speak of the requirements of the cult, and he began to enumerate the things needed for the celebration of the ritual in which he participated. He began to list the persons that had to serve, the branches that had to be arranged and the fowls for the sacrificial offering. He noted the necessity of undertaking a pilgrimage to the Lagoon. Antonio, the priest who was his godfather, asked him to fulfill his *promesa* and Pedro Agustin observed the rituals. He bought four candles for the altar and they started off on the road to the Lagoon. On the road, the party of priests, godparents, and musicians ate the sacred rose. They reached the site, a small pool, and in unison, the priests and godparents asked for rain. Then all experienced the same sensation and perceived the same phenomenon: they heard a rumble of thunder and the approach of a great torrent; the site was darkened and they saw the water in the pool rising. They made an offering of *aguardiente* because they heard *la santa rosa* ordering them thus. On the following day, they gave another offering: they threw birds into the pool. It was an offering for the water. And they returned to the community to eat *la santa rosa* and continue their conversing and their ceremonies.

The effects described by Pedro Agustin are relatively simple in comparison to those related to me, in 1953, about a ceremony officiated by the priest, Antonio, in a small chapel which carried on the religious tradition of the group.

In this pre-Hispanic chapel, the altar had two parts, an upper platform with images of Catholic cult saints, and a lower one, with wooden locked boxes, whose contents were called *los antiquas de la semilla*, "the ancient things of the seed." Two platters containing crystals and archeological fragments were placed on the boxes.

In front of the altar decorated with lemon branches, a greeting to the ancestors and purification of those participating in the rites was taking place. There were certain ritual steps to be carried out before taking *la santa rosa*. The priest distributed flowers among the participants and crouched down to pray. Then he joined the people and proceeded to cleanse them with lemon branches. The musicians played. The priest stood before the altar in a meditative attitude with his hands over his head; he passed the incense burner over the branches with which he brushed the chairs. He set aside six chairs; he and a female priest occupied the two central chairs. From his seat he handed branches and candles to those in the other chairs and prayed holding a candle with his branch. Then he took a whistle and a bell from the altar, making them sound a signal that spirits were arriving from the ancient things, from the ancestors, from the deities. The priestess sang, humming a musical tune. The priest touched the shoulders of the seated ones with his bundle of branches, then cast away the branch, as if it was a further proof of purification. The priestess then brushed the shoulders of the others and the priest placed his wax taper on the altar. Others sat down to receive the same treatment; and the priest ended the act of purification by touching the small bell, recording the presence of the ancestors to whom they presented an offering of bread and coffee. The priest sprinkled *aguardiente* on the earth and lit candles, taking the candles from those who had been purified and from those who came to take communion with the sacred rose.

The act of purification allowed the godfathers and godmothers to take *la santa rosa*. They left the temple to go to a nearby small hut, the habitation of the priest, Antonio, on whose altar was a platter with a bundle of red handkerchiefs. The priest's assistant handed the platter to the *madrina* to carry to the altar of the little chapel, followed by the same group.

From his chair, the priest stretched out his hand to receive the platter, leaving the bundle of red handkerchiefs and revealing a package covered by leaves of *papatla*. He untied this to reveal the sacred plant, and put a small amount in the hand of the priestess. She presented this to the *madrinas* who took portions of the sacred plant between their index finger and thumb. They began to chew it. The priest handed some to the *padrinos*. The music began to sound and the herb eaters gathered in a circle around the two chairs occupied by the priestess and her assistant. They began to dance. Some of the godfathers were kneeling, others remained crouching around their chairs. The priestess sang at intervals and the dancers exchanged branches with her.

The priestess saluted the deities which had come to the altar, and then she moved toward her seat, turning from one side to the other. She joined the others and danced, then returned to her chair and started to speak in an unusual voice, in a very high tone. The women, on one side of the priestess, continued dancing in front of the altar, turning to each side as they danced.

The assistant of the priestess spoke with admirable fluency in a high voice, perspiring as she spoke. She seemed to be an animated orator. The priestess continued turning in her chair, singing and humming to the rhythm of the music; she seemed animated by an inner fire which made her breathe loudly and clench her hands; she revolved in her seat, speaking incessantly.

The priest blew a whistle and rang a little bell because the ancestors were present, as were the spirits of the priest and priestess. The music echoed this sound and the priest sat close to the altar and prayed to the spirits that had come to the ceremony.

The priestess continued moving back and forth; her assistant was possessed, sweating and swinging a branch with her right hand; while her right arm was trembling, the left hand was kept closed, rigid. It was not possible to record her words since I had to be content with the brief commentaries of the translators at the time. The priestess chastised those who did not return to the tradition of consuming the sacred plant and she urged them to return to their traditions. The assistant described the elements they lacked for celebrating the ritual, while the priest remained sitting with a staring gaze.

The priestess stamped both feet on the floor and everyone began to move in the same swaying motion. A midwife fluttered her candle and performed her wheeling turns. She and the priest prayed. Immediately afterwards the priest handed *las madrinas* the two platters with small idols, crystals and glasses, *los antiquas;* and a girl received the package of the sacred plant. They took these things to the patio briefly to sing and dance an *areito* while the speaking pair continued speaking. They returned to the chapel. The priest's assistant who had been speaking to *la santa rosa* had succeeded in communicating with the sacred plant. The music stopped and an hour elapsed while the possessed ones passed from the state of euphoria to tranquil normality. New sounds were heard, and at dawn some participants were still dancing in front of the altar.

SPEAKING EFFECTS

It was apparent that the effect of the sacred plant on the central nervous system provoked both body tremors and the urge to speak. Although various themes were mentioned, the oratory seemed to center on religious matters, as if these were the only vital preoccupation. I would have needed to keep extensive records in their language and to translate them in order to know about what they were speaking.

The course which should follow the celebration of the rites was explained. Pedro Agustin, habitual consumer of the herb, with over ten years experience, indicated that he felt nothing upon eating the sacred plant. He also said, however, that once the effects had passed, the person relaxes, which implicitly means he accepts the fact that changes are induced. He considers that the sacred plant serves only to give ideas: it is a stimulant to thought.

According to the earlier descriptions, one would conclude that the principal effect of the herb is that of stimulating speech. But that is only the most apparent principal effect as one finds another, in the account of the visions experienced at the site of the Lagoon. There may be a predisposition to the phenomenon of hearing the sound of thunder and seeing the rise of water in the pool, since this is a theme of public knowledge. One may speculate that the narration of that experience by a priest was diffused to the community. Having become public knowledge, the priests that come to the site are then predisposed to experience the phenomena. It cannot be considered a spontaneous, unconditional vision, equal to the religious themes which are revealed during the previously mentioned discourses during trance.

Another priest, a disciple of Pedro Agustin, also mentioned that he felt nothing when he ate the sacred rose, except the desire to dance while hearing the music played on ceremonial occasions. His reaction should be considered a response to musical conditioning. He commented that the sacred rose speaks through the music: the music is its language. One of the songs tells us that it is a long time since the plant was created and we do not know when it will end.

If the people who eat it feel the desire to dance, what is the feeling of the musicians? They are simply transmitters of the feelings of the sacred rose, its interpreters. The musical notes are the words of the sacred rose, which touch whoever is moved by the sacred rose which possesses him. This is expressed by the music:

Many thanks,
I am very grateful to whoever touches me,
to whoever touched me,
if they are in harmony with me
I wish that forever we are one
we have one thought,
we have one heart
we have one road.

Every priest knows the music; it is one of the requisites of his profession. He must know the sounds that must be played and the order in which they are played, since the music indicates the sequence of activities. Pedro Agustin gave a demonstration. First he made the sound that gladdens the moment when the sacred plant is taken. The followers ate the plant while listening to the music and hummed the melody without words, while aware that the sounds meant the following:

Today we who have taken it
shout with joy
today we have seen
and we who are taking it
we are rejoicing.

The next sound is the calling or resurrection of the spirits, played so that the spirits gain life, so that they present themselves. Another sound speaks to the sacred plant because it has reached the place where there is an offering, the altar that is the house of its father and mother. "It has come," says the music. Then, the music speaks of the souls, invokes the companions of *la santa rosa*, to ask something of the sacred plant. Another sound is played requesting that it remain, not leave, not depart. Once they have said enough to the gods to whom they have played, in this case the sacred rose, the deity then thanks those who are making the offering, and those who have made offerings.

VISIONS

One priestess takes a position opposed to the verbal effects caused by ingestion of *la santa rosa*. She has been a priestess in the community for over twenty years and is a regular consumer of the herb. She considers that the effects vividly manifested by other diviners are simply theatrical acts of charlatanry. She thinks that some who become "speakers" are fools and some are deceivers, because they come together to speak about the very act they are doing. With the sacred plant one is put to thinking and the one who has eaten the sacred plant should not speak because that would interrupt his thinking, his thread of thought. When this priestess has eaten the sacred plant, she only *sees* things; and, the same happens to her husband who is a priest and to their followers who accompany them to the rituals celebrated in their house.

The first time she took the sacred plant was in San Pedro, the scene of my observations in 1953. She started out early in the morning, with two boxes of small idols or ancient things. When she arrived in the afternoon a crowd was gathered in the hut of Vicente, the priest, their teacher. So many people were there, it seemed that they were awaiting a bishop. The ritual had already started; the musicians were playing and six women were dancing and repeatedly asking themselves why they were there where they were suffering, awaiting their sisters (the ancient ones? the ancestors?). Then the sounds rang out to awaken the ancient one who approached and the music sounded again. Then the priest asked her and her husband if they desired to remain and invited them to try something, that she immediately recognized as the sacred plant. "This is the San Antonio" he told her as he put a small amount in her hand, recommending that she perfume it with the burning incense. He told her to eat it. She ate it. "It did nothing to me," she said. A woman approached her and said, "no, my daughter, do not be ashamed if all the people command you; now that you are on the road, you are not going the other way. Now, don't be ashamed, and forget your embarrassment." She replied that she felt no embarassment. But she did not speak further, she was only thinking about what would be happening.

On the second occasion when she took the sacred plant, she saw some of the participants scattering flowers of all colors. Everyone gathered flowers in their hands or in their hats, not letting them fall, glancing upwards. These flowers were all going to bear good results.

On the third occasion and at subsequent times her field of vision expanded. She saw scenes of *Cerro de Oro*, the Hill of Gold, possibly derived from descriptions by the priests. According to their tales, the Hill of Gold is situated in the East, where all those who have dealings with the supernatural reside. The priestess described it with feeling, as a place where it is always brilliant, "the largest of the hills, where our master god always goes, who always illuminates our world." It is the place of the reunion of all the souls of the priests, priestesses, musicians and midwives; musicians are always playing, while offerings are being brought to the altars of the earth, offerings that are placed on the table presided over by the gods, among which is the *santa rosa*.

When a follower of the *santa rosa* dies, he undergoes purification and is traditionally attended by a musician who has eaten the *santa rosa*. At the purification rite of a follower, women waving small branches danced beside the body. A priest kept swinging the incense burner to the four cardinal points. He gathered in his hands the right hand of the old man to make it tremble, simulating the tremors experienced by the eaters of *la santa rosa*. He passed a branch of the herb along the length of the body, sweeping it from head to foot, so that the deceased would be clean, purified, for his presence in the beyond, in the Hill of Gold where the sacred plant lives.

DIVINE ORIGIN

The herb represents that which is living, "as if it were a small piece of the heart of god," according to the folk saying. The simile is apt because the sacred plant is the mother of the supreme deity. The myth says the following:

A child in gestation informs his mother that he will be born dead and instructs her to bury him in a place close to the site where she usually bathes. The mother buried him in that place and there grew forth a maize plant from which she prepared tamales; but they were bitter and she proceeded to throw them away. The rejected tamales were transformed into a boy who then presented himself to the mother as her son. She tested him and then asked him to accompany her in the direction of the east. On the road they met a lizard lying flat with its face up; the child cut its tongue and gave it to his mother. They arrived at a large house guarded by St. Peter which they entered without alerting the gatekeeper. The boy told his mother to stay near the entrance and prophesied that she would always be worshipped and would find herself clean and fresh, sprouting and giving seed, because she would be the sacred rose. The boy continued along his route; he moved the tongue of the lizard provoking storms. The elders, or thunders, asked St. Peter who had granted him entry; St. Peter, confused, did not know what to reply. The thunders located the boy and promised not to harm him in exchange for his giving each one of them, a piece of the lizard's tongue. That boy was the sun, the supreme deity, who had manifested himself as maize. His mother, the sacred rose, lives at the entrance of the heavenly mansion.

CULTIVATION

The myth seems to dictate the concerns which should be lavished on the plant. Whoever has a herb garden attends it daily and clears the earth, gathering the small leaves and clearing the refuse. His neighbors and priests count on him. The cultivated plants grow to over a meter and a smaller species grows on the banks of the brooks. Access to the garden itself, however, is not possible; it is reserved.

The priests say that every plant has two varieties, masculine and feminine, differentiated by the size of their seeds, the masculine being the one with the larger seeds. When it is eaten, no sex distinction is made; as we observed in 1953 when the priest divided the bundle equally among the men and women, the entire plant was used. Ordinary people speak of the use of the plant with female seeds as malevolent, and they use the male plants to offset such effects.

THE EFFECTS AMONG MESTIZOS

In order to know its effects while knowing that it would not affect me I ate it with a companion, in an informal way, in the hut of the priest, Pedro Agustin. I should mention that I had been invited to eat it at a special ceremony during the maize fiestas in September which the priestess of the visions celebrated.

Pedro Agustin acceded to our request and had beer and bottled refreshments brought to us to purchase. His altar was covered with many dry branches from recent ceremonies, and on a table set before the altar, there was a package covered with a crown of paper flowers to correspond to the sacred rose. The priest took a candle, asked that copal be thrown into the incense and proceeded to pray in a standing position. It should be noted that he had recently begun to lose his sight and had become inactive; perhaps that is why his body trembled, since he had begun trembling a few months before. They said that his father went blind. Another person who went blind is the priestess, Juana, whom I knew for twenty years in San Pedro.

When he finished praying, he sat down, and I opened the refreshments, my companion took the beer and I the soft drink. Then, the priest ordered his niece to bring us the sacred rose; she opened the bundle that contained the crown of flowers. After my companion received it, I extended my right hand and she corrected me, saying that I should extend the other hand. In the hollow of my left hand I received a dose consisting of what she gathered with her tightened fingers. We chewed it.

It was clear that the entire plant was used, since there were some small pieces of the stalk. It was somewhat dry. Later the priest took his violin to demonstrate the music played during the ceremonies, the first sound being that of jubilation on having consumed the sacred rose. After half an hour of hearing the music, I felt nothing. The most I perceived was a slight noise in my ears, and this only briefly. My companion confided to me that it had no effect on him, but thought that a larger dose would succeed, supporting his opinion by the fact that he had taken it in a distilled form a week before.

My friend, then 36 years old, had taken it in the form of tea. After a meal and some drinks, at five in the afternoon, tea was offered to him, to which some green drops had been added. The dose covered the bottom of the cup. Another night, at a supper with friends, in an atmosphere of drinking, drops were put in their drinks. His principal sensation was that of "stopping time." The sounds seemed more prolonged, somewhat like the acoustical sensation on hearing Ravel's *Bolero*. The same friend had had experience smoking it, noting that his pupils dilated a little and he could see images.

I can offer no ritual testimony regarding smoking. Additional information is needed to arrive at definite conclusions. Several accounts by individuals are presented below to indicate the range of reactions to smoking marihuana in secular settings.

A female student from the provinces reported that she did not feel anything the first time she smoked it. The second time she felt great excitement: her senses were more acute — she heard more, saw more, and her sense of taste was keener. She did not smoke it a third time.

Another woman, 23 years old, was initiated in an unfortunate way. At a reunion of teachers and students in Mexico City, where she was born and now lives, she smoked her usual cigarette and was then offered one which made her feel strange. Nevertheless, she smoked it and passed it on to another. When she gave an account of the effects, her companion, who was her quasi-official chaperon, persuaded her to leave and took her home in a bus. She felt a desire to establish contact, to chat — to communicate with the people! — to express herself with someone regardless of sex or economic condition: "I had a desire to chat with them. I knew that they were going to say beautiful things to me. That was my first response." The young woman, who seems shy, is very talkative when she feels confident. "On board the bus I felt the effect of my desire to chat with people but not with the woman who sat near me. I felt a slight headache. Then again the sensation of wanting to talk returned. When I reached my house I said to my sister — 'listen, I believe I smoked marihuana.' My sister was astonished. She ran to make a tea which is an antidote. I said to my father, 'listen I wanted to chat with the people whatever happened. But let's talk I...gua...gua...gua!' Happy! and thus ended my reaction, perfectly content with the world and there was no discomfort."

Her second experience took place in an atmosphere of gaiety, laughter and jokes, an atmosphere conditioned for smoking marihuana. "I took it in a mood of playfulness, without any hesitancy, or concern." But the third time she took it, in the same group, she felt normal and thought possibly, she was more restrained by her conscience. She was disturbed because people were laughing at silly repetitious jokes. It disturbed her to see those people incapable of saying anything more pleasant or, better still, to be quiet and peaceful. Her friends explained that "what happened is that you overcame the marihuana and it has no effect on you; you can overcome on the level at which you open yourself up to the world; you have a dialogue with people; you have no problem, since marihuana does nothing to you." "It does nothing to me!" she said contentedly. She had smoked four or five times, and considers it like any cigarette except for the taste which is richer, like the taste of herbs. She began to substitute for tobacco cigarettes, cigarettes that she made herself by grinding eucalyptus leaves because the smell was like marihuana and she liked the flavor. She believed that people of a "very pliant psyche," those who can act out the role they desire by auto-suggestion, are vulnerable to marihuana. She cited the case of a professional who acted like a young man when using it because that was his concern. In his daily life he tried to act like a young man, not accepting his level of maturity.

My position that reactions correspond to cultural backgrounds was bolstered by another case. A young man of 21, a capable student, in the provinces, told me that marihuana helped him to free himself and that he had been smoking it for a year. He observed that while people feel nothing the first time, everyone is affected by it the second time, and the effects relate to the capacity for imagination. He mentioned an incident when he was walking by a woods one night. The ground was wet since it had just rained and reflected the light from the street lamp. "The lights were like white spheres that seemed to me to be cloaks of *"manifestantes."* Then that image was blurred and on reflection, he recalled that he had seen a photograph of student-like *"manifestaciones"* who wore cloaks. The imagination he added, could frequently surge. My question was, "Can one keep the source of imagination within discretion or does it carry one away?" He told me, "It is not necessary that it play with you, it is necessary that you play with it. And those who cannot restrain themselves, who are of a mind that has problems, they have trouble. This type collapses.

If one controls oneself, one learns new things about psychological processes."

The student wore a white short sleeved shirt, printed with large red mushrooms, and smaller cursive lettering: *Huantla City*, that motivated our discussion about hallucinogens, mushrooms and marihuana. The latter, he deduced, provokes illusions based on something that exists, but he had another reaction with the mushrooms. He ate six that were brought from Huantla. The only effect produced was an identification with nature. I commented that he could have achieved those results through concentration and meditation. He replied that he could achieve that sensation only through the mushrooms. He had no color hallucinations. He thought that the mushrooms did not have sufficient strength; and I agreed with him attributing this to the climate of Huantla, where the mushrooms originated.

My companion also told me of his experiments with hallucinogenic mushrooms. His sensations were of levitation, flying over a flowering woods. He told me about a young man outstanding in knowledge and intelligence who "destroyed" himself with marihuana; "he burned himself out." There is of course no way to determine that marihuana "destroyed" this brilliant youth. He may have been taking various drugs, although marihuana is often called "the monster with green eyes."

Before concluding, I should describe my own experiments, or rather, experiences with the two hallucinogens. Actually, I was not aware of having used marihuana because the name under which it was concealed diluted the aversion to cannabis. I have eaten the sacred rose twice. Once in 1953 during a ritual ceremony where I asked for it; eager to know it botanically, I ate a small quantity. Another time was during the current year also in a ritual context. It did not affect me, surely because of the small doses. With respect to the mushrooms, I ate them in 1966 and they produced no dependency in me, no desire to eat them again in spite of the beauty of my visions. According to the data obtained, there is also a diversity of responses to the mushrooms, affected by the individual temperament and preoccupations. In general terms one can say that with the mushrooms, one invents reality, new situations are created; while with marihuana only images concerning concrete situations are produced, such as those described by the twenty-one year old youth.

Reference to my own visions will further illustrate my point. The mushrooms produced for me some beautiful luminous situations of color in motion. And the most lasting impression is of an intellectual order, surely because it was my preoccupation at the time. I saw a part of a sphere revolving around an intensely brilliant blue base. Around the sphere there revolved a small one, like a satellite, which I identified as the myth. The large sphere was human thought. And my reflection on that world of my hallucinations was to accept it with approbation.

Cannabis and Cultural Groups in a Colombian Municipio

WILLIAM L. PARTRIDGE

ABSTRACT

Data, drawn from field work in progress in Colombia, South America, are presented on the cultivation, marketing, and consumption of cannabis. The analysis is an effort to liberate cannabis from the individualistic, idiosyncratic thinking of past studies. Emphasis is placed on the structure of the community of which cannabis is a part. Subcultural groups related to various stages of the cannabis cycle are discussed with reference to their position and function in the larger community, their histories, socioeconomic characteristics, and relationships to each other. Data on cannabis use are presented on the types of social groupings characterized by participation in the cannabis cycle versus those which are not.

The anthropological contribution to an understanding of cannabis seems to lie in three distinct but related areas: (1) studies of the nature of the culture and community in which the phenomenon is present; (2) translation of concepts, models, and methods into applicable forms for testing in the field of social and cultural realities in which the phenomenon is immersed; and (3) ethnohistorical study. The work reported here falls mainly within the first of these three divisions, a community study in the tradition of social anthropology (Arensberg and Kimball 1965).

The objective of the study, begun in July of 1972 and still in progress in a *municipio* on the north coast of Colombia, South America, is the description and analysis of the subcultural units connected to the cannabis cycle, cultivation, marketing, and consumption. The paper will focus on the subcultural groups associated with cannabis in relation to their position

The research is supported by the National Institute of Mental Health Predoctoral Research Fellowship number 1FO1MH54512-01 CUAN and the supplementary grant number 3F01DA54512-01S1 CUAN.

and function in the larger community, following a brief ethnohistorical review.

I. ETHNOHISTORY

The introduction of cannabis into Spanish South America is not well known. Patiño (1967, 1969) indicates that hemp was introduced not once but several times by the Spanish: experiments were attempted in Peru, Mexico, Chile, and Colombia, but only Chile developed the capacity to export hemp to Spain (Patiño 1969). In Colombia reports from 1607, 1610, 1632, and 1789 indicate that repeated introductions failed to produce a hemp industry for the rigging of the Spanish fleet (*Ibid.*). Silvestre (Vergara y Velasca 1901) in his 1789 description of the viceroyalty of Santafé de Bogotá indicates that hemp was introduced in the savanna of Bogotá, but failed so completely that no seed was available for further experimentation. He urged the reintroduction of hemp cultivation near Santa Marta or Cartegena and urged that seed be shipped from Spain (Vergara y Velasca 1901). In Silverstre's opinion hemp could replace *cabuya* or the fiber of *Fourcroya foetida* (Patiño 1967) in Colombia, indicating the most telling reason for the former's failure in South America. *Fique, pita*, or *cabuya* was collected in tribute from the indigenous peoples of Colombia by the first Spanish colonists (Reichel-Dolmatoff 1951). As late as the early 1800's *cabuya* was a Colombian export (Vergara y Velasca 1901). *Cabuya* replaced hemp in the manufacture of such items as sandals, rope and cordage, sacks, harnesses, and fish nets (Patiño 1967). Another native fiber, cotton, replaced hemp in even such basic items as candle wick, used in huge quantities in the mines of South America, which in Europe had been made of hemp or flax (*Ibid.*). It appears that native fiber producing plants acted as a barrier to the diffusion of hemp. As late as the present century experiments continue in Colombia (Patiño 1969), but no hemp industry has ever existed in Colombia compared to that which existed in North America (Seale *et al.* 1952).

The use of cannabis products as intoxicants is still another question. Linguistic evidence indicates West African slaves brought cannabis to Brazil as the earliest route of diffusion (Patiño 1969; Aranújo 1959). The adoption of cannabis smoking by indigenous people of Brazil seems to confirm the antiquity of diffusion in that part of South America (Wagley and Galvão 1949), but the spread of the custom to Spanish America is less well known. It should be noted that cannabis competed with available indigenous intoxicants, narcotics, and hallucinogens.[1] Of these, only tobacco was adopted by Spanish colonists, which with coca had the widest distribution and popularity in the New World. Tobacco was snuffed for headache, chewed for toothache, smoked for "cold humors," and mixed with rum and *aguardiente* and applied to mosquito bites (Patiño 1967). Negro slaves and Spaniards were reported to use it for working because it reduced fatigue (*Ibid.*). Due to this property tobacco was allotted as part of the workers' rations on a Jesuit *hacienda* (*Ibid.*). Perhaps we have here another barrier to diffusion of cannabis in South America.

It seems certain that smoking cannabis is a relatively new innovation in the region with which we are concerned. Ardila (1965) and Patiño (1969) suggest the Magdalena River valley as the route of penetration into Colombia, from the ports of Santa Marta, Barranquilla, and Cartegena, originating in the Antilles and Panama. Specifically, Ardila (1965) suggests that the spread of the use of cannabis as an intoxicant dates from the work on the Panama Canal and the "intense human interchange" which resulted among Circum-Caribbean countries. This interpretation is given weight by the observation that both Costa Rican and Colombian laws concerning marihuana date from 1927 and 1928 respectively (Patiño 1969; Ardila 1965; Torres 1965), when the movement of *braceros* and *marineros* was a fact. Nevertheless, it was not until around 1945 that the Colombian press began reporting clandestine marihuana plantations on the Atlantic coast and in the Cauca valley (Patiño 1969).

II. RESEARCH COMMUNITY BACKGROUND

The *municipio* lies at the base of the western slopes of the Sierra Nevada de Santa Marta, between two of the six rivers which flow to the Ciénaga Grande. Within its boundaries are found vast swamplands and the highest mountain peak in Colombia. The town in which the research was based is the *cabacera* of the *municipio*, at a distance of about 90 kilometers from the city of Santa Marta. The areas of dense settlement are the nonflooding lowlands at the base of the mountains and the highland valleys of the rivers. The two areas are ecologically and culturally distinct, each inhabited by a distinct subcultural population, although each is articulated politically, economically, and ritually with the *cabacera* of the lowlands.

Neither of the ecological-cultural zones was of much interest to the

---

[1] *Erythroxylon coca, Banisteriopsis* spp., *Phyllanthus mexiae, Opuntia* spp., *Datura arborea, Methysticodendron amesianum, Nicotiana tabacum,* and *Clibadium surinamense.*

Spanish colonists of the 16th century: Spanish efforts on this part of the coast consisted mainly in exterminating the native population. A high price in blood was paid for a territory left uncolonized until the present century (Alarcon 1963).

The *municipio* is an excellent example. Governor Garcia de Lerma instituted a scorched earth policy in the region in 1529, burning towns and fields between Santa Marta and the river Magdalena. By 1600 there was no native population in the region. The land was mostly swamp. As late as 1898 a Colombian geographer notes that the region is densely forested, subject to frequent floods, and sparsely populated (Vergara y Velasca 1901).

Beginning in 1896 however, this picture started to change dramatically, when the United Fruit Company began operations in the future *zona bananera*. By the second decade of the twentieth century, banana plantations blanketed the lowlands from the mountains to the Ciénaga Grande. The *municipio* was a center of this development. The Company put in production some 10,000 *hectáreas*, and at the height of productivity a total of 30,000 *hectáreas* were under cultivation (Kamalaprija 1965; Comisión de Planificación 1964).

Development was spectacular. By 1938 the *municipio* had sprouted a population of 15,861 persons. United States capitalists, French, English, and American engineers, and a work force recruited from all over the coast founded several such towns, straightened the course of rivers, built a drainage and irrigation system, paved roads, installed bridges, completed a railroad from the docks in Santa Marta to the southern limit of the banana zone, and built work camps and employee housing on vast banana estates. Church records from 1914 to 1925 indicate that about half of the marriages performed united persons from distant regions of the coast. This pattern continues to the present.

The influence of the banana company upon the organization of life in the region was felt in four ways: (1) the local elite composed of original settlers was transformed into a wealthy elite; (2) a middle sector was created by recruitments of employees from the coastal cities; (3) the traditional social relationships among landowners and laborers were altered; and (4) the nature of the social relationships among laborers themselves was changed.

Landowners who were operating tracts of cattle and sugar cane quickly converted to bananas. Some sold their land and moved to the cities, but many built fortunes selling bananas and purchased homes in the coastal cities. They sent their sons and daughters to the capital, to Europe, and to the United States for education. They held political offices at the departmental and national levels where the aristocratic cattle barons of ancient Spanish towns had previously dominated political life.

The middle sector was comprised of employees of the Company: estate managers, clerks, commissary directors, secretaries, fruit selectors, and labor supervisors. They received single family dwellings with running water and indoor plumbing, furniture, mules and horses, coupons for shopping at the Company store, medical treatment in hospitals staffed by United States physicians, and a monthly salary. Their sons and daughters were given scholarships to study at universities. Several of these families also built fortunes during the banana heyday.

Workers were provided with three rooms of a row house, running water and indoor plumbing, reduced train rates, hospital services deducted from their pay (2%), a machete, work clothes and boots, coupons for shopping at the Company store, and a cash wage higher than that paid to workers on the coast today.

Traditional patron-client relations existed among landowners and their laborers. On the coast this relationship entailed the following responsibilities for the landowning employer: lending several *hectáreas* to his client to plant crops, credit reference at a store in town or an estate commissary, providing a degree of security in times of life crisis or illness as well as small cash gifts. Wage labor destroyed this relationship; workers demanded money in return for labor on the model of the Company relationship with workers, rather than the beneficence of a patron. Landowners charged the Company with "ruining the workers."

Among the workers themselves the industrialization of agriculture naturally included industrial forms of organization. The workers became quite specialized, working in groups at specialized tasks. Significantly, there were no peasants in the *municipio* during the development of the banana zone[2] as all land was devoted to the plantation production of bananas.[3]

Other subcultural groups present in the *municipio* during the early 20th century included Middle East immigrants who opened stores, bars, and brothels, a small number of West Indian immigrants who worked as day laborers, and Americans living in the *quinta* or group of manor houses on the other side of the railroad tracks.

[2] This pattern changed during World War II with the invasion of the lands of the United Fruit Company by landless workers who then became peasants exploiting a few *hectáreas*. These peasants are now being offered title to the land by INCORA, but many refuse as they wish to avoid taxes. Still others desire title so as to qualify for loans with the Caja Agraria for cash crops, animals, or more land.
[3] Original maps used by the United Fruit Company were kindly made available by the offices of INCORA in Sevilla, Magdelena.

The picture painted by Gabriel García Márquez of this period in his novel *Cien años de soledad* is for the most part accurate. The small hamlet was indeed transformed into a boom town, with accompanying street brawls and deaths by machete. Many informants repeat the tales of "happy drunks" on Saturday nights burning pesos to light their cigars. The elite founders were the prime movers and beneficiaries of the boom; they drank Scotch, played poker, and grew rich with the Americans.

From 1915 to 1943 the Company exported to the United States all the fruit it could buy or produce. In 1928 the first labor strike in Colombia began in the banana zone resulting in the massacre of thousands of workers by the Colombian army, on the morning of December 6th, 1928, a fact often cited as the reason for the ultimate departure of the United Fruit Company (Montaña 1963; Fluharty 1956). On the contrary, production rose after the strike, reaching a high in 1930 and levelling off at pre-strike levels. Production continued high until 1943 and only then fell drastically. During the World War no ships called for bananas at the port of Santa Marta. When the Company reopened its operations in 1947, it found the land had been invaded by both wealthy private producers and landless laborers (Kamalaprija 1965).

The elaborate road system constructed by the Company provided channels for invading workers, who founded several small hamlets that exist today, and colonized small holdings nearby. In like fashion, but on a grander scale, wealthy landowners annexed lands. The company negotiated a new policy with the Colombian government. Contracts were signed which gave the wealthy squatters the status of *arrendatarios* or tenants; the peasants were simply ignored. The tenants in turn agreed to sell all bananas produced to the Company and to pay US $ 1.00 for each *hectárea* not producing bananas. By the year 1949 exports were higher than the highs of 1930.

But at this time the Company began liquidating its holdings in Colombia as a result of the changed world market. The Company landholdings were reduced until by 1964 it owned no banana-producing land (*Ibid*.). They were concentrated to the north and the banana industry of the town and *municipio* died.

With the exit of the Company the *municipio* saw the exit of wealthy plantation owners, much of the middle sector of employees, and hundreds of workers. Many families of the elite and middle sectors were ruined. The workers lost an income that provided the impetus for migration, an income that was high compared to today's wage.[4]

[4] At the exchange rate of 1.02 pesos to the dollar in 1925, the worker earning 1.30 pesos a day received about US $1.30 a day. Today the worker makes 25 pesos a day

Today the lowlands are devoted primarily to rice, cattle, and cattle products. Some 48,964 *hectáreas* are devoted to pasture while only 23,195 are in agricultural crops (Departamento Administrativo Nacional de Estadística 1971:23). Of the lands in agricultural production perhaps only 3,000 *hectáreas* are in *pan cojer* or maize, manioc, and *plátano*, the staple foods consumed by the population (Comisión de Planificación 1964:99). Of total lands being exploited 683 persons own farms of between 1 and 50 *hectáreas* (Departamento Administrativo Nacional de Estadística 1971:12).[5] In short, the *latifundia* devoted to cattle dominates the landscape, a cultural value with an ancient pedigree in this region of Colombia.

Concomitant with the departure of the Company another process of change was set in motion. In 1948 the civil war called *la violencia* began in the interior regions of Colombia (see Dix 1967; Fluharty 1956). The effects of this bloodletting, which Hobsbawn (quoted in Dix 1967:361) has characterized as "the greatest armed mobilization of peasants in the recent history of the western hemisphere, with the possible exception of some periods during the Mexican revolution," are many and varied. The one that concerns us here took place in the *municipio*. Families of Andean peasants, mainly from the departments of Santander, Norte de Santander, and Cundinamarca, fleeing the spreading mania migrated to the foothills of the Sierra Nevada, an area similar ecologically to the ones they had been forced to abandon. Study of the origins of these families indicates that the move was generally made between the years 1950 and 1953. Most of them directly cite *la violencia* as their motive for moving. They brought their wives, children, parents, siblings, and other relatives and staked out 50 to 200 *hectáreas* of land in the low altitude valleys at about 400 to 500 meters. The coastal label for these new colonists is *cachacos* meaning persons from the interior of Colombia. With them came *cachaco* storekeepers buying up stores, bars, and brothels.

(some as little as 15 or 20), and at the exchange rate of 23.00 he earns the equivalent of US $1.05 a day. (Wage levels collected from former workers for the United Fruit Company. Exchange rates taken from Kamalaprija 1965.) It should also be noted that food and goods available in Company stores were much cheaper than that available for persons not working for the Company.

[5] These figures are based on the Department of Statistics' concept of a "unit of exploitation" which is all the land within a *municipio* exploited by a single producer, individual, or corporation. It should be noted, however, that the land use pattern in this region of Colombia is different from that observed in other regions (e.g. Fals Borda 1956; Fluharty 1956) where holdings are widely scattered. Land holdings in this region tend to be concentrated in a single farm. Exceptions are generally *latifundistas* who have holdings scattered over the *municipio* and often in several *municipios* and departments.

Between 1947 and 1964, therefore, the entire fabric of community life underwent dramatic change, affecting every element of the community. The transition was not easy or peaceful.[6]

III. SOCIAL GROUPS AND PARTICIPATION IN CANNABIS CYCLE

The *cachacos* and *costeños* form the major division within the community; foreign nationals have departed, except for the *turkos* or Arabs who have been incorporated through marriage. Each subculture has a distinct social and economic organization, a distinctive heritage, and interacts socially and ritually apart from the other. Within each subculture there are further subdivisions.

The *cachacos* are composed of the highland peasants living on dispersed individual family farms and the storekeepers who live in town and are gradually acquiring large herds of cattle; the two groups form an interdependent relational system. The peasant subsists mainly upon crops he himself produces (corn and yucca or sweet manioc being the staple foods), in addition to which cash crops, rice, beans, and corn, are sold to storekeepers in town. The storekeepers grant clients credit and contracts for raising cattle on the highland farms. The peasant can therefore acquire two sources of income: cash crop sales and from the share of cattle he may fatten for a storekeeper patron. But the majority of Andean peasants have only the former option, as there are a limited number of *cachaco* patrons and cattle.

An additional source of income is provided by the cultivation of cannabis. The sparse settlement of the Sierra Nevada and the rugged terrain permit some protection and the legend of *cachaco* violence prevents too many inquisitive intruders. Cannabis is grown as a cash crop; it is not consumed by the *cachacos* who cultivate it, nor by those neighbors who do not. The sale of the crop is arranged through coastal middlemen who live in the towns and cities. *Cachaco* storekeepers do not deal in cannabis. Contracts are often made before the crop is planted and buyers sometimes treat their clients in traditional paternalistic fashion, giving gifts of rum,

---

[6] The legend of *cachaco* violence persists to the present. Some *Antioquia cachacos* migrated into the *municipio* at the start of this century to work for the Company and were responsible for the deaths of several coastal men in razor fights, according to informants. One night in 1914 the coastal townspeople dispatched the entire immigrant group with machetes. No other *cachacos* came to the *municipio* until the 1950's. While no incidents occurred at this time, the *cachacos* are perceived as violent and dangerous as evidenced by *la violencia* in the interior departments from 1948 to 1968.

aguardiente and money. But such contracts seldom bind either party for more than one growing season. Cash cropping of cannabis appears to be the best of all possible incomes for a peasant: a kilo of coffee, the best of cash crops in Colombia, brings 12.50 pesos whereas a pound of cannabis will net from 100 to 300 pesos, depending on the quality. But it is a business that takes *pateloncitos* or guts as one farmer said. Yet at the time of this writing no peasant in this region has been bothered by police investigation or arrest. Most highland peasants are aware, however, that pressure from the United States has produced arrests for cultivation of cannabis in other regions of Colombia.

The *cachaco vereda* or rural neighborhood is an ethnocentric homogenous, politically cohesive unit (Fals Borda's 1955 definition applies equally well to these immigrants as it did to peasants in Boyacá). The various highland *veredas* are linked together by filial and affinal kinship ties of ritual obligations and ties of common origin. The work unit which exploits the land is composed of male members of the extended household, a man, his oldest sons, sons-in-law, and any other male relatives present. The household head directs all farming activity and even adult sons will consult with him before setting out to the field to work. Few residents of the *vereda* have family in the town or in the rural areas of the lowlands, but all have family in their *municipios* of origin. When a death occurs relatives and neighbors of the *vereda* come for the nine-day wake and the first anniversary wake. In several cases, families living in the highlands have migrated from the same *municipio* in the interior and settled near each other. But the males of different families do not work cooperatively, except in hunting *ñeke* and other wild meat. Wage labor is absent from the highland *vereda*, excepting the police commissioner who is recruited from among the peasants. The current officeholder cultivates cannabis for cash sales. Aside from his familial and friendship ties, this may be another reason he has never arrested anyone for cultivating cannabis.

The *cachaco* storekeepers are an important economic force in the *vereda* and the town, and are clearly part of the *cachaco* subculture. They willingly sell rum and *aguardiente* for coastal fiestas such as Carnaval but do not themselves participate. Although they are part of the highland *vereda*, they play no role in the cannabis cycle.

The coastal subculture is more complex in structure and is perhaps best described as a series of subsystems. The first of these is the estate system, including landowners, estate managers, estate employees, and wage laborers. The employees on the estate sometimes live in outbuildings left by the Company, but frequently they live in the better town *barrios*.

They receive only slightly higher wages than the day laborer, but they have the security of steady employment, often the use of 2 or 3 *hectáreas* for planting, and the higher status of machinery operators. It is the estate employee who drives the tractors, combines, trucks, and other farm equipment. When landowners have estates in several different parts of the *municipio*, or in other *municipios* or other departments, the employees usually work on all of his holdings and thus travel widely. The day laborers, on the other hand, are recruited from the landless poor of the town and country. None live on the estates where they find work. The day laborer obtains work on a contract basis and is often called a *contractista*. He is hired by the job, for a certain task over a certain period of time, and then released: to clean an irrigation canal, to cut and clear brush from a field, to dig ditches that carry water to the crop, to fumigate a field to keep weeds down, to herd cattle, etc. Thus, the work group in the coastal subculture is composed of male nonkin. It is from this group of day laborers that the cannabis consumers come. Cannabis in the form of cigarettes is consumed among groups of day laborers while working; it is generally purchased as they have no land on which to grow their own.

The landed gentry live in the coastal cities, in contrast to the days of the banana zone when they constituted a town landed gentry. An estate manager has the responsibility of running the estate, including hiring and firing workers, directing day to day operations, operating a commissary for employees, and traveling to the city to consult the owner and receive money for paying workers and expenses. The managers form a minor elite in the rural lowlands and are generally recruited from an educated minority in this and other coastal towns. In many cases they are the offspring of former employees of the United Fruit Company.

Identification of commercial buyers of cannabis is a tricky and dangerous process. Contacts are difficult to maintain when one is not buying. But those who are known are drawn entirely from the upper sector of the community. Given the crisis which enveloped many of these families upon the departure of the Company, it is logical that they would be drawn into lucrative trade activity in an effort to retain their newly won status and income. Not only in the case of cannabis but in the bustling contraband trade with Venezuelan black marketeers, members of the upper sector play principal roles. It is they who staff the patronage government customs posts and the smuggling operation. Cannabis traffic has been accepted as merely another contraband activity, one of the more lucrative specializations. Members of the best families are involved in contraband activity and in the towns and cities the upper sector families are avid consumers as well. Thus, professionals, landowners, and businessmen of the coastal subculture form the commercial buyers of cannabis.

The third subsystem of the coastal subculture is that composed of coastal peasants and coastal shopkeepers. The Arab-owned shops on the market square are the focus of this subsystem, just as the highland shopkeepers of the town are the focus of the *cachaco* subculture. Credit is granted the coastal peasant and he markets some of his produce to pay his bill where he has credit. Similarly, coastal peasants sell fruit and vegetables to street vendors. The coastal peasant generally has less land than his Andean counterpart, sometimes only 2 or 3 *hectáreas*. The coastal peasant also raises fewer cash crops than his *cachaco* counterpart, and depends upon *plátano* as his staple food more than on corn or manioc. He frequently lives in a poor *barrio* in town, commuting by burro or by foot to his farm where he may stay for several days. Typically, the coastal peasant has had years of experience as a wage laborer on other people's land. Through saving, establishing a good reputation as a *padre de familia*, and obtaining credit through a *fiador* or cosigner he has been able to purchase his own land. He himself and his neighbors consider him a successful man.

Unlike the highlanders, the coastal peasants are consumers of cannabis, which they frequently grow for their own use and for petty trade with landless day laborers. Cannabis grown in small quantities in the lowlands is used by the long-term cannabis user. Highlands commercial growers produce for the urban internal and international markets in large quantities on a *hectárea* or more whereas the coastal peasant often grows no more than a few plants.

In summary, the cannabis production-distribution-consumption cycle involves groups drawn from both the major subcultures of the community. Andean peasants in the lower altitude valleys of the Sierra Nevada are the commercial cultivators. Consumers are drawn from the wage laborers and coastal peasants; the latter also being small-scale cultivators and the former frequently petty merchandisers. Large scale merchandisers are members of the upper sector of the coastal subculture and among the most respected of townspeople. The place of these groups in the organization of community life is best demonstrated by Figure 1. It is important to note that these groups are not drawn from deviant, parasitic, or marginal elements of the community.

IV. CANNABIS CYCLE

Cultivation:

Today cannabis is farmed in secret; the peasant generally plants his

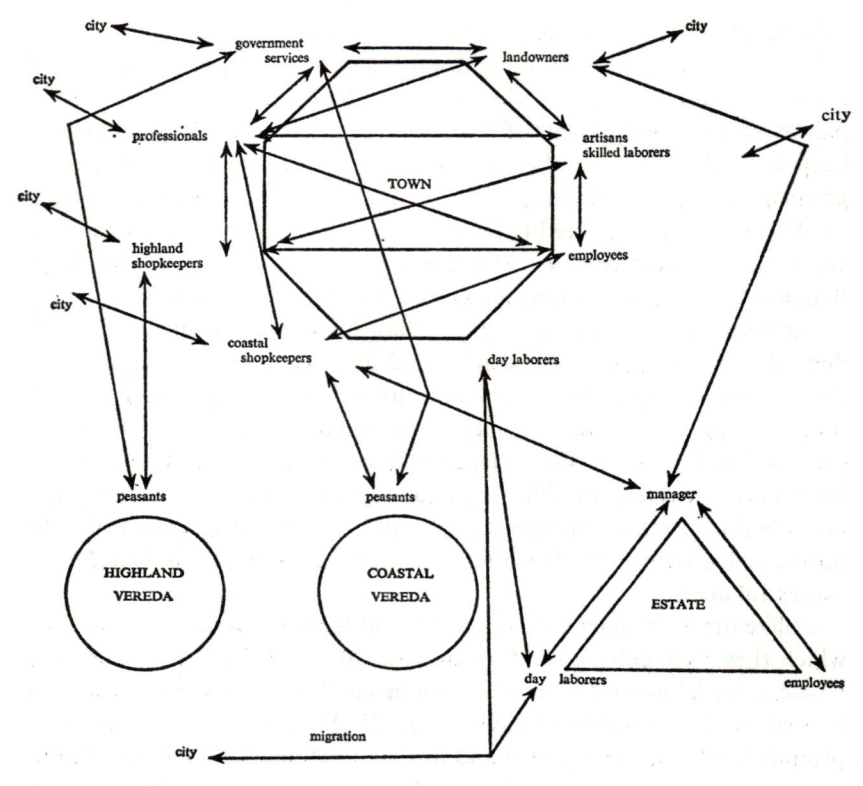

Figure 1. Reciprocal social and economic relations between town, estate, highland *vereda,* and coastal *vereda* (including the exchange of personnel, goods, money, and services)

seeds just as the March rains begin, usually on an isolated part of his farm hidden by dense underbrush. Commercial growers in the highlands first germinate their seeds in a germination box made of four logs placed in a square surrounding well cleaned and mixed soil. Seeds are simply scattered on the surface of the prepared soil. A thick layer of commercial ant-killer is spread around the perimeter. The plants are thinned, selected, and transplanted in about 15 or 20 days to the peasants' *rosa*. The *rosa* is a mixed garden plot, always located on the steep hillsides, and moved every few years in the pattern of swidden land use. When cannabis is included in the *rosa* it is planted at the lowest point on the hillside, below the tall corn plants, far from the numerous paths which criss-cross the ridge tops, to conceal the growing crop.

Coastal peasants do not utilize the germination box; they simply plant cannabis seeds in the same way they plant corn. A hole is poked in the prepared soil with a machete and covered with the foot after several seeds are inserted. Several weeks later the smaller of the plants are thinned out, leaving the healthiest looking plants to grow to maturity. When asked about this difference in planting techniques coastal informants explain that the *cachacos* use a germination box because they are all from Norte de Santander. In that region tobacco is an important cash crop, and since tobacco seeds are quite small a germination box is needed. But there is no need for this with cannabis. The coastal peasants conclude that *cachacos* plant as they do out of habit.

Peasants classify the parts of the plant in two categories: *la mona*, a mixture of resin and small leaves from the tops of the mature female plants, and *la hoja*, the larger lower leaves of both male and female plants. *La mona* is sold for around 200 to 300 pesos a pound and *la hoja* brings about 100 pesos a pound. The merchandiser usually doubles the prices paid to the peasant when the product is retailed. The growing season runs from March until August or September, or five to six months to obtain *la mona*. Consumers universally prefer *la mona* for smoking.

It should be noted, however, that *la mona* is a generic term for cannabis as well as the terms *la amarilla* and *marihuana*.[7] Consumers usually refer to cannabis simply as *la mona* or *ella*, regardless of the category being consumed. One never hears the Spanish *cáñamo* or hemp applied to cannabis in the *municipio*; *cáñamo* signifies a lasso of *cabuya* fiber in this region of Colombia.

Harvesting the cannabis crop takes several days of intense labor. The plants are first girdled by cutting off a ring of bark around the circumference of the trunk. In a few days the leaves begin to fall off. These are either gathered and packed for sale as they fall or are picked just before falling. When all the leaves have fallen the tip of the female plant, called *la mota*, is harvested. In this fashion the leaves are air and sun dried before sale or consumption. This process of harvesting is believed to increase the potency of the marihuana: by girdling the trunk, informants state, one conserves the *leche* or sap of the plant and this is believed to rise to the tip of the plant since it cannot flow to the roots.

At least two varieties of cannabis are recognized by highland commercial growers and lowland consumers and petty merchants. Samples of

[7] The word cannabis is frequently heard among the offspring of upper sector families who experiment with cannabis and other drugs. A discussion of this group is omitted here, since the phenomenon is related to the influence of American and European hippie groups and clearly not related to customary patterns of long-term use in the lower sector of the *municipio*. For similar reasons, a discussion of cannabis smoking by lawyers, dentists, agronomists, and other professional people in the urban centers is also omitted.

these varieties have been collected for botanical and chemical analysis.[8]

Some commercial growers report a variety of cannabis they call *patagallina* or chicken foot. This is said to be an inferior grade, but in reality appears to be *Hibiscus cannabinus* L. or *kenaf* (Pate *et al*. 1954). During the 1950's a landowner in the *municipio* operated a fiber industry under contract with the United States Department of Agriculture. This operation was closed down in 1961, but plants can still be found in the area. *Patagallina* seems to resemble cannabis in leaf form and stature only, which does not preclude its sale as cannabis. This mistaken identification of *kenaf* as cannabis and the inappropriate cultivation techniques imported from the interior of the country both point to the *cachaco* cultivators as relatively new innovators. While the presence of cannabis among coastal people seems traditional, it is probably a market-induced phenomenon among the highlanders.

Distribution:

There are two separate distribution systems which correspond to the two systems of cultivation. The first is the market induced system, involving highland commercial growers and wealthy coastal buyers and retailers. This system moves large quantities of marihuana to the cities of the coast, often for export to the United States.[9] The second or local system involves no wealthy upper sector middlemen but is specific to lower section day laborers and coastal peasants. The coastal peasant produces cannabis in small quantities and day laborers who are consumers also purchase some for resale to fellow day laborers in the town and countryside. A single plant may produce two pounds of *la mona* and up to twenty pounds of *la hoja*, so that a peasant who grows around 10 plants will frequently be able to sell several pounds and still conserve enough for his own needs.

The homes of day laborers who act as distributors are often centers where users assemble to smoke marihuana, talk and gossip, and make small purchases. Such sites are called *caletas* which means small bays or coves in nautical terminology. Since these sites are frequented by a number of people, informants were asked how secrecy and some degree of security from law enforcement officials was maintained. They explained

---

[8] Professor Richard Evans Schultes, Harvard University, has agreed to examine samples collected by the author from the plantations in the Sierra Nevada de Santa Marta. Chemical studies of these plants will also be undertaken in the near future.

[9] Quantities of marihuana are confiscated by the police in the major cities of the coast as reported by *El Tiempo*, May 8, 1973, *El Espectador*, April 12, 1973, *El Espectador*, January 5, 1973, *El Espectador*, November 19, 1972, *El Tiempo*, June 13, 1973, *El Diario del Caribe*, May 26, 1973.

that the police are frequently consumers of cannabis, and that those who are not accept bribes quite readily. Secondly, the petty merchant usually gets on well with his neighbors because he gives them small loans of perhaps 5 or 10 pesos, which are seldom repaid. Such a good neighbor policy is considered a business cost to be absorbed.

Consumption:

Figure 2 shows the varieties of cannabis use in the *municipio* and the groups in which each form occurs. These will be discussed separately.

Figure 2. Forms of cannabis use in the *municipio*

Forms of cannabis use	Subcultural groups
Mixed with rum or *aguardiente* and applied to the skin for pain of joints and muscles	All groups of the coastal subculture
Smoked to reduce fatigue during work Smoked to relax and socialize with friends Smoked to augment sexual intercourse Smoked in a program of health maintenance Green leaves crushed and rubbed on the skin for treatment of pain Boiled with water and raw sugar and given to infants for excessive crying	Day laborers and peasants of the coastal subculture
Not used in any form	Highland subculture

There is widespread belief in the efficacy of cannabis mixed with rum or *aguardiente* and applied to the skin for pain of joints and muscles. The practice is present throughout the coastal subculture. A puzzling fact is that this mixture and its use for relief of pain is absent from the treatments reported by coastal *curanderos* or herbalists. The practice of mixing various plant parts with rum or *aguardiente* is common for the treatment of pain, snake bite, and to stop bleeding; but in all cases the mixture is to be drunk, not applied to the skin. Perhaps the explanation is to be found in the fact that herbalists are specialists, for example, in snake bite treatment or protection from evil curses. In contrast, the knowledge that cannabis can be used for treatment of pain is widespread and not the unique property of the *curanderos*. *Curanderos* normally keep their formulas secret. And it will be remembered that the use of tobacco in this form is quite old on the coast, and the medicinal use of cannabis might derive from this practice (Patiño 1967).

The use of cannabis for health maintenance is also reported (Fabrega and Manning 1972). Cases cited involve men of advanced age who smoked all their lives and have enjoyed excellent health; they state that smoking marihuana is generally good for one's health. The green leaves are crushed and rubbed on the skin for treatment of minor pain and cannabis is mixed with water and raw sugar and brewed as a tea given to infants to stop excessive crying.

Smoking cannabis is restricted to the lower sector of the coastal subculture, composed of landless day laborers and peasants as reported for the Caribbean (Rubin, Comitas, this volume). In all cases cannabis is smoked in cigarette form. It is first air and sun dried; green cannabis is said to "inflame the head." It is smoked pure, unmixed with other substances. The cigarette is rolled in commercial tobacco cigarette paper, other kinds of paper burning too hot, and it is generally short and thin. Probably no more than a gram is contained in these cigarettes.

The coastal group is composed of unrelated males, the exact composition of which may change from week to week; it is in this group that marihuana is consumed. A group contracted to clean an irrigation ditch, for example, will assemble in the morning on the estate after catching rides or walking from town. They assemble to sharpen their machetes, talk about girls, dances and drunks, and to smoke a marihuana cigarette.[10] The cigarette is shared among the men just as tobacco cigarettes are often shared. They receive work directions from the estate manager and set about their task. Around 10:00 o'clock in the morning they may pause again for another marihuana cigarette, they continue working until noon. They bring with them in their *mochilas*, or woven carrying bags of *cabuya*, several nesting aluminium pots with a hot stew prepared in the morning by wives, sisters, or daughters. After lunch they stretch out under the branches of a tree for siesta. Work resumes around 2:00 p.m. and another marihuana cigarette is smoked. Around 4:00 or 5:00 p.m. they will start for home. In the evening they may meet neighbors and friends at a bar for beer, rum, or *aguardiente*. But the friends with whom they drink may or may not be the same with whom they spent the daylight hours working.

Marihuana cigarettes are not always consumed by the workers, de-

---

[10] The marihuana cigarette is called a *cigarrillo* just as are tobacco cigarettes. There is little evidence of a special argot among cannabis consumers.

pending upon the availability which in turn depends upon limited resources. But some informants report that they are unable to work without smoking marihuana; they have no *fuerza* or force and they lack the necessary *ánimo* or spirit for working. Not all workers smoke, nor are they encouraged to do so. I have never heard disapproval of the practice expressed in work groups: "he is an addict" nonsmokers will say, but they do not avoid smokers in town or treat them in any special fashion. At work it is impossible to tell one who is a smoker from one who is not, unless consumption is observed.[11]

On the basis of interviews and observations, from 5 to 7 marihuana cigarettes are consumed in a day, only one is smoked at a time. These are not passed from person to person, but each individual smokes the same way he normally smokes a tobacco cigarette, no effort apparently being made to retain the smoke in the lungs (Partridge 1973). Coastal peasants consume cannabis in the same manner and in the work context, but they smoke alone on their farms since they are no longer working in a nonkin male group. One old man is locally known as the *Rey de la marihuana*. He is an adobe brick maker who uses cannabis during his work; he is said to be the best brick maker in town by consumers and nonconsumers alike, turning out more brick faster than any other brick maker. Smokers credit this to the effects of cannabis to *quita el cansancio* or reduce fatigue, to increase *fuerza* or force, to make a man *incansable* or tireless, and to give *ánimo* or spirit for working. Such words and phrases are the most frequent responses to questions regarding the effects perceived by the user. A few informants report that they smoke marihuana to relax, to think about and resolve some problem that is troubling them, or to go to sleep at night, but these are not mentioned as frequently as those connected with work. Laborers on construction sites in coastal cities are also reported to smoke marihuana in the morning before going to work and during their *agua de panela* (water mixed with raw sugar) breaks during the day.

While most informants also report using marihuana for leisure activities such as fiestas, I have not observed this with any frequency. Several informants who live and work in the *municipio* confirm the report that in Cartagena where they were born, there are social clubs for smoking marihuana and leisure activity (U.S. Department of Health, Education, and Welfare 1972). And in fact all the female smokers interviewed were

---

[11] Dr. Joseph Schaeffer has pointed out that detailed study of video tapes made of smokers and nonsmokers in Jamaica reveal that there are subtle behavioral modifications among the smokers. But this can not be detected by the observer (Schaeffer, this volume).

born and grew up in the city of Cartagena or in the department of Bolívar. In the department of Magdalena, in which the *municipio* is located, the incidence of female smokers is quite low, and there are no social clubs where cannabis is smoked during leisure activities.

In reality, alcohol is the drug of choice on festive days in this region of Colombia, being an essential element in the reciprocal relationships among male laborers (Gutierrez de Pineda 1958). Informants mention that cannabis is cheaper than alcohol and is preferred for this reason. They also report that cannabis is better than alcohol for sexual relations because the former does not inhibit sexual desire or capability in contrast to alcohol, but the same informants can often be found drinking at the stores and bars in town.

Female smokers are rare in Magdalena; however, one female informant reports that women habitually smoke greater amounts of cannabis than do men. She informed me she smoked up to twenty marihuana cigarettes, each day, every day. Little information is available at present concerning the socialization of females into cannabis use patterns.

Males are socialized into use during late adolescence, with the initiation of adult work patterns. Informants report learning to smoke in the male work group; only one learned in the context of a fiesta activity. Such learning seems to depend largely upon individual interaction patterns and friendships, since most informants are the only adult males in their families who smoke cannabis. No informant reported that his father used the drug. This is not surprising given the nonkin composition of the male work group where socialization takes place.

Informants began smoking cannabis between the ages of 12 and 22, and have between 11 and 31 years of experience; all are male heads of households which they support entirely. Those informants who are coastal peasants are all former day laborers, as is typical of the group. Through saving and obtaining a cosigner they have been able to establish credit and buy a piece of land or they are *colonos* who for years have sucessfully supported a family from the land they took over and planted. For these peasants, socialization into cannabis use patterns began in the nonkin male work group. Cannabis consumers are thus best described as nonkin networks of landless day laborers, some of whom eventually obtain land.

Informants report that a person who is *debil en la cabeza* or weak in the head should not use cannabis. They observe that the drug often "turns people crazy," but these are said to be people with "weak heads." Only one informant reported experiencing negative effects which he described as a feeling of sleepiness; he recommended cold water poured over the head, eating green bananas, and drinking hot black coffee as remedies.

No informant reported visual distortion, seeing strange things, or having hallucinations while smoking cannabis. This is remarkable given the belief, common in the United States, that cannabis grown in this region of Colombia is one of the most potent varieties. One informant reported that the novice often feels hunger, as if he could eat a "whole cow." But this passes when one learns the effects of the plant.

Consumption patterns of other drugs should also be considered, given the high correlation reported in the United States between the use of alcohol and tobacco and cannabis (U.S. Department of Health, Education, and Welfare 1971; U.S. National Commission on Marihuana and Drug Abuse 1972). Alcohol is easily the most popular of all drugs used by all subcultural groups in the *municipio*. There are four patterns of use: (1) reciprocal buying and mutual consumption among friends and business associates at cockfights, during the sale of animals, at leisure at stores and bars, etc.; (2) individual consumption by peasants and coastal day laborers in the morning before going to work, and to a lesser degree during working hours; (3) two-to three-day *borracheras* or drunk feasts during fiesta days, family celebrations, or on a whim; and (4) ritual drinking at the point of stupefication at weddings, during the nine-day wake, and at other life crisis events.

The first pattern is part of a wider system of social and economic reciprocal relationships. The sale of a cow by a storekeeper to a peasant demands that the former buys drinks for the latter. A landowner attending a cockfight who meets an employee of his, will purchase drinks for both as part of the patron-client relationship. A peasant who had been given good manioc or corn seed will partly repay his peer with a bottle which they can share at a store.

The second pattern is largely confined to agricultural workers and peasants. Alcohol is consumed with the morning black coffee. Infrequently laborers will consume a bottle during the day while working, this is shared among their fellows who are expected to reciprocate later. And a few laborers are so fond of *aguardiente* that a ration of it is part of their contract with an employer.

The third pattern of use is confined to the upper sector of the coastal subculture, since the poor have few resources for binges. The wealthy are famous for drunken feasts; stories are told and retold of conspicuous alcohol consumption, pranks such as chicken stealing and putting soap in food for a wedding party, and extended stints in local brothels.

The fourth pattern is present throughout the highland subculture. Life-crisis events are generally drunken affairs; the wake and the first year anniversary observation of the death of a relative are the most outstanding, calling for the consumption of quantities of food, *chicha* or maize beer, and *aguardiente*.

Tobacco is also consumed by all groups but it is seldom used habitually as in the United States. Rather, cigarettes are frequently purchased one or two at a time. One may go for days smoking only once or twice and then at a fiesta or during an evening of drinking, consume an entire pack with friends. At upper sector feasts tobacco cigarettes are provided together with food and drink for the guests, and on such occasions persons who normally do not smoke tobacco may indulge. Females of all groups in the *municipio* use alcohol and tobacco only rarely; upper sector females take both during fiestas and private parties at home. Females of advanced age in all groups of the coastal subculture smoke tobacco cigars, with the burning end inside their mouths as is the coastal custom.

V. LEGAL PROHIBITION AND SOCIAL VALUES

There are legal and social sanctions against the cultivation, sale, and use of cannabis in Colombia. Decree 1699 of 1964, Article 23, dictates from 2 to 5 years of incarceration for cultivation, elaboration, distribution, sale, use, or possession of cannabis. Article 24 prescribes 1 to 4 years of incarceration for the same offenses regarding any kind of *estupificante* (Torres Ortega 1965). In the *municipio* it is recognized that cannabis is totally prohibited by law. Moreover, social tradition conceives of a *marihuanero* as a lazy, often criminal, vagabond. To be called such is to be called a bum. Neither of these sanctions seems to deter cultivation or use.

Most townspeople, public officials, and growers simply wink an eye at cultivation and say that it brings United States dollars into Colombia. Cannabis cultivation and marketing are placed in the same class as contraband, in which most upper sector persons play some role. As one upper sector woman laughingly told the observer, "[name of *municipio*] produces the best marihuana in the world." Contrary to what might be expected, the commercial growers are drawn from among the most well off and prosperous of the *cachaco* peasants. Some cultivators are youthful adults, but most are well advanced in age, well established, and highly respected household heads.

Consumption of cannabis is another matter. Smoking is a lower sector activity. All instances in which I have heard persons called *marihuaneros* have involved upper sector families reprimanding their offspring or gossiping about other families. One never hears the word in lower sector families. This label appears to be a stigma applied to poorer persons in general by upper sector families, since the people they gossip about and label *marihuaneros* are often not cannabis consumers. And the true identities of long-term users are well known in the *municipio*, by everyone from the mayor to the police.

Such negative stigmas, however, tell us little about what people actually value. For this reason the anthropologist examines values as they are reflected in social interaction, rather than ideology, spoken and written words, and formal law (Kluckholn 1954). We have seen that many lower-sector males value cannabis as a supplement to work, leisure, sex, for the treatment of pain, and in health maintenance.

Analysis of the interaction patterns typical of each subculture brings into sharp focus the significant differences between them. The subculture in which the consumer lives is characterized by a mobile subsistence pattern, nonkin male work groups, stem family structure, and wage labor. The subculture which does not contribute consumers (although there is ample opportunity since they produce tons of cannabis) is characterized by a sedentary subsistence pattern, the kinbased male work group, the three-generation extended family structure, and swidden agriculture.

These are only the central differences, many others exist. Perhaps the most telling difference is that of mobile versus immobile settlement patterns. The coastal subculture concentrated in the towns and cities is an urban oriented population. Even when living in the rural area geographical mobility is normal and urban work experience is common. The nonkin male work group, adolescent peer groups, and the stem family are all structures which conform well to the migratory subsistence pattern. In contrast, the highland subculture scattered about on dispersed individual family farms offers little opportunity for mobility, cooperation among nonkin, the formation of adolescent peer groups, or the budding off of nuclear units. Mobility data from the *municipio* confirm this pattern. In a rural hamlet surveyed only 2 of 25 male household heads and only 5 of 25 female mates were born in the *municipio*. Only 4 household heads had worked solely in the *municipio*, whereas 21 had worked in other *municipios* and other departments. Of the latter, 10 had worked in cities of the coast. In a town *barrio* surveyed, 23 of 76 household heads were born in the *municipio*, and 36 of 76 mates were born in the *municipio*. Of 76 household heads, 26 had worked in other departments of the coast and 33 had worked in the cities.

The process of migration begins in the late adolescence or at about the age of 18 when a young man frequently leaves home and obtains wage labor where his travels lead him. Typically, the worker settles down with a mate some years later. He is brought in and out of contact with his family members, reciprocal relations with nonkin evolving as he travels. Almost always he will come home for fiestas and holidays, traveling 100 or more kilometers.

Socialization to cannabis use takes place during this migratory phase in the life of a coastal worker. All informants have histories of wage labor in other departments and cities. Several have had a few years of experience working in the banana zone; some have been able to save money, maintain a good reputation, and obtain credit and are now landowners living a sedentary existence. Others merely acquired mates and children and settled in one of the towns discovered during their youth. They all learned to smoke cannabis as young wage laborers.

Since not all coastal peasants and day laborers consume cannabis we must ask what are the differences observed among users and nonusers. Briefly, none have been observed. Studies of other Colombian user populations have pointed to factors such as mobility, single marital status, marginality, unemployment, concubinage, criminality, lack of housing, lack of children, low salary, low productivity, illiteracy, family disintegration, and segregation from the larger society as characteristic of cannabis users (Ardila 1965). Interestingly enough, nonusers and users of the day laborers and coastal peasants are more alike with regard to these factors than different. About half of all day laborers live in concubinage, more than a third are illiterate, and the rest have only 1 to 3 years of primary schooling; all earn low wages and have no resources of productivity aside from their backs. All workers in the coastal subculture are mobile early in life, unemployment is generally confined to the aged and is absent among cannabis informants; criminality is rare and no cannabis informant has ever been in jail; and cannabis consumers are no more segregated from society than are nonusers. Lack of housing is atypical of users and nonusers and some users have more than one house. Single marital status is not typical of any group in the *municipio* and a lack of children is unheard of. "Marginality" and "family disintegration" are concepts that cannot be compared among populations without definition. If marginality means an absence of the social and economic reciprocal relationships typical of the community, then cannabis consumers are not marginal. If family disintegration means some form of family life other than that typical of the community, cannabis consumers do not live in disintegrated families. In short, cannabis consumers and nonconsumers have more in common than in contrast by the light of these characteristics. The fact is that Ardila (1965) depends mostly upon Colombian police records, since there has been no scientific work on cannabis in Colombia.

Some investigators in the United States have posited a relationship between social and psychological stress and cannabis (Ausubel 1970; Partridge 1973). Since the community discussed in this paper has experienced significant social and economic changes that are generally stressful, we should consider this interpretation. Abandonment of the banana zone produced a grave economic crisis throughout the coastal subculture; upper sector families were probably the hardest hit, since they had developed considerable wealth and status due to the presence of the United Fruit Company. It is likely that this crisis is a factor in explaining their present involvement in the internal and international drug traffic. The workers, on the other hand, experienced no dramatic social mobility. It is true that the worker is worse off than at any time during this century, but he did not experience the relative deprivation of upward mobility followed by economic crisis. Moreover, about 11 of 25 families in a rural hamlet had some member working for the Company, while in the town *barrio* only 16 of 76 families had a similar experience, and most day laborers and peasants had worked with the Company for only 1 to 5 years, unlike the grandparental generation in which 30 and more years experience is not uncommon. Cannabis users frequently have had work experience with the Company, but never unbroken by other employment and never for more than a few years. We might relate cannabis consumption to stress if the exit of the Company affected the present generation of coastal workers in general and cannabis consumers in particular, but work histories are varied and rarely dominated by experience with the Company.

In conclusion, the following generalizations are supported by the data:[12]

1. Cannabis cultivation, marketing, and consumption seem to be relatively recent innovations on the north coast of Colombia.

2. Cannabis cultivators, merchants, and consumers, are integral members of the community in which they live, involved in typical community systems of social and economic reciprocities.

3. Long term cannabis consumption (more than ten years) is not observed to engender indolence, parasitism, or marginality, in that the oldest and most experienced consumers have often bettered their social and economic position during their lives.

4. Cannabis consumption is related to mobile patterns of subsistence early in the life of the coastal day laborer, in which there is contact with users and socialization to cannabis use.

---

[12] These conclusions must be considered preliminary, as full analysis will not be possible until all data collection has been completed.

5. Cannabis consumption occurs in the context of the nonkin work group, although users continue to consume the drug alone when patterns of subsistence change.

6. Cannabis consumption does not appear to be related to stressful conditions produced by severe social and economic change in the history of the community.

7. Cannabis merchandising does appear to be related to stressful conditions produced by severe social and economic change in the history of the community.

8. Cannabis merchandising is governed by two distinct systems of distribution, a market induced system involving Andean peasant growers and wealthy upper sector coastal buyers, and a local system involving small vendors among the day laborers and peasant growers of the coastal subculture.

9. Alcohol is the traditional and actual drug of choice for business negotiation, social relations, and religious celebration. Since a bottle of alcohol costs a full day's wage for a day laborer, cannabis may be related to economic deprivation resulting from exploitative wage levels.

10. The use of tobacco for treatment of pain and reduction of fatigue are traditional, and cannabis has been adopted to serve these same functions; this suggests that cannabis use may be related to tobacco use in the coastal subculture, and may have been substituted for tobacco at some time in the past.

REFERENCES

ALARCON, JOSÉ C.
  1963 *Compendio de histoíra del departamento de la Magdalena de 1525 hasta 1895.* Bogotá: Editorial El Voto Nacional.
ARANÚJO, ALCEN MAYNARD
  1959 *Medicina rustica*, Brasiliana, V. 300. São Paulo: Compañia Editora Nacional.
ARENSBERG, CONRAD M., SOLON T. KIMBALL
  1965 *Culture and community.* New York: Harcourt Brace Jovanovich Inc.
ARDILA RODRIGUEZ, FRANCISCO
  1965 *Aspectos médico legales y médico sociales de la marihuana.* Thesis Doctoral, Universidad de Madrid, Facultad de Medicina.
AUSUBEL, DAVID P.
  1970 "The psychology of the marihuana smoker," in Erich Goode (ed.), *Marijuana.* New York: Atherton Press.
COMISIÓN DE PLANIFICACIÓN
  1964 *Plan de desarrollo económico y social del departamento de la Magdalena.* Santa Marta.

DEPARTAMENTO ADMINISTRATIVO NACIONAL DE ESTADÍSTICA
1971   *Censo agropecuario*, 1970–1971, Tomo II. Bogotá: Centro Administrativo Nacional via a Eldorado.
DIX, ROBERT
1967   *Colombia: the political dimensions of change*. New Haven: Yale University Press.
FABREGA, HORACIO JR., PETER K. MANNING
1972   "Health maintenance among Peruvian peasants." *Human Organization* 31 (3):243–256.
FALS BORDA, ORLANDO
1955   *Peasant society in the Colombian Andes*. Gainesville: University of Florida Press.
1956   "Fragmentation of holdings in Boyaca, Colombia." *Rural Sociology* 21 (2):158–163.
FLUHARTY, VERNON LEE
1956   *Dance of the millions: military rule and the social revolution in Colombia, 1930–1956*. Pittsburgh: University of Pittsburgh Press.
GARCIÁ MÁRQUEZ, GABRIEL
1970   *One hundred years of solitude*. New York: Harper and Row. (Original title *Cien años de soledad*.)
GUTIERREZ DE PINEDA, VIRGINIA
1958   "Alcohol y cultura en una clase obrera," in Paul Rivet (ed.), *Homenaje*. Bogotá: Editorial ABC.
KAMALAPRIJA, V.
1965   *Estudio descriptivo de la estructura del mercado del banano Colombiano para la exportación*. Bogotá: Instituto Latinoamericano de Marcadeo Agrigola.
KLUCKHOLN, CLYDE
1954   "Values and value orientation in the theory of action," in Talcott Parsons and Edwards Shils (eds.), *Toward a general theory of action*. Cambridge: Harvard University Press.
MONTAÑA CUELLAR, DIEGO
1963   *Colombia: país formal y país real*. Buenos Aires: Editorial Platina.
PATE, JAME B., CHARLES C. SEALE, EDWARD O. GANGSTAD
1954   Varietal studies of *kenaf*, Hibiscus cannabinus L., in South Florida. *Agronomy Journal* 46 (2):75–77.
PATIÑO, VICTOR MANUEL
1967   *Plantas cultivadas y animales domésticos en América Equinoccial: plantas miscelaneas*, Tomo III. Cali: Imprenta Departamental.
1969   *Plantas cultivadas y animales domesticos en America Equinoccial: plantas introducidas*, Tomo IV. Cali: Imprenta Departamental.
PARTRIDGE, WILLIAM L.
1973   *The hippie ghetto: the natural history of a subculture*. New York: Holt Rinehart and Winston Inc.
REICHEL-DOLMATOFF, GERARDO
1951   *Datos historico-culturales sobre las tribus de la antigua gobernación de Santa Marta*. Bogotá: Banco de la Republica.

SEALE, C. C., J. F. JOYNER, J. B. PATE
   1952   *Agronomic studies of fiber plants: jute, sisal, henequen, fureraea, hemp, and other miscellaneous types.* Gainesville: University of Florida Agricultural Experiment Stations Bulletin 590.

TORRES ORTEGA, JORGE
   1965   *Código penal y código de procedimiento penal.* Bogotá: Editorial Temes.

U.S. NATIONAL COMMISSION ON MARIHUANA AND DRUG ABUSE
   1972   *Marihuana: a signal of misunderstanding.* New York: Signet.

U.S. DEPARTMENT OF HEALTH, EDUCATION AND WELFARE. NATIONAL INSTITUTE OF MENTAL HEALTH.
   1971   *Marihuana and Health: a Report to the Congress from the Secretary.* Washington: U.S. Government Printing Office.
   1972   *Marihuana and Health: Second Annual Report to Congress from the Secretary.* Washington: U.S. Government Printing Office.

VERGARA Y VELASCA, F. J.
   1901   *Nueva geografía de Colombia,* Tomo I. Bogotá: Republica de Colombia.

WAGLEY, CHARLES, EDUARDO GALVÃO
   1949   *The Tenetehara Indians of Brazil.* New York: Columbia University Press.

Patterns of Marihuana Use in Brazil

HARRY WILLIAM HUTCHINSON

ABSTRACT

The paper examines the type and sources of data concerning *Cannabis sativa* in Brazil, and presents the terminology used in the various regions of Brazil. The types of users of cannabis, methods of use, and a brief examination of the reasons offered for the use of cannabis are presented. The paper ends with suggestions and observations concerning future research in Brazil on this topic.

In a recent article Schultes (1973) pointed out that *Cannabis sativa* has been used throughout its history for five principal purposes: for hempen fibers; for its oil; for its achenes, or "seeds," which man has consumed as a food; for its narcotic properties; and as a therapeutic agent in folk medicine and modern pharmacopoeias. (Ten of the papers in the first session of this conference mentioned cannabis use for pleasure-escape, therefore I think we can add this to Dr. Schultes' list.) In its 400-plus years' history in Brazil it apparently has served primarily for fiber, its narcotic properties and in folk pharmacopoeia as well as pleasure-escape.[1]

Before going any further, I must make a few remarks concerning the data on *Cannabis sativa* in Brazil. There are two striking factors here: 1) the paucity of data concerning the relationship of *Cannabis sativa* and the indigenous population, i.e., Tropical Forest and Marginal Indians: the entire Colonial and Imperial Period, 1549 through 1899; and contemporary Brazil, 1899 to the present. 2) the types of data available: these consist of medical, psychiatric, botanical, and "law and order" data. There is a

This work was supported by a grant from NIH # Sub 4, 5 SO5 RR07022-07.

[1] Although I have found references to use of cannabis in folk medicine, I have found none to indicate its use in modern medicine. However, it might still be a component in the prescriptions of Homeopathic Drug shops, an aspect I suggest be investigated.

conspicuous lack of social science data, written by either Brazilian or foreign authors. Furthermore most of the data is prejudiced against cannabis.

Let us first look at data concerning the use of cannabis by indigenous peoples. There is a general consensus that cannabis was imported to Brazil sometime in the early sixteenth century, probably by slaves brought from the west coast of Africa and particularly from Angola. This would indicate, and many authors have substantiated the fact, that cannabis is not a plant native to the New World, at least to South America. However, it must not be forgotten that South American Indians had a wide range of hallucinogenic drugs, especially tobacco, which they used in ritual and medicinal instances. There is very little mention of Tropical Forest Indians having adopted cannabis even much later on in the acculturation period. An examination of the Human Relations Area Files reveals little or no mention of cannabis use amongst Indians living in what is now Brazil. The same is true for the *Handbook of South American Indians*. One mention of the use of hashish is made by Wagley and Galvão (1949) in their study of the Tenetehara. For the remainder of this paper, we will have to disregard the use of cannabis among Brazilian indigenous peoples.

As for the Colonial and Imperial Periods, the data although scarce is interesting from a diffusionist point of view. The major stream of thought held by Brazilian authors on the subject, as exemplified by Rosado (1958), indicates that cannabis was brought to Brazil from Africa starting at approximately 1549, if not before. 1549 is the outstanding date used by most authors because of a decree issued by Don João III of Portugal authorizing newly established sugar cane planters to import to up 1200 slaves per sugar mill. Rosado (1958), quoting Pio Correa, indicates that cannabis seeds were brought to Brazil in cloth dolls which were tied to the rag tag clothing worn by the slaves. He further states, that cannabis was planted and adapted itself well to the entire area from the state of Bahia all the way up to the state of Amazonas. (This is, in part, because slaves went to the states of Bahia, Alagoas, Sergipe, and Pernambuco in great numbers. No explanation is offered for the implantation of cannabis in the states of Ceará, Rio Grande del Norte, Maranhão, Pará and Amazonas. It should be noted that Maranhão, Pará and Amazonas had exceedingly little African influence through the medium of slavery.) Most authors disclaim cannabis use in southern Brazil until this century, in spite of evidence to the contrary.

There are two other scraps of information pertaining to the Colonial Period which are of interest. The first is a brief piece of information cited by Lucena, Ataide and Coelho (1958). This concerns the work of one Garcia de Orta, a Portuguese writer who made one of the first descriptions of cannabis use in India as early as 1556. (I do not know where this was first published, however a second edition of his works was re-edited in 1872 by the National Press, Lisbon, Portugal.)

A second scrap of information is even more interesting. It concerns the use of cannabis in the Portuguese Royal Court in Rio de Janeiro and in Lisbon. The reference is brief; it concerns Dona Carlota Joaquina, the wife of Emperor Don João VI, King of Portugal and Brazil. In 1808, the Portuguese Royal Court, threatened by Napoleon's invasion of the Iberian Peninsula, escaped to Brazil, settling in Rio de Janeiro. The court spent approximately six years in Brazil, returning to Portugal at the end of the Napoleonic Wars. Queen Carlota Joaquina was dying in 1817. Her favorite Negro slave, Felisbino, who had accompanied her to Portugal, usually provided her with cannabis. On her death bed, she asked Felisbino to "bring me an infusion of the fibers of *diamba do amazonas*, with which we sent so many enemies to hell." Felisbino made an infusion of cannabis and arsenic and gave it to her. It is recounted by Assis Cintra (1934) that upon taking the infusion, Dona Carlota felt no pain because of the analgesic action of *diamba*, "thereupon taking up her guitar and singing," later dying. (Her slave Felisbino had the same end, drinking *diamba* infusion with arsenic.)

Another interesting piece of information during the Colonial Period concerned the prohibition of "the sale and use of *pito do Pango* as well as keeping it in public establishments." This was an edict of the Municipal Council of Rio de Janeiro issued in October, 1830. Although most authors point to the concentration of cannabis use in northeastern Brazil, it would appear to have been in considerable use in Rio de Janeiro to have had the Municipal Council pass restrictive measures. The Edict of 1830 in Rio also prohibited the importation of marihuana but whether from other countries/colonies or Brazilian provinces isn't clear.

A last indication of the use of cannabis in Brazil during this Colonial Period is offered by Gilberto Freyre in his book *O nordeste*. He points out that throughout the northeast of Brazil in the principal period of the sugarcane *engenho*, during the yearly periods of inactivity between harvests, "the White man filled his empty days with perfumed cigars while the Black man smoked *maconha* for its dreams and torpor!" The *senhor de engenho* allowed the Blacks to plant and grow *maconha* in between the rows of sugarcane (Moreno 1958).

At this juncture, I would like to propose that cannabis perhaps had two routes of entry into Brazil rather than only one. It may well be that

African slaves brought cannabis seeds to Brazil; perhaps even the Portuguese sailors brought it as well, and perhaps the habit did grow among slaves and spread to the free peoples in the northeastern part of Brazil.

Perhaps, however, the Portuguese themselves brought cannabis from India either directly to Portugal where it was already in use by the Portuguese Court; or else the Portuguese took it to Brazil and introduced it to the Court during its short stay in Brazil. If not, they probably would not have referred to is as *diamba do amazonas*.

In terms of what I'm calling contemporary Brazil, i.e., the twentieth century, the amount of data increases and becomes somewhat more specific. If we attempt to group the data for this latter period it seems to fall into four categories: 1) botanical, 2) medical, 3) psychiatric, 4) law and order.

The major source of data for this period is "A collection of Brazilian writings on Maconha," a compilation of original research and reports dating from 1915 through 1956. This collection was re-edited in 1958. The collection consists of 29 reports. Three things should be pointed out about this outstanding collection of materials:

1. It spans a long period during which *maconha* was taken for granted as being a "vice." The adjectives most used are "viciados," "criminosos," "vagabundos" and "maloqueiros" (crazy people).

2. A second trend demonstrated by this particular collection is that the works spanning the period 1915 through 1956 tend to be highly incestuous: i.e., to a great extent the authors of succeeeding articles quote almost verbatim the authors who preceded them, each adding only a little to the gradual accumulation of knowledge.

3. A third phenomenon demonstrated by this collection of data is that interest in activities surrounding the growth and expansion of cannabis use has always come in cycles. We can see this starting in 1830.

Coming up to this century, there have been several cycles of interest in the phenomena surrounding cannabis. The cycles can be dated at 1915, the late 1930's, the mid-1940's and the 1950's. (Late materials available to us from the sixties and the early seventies follow the same pattern.) The cycles alluded to tend to follow periods of culture stress, such as war, depression and its aftermath, and rapid socio-economic development.

At this point, I would like to move on to a list of the terminology for cannabis found in contemporary Brazil. A list of thirty major synonyms follows, some of those synonyms carrying variations in spelling, such as a change from 'd' to 'r' to 'l' or to 't,' etcetera. These minor changes I would suggest are local dialect changes.

Local Brazilian Terms for Marihuana or Cannabis sativa

maconha (maconha and makiah in West Africa — maconha in Brasil)	moconha	cangonha
fumo d'Angola	maconha-fumo de Angola	
diamba − r − L	Tiamba	
riamba		
liamba		
pango −	pungo	
cânhamo −	cânhamo da India	
planta da felicidade		
dirijo		
birra −	cha de birra or bilra	
Tiquira		
umburu −	umbaru	
atchi e erva		
mariguana		
rafi		
fininho		
basiado		
morrao		
cheio		
entorpecente		
erva		
fumo brabo		
gongo		
malva		
fêmea		
maricas		
Rosa Maria		
D. Juanita		
bang		
Kif		
Haschich		
fumo de caboclo		

Here I must add a personal anthropological note: I was a member of the "foreign" group which allegedly used marihuana in the mid-forties, while I was in the northeastern part of Brazil with the U.S. Navy. (See below for further discussion.) Never during those two years was I approached nor introduced to cannabis use nor the vocabulary concerning it.

My first piece of anthropological fieldwork was done in a rural sugar-cane planting community in the state of Bahia in 1950–1951. I have gone back over my original field notes and have found no mention of any of the synonyms used for cannabis in any of the folk pharmaceutical recipes which I collected. Nor did I knowingly smoke nor see anyone else smoke cannabis.

However, on the basis of the research for this paper and thinking back to my first field trip as well as to subsequent field trips, I now understand why the inhabitants of the interior regions of the state of Bahia and other northeastern states used to smile knowingly at my constant smoking of a pipe. In fact, the pipe was consistently referred to as "um pito." Little did I know! (Pipe smoking of tobacco was most unusual.)

Earlier this year, while in Brasil on a short field survey in connection with the preparation of this paper, I specifically asked informants in the community which I have been studying for 23 years whether they knew of, about, or used cannabis in any form or under any circumstances, i.e., either medicinal or ritual (Afro-Brazilian cultism). The answer this year always consisted of a horrified "no!" It appeared this year that everybody questioned knew or had heard of cannabis but no one in "my community" ever used it. I should point out that denial would be the expected answer this year in view of the extraordinarily restrictive measures being taken by Brazilian law enforcement agencies.

Now let me pass to patterns of use of cannabis in Brazil. Here there are two categories of information: who and how. Who – we have already seen during the Colonial Period that marihuana had penetrated to the top-ranking social strata, i.e., the Royal Court. From that particular period up until the second half of the twentieth century, there is little or no information available. However, during the past few decades, it has been pointed out that upper class Brazilians have used cannabis. For example, the intellectual elite is obliquely charged with the use of cannabis. However, there seems to be little proof in terms of the research done. And, in fact, Dr. de Pinho has pointed out that in the late fifties he was indeed unable to gather data on cannabis use from this particular group.

Another group of "upper class" individuals who have used cannabis consists of those scientists interested in research on cannabis. In this century, a number of Brazilian scientists have experimented with cannabis, following the works of French, British, and American scientists in this particular phase of their activity.

Surprisingly enough (at least to me) at one point, i.e., primarily the forties, it was felt that "foreigners" of two types in Brazil were using cannabis: The first type were those foreigners who lived more or less permanently in Brazil (Cordeiro de Farias 1958). The second type was considered to be composed of those servicemen who were stationed in Brazil during the Second World War (Cordeiro de Farias 1958).

In contemporary times, the major use of cannabis is assigned to the lower class. By lower class is meant those who are unemployed or who are employed in certain specific physically difficult occupations, such as canoemen, fishermen, stevedores, as well as vagabonds, and "disturbers of the peace." The list can also be extended to include prostitutes (Moreno 1958). It is interesting to note that throughout all the articles in the collection, it is pointed out that women are not major users of cannabis. This is somewhat in contradiction to the star case of Dona Carlota and to a rather numerous population of prostitutes. Apparently outside of the nobility and the prostitutes, women do not use marihuana: is this simply *machismo?*

At least two processes concerned with cannabis use seem to be at work here: pleasure (or escapism) and pharmaceutical use.

Marihuana is smoked, according to the literature, in the military barracks and in prisons, to alleviate boredom and despair. Other accounts talk of the *Club de Diambistas* (Pereira 1958) wherein individuals, not specified as to class, gathered weekly to enjoy the delights of marihuana. (The bibliographic insinuation is that these individuals are of lower class.) They functioned much in the way the French Club des Hachichins did in the middle of the last century in France. No explanation is offered in any of the literature for this particular phenomenon.

The use of cannabis in Afro-Brazilian cultism (variously known as *Candomblé, Xango, Macumba,* and *Umbanda*) is disputed. Early accounts assumed it was used, even though cult leaders disclaimed it. Dr. Rubim de Pinho (see paper in this symposium) points out that it is not used in Bahian cultism. To this, I must add my own field experience, which indicates non-use of cannabis in cultism at least in Bahia, whether ritualistically or for pleasure.

Now let us move on to the methods of use of cannabis in Brazil. During the last century, in the northeastern part of Brazil, apparently the most common method of use of marihuana was in the *pito,* meaning at that time an adapted version of the water pipe, i.e., either using a calabash or a glass bottle as a water container which filtered and cooled the smoke from the marihuana going to the smokers' mouth. In this century, the *pito* or water pipe is less common, if at all existent. This observer has never seen one in more than twenty years in Brazil.

Today, the most common form is either a regular type with a single stem, in which marihuana is mixed with regular tobacco and smoked, or else the marihuana is rolled into a cigarette. In some instances, marihuana is actually chewed; however in the form of snuff it is almost unknown in Brazil.

When cannabis is used for medicinal reasons, the most common method of preparation is an infusion of tea, i.e., a mixture of marihuana leaves, in hot water which is then stirred and swallowed by the patient. Such an infusion is taken to relieve rheumatism, "female troubles," colic and other common complaints. For toothache, marihuana is frequently packed into and around the aching tooth and left for a period of time, during which it supposedly performs an analgesic function.

Another, and most pleasant way, of taking marihuana is in the form of a *licor*. This is simply placing marihuana leaves into a bottle of *cachaça* and letting it "set." I do not know the extent, at the present time, of this mode of ingesting marihuana. I can report, however, that many who "play at" taking marihuana use this method and are quite apt to spring it on unsuspecting friends and relatives. One becomes "stoned" before one realizes that one has not consumed plain *cachaça*.

I would like to touch on one other point concerning contemporary Brazilian use of marihuana. That is the cultural pattern of the hallucinogenic visions as expressed by those who indulge in marihuana. After a thorough search of the literature, I find two differently patterned cultural responses to the hallucinogenic effects of marihuana among certain classes of Brazilians. First of all are those medical doctors, psychiatrists, and others who have themselves experimented with marihuana and have recorded their observations while under its influence (or rather I should say had others record their experiences). It would seem that the "scientific" circumstances of experimenting with marihuana lead the experimenter to experience hallucinatory states which previous experimenters have already outlined in the literature.

On the other hand, those same investigators interested in marihuana, observing the effects of marihuana on specific populations (meaning in Brazilian terms, individuals interned in prisons or mental hospitals) tend to see or to interpret the hallucinogenic "trip" of the patients or wards as being one which consists of a state of hilarity, disassociation from an overwhelmingly real (poverty) situation, a configuration which suggests it to be an adaptive mechanism employed when the total sociocultural conditions become too much to be borne by those individuals. Here, the lines of interpretation are split: either one calls these people depraved (*viciados; maloqueiros*) or one admits that they are not depraved but are "using" marihuana as a mechanism for survival.

The important point in this section is that I am suggesting that, depending upon the sociocultural status of the individual taking marihuana, the hallucinogenic visions which he or she will experience are quite definitely culturally patterned. I must admit that this statement will require considerable research in the future to see whether it stands up under systematic scrutiny.

In closing, I would like to attempt to make several tenuous points. Marihuana is just one of several crops which seem to have moved from restricted ritualistic and/or medicinal use to "consumer" use, during the history of mankind. Others are sugar, coffee, tobacco, heroin, coca, and alcoholic beverages. So far, only some of these products have been prohibited at certain times. Those are alcohol, cocaine and derivatives, heroin, more recently tobacco, at the present time marihuana, and most recently of all coffee (Maugh 1973). These have been singled out as either health and/or social problems and some escalated into the realm of law and order.

Earlier in time, these products have been labeled as producing craziness, vice, or criminality. Most recently, and especially in the case of stronger hallucinatory drugs, the argument most used against them is that organized crime (and sometimes even "Communism") is responsible for the spread of these agents and their deleterious effects. That is, looked at historically, the reasons for repression of certain plant and/or technological processes have been damned in the name of health, mental health, vice, law-breaking and general societal disintegration.

One wonders about the reasons advanced for the repression of most of these agents. It is difficult to make any sense out of what is presented to us by the various health-law enforcement agencies since their stance is usually strongly biased. We must ask not only the question of why the repression but also why the cyclism of use involved. In the case of marihuana, which has been part of mankind's baggage for a very long time, the cyclism seems to be related to periods of cultural stress, at least in historical periods. For example, certain sectors of populations tend to increase their use of marihuana or other hallucinogenic drugs when the going gets rough. It is quite possible, as Emboden (1972) has pointed out, that the conservative elements of the countries affected by such use realize the potential threat to authority in a liberated younger generation given over to using the exudate of hemp, and for this reason they inveigh against it.

In any country, it is difficult to know the parameters of drug use. For example, Parreiras (1958) points out that usually only those in health or penal institutions are countable. However, it is not difficult to know that periods of stress are upon us. There is, however, no specific link, statistically visible, between drug use and stress. I would hypothesize, however, that any governmental agency or inter-governmental agency, aware of the fact that the system is under stress will declare that drug use is on the increase, is deleterious, and therefore will take steps against it.

To bring this short paper to an end, I would like to suggest further research among populations which are habitual drug users and among populations which are simply "toying with drugs" (i.e., the most recent phenomenon, well described by Dr. R. de Pinho).

At the same time, I must point out the difficulties of unbiased research during a period of cultural stress, at which time forces of law and order seem to be in the ascendancy. Field research is extremely difficult if not impossible. One final note to this paper: I refer again to Schultes' article (1973) in pointing out that man and cannabis have had a very long period of interaction. My own feeling is that cannabis has been with us in spite of many cultural repressions at different historical periods and that because of its long association with man will always be with us as long as there is mankind.

REFERENCES

CINTRA, ASSIS
   1934   "Escândalos de Carlota Joaquina," ed., Civilizacão Brasileira. Rio de Janeiro, cited by Heitor Perés, 73.

CORDEIRO DE FARIAS, R.
   1958   "Relatório Apresentado aos Srs. Membros da Comissão Nacional de Fiscalizacão de Entorpecentes," 108, 112.

EMBODEN, WILLIAM A., JR.
   1972   "Ritual use of Cannabis sativa: a historical ethnographic survey," in *Flesh of the gods*. Edited by Peter T. Furst, 218. New York: Praeger Publishers, Inc.

FREYERE, GILBERTO
   1967   *O nordeste*, 4th edition. Rio de Janiero: Olympio.

LUCENA, JOSÉ, LUÍS ATAIDE, PEDRO COELHO
   1958   "Maconhismo Crônico e Psicoses," 187.

MAUGH, THOMAS H., II
   1973   Coffee and heart disease: is there a link? *Science* 4099 (181):534–535.

MINISTÉRIO DA SAÚDE
   1958   *Maconha, coletânea de trabalhos Brasileiros*, 2nd edition. Rio de Janeiro, Brazil.

MORENO, GARCIA
   1958   "Aspectos do Maconhismo em Sergipe," 156.

PARREIRAS, DÉCIO
   1958   "O Problema Nacional do Canabismo," 387.

PEREIRA, JAYME R.
   1958   "Contribuicoes para o Estudo das Plactas Alucinatórias, particularmente da Maconha," 129.

ROSADO, PEDRO
   1958   "O vício da Liamba no Estudo do Pará-Una Toxicose que ressurge entre nós," 90.

SCHULTES, RICHARD E.
   1973   Man and marihuana. *Natural History* 7 (LXXXII):59.
WAGLEY, CHARLES, EDUARDO GALVÃO
   1949   *The Tenetehara Indians of Brazil*, 41–42. New York: Columbia University Press

The Economic Significance
of Cannabis sativa *in the Moroccan Rif*

ROGER JOSEPH

ABSTRACT

Cannabis sativa, or *kif*, grown in large quantities in the Rif Mountains, is one of the chief cash crops in the area; although illegal, cultivation has flourished as a result of ecological and political factors that delimit the economic potential of northern Morocco. Cannabis serves as a stimulant among the Rif tribal groups and as a means of relieving daily pressure. Unlike drinking alcohol, smoking *kif* does not violate religious sanctions and the use of *kif* remains an integral part of the culture.

In his 1966 paper in *Economic Botany*, Mikuriya discussed the cultivation of *Cannabis sativa* or *kif* in the Rif Mountains of Morocco. The present paper will amplify his statements concerning *kif*, particularly within an economic context, based upon data gathered during a year and a half of anthropological field work in Northern Morocco. Grown in large quantities in the Rif and smoked by a fairly high proportion of native adult males, *kif* ranks, along with citrus fruits, lumber, cotton, and palmetto fiber, as one of the area's chief cash crops.[1] Unlike the other crops, it is illegal, but for various reasons to be developed, it continues to flourish.

ETHNOGRAPHIC SKETCH

The northern part of Morocco is perhaps the poorest agricultural area

Field work for this paper was sponsored by the Wenner-Gren Foundation of Anthropological Research. I wish to thank Professor Marlene Dobkin de Rios for comments and suggestions. Responsibility for interpretation and inaccuracies are, of course, entirely my own.

[1] Mikesell, in his very excellent study of the cultural geography of northern Morocco, makes only occasional mention of *kif*. He does, however, acknowledge the plant as an important cash crop (1961:82).

within the regime. This fact is due to two conditions, the first of which is basically ecological. Lacking any stable water source except that along the banks of Wad Ghis and Wad Nkqur, subsistence agriculture depends on the dry farming of grains and fruits, necessitating an adequate rainfall. When sufficient precipitation is available, the peasantry manage a livable existence. However, when drought occurs, survival becomes more hazardous. Occasionally, as in 1947, famines have been recorded. The ecological situation is further complicated by land denudation through destruction of the natural forests. This has been due in part to local consumption of wood for building houses, burning to clear fields for cultivation, and the use of wood and charcoal for fuel. However, the major agents in the deforestation process were the Spaniards, who held this part of Morocco as a protectorate. This period of Spanish "custody," which lasted from 1912–1956, was one in which massive amounts of timber were cut and exported. Although the period was relatively short, Spain managed by using modern equipment, according to Mikesell (1961:101), to "cut more trees in a decade than the local tribesmen could destroy in a century." The process, which has been somewhat reversed by government programs in planting new trees, has left large sections of mountainous area without any natural protection against water runoff and further soil erosion during the rainy season.

The second factor in northern Morocco's poverty is political. Spanish colonial policy sought extraction of whatever economic value was to be found in the Rif mountains, while contributing little to the country's economic condition. To a certain extent this was due to the very low base line of economic potential which existed in the Rif. Of equal importance was the fact that Spain itself was poor, and spent much of the period between 1912 and 1956 either fighting rebels within the Rif led by Abdel Krim, or fighting internal wars within its own boundaries. Unlike France which held control over the larger part of Morocco, Spain was unable to make many economic improvements.

Given these ecological and political factors, *kif* remained an important cash crop as well as stimulant among Rif tribal groups. The center for *kif* cultivation is in the mountainous region around Ketama, a small *ville* located within the province of Alhucemas and administered by a government appointed *caid* at the *ville* of Targuist. He, in turn, is under the political jurisdiction of the Governor of Alhucemas Province, located in the city of the same name. Although *kif* could be grown in other areas in northern Morocco, its cultivation is centered almost exclusively in the tribes (*qabilas*) of Ketama and Beni Seddath. The *kif* from other areas is regarded as inferior in strength and texture. The Berbers have a saying that "the land of Ketama likes only *kif*," referring not only to the fact that most other crops do not grow well there, but also to the superior quality of the *kif* product from this area.

ECONOMICS

The mature female plant, as harvested, consists of brownish stems and golden leaves. The leaves are stripped off by hand and the stems are either thrown away, or retted by submerging in water for a period of time, after which the fibers are separated and used for making hats, baskets, shoes, and the like. The leaves are separated from pods or seeds, then cut up by a small hand sickle into very minute particles. The *kif* is then mixed with uncured tobacco. Since there is a government monopoly on tobacco, it is necessary for the producers and distributors of *kif* to provide their own tobacco. In the economics of *kif*, tobacco plays an important role. Uncured tobacco is ground up and mixed into any quantity of *kif* prior to smoking the drug in a ratio of .3 tobacco to .7 *kif*. Mikuriya's data on this admixture of .5 and .5 is, to the best of my knowledge, inaccurate. The Berbers maintain that without the tobacco, *kif* "doesn't have salt."

Tobacco, oddly enough, costs more in bulk than does *kif*. Prices fluctuate according to the product's availability. Within the province of Alhucemas, during the years 1965–1966, uncured tobacco in leaf form cost approximately 40 dirhams (one dirham equaled 20 cents American) a kilo. The natural *kif* plant during this period was marketed at between 12 and 30 dirhams a kilo within the same province. A kilo of *kif* ground up and mixed with tobacco would fetch about 70 dirhams, the additional cost stemming from the labor input. Higher prices in urban areas were due in part to additional middlemen in the distribution system, as well as the added risk of marketing under closer police surveillance. Tourists and persons uninitiated in the price structure paid considerably more.

Kif is usually smoked in a pipe called *sibsa*. The long stem can be dismantled into two connecting parts and presumably offers greater security to the carrier, in addition to a cooler smoke. Stems are made from the wood of the walnut tree, and a small bowl made of baked clay is fitted at one end of the *sibsa*. It is reputed that a clandestine factory exists in Tetuan Province to manufacture such pipes, although I was unable to get further information on this matter. The price for a simple *sibsa* in local *suqs* or marketplaces was 3 dirhams, although again tourists and strangers were charged more.

The *kif* and tobacco plants are distributed directly to middlemen from the farms in the Ketama region. Since, at this point, *kif* as an economic commodity becomes illegal, it is extremely difficult to gather information on the complexity of transportation to urban markets and buyers or middlemen outside Morocco. Mikuriya's presumption that large vehicles are used to transport *kif* to outside markets is probably valid, although in order to do this, merchants would need some influence with segments of the national police. Too careful questioning along these lines, however, is discouraged by everyone involved directly or potentially in *kif* traffic. During the period of field work in the Rif, it was made explicit to me that if I wished to remain in the country or, for that matter, preserve my health, it would not be wise to investigate this problem too closely.

With regard to crop yield, I was equally unable to obtain much information. Mikuriya stated that he was informed that the average yield was two kilograms of dried tops and stems (excluding leaves) per square meter. While I cannot confirm this, I do have figures on the amount of profit per man hour of labor. Informants estimated that to realize a net income of 1,000 dirhams for a crop of barley, six months of labor would be required; the same amount of profit that could be derived from a *kif* crop necessitates only five day's labor.

While I was unable to obtain information about kif traffic outside the Rif, it was fairly simple to acquire data about distribution and price structure within the area itself. This can be attributed to the fact that most *kif* merchants inside the Rif are relatively low-level middlemen, who are marginal and are neither as protected nor endangered as large producers. Because of their marginality and intimate knowledge of the distribution system, these middlemen do not have to bribe officials. Their customers are located in such remote areas that it is impossible to police their activities.

These middlemen transport their product on their backs or on donkeys in specially made bags of cloth which contain up to 40 kilos each. Supplies are picked up at night. Staying on isolated dirt paths, these individuals branch out to their regular distribution points. Unlike large-scale distributors who operate from primary markets such as cities and abroad, these rural points can be viewed as secondary links in a market system indigenous to the area. They are generally located in small cafes in the local *suqs*, market centers in the province of Alhucemas. Rif market systems are cyclical, with a market (*suq*) held once a week at a permanent location within each tribe or large tribal section. By holding their markets on separate days, tribes have produced a weekly staggered system of markets all across the Rif. Thus, a merchant selling any commodity, including *kif*, can travel to a different *suq* every day of the week, except Friday, the

Muslim sabbath. The marketplace itself, except on market day, is usually rather deserted, with the exception of a few cafes that remain open all week long. These cafes generally serve as terminals for secondary distribution. A cafe owner occasionally may also serve as a middleman, but he is more likely supplied by a relative or friend. It is also rare for a *kif* producer to serve in any role other than producer. This accords with other cash crop activities in the Province, since the farmer's role terminates once he meets his middleman who then acts as distributor. Once *kif* plants reach the cafes, the owners grind up a certain amount for sale in small lots, which are generally packaged in small empty match boxes and sold for 70 or 80 francs[2] per box. Regular *kif* smokers prefer to buy the unground, unblended *kif* and tobacco because it is easy to process into smokable form. Hence, they save on labor charges by doing their own work. However, the occasional *kif* smoker finds it more convenient to purchase a small match box or two of the drug.

There are at least ten cafes in the city of Alhucemas that cater to *kif* smokers, and one or two depots operated by local large-scale distributors. They are well known and presumably pay for protection against prosecution. In addition, at least one cafe in every market center deals in kif. These cafes, both within the city and at the rural markets, are terminal points for distribution within the secondary *kif* market. No one buys at a cafe to resell later, since this would involve two middlemen transactions, thereby placing expenses outside the normal competitive range.

NATIVE ATTITUDES

Although the socio-cultural significance of *kif* is somewhat outside the scope of a study such as this, treating mainly economic aspects of this plant, we can obtain some insight into the lack of restrictive mechanisms on *kif* distribution. Not regarded as particularly evil among Berber males, it is, unlike alcohol, not prohibited by any religious stigma. This is explicitly recognized by the judicial sanction system. A person caught smoking *kif* is generally ignored or placed in jail overnight, whereas a Muslim can receive from three to six months in jail for drinking alcohol. Some informants explained to me that this rather lenient attitude was

---

[2] One hundred Moroccan francs are equal to one Moroccan dirham. The monetary value of the dirham is pegged roughly at the same level of the 1965 French franc, although this value is maintained artificially. There is a considerable black market in Moroccan currency.

based in part on the fact that a high percentage of the soldiers and local police smoked *kif*.

Kif is regarded by the educated literate elite as an evil, as they themselves have become accustomed to emulating western customs. Many of those who decry the use of *kif* drink alcohol. To a certain extent, a stigma is placed on the *kif* smoker, as poor, illiterate, and backward. On the other hand, *kif* smokers regard the urban elite who frown upon the use of kif as bad Muslims, since they accept to much of western culture, including alcohol drinking. In 1959, *kif* cultivators argued in a confrontation with the government that if the production of *kif* were to be eliminated, the import and export of alcohol must also be banned. Since Scotch has become a favored drink among some elite circles, and inasmuch as considerable revenue is derived from the exportation of wine, such a policy was not instigated and *kif* growers won something of a moral victory.

Another element to be considered from a socio-cultural point of view is that within the mountain area, *kif* is largely restricted to men of middle age or older. Unlike many industrial nations where marijuana smoking is regarded as a rebellious act against an older generation, *kif* smoking in the Rif is regarded as part of the older establishment. Young men who fancy themselves poets or moderns are more likely to drink beer or wine as a sign of rebellious feelings.

A third factor in the use of *kif* is that it is not generally associated with any ritual or mystical features. Users may employ *kif* in order to induce what they consider a transcendental experience, but *kif* smoking seems to be completely disassociated from mystical searches, and is not encouraged by any of the local *sufi* organizations. In fact, it is somewhat frowned upon by most prominent religious brotherhoods in the area. *Kif* smoking seems to be motivated more by the pleasure it brings or the depression and anxiety it alleviates. One can therefore say that the use of *kif* in this area is not regarded as a manifestation of a "sick" society but rather as a means of relieving everyday pressure. At the same time, it is not irreligious to smoke *kif*, as it is to drink alcohol, and *kif* is considerably cheaper.

In a society where social structure is devoted primarily to relationships between social groups, personal behavior that does not affect traditional mechanisms of social order is not regarded as a dereliction. The use of *kif* remains an integral part of the culture and is regarded as no great threat to community or group relationships. Since *kif* smoking is considered to be outside traditional legal and religious structures, its use becomes a matter of personal disposition and economic ability.

HISTORY

The origins of *kif* use in Morocco are too hazy to attempt any precise reconstruction. The plant may have been indigenous to the area, but equally possible is that it was accidently introduced during one of the Arabic invasions of Morocco or else transported to the region by an individual returning from a pilgrimage to Mecca. It is also possible that it came to Morocco from the south carried by slaves imported from West Africa. Whatever route its introduction took, its cultivation and use became firmly established by the 19th century.

Informants insist that their great grandparents smoked *kif*. To the best of my knowledge, however, Spanish chroniclers of the early days of the Protectorate make no mention of its use. I was told by veterans of the Spanish Civil War that when Franco enlisted Berbers from the Rif to support his cause, he paid them in part with *kif* supplies. Whether this is true or not, the drug was available to them in Spain; the Spanish in fact took a lenient position toward *kif*-use among the Berbers, both during the Civil War and within Morocco itself.[3] Spain made no attempts to suppress the cultivation of *kif*, and very little effort was made to halt its distribution within the Rif. This is interesting in view of the fact that the Spanish government is not favorably disposed toward the use of *Cannabis* and has stringent laws within its own boundaries governing the possession and use of the plant.

To a certain extent it is possible that Spain inadvertently encouraged the spread of regular *kif* smoking. This conjecture arises from the fact that Spain created a special social class which regularly used *kif*, namely the native Moroccan soldier. While *kif* smoking was never associated with any particular group or institution, the rise of a full-time militia also gave rise to a social group that regularly engaged in using the plant.

The Rif is regarded as part of the land of *siba*, an area outside the administrative boundaries of the traditional Moroccan Empire. Although the Riffian had always been a warrior, prior to the advent of the Spanish Protectorate he was never really a soldier. There is, I think, a basic difference between these two activities. Tribal warriors operate within a specific context of family and kin communities. They are called together only as temporary congregations. They are not full-time specialists in war. Rather, they devote only a portion of their time to war, another

---

[3] An army which fights under the influence of marijuana is not necessarily an inefficient army. Berber soldiers were more feared by the Republican army than even Franco's German Axis troops.

parcel of time to cropping, and still another to their community's social affairs. They are rarely burdened with the repetitiveness of police activity or garrison life. The business of warfare takes up only a small portion of the time of the professional soldier. There are long breaks between the time he is fighting. These breaks are filled with routine activities, which are divorced from his usual occupations and amusements. The soldier's social life is a good deal different from that of tribal warrior, in that the former is placed in an all-male society that has a professional rather than a community basis for existence. His new social group sets up a different sort of social and personal relationships. His orientation is changed from one of family and neighbors to one of professional peers. It is within this latter context that *kif* became an accepted part of everyday life.

The Spanish point of view showed limited concern toward the native use of *kif* because within their cultural mapping it reflected an attitude and behavioral pattern which they considered barbaric. This lent an additional self-justifying motive for their "civilizing" venture into Morocco. It is equally likely that the Spaniards found themselves in the same position as that of the present independent Moroccan government, inasmuch as it is practically impossible to control the cultivation of *kif* in the Rif.

From time to time, the current Moroccan government made attempts to halt the cultivation of *kif*, although this has met with complete lack of success. Mikuriya pointed out that the Moroccan army mounted a campaign to eradicate the Ketama *kif* fields in the early 1960's, but because of the poor communication systems, rugged terrain, and armed resistance this attempt failed. I suspect that any army attempt would be more in the nature of a dramatic charade to placate world opinion. Morocco, like other countries, such as Turkey, China, etc., faces occasional censure from international organizations such as WHO, if it makes no attempt to eradicate illegal plant supplies. However, producers are not only well entrenched in their environment, but also wield considerable political power. While I doubt the accuracy of Mikuriya's conjecture that Ketama is "reputedly producing the most kif in Asia," the *kif* growers have not only a large indigenous market, but as a result of proximity to Europe and an increasing market there, the commodity has an expanding demand curve in which huge amounts of money are involved.

While no slur against the Moroccan government is intended, to a large extent public officials here as elsewhere are susceptible to bribes. The collusion between some officials and producers, the awareness that the crop provides Rif inhabitants with possibly their only familiar alternative to starvation, as well as the resulting inflow of hard foreign currency, makes it problematic that effective control can or will be established over the production and sale of *kif*. The present government position is a paradox that can be explained in terms of the above factors. The government prohibits the sale of *kif* but does not prohibit the production of *kif*. When I was first told of this situation, I feared my translating of Berber into English was faulty. Repeated statements of this nature lead me to believe that it is true. I only conjecture that this situation is a rather ingenious way of keeping external pressure off the Moroccan government, while at the same time allowing for the continuation of a *kif* market. Occasionally, small lot dealers of *kif* are arrested and sentenced to short prison terms. While such arrests are widely publicized in Moroccan Arabic, French and Spanish language newspapers, they are really fictions in that they do not reflect any comprehensive campaign on the part of public security officials to terminate *kif* supplies. They serve as announcements to the external world that Morocco holds an anti-*cannabis* position, but at the same time production, distribution, and consumption of *kif* go on at an unabated rate.

REFERENCES

MIKESELL, MARVIN W.
   1961   *Northern Morocco, a cultural geography*. University of California Publications in Geography 14. Berkeley: California Press.

MIKURIYA, TOD H.
   1967   Kif cultivations in the Rif Mountains. *Economic Botany* 21 (3):231–234.

Traditional Patterns of Hashish Use in Egypt

AHMAD M. KHALIFA

ABSTRACT

On the basis of data derived from a major research project conducted by the National Center for Social and Criminological Research in Cairo on the use of cannabis in Egypt and several minor studies dealing with the same subject, this paper outlines traditional and current patterns of hashish consumption in Egypt. General observations and impressions are presented where no scientifically tested data are as yet available.

Along with the presentation of a particular pattern, the paper touches upon possible similarities or dissimilarities to other patterns of cannabis use, particularly in highly industrialized societies.

The main assumption is that in the case of drug consumption, we are faced with a broad diversification stemming not only from the type of the drug but from the varying cultural context of the phenomenon.

The aspects of drug abuse are so widely diversified that to achieve any understanding or insight, the problem should be studied within its cultural context. A cross-cultural approach is indispensable to determine and interpret the epidemiological characteristics of a given drug in any given society and to identify the rationale behind its incidence. Against so many different sociocultural backgrounds, one must expect to find dissimilarities and differences in the underlying values and manifestations involved.

This assumption is plausible particularly in the case of mild levels of drug consumption where the practice tends to be culturally conditioned. This is not exactly the case, however, when we consider more serious levels of consumption where underlying individual inadequacies are generally responsible for drifting into addiction, whether through addiction-producing drugs or through heavy and frequent doses of milder drugs. Character and personality factors are probably more at work in the selection of addicts as well as other environmental circumstances.

Beyond the relatively limited scope of addiction, drugs have played an important role in man's life throughout known history. Man has always used some "substance" whether in relation to spiritual or ritualistic experiences or to induce changes of mood, feelings or perception. The choice of the substance depended on its availability and the nature of the change desired. The idea, in fact, behind many pharmacologically unrelated substances is the same: to induce an artificial sense of satisfaction derived from feeling "up" or "down" or bringing about a change of perception.

In this sense, it is a safe assumption that drug use or abuse has always been functional. This supposition could be sustained by the concept of anomie advanced by Merton who maintains that people who are denied access to the goals society values, who are given little or no opportunity to achieve those goals may withdraw and retreat from these goals and have recourse to deviant substitute activities such as drug use. Merton has stressed the need to alleviate the strains between the cultural goals and the unequal means for achieving them, which constitute a constant pressure toward deviancy (Brill 1966).

We could cite, for example, the case of chewing coca leaf, which probably has the effect of alleviating thirst and reducing sensations of hunger. The rationale behind coca-leaf chewing could be basically utilitarian in the sense that it provides a means to overcome unwillingness to work, or enables adequate functioning in socioeconomic conditions where work is an unpleasant or arduous experience.

As regards cannabis, the studies on habituation to hashish consumption undertaken by the National Center for Social and Criminological Research in Cairo which have been going on for several years,[1] indicate that there is a popular close association between hashish and feelings of elation and relaxation, good highs, improvement of personal communications and relatedness and a deep sense of togetherness. The research findings also indicate that under hashish a more pleasurable sex experience is believed to be attained. Of course, the objectivity of this observation is debatable but certainly, in a matter based so much on imagination, it is quite important.

There are some clues which could support the assumption that drug intake is indeed functional especially when viewed in broad cultural perspective. Cultural beliefs define to some degree the situation of any drug use and by far condition its effects. With this functional character

---

[1] In November 1957, a committee was set up to carry out the enquiry under Professor Zeiwar. In June 1966, Professor M. I. Soueif took over from him. Professor Soueif, who was on the first committee, was responsible for writing up the successive reports published by the National Center and the English summaries, some of which were published in the *United Nations Bulletin on Narcotics*.

in mind, society, which seems to have always lived with drugs, should learn to live with the fact that drugs are here to stay and their use may even be expected to increase. This licit expectation of a human society more involved in drugs could find a strong argument in our gradual development into a leisure society looking increasingly for mind-expanding experiences.

To turn to the more recent manifestations of drug misuse, a close review of the drug scene discloses disturbing trends which have become apparent in the past decade, mainly the increasing resort to drugs by younger age groups and the popularization of psychotropic drugs. These are usually classified into three groups: hallucinogenic mind-expanding drugs, e.g., cannabis and LSD; stimulants, e.g., amphetamines and cocaine; and sedatives. In the present order of popularity, cannabis seems to come first. While the misuse of heroin and other opiates seems to remain comparatively static, the psychotropic drugs, the so-called pop-drugs, are gaining more popularity. This thesis is apparently sustained by Interpol reports that the volume of illicit traffic has increased by thirty per cent in 1968 as reflected by seizures, and that except in the case of opium the quantities of drugs seized appeared to be on the increase. In this connection, we might observe that the popularization of psychotropic drugs has taken place in developed and industrialized parts of the world while it was almost traditionally limited to less-developed regions.

We, therefore, seem to be confronted now with a problem of a dual character, sometimes described as two subcultures of drug use, the narcotics subculture and the psychedelic subculture. Research in the United States where the two types coexist tends in general to indicate that "junkies" (narcotic users) represent a cross-section of socially, economically and culturally deprived Americans while "hippies," the most outstanding or visible group favoring psychedelic drugs, are middle-class Americans. The maximum cluster among hippies falls within the ages of 18 to 21, while junkies range from the mid-teens to older citizens age groups (Hamburger 1969).

Without going as far as assuming the existence of two drug subcultures, we are of the opinion that the drug wave should not be viewed as a unique phenomenon revealing identical traits. Putting aside for more detailed consideration the traditional use of some drugs in many parts of the world that could not be ascribed to the modern drug wave, we have on the one hand the most socially and economically deprived neighborhoods with the highest rate of juvenile delinquency and crime which have always developed a special cultural climate favorable to drug abuse and addiction; on the other hand we have the angry or apathetic young generation disillusioned by what they believe is the evident failure of the establishment or the "system." On the whole, these are experimenters looking for new experiences rather than desperate life-deserters squeezed by the life machine. Generally, unless they drift to heavy doses and addiction, they experience no serious side effects and are often able eventually to break the habit. Glorifying justification is sometimes given to these experimenters; their indulgence in drugs is not viewed as a case of acting out internal problems or as a consequence of failure in legitimate or illegitimate social endeavor; they are seen rather to be playing a conscious active role by striving toward the high status of protest or rebellion, while at the same time, feeling fatherless in modern society, they find common bonds and a sense of belonging through a peer group of drug users.

Coming back to traditional patterns, we realise that habitual consumption of cannabis assumes a different character in those countries where it constitutes a traditional habit practiced for hundreds or even thousands of years. In these countries many otherwise normal people consume cannabis with the same attitude as people who consume alcohol in a normal social manner. In some North African countries with a long established pattern of use among lower-class males, there appears to be no upsurge among youth or middle-class groups. In Morocco there are indications of an overall decline in cannabis use, associated with an increase of the use of alcohol.

In India, there is a well-known long history of cannabis use in religious practices, both in celebrating various religious holidays and in use by priests and other religious figures. As regards the use of cannabis in indigenous systems of medicine in India, eighty per cent of the population lived in villages which had no access to modern medicine and traditional systems of medicine employing cannabis were essential for the treatment of a number of illnesses. The introduction and supply of modern medicines to a huge population was a gigantic task which could only be accomplished over a period of time.

Egypt has a long history with hashish use that probably goes back several hundred years. It is usually maintained that this may be the result of religious sanctions that prohibited the consumption of alcohol. While there may be some justification in this assumption it would be an oversimplistic interpretation. Maqrizi, an Egyptian historian (1364–1442 A.D.), reports how the Sultan Nigm Al Din Ayoub ordered Prince Gamal Al Din Fath Moussa Ibn Aghmour to prevent the plantation of hashish in the Regouri Gardens. One day, when the Sultan went to the gardens, he observed that there were yet great quantities of hashish left intact, consequently, he ordered that the plants be collected and burnt.

Maqrizi also maintains that, at the turn of the fourteenth century, the Sultan punished eaters of hashish by pulling out their teeth. Despite the harsh punishment, a quarter of a century later, hashish consumption was a public matter; eating the plant was quite fashionable and talking about it became most uninhibited.

According to modern Arabic historians, cannabis came to be planted and used in Egypt around the mid-twelfth century during the reign of the Ayyubid dynasty, as a result of the emigration of mystic devotees from Syria. Poems published in the twelfth and early thirteenth centuries describe the desirable behavioral changes attributed to cannabis consumption. They are: euphoria, acquiescence, sociability, carefreeness, feelings of importance, meditativeness, activation of intelligence, jocularity and amiability. By way of comparison with alcohol the following qualities were attributed to hashish; it was cheap and not prohibited by the Islamic religion, a comparatively small quantity was enough to get the desired effect; it did not smell like alcohol and, therefore, was not easily detectable; and lastly, that it was not pressed by the feet in preparation for consumption. On the other hand, the adversaries pointed out five undesirable effects resulting from hashish use: submissiveness, debility, insanity, some sort of organic brain damage, and prostitution (Hussein 1957). This poetry reflects the poets' diagnostic practices supposed to draw upon popular wisdom.

As far back as 1879 Egyptian authorities attempted to enact laws for the prevention of hashish consumption. The first piece of legislation in fact only prohibited the cultivation of cannabis. Since then harsher penalties have gradually been set: Law 182/1960, amended by law 40/1966, punishes by the death penalty and a fine from three to ten thousand pounds the illicit import, export, production or manufacture of drugs. To possess, buy, sell, transport or offer drugs for illicit traffic is an offence punishable by the death penalty or hard labor for life and a fine in the above amount.

An Egyptian researcher who conducted a study of the consumption of hashish in Egypt in the 1950s explains the stigma attached to hashish by the fact that consumption was associated with the poor and lower classes who were subject to the contempt of the upper classes. The results of his work point to the fact that while hashish consumption is not exclusively a one class practice, it is more widespread among the poor working class. Next on the social scale are the middle class followed by the wealthy, who consume the least (Al-Magraby 1963).

Here we might note that cannabis use in the United States heavily involves college youth, the educated and the middle class which supports the assumption that we are faced with diversified cultural patterns of consumption.

The most thorough and comprehensive study on hashish consumption in Egypt to date has been undertaken since 1957 by the National Center for Social and Criminological Research in Cairo. A series of reports on the research findings have been issued by the research team headed by Professor M. I. Soueif. A recent publication reports the results of the administration of the interviewing schedules to 850 hashish takers and 839 non-takers (Soueif 1971).

The experimental group included the whole population convicted exclusively for hashish use and detained in Egyptian penal institutions during the period from June 1967 to March 1968 who admitted using the drug at least once per month throughout the year preceding imprisonment. Ages ranged from 15 to slightly over 50 years with an average of 39 years. Four hundred sixty subjects were in prisons in big cities intended for urban offenders, while 390 subjects were villagers detained in rural prisons. Seventy-two per cent of the group were married, 21% bachelors, 6% divorced and about 1% widowed. Sixty percent were illiterate and the rest distributed among various levels of education with only six subjects having completed high school. None were university graduates. Approximately 25% of the group were skilled laborers and the rest were unskilled workers.

Controls were selected from among the convicts detained in the same prisons as the experimentals. The control group is fairly well matched to the experimentals in regard to age, urban or rural background and percentages of skilled laborers. The experimentals have a better position as to income while the opposite is true concerning literacy.

Smoking was found to be the prevalent route of administration (89.4%) either by *josah*, a smoking pipe (61.7%); or cigarettes (10.5%); or a combination of both (17.1%). Very few habitues (1.3%) take the drug orally only, and the rest (9.3%) combine smoking with some method of oral administration.

It is interesting to note in this connection that the literature on hashish consumption in Egypt indicated that the drug was eaten rather than smoked, and that hashish was eaten in its purest form. Methods of mixing the drug appeared later. In modern times, however, smoking is the usual manner of consumption, and smokers have often been viewed as being more refined than eaters of hashish.

Smoking as a preferred way of drug use was found to be related to the number of times per month the drug was taken. Thus, 87% of heavy users (those who take the drug more than 30 times) versus 93% of moderates (those who take it 30 times or less) invariably smoke the drug.

The majority (82.5%) take hashish in groups, and only 17.5% consume it alone. Heavy users do not differ markedly from moderate ones in this respect; city dwellers, however, have a significantly higher percentage of lone-takers (23.9%) than the users from rural areas (10%).

A significant relationship was found between frequency of hashish use and age of onset; the earlier the onset the higher the frequency. When the group was divided into those who started taking the drug regularly before the age of 22 (N = 488) and those who began at 22 or after (N = 354) the relationship was very striking. Whereas 76% of those who started before the age of 22 were heavy users, only 56% of the beginners after 22 were in the same category. The discrepancy between the two percentages is highly significant.

Heavy users did not differ markedly from moderates as regards the situation (i.e., the external circumstances) which occasioned the onset of use. When asked about their conscious motives for starting hashish use, more heavy takers than moderates mentioned imitation (62.5% v. 53.4%, respectively), trying to behave in a "manly" manner (78.4% v. 58.9%) and seeking euphoria (86.3% v. 79.1%).

Nearly a third (31.6%) of the group admitted that they used to take opium. More heavy takers (34.3%) than moderates (25.7%) tend to take opium. Opium taking was also found to be slightly more prevalent among urban habitues (34.5%) than among the rural group (28%).

More hashish users (22.7%) than controls (9.1%) (regardless of urban or rural background) were found to be alcohol drinkers. The difference is highly significant. As in the case of opium, more alcohol drinkers were found among heavy hashish users (27%) than among moderate users (13.5%) and the difference was again highly significant.

Forty-two per cent of the group started to take cannabis before the age of 20. Out of this subgroup 32.8% had their first experience with the drug before completing 16 years of age (early beginners). On the other hand, 17.6% of the total group did not start before the age of 28 years (late beginners).

More early beginners (61.2%) than late ones (24.7%) reported some family member or members using cannabis. Again more early beginners (36.4%) than late ones (17.6%) with one parent reported dead, stated that the remaining parent was remarried. The difference is significant. Early beginners reported more incidence of separation and/or divorce between parents (15%) than the late beginners (7.8%).

Thus, early onset of cannabis use is associated with exposure to the influence of a drug consuming example within the family circle, combined with the effect of the loss of father or mother and the intrusion of a stepparent.

Asked about their conscious motives for taking hashish for the first time subjects stated numerous motives, ranked in the following order: conformity to a group of personal friends (87.8%); seeking euphoria (86.6%); behaving like "real men" (72.5%); imitating others (59.5%); curiosity (75.5%); forgetting personal problems (42.8%); alleviating a mood of depression (40.5%); medicinal use (27.3%); and lastly, for the enhancement of sexual enjoyment (23.8%). This ranking of conscious reasons for taking hashish for the first time was found to prevail among the experimentals irrespective of urban or rural background, heavy use or moderation and early or late onset.

Of the group, 27.3% stated they had interrupted cannabis taking once or twice. Only 17.1% of the early starters did so compared with 31.7% of the late ones.

When asked about their conscious motives for resumption they stated three main reasons, in the following order: the impact of the occasion; to be able to bear their troubles; and having leisure time to spare. Almost the same pattern emerged when early beginners were compared with late beginners, and again when comparing heavy users with moderates.

When asked whether they still wished to stop taking hashish, 78.5% of the total group answered in the affirmative with a marked difference between early (60%) and late beginners (93.2%). A difference was noted between heavy users (75.1%) and moderates (85.6%). The reasons, in their order of frequency, were as follows, irrespective of heavy taking versus moderation and/or early versus late onset of the habit: financial reasons, fear of punishment, health reasons, and lastly, concern about social status.

It is safe to assume, as a result of research and observation, that cannabis more than any other intoxicant is used to achieve a sense of belonging to an intimate group. It is widely believed that a hashish session creates an atmosphere of joy and fun-loving causing the participants to be amused by the slightest matters, to exchange jokes and repeated greetings and words of endearment combined with a tendency to forget one's troubles and enjoy the moment. Smoking hashish in a water pipe, as a folk song points out, has the function of "grouping" the "beloved."

An in-depth study of the "togetherness" of hashish consumers could shed light on the factors of attraction and the manner in which newcomers are initiated. The reason for initiation is usually to conform to the general atmosphere of one's friends and to avoid their criticism and insinuations that non-participants should leave.

A hashish session usually brings together people from different professions, classes and educational standards, who meet in an atmosphere of brotherhood and equality as well as freedom fron social norms that prescribe certain modes of behavior. Furthermore, these sessions follow particular rituals. There is a supervisor usually called *The Sultan* who has the honor and privilege of having the first "drag" from each new "load." The water pipe is then passed around to the participants who sit in a circle. The person who is in charge of the pipe changes the water, feeds the fire and loads it with hashish.

It is reported that hashish consumers feel superior to alcoholics and to consumers of other drugs such as opium and cocaine. They believe that alcohol and other narcotics are addictive and could lead to insanity and loss of respect and identity. Hashish consumers in Egypt have always insisted that the practice was not prohibited by Islam despite the fact that the Egyptian Islam Mufti issued a Fetwa in 1940 that prohibited the consumption of hashish or any other drug, equating it with alcohol.

If society has lived with drugs, it has always also lived with some sort of social control related to drug use. Drugs have been a subject of legislative regulation all over the world reflecting local conditions and underlying legal philosophy. The legal-thought impact has had great influence in the shaping of popular ideas. The drug offence is the creation of a legal norm set out by legislation; and it is safe to assume that the law has largely acted upon the premise that drug addiction was largely a vice which could be conquered by an effort of the will.

Setting aside the evident case of compulsive addiction, some sort of legal philosophy is at the base of incrimination of drug offences. In the light of the prevailing thesis of the protection of social interests, some would wonder if the law has often gone too far in incriminating drug offences and enacting severe penalties. It is necessary to determine precisely what interest society wishes to protect. Indeed, one is somewhat confused about the thin line which cross-cuts the use of such substances and divides it into permitted and prohibited substances.

Needless to say, however, illicit traffic in and production of dangerous drugs should remain a criminal offense or even be regarded more severely. On the other hand, if private moral conduct should not be criminalized there always remain the social effects which could have more drastic consequences on those using drugs, especially the young. If the use of narcotics hardly needs to be argued, psychedelic drugs are seen as giving rise to major undesired social consequences such as psychological dependence, drug-seeking behavior, leaving little room for other activities, restriction of stimuli conducive to social apathy and marginality and irresponsible behavior.

Marihuana is generally agreed to be the mildest, least dangerous of drugs. Yet it is classified as a narcotic along with morphine and heroin, and long terms of imprisonment are imposed for its possession and use. These laws governing marihuana are an example of the irrationality of legislation and are completely out of proportion to the actual dangers and constitute social hypocrisy regarding drugs and alcohol.

Some recommend legal reform through a new classification of drugs by danger, with offences scaled accordingly. Cannabis should be removed from its present category to a lesser one. Offences relating to cannabis should be set according to the quantity involved, with higher penalties for trafficking and more modest ones for possession of quantities intended for personal use. On the whole, the laws in a great number of countries have failed to act flexibly on the differentiation related to the type and quantity of drugs. Perhaps possession for personal use or for trafficking has been the most popular basis of differentiation.

In Egypt, Act 182/1960 amended by Act 40/1966 makes no distinction between drugs as to type or quantities, and does not subscribe to differentiation in punishment between hard and "softer" drugs like cannabis. Egyptian law only distinguishes between types of offences. The import, export, production or manufacture of drugs for illicit traffic is punishable by death and a fine of 3–10 thousand pounds; other acts of commerce are punishable by death or hard labor for life and a fine as mentioned above; penalty for possession for personal use is imprisonment for 3–15 years and a fine of 500–3000 pounds.

Strict law enforcement — if ever totally or partially attained — and severe penalties are not the easy answer to problems of drug addiction and misuse. It is a fallacy, though, that law enforcement is the best method to deal with social evils. We must look for a rational drug control program based on a thorough understanding of the phenomenon.

REFERENCES

AL-MAGRABY, S.
    1963   *The phenomenon of hashish use*. Cairo: Dar-el-Maaref.
BRILL, LEON
    1966   Drug abuse as a social problem. *The International Journal of the Addictions* 1:2, 10.
HAMBURGER, E.
    1969   Contrasting the hippie and junkie. *The International Journal of the Addictions* 4:1, 133–134.

HUSSEIN, M. K.
1957 *Studies in poetry during the Ayyubid dynasty.* Cairo: Dar al-Fikr el Arabi.
SOUEIF, M. I.
1971 The use of cannabis in Egypt, a behavioral study. *Bulletin on Narcotics* 33:17–28.

The Traditional Role and Symbolism of Hashish among Moroccan Jews in Israel and the Effect of Acculturation

PHYLLIS PALGI

> We can assume ... that any feature of culture once established will automatically tend to spread to the cultures of other societies, just as it will tend to persist in its own.... The principle is empirical, but so great is the mass of experience, both contemporary and historical on which it is based that it has the force of an axiom.... Roughly, we can assume that culture traits will spread unless there are specific factors to prevent spread....
>
> A. KROEBER

ABSTRACT

The paper examines the factors involved in resistance to hashish use by the traditional Jewish community in Morocco where hashish use was an accepted custom and the factors involved in their selective receptivity to the custom, paradoxically, after emigration to Israel where the environment is not conducive to drug use.

INTRODUCTION

All modern societies view the use of drugs with much alarm precisely because of their assumed natural potential to spread like an infectious disease. This paper is a case study illustrating resistance to diffusion, due to the existence of specific factors. With changed circumstances, when those specific factors no longer fulfill the same function for the particular society, resistance to diffusion becomes substantially weakened.

In concrete terms, the discussion of resistance to diffusion deals with

---

I wish to thank Dr. M. Ritter and J. Teich who allowed me to participate in their group meetings with drug and ex-drug users at the Community Mental Health Center, Jaffa. Special thanks to all the informants.

the rejection of the custom of hashish smoking or eating by the traditional Jewish community in Morocco while it was living in an environment *prima facie* favorable to its adoption. The second part of the discussion deals with a certain selective readiness to accept the custom by the Jewish community after undergoing a major social upheaval prior to emigration to Israel. Paradoxically, the cultural setting in the new Israeli environment would appear on the surface to be non-conducive to drug-taking.

THE TRADITIONAL ROLE OF HASHISH

The use of intoxicants is proscribed by the Islamic religion in general terms. The Quran makes no special reference to cannabis, or to any other of the drugs known at the time. While there are a number of local differences, the use of cannabis with varying intensity has had a time-honored role in many Muslim countries. This is in contrast to the use of alcohol which, from the religious point of view, became the prime forbidden intoxicant.

While it is difficult to distinguish between legend and fact, due to the lack of accurate documentation, by the 11th century a very special type of imagery was apparently associated with hashish, the Arabic term for cannabis. Through the colorful writings of Marco Polo the story became popularized that the Assassins, a fanatic Muslim religious order located originally in the hills of Persia, gave their disciples hashish to induce wonderful visions of Paradise with gardens, fountains and beautiful maidens. The effect, it was claimed, was to give them the moral strength to kill, to carry out suicidal missions. In this way they could insure their place in Paradise. The etymology of the word "Assassin" is said to come from Hashishin, i.e. hashish-taker. It was transmitted through the Romance languages by the Crusaders who in the 12th century, fearful of this sect, associated their daring killings with the power of the drug.

In the 13th century the physician Ibn-al-Baitar described the intoxicating effect of *Cannabis indica* which grew in Egypt. There are many reports from that period onwards that hashish was also used in medical preparations. Levy has suggested that the interpretation of the Quranic law on intoxicants might have been more tolerant toward the use of drugs such as opium and hashish because of the paucity of means of relieving pain in the medieval Muslim world (Levy 1957).

The Traditional Role of Hashish among Jews in Muslim Countries

The indigenous Jewish communities which had been living in the Middle East and North Africa since ancient times, came under Muslim rule from the 7th century onwards. Like all Jewish minorities the world over, their life style was influenced by their co-territorialists. With regard to intoxicants, however, the traditional Jewish cultural pattern was always different, if not completely contrary to that of the Muslim population. The first fundamental difference is that the Jewish Law, in contrast to that of Islam, does not forbid the use of intoxicants. There are many references in Biblical and other Jewish sources to the use of alcohol, which is closely associated with religious and family ritual. With regard to "Kanbus," the talmudical term for hemp, it was referred to only because of its particular religious significance, that it was forbidden to weave it together with wool.

Despite the fact that cannabis as a drug must have been known to the ancient Jews, it was apparently not used by them. Herodotus (*Historia* 4:75) for instance, mentions that the Scythians scattered hemp seeds on heated stones and inhaled the fumes. In broad terms, with regard to intoxicants, the traditional Jewish communities prior and during the Muslim period were characterized by avoidance of hashish smoking and approval of the use of alcohol, provided the latter was taken at the appropriate time and according to socially sanctioned quantities. If Weil is correct in his theory that every society offers its members some external means of altering the state of consciousness, possibly alcohol fulfilled that role for the Jews as hashish did for the Muslims (Weil 1973).

Hashish Use in Morocco

There are many differences to be found among the three main Islamic areas with regard to the interpretation and practice of the religious laws by the Muslim community. As the Jews and Muslims lived together for centuries in a symbiotic type of relationship, many differences were also to be found between the respective Jewish communities. The Moroccan Jewish community has been singled out for the purpose of the discussion in this paper for two main reasons. First, due to their long history in North Africa they have for centuries known about and thus have been exposed to the custom of hashish smoking. Second, they constitute today the largest single group in Israel which migrated from the Muslim world (approx. 300,000 in 1973). The Egyptian community will be referred to so as to highlight, through comparative data, the significance of those factors which work against the diffusion of the custom of hashish use.

In North Africa, the mixed Arab-Berber Empire of Morocco developed historically along lines peculiarly its own. There, the explicit prohibition of the use of intoxicants in the Quran was more severely interpreted and observed than in Egypt: even the smoking of tobacco was frowned upon by the extreme orthodoxy. However, in spite of the disapproval of the small group of "the Learned of the Faith," hashish, or *kif* as it is known locally, was grown in the southern mountain region and its use was regarded as an accepted custom particularly among the less educated and poorer classes.

As a rule, the *kif* was smoked in a pipe made of a long, hollow piece of wood to which was attached a clay container for the chopped cannabis leaf. This pipe was passed round and each participating member of the group awaited his turn for the puff. *Kif* was also cooked with a syrup or in the form of jam and was sometimes made into a paste or eaten as a small cake.

From various reports and also from a recent analysis of *kif* grown in the Atlas mountains, the intoxicating quality is relatively weak compared with the Lebanon-grown hashish used in Egypt. Among the upper classes its use was sanctioned for medical purposes, sometimes mixed with opium. There are also hints in the literature that in the late 19th century, in the town of Fez, for instance, wives and concubines of the rich obtained hashish from their servants and smoked it secretly in their quarters. It was always officially illegal, but in fact, apparently, tolerated by the authorities, as long as it was institutionalized as lower class male behavior. It is relevant to point out that Morocco for centuries was an extremely poor country with a very small wealthy elite.

In Morocco, the entire drug scene was considerably more constricted and much less elaborate in erotic imagery as compared with that of Egypt. They did not have the "wit" i.e. the "hashish," the regular heavy smoker who kept the company entertained by jokes, puns and clever sayings. This does not mean, however, that the use of hashish in Morocco was free from sexual overtones. They were inclined to be a little more covert, compared with the open ribaldry about male potency heard in Egypt, particularly among the lower classes. In Morocco the emphasis was on "kef," namely elation. Hashish was regarded as having relaxing and uninhibitory powers: the individual was not really responsible for his actions while under the influence of hashish. He might talk or behave foolishly but he would feel happy and possibly sexually stimulated. It was thought that a female under the influence of hashish would have complete sexual abandonment; the association of loss of control particularly with regard to women was a major threatening feature to the Jewish community, as will be seen later.

The Moroccan Jewish Reaction to Hashish

There was full consensus among Moroccan Jewish informants in Israel that hashish smoking or eating was not an accepted or practiced custom within their community. It was never part of their social tradition. This information was confirmed by Israeli and other Jewish representatives: doctors and educators who worked among them prior to their emigration to Israel. When the question was put to Moroccan informants as to the reason for their rejection of the custom, they all answered "it was not Jewish behavior." The answer was reminiscent of the traditional attitude of Eastern European Jews toward drunkenness, which was regarded as Gentile behavior. When pressed for further elaboration the answer was invariably that Jews conducted their community life separate from that of the Muslim community. There were numerous contacts but they were always on a formal level — economic, legal, etc., but never social. In their eyes, hashish smoking would have brought the Jews into the Muslim social network, a situation which they viewed as threatening. At no time was the drug, *per se*, presented as a danger because of its particular chemical properties. Its rejection was always discussed within the framework of Jewish-Muslim relations in Morocco.

THE PLACE OF THE TRADITIONAL JEWISH COMMUNITY IN MOROCCO

The history of the Jews in Morocco is a history of a minority group which struggled with unusual tenacity, suffering severe hardship to maintain its identity. From time to time they enjoyed an attitude of tolerance toward them depending on the degree of benevolence of the particular ruler. It was in these periods that there was usually a burst of cultural and economic activity. Chouraqui sums up the history in a sentence: The Jews who retained their own identity arrived with the victory of the first conquerors the Phoenicians, and left twenty-five centuries later, after the defeat of the last (the French) to return to their starting point in the Holy Land of Israel. But it was the Arab-Berber regime which ruled Morocco from the 7th to the beginning of the 20th century which left a permanent mark on the Jewish community. As in all Muslim countries of the Middle East and North Africa, the Jewish communities were accorded the *Dhimmi* status (Quran 9^{29}) which formalized their inferior position, with the addition, however, of certain rights of protection from the Sultan. The interpretation of this law differed according to the country and period but the principle remained that the Jews were a separate and inferior community. In Morocco, for example, they were forced to wear distinctive clothes, had to pay special taxes, could not give evidence against a Muslim, etc. At the same time, throughout the centuries of either suffering or precarious quiet, the position of the Jews in the Muslim countries as opposed to that in medieval Christian Europe was basically more sound because they were legally recognized as the "People of the Book." This attitude reinforced the worthiness of their own identity and helped them retain their link with the Holy Land which was more on a mystic plane than an actuality. Due to their minority position, and not necessarily because they were Jews, they became the natural victims during inter-tribal and inter-dynastic warfare which characterized North Africa.

Kroeber (1948) has described the development of defensive behavior such as the blocking of diffusions when societies find themselves in a weaker position or inferior status *vis-à-vis* a more aggressive culture. He cites as examples China, Tibet, Korea and Japan that tried for two or three hundred years to shut out all occidental contacts. In the same way, the Jews in Morocco became fanatic about the preservation of their identity. A single conversion of a Jew to Islam was considered a calamity of enormous proportion and, in fact, happened only rarely. The smoking of *kif* was thus regarded as a dangerous blurring of borders between the Jewish and Muslim communities. Again, in view of the association of sensuality with *kif*, the drug took on an additional quality of danger, namely the weakening of sex control. The Islamic culture includes many puritanical elements but, in contrast to Jewish and Protestant tradition, sexual behavior is notably free from puritanism.

THE SOCIAL UPHEAVAL AMONG JEWS UNDER FRENCH RULE (1912–1948)

With the social upheaval following the French occupation of Morocco in 1912, a stream of Jewish migration began flowing, from the small towns particularly, to crowded Casablanca, where there was no formal Jewish ghetto with the characteristic high walls. Among the many consequences of this large-scale mobility, kinship ties weakened, social control lessened, and in some instances poverty became even worse. By the 1940's more and more Jewish girls began working outside the home and thus contact was possible with Muslim males. During this period there were a few cases of marriages between Jewish females and male Muslims, but in particular it was the period of the growth of Jewish prostitution. One of the cultural explanations for this was that the girls were lured into a situation where it was possible to place hashish in their food or drink without their knowledge and in their drugged condition they were seduced or abducted.

During this period of rapid social change, the Moroccan Jewish community in an active and organized manner, sought to prevent prostitution. If it did occur, however, they devised all sorts of means to try and bring back the deviant girl to the community. However, the hardships imposed by the Vichy government during World War II and the subsequent arrival of the Allied troops was a further encouragement for prostitution. Prostitution was like a recurring nightmare within the culture reminding them of their struggle to maintain their proud ethnic identity throughout the ages. There is a famous folk tale about a Jewish girl who sacrificed her life rather than accept concubinage in a Muslim harem. It should be pointed out that prostitution was legalized in Morocco only provided it fell under the control and jurisdiction of the authorities. In Casablanca, for instance, there was a separate reserve set aside for prostitutes whose freedom of movement was strictly controlled.

As to those Jewish males who began to use *kif* openly in this period, they were regarded as outsiders or deviants who brought shame on the community. Usually they attempted to keep it secret and would smoke the hashish rolled in a cigarette because it was less obvious and was not Arab in style.

To sum up, the rejection of hashish smoking had the function of strengthening the positive Jewish identity and internal solidarity *vis-à-vis* the Muslim majority. The Jewish community was capable of resisting its use because its inclusion with its specific symbolism would have clashed with the Jewish ethos. When traditionalism weakened under the influence of the French, there were indications of change.

ISRAELI SETTING: POST-EMIGRATION PERIOD

Moroccan Jewry disillusioned by French rule and buoyed up with the hope of freedom and a better economic life in the newly established State of Israel, began to pour into the country particularly during the years 1948–1951. In Israel, at the time of the advent of the State, hashish smoking was non-existent among veteran settlers of European origin. It existed to a small degree among urban Arab workers. There was also a hard core group from Turkey, Iran, and Salonika, who brought with them the habit of opium smoking and an even smaller group of addicts from Europe, morphinists in the main.

Between the years 1948-1970 more than 600,000 immigrants came from the Muslim world. The large majority of these immigrants continued to avoid the use of hashish in the new country and there is evidence that many mild opium users, particularly from Persia, dropped the habit. However, among the large masses of these immigrants, there was a segment which did not find a place for itself either socially or economically in the mainstream of modern Israeli life. This group included a number of single young persons who left their parents in their early teens seeking a better life in Israel. Many of them came from poverty-stricken homes in overcrowded Casablanca where social control had already weakened. Drifting into the slum areas, lonely and feeling rejected, these Moroccans made contact with others from the Middle East who found themselves in the same position. They met those who were either delinquents or who felt less strongly on the issue of hashish than they did.

Some Egyptian Jews, for example, who had lived in close and harmonious contact with the Muslim working class, had adopted hashish smoking, prior to immigration to Israel. In the early days of the State there were many instances where they passed the pipe around at weddings and at circumcision parties, reminiscent of the custom in Egypt where hashish smoking was part of an ordinary social occasion, with plenty of sweetmeats, fruit and laughter. On the whole, however, until the Six Day War in 1967, hashish smoking was on a very limited scale, almost completely identified with unskilled or socially marginal groups among Eastern Jews and the urban Muslim population.

ISRAEL — POST SIX DAY WAR

The Six Day War brought in its wake a number of unexpected consequences. Israel became a haven for the hippie population of the United States and Europe and they formed a bridge for the local population when they made easy contact with the urban Arabs of East Jerusalem. Down south, in the desert town of Beersheba, delinquent groups, mainly linked to prostitution, obtained supplies from the Bedouins who traditionally transported hashish in their caravans across the Sinai. The active drug scene in the United States, particularly among students, gave impetus to the curiosity about drugs of the Israeli-born population of European origin and added prestige by its use to the poorer sections of the population.

This led to increased use of the drug in general and spread to small groups in high-schools and universities. It also became incorporated into bohemian artists' circles. The reaction of the majority of Israelis, particularly those from Europe, was one of horror. There were many panic reactions arising from the fear that a nation with the self-image of physical strength and high motivation could become morally weakened by the drug and thus militarily vulnerable. However, for the majority of those using it, the avoidance of hashish no longer fulfilled the function of maintaining Jewish identity — on the contrary, it brought together those who felt either alienated or on the periphery of the society. The artists' society and the small group of middle-class students who smoked hashish adopted the same symbols as found in the United States. They referred to the use of "hash" as a necessary anti-establishment measure or as a self-realization mechanism.

At the present time, 1973, there is clearly a decline in middle-class usage and a loss of interest in the drug among the student population. The zeal of the authorities in clamping down legally on the use of hashish might, however, be a contributory cause for the apparent increased use of opium and pills, notably among marginal and delinquent groups. To the small extent that performers and those of higher educational background are hashish users they will be in contact with the marginal uneducated group only for the purpose of obtaining the drug which they use mainly on party occasions.

In summary, Moroccans or their Israeli-born children who smoke hashish are most likely to belong to the unskilled, living on welfare or if young, to be school drop-outs. Wives object to the drug because they resent the money spent on it and attribute their husbands' irregular work habits to the effect of the drug. As for the actual users, they tend to see themselves as victims of circumstances due to their cultural maladjustment in the new country. They claim they use drugs, whatever kind, to counteract their feeling of failure in not having been given respected standing in the dynamic work-oriented Israeli society.

Contrary to the pattern in traditional Jewish society in a Muslim world, the use of hashish in Israel has been a socially unifying force for alienated adults and youth from the various Eastern ethnic groups together with those urban Muslims who traditionally have been exposed to the drug. Few of those from the Middle East believe that hashish is harmful as a drug; they feel that hashish use indicates their lack of success in life and their lack of finding better means of social amusement or enjoyment. This is contrary to the beliefs held by Western Jews, particularly the older generation who feel that hashish affects the mind and the moral fibre of the person.

The amount of hashish smoking has increased among the Moroccans since emigration to Israel. My main thesis is that the need to be differentiated from the Muslim population in a Jewish state became irrelevant. In addition they could now associate hashish with the modern Western world. In the new setting, its use apparently served as a certain type of communication shared by the delinquents and non-prestige "outsiders" in Israel, and is considered as a helpful means of fighting mental depression arising out of lack of self-esteem.

REFERENCES

CHOURAQUI, A.
   1968 *Between East and West: history of the Jews of North Africa.* Philadelphia: Jewish Publication Society.

HERODOTUS
        Historia 4:75.

KROEBER, A.
   1948 *Anthropology: race, language, culture, psychology, prehistory.* New York: Harcourt, Brace & Co.

LEVY, R.
   1957 *The social structure of Islam.* Cambridge University Press.

WEIL, A.
   1973 *The natural mind.* Boston: Houghton Mifflin Co.

The Social and Cultural Context of Cannabis Use in Rwanda

HELEN CODERE

ABSTRACT

Data collected in Rwanda in 1959-1960 show cannabis in its social and cultural context. Cannabis use has its place in a socio-cultural system that determines its character and extent and that is in turn affected by the nature of cannabis use.

The use of cannabis was virtually confined to the men of a miniscule, despised and backward social group, the Twa, constituting less than one percent of the population. The expectation of strong effects causing violent behavior, methods of smoking cannabis designed to produce such effects, and the connection of Twa cannabis use with the social status, role, and culturally assigned "character" of the Twa, all combined to restrict use to the Twa and to prevent its spread to the non-Twa, 99 percent of the population of Rwanda.

THE TWA IN RWANDA

The basic fact of Rwanda social and political structure before the 1959-60 revolution was the dominance of the Tutsi minority caste over the Hutu majority. The Tutsi made up 16 percent of the population, the Hutu 83 percent, and the third caste, the Twa, who were attached to the Tutsi by bonds of loyalty and economic and political advantage, less than one percent. The traditional society had been an oppressive Tutsi state (Codere 1962; De Laeger 1939; d'Hertefelt 1962, 1965; Maquet 1954; Pages 1933). Under the League of Nations mandate and later United Nations Trusteeship the abuses of Tutsi domination had largely been eliminated, but as the traditional ruling caste and the one to have been given a head start in attaining European educational qualifications, the Tutsi before 1959-60 still held the vast majority of all governmental positions and well-paid European jobs. The economic and educational situation of the Hutu majority had improved to the point of enabling them to mount what

For Plate, see p. x, between pp. 266-267.

proved to be a thoroughly effective challenge to the altered and weakened form of Tutsi domination, as subsequent events leading to the Hutu Republic of Rwanda were to prove, but the condition of the Twa remained much the same as it had been traditionally. Few Twa had received any schooling whatsoever. They were parasitically attached to the royal court and the households of rich Tutsi of the traditional nobility; some still hunted in the forests sporadically, and others still made clay pipes and pots. Their services were mostly rewarded in kind and the goods they produced were bartered, so they had almost no cash income and had least to do of any Rwandans with the developing money economy. Their role as courtiers no longer required the tasks of torturer and executioner, as it had in the days of Musinga, who was deposed in 1931, but it still included those of dancer, musician, body-guard, buffoon, messenger, and in the 1959–60 revolution, they were once again involved in armed raids and political assassinations.

A myth embodying a stereotype of the character and capacities of the three castes justified their roles and relations in traditional Rwanda society. It stated that the Tutsi, Hutu and Twa were each descended from one of Kaynarwanda's three sons, Gatutsi, Gahutu, and Gatwa and that the character of each of these three eponymous ancestors was perpetuated in their lineages. Accordingly, from the beginning, the Tutsi supposedly had the qualities of rulers: intelligence, aristocratic sensibilities, political sagacity, and the capacity for cruelty. Their physique, tall and willowy, was thought to suit them well enough for ruling and warfare, but not for heavy unremitting physical work which was the appropriate lot of the sturdier Hutu. The Hutu were supposedly born serfs, dull of mind and in need of rule and direction for their horticultural labors and other heavy, rough and steady work. The Twa, though as a pygmoid people they were the smallest in stature of the Rwandans, were considered to have fantastic physical strength. The other qualities assigned them were also exaggerated and more animal-like than human: the capacity of utter loyalty and devotion, great courage, and lack of any self control in their gluttony and inordinate drinking whenever the opportunity arose, and in an unruly spontaneity in talk and manners.

Social facts supported much of the stereotypic picture. It would be difficult, for example, to deny the qualities of rulers to those who always ruled, or the capacity for unremitting service at hard labor to those who regularly performed it. Only the Tutsi, however, would seem to have accepted the version that has been presented. In Tutsi eyes the qualities of the Twa were those of quasi-domesticated pets who could perform some valued special services for them as their masters and afford them amusement. The Twa did not see themselves as tolerated in an essentially contemptuous way, but as socially elevated far above the Hutu because of their association with the Tutsi who valued their special qualities and capacities. They despised the Hutu for what they considered their cloddishness compared to their own cleverness and knowledge of the ways of the aristocracy and would have nothing to do with them. In their turn, the Hutu despised and avoided them, principally for their parasitism. They saw them as non-workers who mostly lived off the food and goods the Tutsi gave them, but which they, the admirably hard-working Hutu, had actually produced.

By 1959–60 the traditional situation and relation of the Hutu and Tutsi was quite changed and traditional stereotypes challenged by the new social and political facts of a democratic movement and revolution. However, little had occurred to alter the views the Twa held about themselves and those the Tutsi and Hutu held about them. The social position of the Twa in Rwanda had actually deteriorated. The traditional enclave in which, with few exceptions, they remained was sealed off from everything new that was affecting welfare and relative social status by making it in larger and larger part dependent upon the acquisition of European education and goods. In the field research in 1959–60 both some Tutsi and Hutu expressed sympathy for the unimproved and backward condition of the Twa, but, although this was far more humane and sophisticated than reiterating the old stereotype as many others still did, it amounted to about the same thing when it came down to a view of Twa social position.

1959–60 DATA ON CANNABIS USE IN RWANDA

Data on cannabis — called *injaga* in Kingarawanda — were not directly sought or elicited in 1959–60. They are to be found among the responses made by 252 Rwandans to one of six photographs showing Rwandans in traditional and modern scenes. The characteristics of the 252 respondents made up a matrix in which the key variations in Rwanda society were represented. There were men, women and children of the Tutsi, Hutu and Twa castes in a range of ages, levels of schooling and in traditional to modern occupations. (See Table 1.) The photograph that yielded commentary and information on the use of cannabis from 113 of the 252 respondents was that of a Twa man holding the gourd water-pipe that is special to cannabis-smoking. As in the case of the other five photographs,[1] the respondents were simply asked to say whatever they wanted about each

---

[1] The other photographs were: 2) a Hutu mother giving beer to her child. 3) a Tutsi

Table 1. Photo-questionnaire responses concerning cannabis

			Depositions on cannabis			Total number
			Favorable Mixed	Against	Non-committal	
TWA						
ADULTS						
Male	16		1	2	2	
Female	5			3		
		21				
*CHILDREN						
Male	8				2	
Female	1					
		9				
		—				
		30				
TUTSI						
ADULTS						
Male	63		3	48		
Female	30		4	9		
		93				
CHILDREN						
Male	8					
Female	6					
		14				
		—				
		107				
HUTU						
ADULTS						
Male	60		5	28	1	
Female	35		1	8	1	
		95				
CHILDREN						
Male	15					
Female	5			1	1	
		20				
		115				
		252	1	13 99	7	113

* Children were defined as eleven years old or under that age.

diviner receiving two Hutu clients. 4) a Tutsi chief with traditional clothing and hair-crests looking at laboratory equipment. 5) a group of Rwanda in front of a modern store, and 6) a Tutsi reading a book.

picture. The purpose of the study, which was conducted during Rwanda's revolution under conditions of great social tension and the necessity for neutral and unalarming field procedures, was to get open-ended and freely expressed political views of the Rwanda, and especially the views of Tutsi, Hutu and Twa Rwanda, toward members of their own and the other castes.

These data specify the users of cannabis or *injaga*, as it was called by the Rwandans. They detail the methods of *injaga* growing and use, reported internal and external physical effects and reported behaviors following *injaga* smoking, along with attitudes toward the use of *injaga* held by the Rwanda men, women and children of all three castes who had something to say on the subject.

INJAGA USE AND THE TWA

With few exceptions the questionnaire respondents associated *injaga* use with Twa men and with them alone. A few responses state that the Congolese and the Bashi used it, but not Rwandans other than the Twa. There is one note that Twa women smoked it as well as Twa men, but that the women used a different method. There are several statements that, although they are the rare exceptions, there are *injaga* smokers among the Hutu and Tutsi, and there is also mention of its occasional medicinal use among the Hutu and Tutsi in ways differing, however, from the method of taking it used by Twa men.

INJAGA GROWING AND METHOD OF SMOKING

Injaga was grown concealed in the middle of patches of tall crops such as maize or sorghum. After harvesting it was dried and powdered. It was generally smoked in a special gourd water-pipe called *urumogi* (Plate 1). The tube of the pipe was filled first with *injaga*, often mixed with powdered charcoal, then little pebbles which were topped with glowing coals. The pipe was set into a gourd partly filled with water. (Twa dancers are said to sometimes use a small clay pipe like a tobacco pipe, and Twa women to smoke it by emptying out half the tobacco in a cigarette and refilling it with *injaga*.) It was smoked in the old days before fighting and hunting, especially elephant hunting, but its use was not restricted to such special occasions. Mornings and evenings were the times for smoking it. The Twa are reported as having a ritual to make the *injaga* as powerful as possible, and in smoking it they are reported as taking in deep frequent inhalations causing the water in the pipe to bubble with a loud noise and producing clouds of smoke.

The Physical Effects of Injaga *Smoking.* The physical effects reported by those who claimed to be eyewitnesses are that the smokers' faces poured with perspiration and that their eyes became very red soon after smoking. There is no data on the strength of the cannabis used, but it is clear that strength was desired and that the smoking method aimed at the taking of a heavy dose within a brief time-period. The reported internal effect of cannabis-smoking cannot be tied to individuals known to be talking of their own experience and may be merely hearsay, deductions from the character of the behaviors attendant on cannabis-smoking, or repetitions of stereotypic notions about the Twa who are thought to have great physical strength. It is said that *injaga*-smoking confers a feeling of remarkable courageousness and physical strength. It is said also that it banishes fatigue and physical pain when taken in much smaller amounts than what has been described in the method used by Twa men.

THE BEHAVIORS FOLLOWING *INJAGA*-SMOKING

A number of individuals who claim to have been eyewitnesses report that the usual outcome of *injaga*-smoking is that the smoker becomes physically violent toward others. Acts of violence are described as wild, mindlessly fearless of receiving any hurt in the fights that ensued, and wholly undiscriminating in their object which might be a wife, a friend, a Tutsi protector and patron, or whoever was about.

ATTITUDES TOWARD *INJAGA*-SMOKING

The photo-questionnaire responses are rich in judgments about *injaga*-smoking which was quite overwhelmingly condemned. (See Table 1.) Most of the other data of an ethnographic character, data on *injaga* growing and smoking methods and so on, were presented to explain and justify the generally condemnatory opinions that were advanced. (Giving reasons and background for their opinions was a widespread Rwanda practice which not only deserves some general anthropological recognition but also the special blessing of the writer whose work in the Rwanda of 1959–60 required many informants drawn from every social category and group.)

One hundred and thirteen Rwandans gave an opinion about *injaga*-smoking in commenting on the photograph of the Twa man. Of these responses 99 were wholly against it, only one, a Twa man, made an unqualifiedly favorable statement, and the remaining 13 gave mixed opinions.[2] (See Table 1.) Reasons given in favor, or partial favor of *injaga* were: that it gave great strength and courage, that it dispelled fatigue, was good for rheumatism, and that it was all right, if used in very small quantities. The mixed opinions pointed out, for instance that *injaga* conferred courage because its use deprived a man of the sense to know real danger when he faced it or that it was all right for the Twa but not for anyone else. Reasons against the smoking of *injaga* centered on the violent behavior it produced and labelled it as crazy and senseless. A sampling of these depositions follows, since it is from the words of the Rwandans themselves that it is possible to get the full impact and tone of their views:

Twa man of 35 with no schooling. This man is smoking *injaga*. It is good to smoke *injaga*. *Injaga* is strengthening. The Twa are very strong, because they smoke it. (This is the only unqualifiedly favorable deposition.)

Twa woman of 28 with no schooling. It is a man smoking *injaga*. I see it well. When the Twa men finish smoking *injaga*, they come to bother us and beat us. I would like once and for all to keep our husbands from smoking that terrible tobacco. It is very bad. Once my husband nearly died from a lance wound he received from a man he fought with after smoking *injaga*.

A Tutsi man of 36 with five years of schooling. It is a Twa smoking *injaga*. I know about the scenes *injaga*-smokers make. On my hill (which is to say neighborhood) after a ceremony connected with a new house the Twa smoked *injaga* when they were drunk, and then fought one another so viciously that they left two corpses there. Then, I know that at Nzega the Twa smoked *injaga* and attacked all the shops wanting to kill a Hindu named Merali and a Swahili. Chief R. intervened or they would have.

A Tutsi man of 29 with five years of schooling. This is a Twa smoking *injaga*. I have seen them smoke it many times, especially in these days recently when the Twa have to build up their strength by alcohol or *injaga*. They smoked and one of them in my neighborhood became half crazy and just missed killing us though all the while he was proclaiming "Defend the Tutsi!" When people smoke *injaga* they lose all power to reason.

A Tutsi woman of 28 with eight years of schooling. It is certainly a Twa smoking *injaga*. I have seen them at our place many times. Besides during the month of

---

[2] The 132 Rwanda who gave no deposition on *injaga*-smoking included many who had probably never seen it smoked and who did not recognize the photographic clue, the water-pipe. This was certainly the case for many of the children of whom only four had anything to say about *injaga*. Many adults as well clearly did not recognize the water-pipe, since they made some inaccurate identification of it. Many others simply talked about other things in the photograph or other subjects the photograph stimulated them to respond to and made no mention of *injaga*.

December the Twa of our neighborhood did nothing but smoke it in order to get courage and strength. After they smoked they ran about on the hillside saying they were going to kill all the enemies of the Mwami.

A Tutsi woman of 24 with four years of schooling. Here is a Twa smoking *injaga*. The Twa are the Tutsi's friends and the Hutu's enemies. The Twa are true courtiers. A Twa vassal is loyal and loves his Tutsi master. But when they smoke they no longer have the right spirit. So that is how *injaga* is bad.

A Hutu man of 38 with three years of schooling. A Twa man smoking *injaga*. After he has smoked it he will be seized with madness and he will begin fighting and doing all sorts of bad things. Near where I live there are no longer many Twa, but there are always some, and when one or more of them have been taking *injaga*, the whole neighborhood stays on guard.

A Hutu man of 39 with no schooling. It is a Twa smoking *injaga*. After they have smoked they become almost completely crazy and fight with one another. Others of them sing or cry. It is an evil tobacco that I have never tried. It makes a man irrational and an idiot.

A Hutu woman of 32 with no schooling. That is a Twa smoking *injaga*. Look at the pipe for *injaga*. *Injaga* is peculiar to the Twa. Anyone else who took it would die on the spot. *Injaga* is for a strong man. The Twa smoke *injaga* to be strong — so they say. I think *injaga* is very bad. The wives of *injaga*-smokers know very well what the effects of *injaga* are, for they are almost always beaten. The *injaga* addict will give everything he has to get that poison. You know a Twa who has smoked it is like a hyena. His acts are those of a cruel beast.

Alcohol in Rwanda. Cannabis use in Rwanda must be considered in relation to the widespread and routine use of alcohol.

Alcoholic beverages were of outstanding importance in Rwanda life as an indispensable accompaniment to all sociability, a necessity for all working-bees as well as all social occasions, and, formerly, before the use of money, the most acceptable of gifts and payments for all the lower range of exchanges in which cattle had too great a unit value to be useful.

The strongest native alcoholic beverage was a kind of mead, a drink made from honey, and it was rarely available to any but the wealthy, which is to say, the Tutsi. Beers of sorghum or millet and bananas made according to a variety of recipes were the staple beverages. Most were weakly alcoholic.

The low level of living of most Rwandans in 1959–60 as in traditional times guaranteed moderation, if not downright sobriety, much of the time. Frequent drunkenness was possible only for the wealthy, and the state of drunkenness was not disapproved of as was the state of cannabis intoxication, although the drunk or the man so fond of drink that he spent overmuch time going about trying to get it, was disapproved of.[3]

All the Rwandans liked and used alcohol in the form of the native

[3] The photograph of a Hutu mother giving beer to her small child yielded many comments and opinions about beer and about drinking.

beers. Even children were given some beer, especially sorghum beer which was held to be "the milk of the poor" who had no cows. The Twa, since they were often attached to the households of wealthy Tutsi, were better supplied with liquor than the Hutu and were considered to have a great liking and capacity for it. Some of the questionnaire depositions indicate that Twa behavior was particularly violent when *injaga* was smoked after drinking a good deal.

Cannabis use by the Twa, was then merely in addition to their use of alcohol, which, in the eyes of all Rwandans, was among the good things life had to offer.

The Social and Cultural Context of Cannabis Use in Rwanda. The data presented show that cannabis use and attitudes toward its use follow the lines of the caste social structure of traditional Rwanda. The nature of Twa cannabis use is wholly in accord with the place given the Twa in the traditional society and the character assigned them in the traditional culture.

Injaga smoking is on the list of Twa practices and behaviors that the Tutsi and the Hutu consider to be uncontrolled or excessive to the point of being more animal-like than human, although for the Twa, themselves, the same list consists of items relating to the particular talents and the stronger appetites and greater capacities, compared to the Tutsi and Hutu, that make them specially and distinctively Twa.

The reported details of the methods of Twa cannabis use indicating heavy dosage, the strong effects that are expected and sought after, and the violent behaviors attendant on its use are all consistent and mutually reinforcing.

The sociocultural system confines cannabis use almost exclusively to the Twa and insulates the remaining 99 percent plus of the population from its use. It is linked with all that sets the Twa apart as a social group, and the Twa obligingly — from the point of view of a working and nearly water-tight system — see cannabis in ways that could have little appeal to other Rwandans, who, whatever their other dissatisfactions, remain quite content with their beer and with not being Twa.

Cannabis use in Rwanda is, therefore, seen to have its specific definition and character because of the sociocultural system in which it is embedded and to which it contributes its, to be sure, not very large but, nevertheless, concordant share of all that determines the system's character, workings and continuity.

REFERENCES

CODERE, HELEN
 1962 Power in Rwanda. *Anthropologica.* N.S. IV (1):45-85.
DE LAEGER, L.
 1939 *Ruanda.* Kabgayi.
D'HERTEFELT, MARCEL
 1962 "Le Rwanda," in *Les anciens royaumes de la zone interlacastre méridionale. Rwanda, Burundi, Buha.* Edited by M. d'Hertefelt, A. A. Trouwbirst, J. H. Scherer. Tervuren: Musée Royale de l'Afrique Centrale; London International African Institute (Ethnographic Survey of Africa).
 1965 "The Rwanda," in *Peoples of Africa.* Edited by J. L. Gibbs, 405-440. New York: Holt, Rinehart and Winston.
MAQUET, J. J.
 1954 Le système des relations sociales dans le Rwanda ancien. *Annales du Musée Royale du Congo Belge. Science de l'Homme. Ethnologie* I. Tervuren.
PAGES, A.
 1933 *Un royaume hamite au centre d'Afrique.* Institut Royal Congo Belge. Brussels.

Réunion: Cannabis in a Pluricultural and Polyethnic Society

JEAN BENOIST

ABSTRACT

The Island of Réunion, presently a French Department, in the Indian Ocean, has a polyethnic population of diverse origins: the descendants of African slaves and indentured laborers from India (principally from the south); Chinese and Europeans (principally from metropolitan France).

Cannabis, known as *zamal*, grown in cane fields and gardens, has been used ritually and medicinally, but these usages appear to be disappearing. Traditional secular use continues clandestinely among certain ethnic groups. Contacts with metropolitan France and the changing social structure have introduced "modern" uses of *zamal*, as a narcotic, among literary circles and groups of young people. The man-plant relationship differs in the ritual and narcotic uses.

Cannabis grows very well on the island of Réunion; it is relatively widespread in several regions, particularly in the mid-altitude zones of the western part of the island. Its use is rare but apparent in a wide variety of forms and in multivaried contexts related to the close articulation between the plant and the social and cultural diversity of the island. The multiplicity of current social changes is particularly well illuminated by the varied significance that the plant assumes in different contexts. The coexistence of different patterns and cultural traditions of cannabis use in such a small territory, within a polyethnic society, affords a grasp of the major values and functions attached to the plant in terms of individual and social consequences of its use.

The introduction of cannabis to Réunion is apparently quite ancient, but there is no precise documentation on this subject. The name most often used to refer to cannabis is *zamal*, which seems to be of Malagasy (Madagascar) origin, but is not found in present-day Malagasy vocabulary. Chaudenson (1973) notes that the word *jamala* is mentioned by R.

For Plates, see pp. xi–xii, between pp. 266–267.

Drury in his *Vocabulaire de la langue de Madagascar*, published in 1729, in the western part of Madagascar, at a time when the peopling of the island of Réunion, previously a desert, had only just begun. Regarding a crime committed on Réunion in 1830 by a Malay, an historian of Réunion (Meerlsman [1895?]) writes that the assassin "had smoked Amale to get his head high" before committing the crime.

It is probable that *zamal* was introduced to the island along with the slaves brought in from Madagascar. Consequently, the term *"zamal"* became current in Réunion, and seems to have been rediffused to Madagascar through immigration from Réunion. The term is not found in Mauritius, however, though this island is quite close to Réunion; the Mauritians use the word *ganja*. In Mauritius, traditional social functions of the plant are related exclusively to the Indian domain, the significant Indian presence provides a contrast to the situation in Réunion where African and Indian cultural currents meet.

I. ETHNIC GROUPS AND USE OF CANNABIS

The ethnic composition of Réunion is quite complex. On two thousand square kilometers there are more than 450,000 people, descendants of waves of migrants who began to intermarry at the end of the seventeenth century. The colonists came from Europe, their descendants, numbering several tens of thousands, occupy the highlands principally. The ascendancy of sugar cane cultivation at the beginning of the nineteenth century created a demand for manual labor that increased the importation of African and Malagasy slaves, and later of indentured laborers from the south of India. While the rate of European immigration was slowed down, it never actually ceased, and is now on the rise because of the status of Réunion, which has been a French department since 1946. Paralleling the migrant waves of population, other diverse groups, mostly minorities, were formed. Chinese immigrants spread throughout the island, taking over almost all of the food-trade business; Muslim Indians still closely attached to their region (Surat, in the Marastrya), have for three or four generations formed solid urban business communities; laborers from the Comores, more recent arrivals, constitute an urban sub-proletariat.

Outside these minorities, the different subgroups do not constitute a clearly contrasting society. Both legislation and official ideology, to the contrary, favor the integration of ethnic groups into the dominant culture, which is Creole and French. Without doing away with differences, this situation often masks them, and ensures transitions through which cultural particulars can be easily diffused. Each group — Indian (*Malbar*), European (white and *Zoreil*), African and Chinese — is thus open to influences from its neighbors, while still retaining certain ethnic and cultural traits.

While the use of *zamal* thus follows different patterns, associated with the origins of the different cultural components of the island, it also undergoes transformations through inter-ethnic contacts and contemporary social change.

(a) *Ritual uses.* It is in ceremonies related to Indian and Malagasy religions that the use of cannabis has retained some of the traits closest to those that characterized it in the societies of origin. But these uses are now quite limited and are gradually disappearing.

The Malagasy of Réunion, quite small in number, have intermarried with the colored creole population on a considerable scale, and in no way form a community. But certain magical activities and, more and more rarely, annual feasts marked by the sacrifice of cows, bring together people who have Malagasy ancestors, and thus call themselves "creoles" and "cafres" (Kaffir) with whom they are often confused. During these feasts, cannabis cigarettes are smoked communally. In the eyes of the creoles, this activity leads to violent behavior and gives the Malagasy people a reputation of brutality. The creole expression, *son zamal y monte* [his zamal is rising] signifies "he is getting angry."

In the few areas where the population of Malagasy origin is relatively numerous, the use of *zamal*, while clandestine, seems to be rather regular and provides a source of supply for other ethnic groups who pass through the area.

The Indians of Réunion lead a very active religious life. There are numerous temples throughout the island; however, while the faithful are mostly of Indian extraction, they come from all of the other ethnic groups on the island as well.

These Indians who are mostly from South India, practice beliefs profoundly marked by Tamil-Nadu village traditions. While the principal Hindu divinities (Shiva, Vishnu) are rather insignificant in local cults, the divinities that are strictly south-Indian rank quite high (Mariama, Madurai-veran, Karupuswami, and various forms related to Shiva, the Muni or Mini). The cult of Kali also has some following. It may, therefore, be concluded that we are dealing with Dravidian cults associated with the Sivaite trend of Hinduism. The priest-healer is possessed during certain ceremonies, and it is at this point that cannabis intervenes.

The religious role, as well as the social functions of cannabis, differs profoundly from what has been observed in the north of India. Only the possessed priest, in the course of specific possessions, is allowed to use the plant. He does not use *zamal* to initiate possession but, on the contrary, only after possession has occurred. The first words of "the spirit" spoken through his lips are to acclaim "candia." At this point, an assistant quickly places in the mouth of the priest one to three tobacco cigarettes, which he smokes at a very rapid rate. Only in certain circumstances (possession by Madurai-veran or by Mini) is the cigarette, the "candia" actually made from *zamal*. It is then called "ciga."

The terminological change that brought about, in Réunion, the naming as "candia" any cigarette offered to the gods or to the spirits and the subclassification as "ciga" any "candia" containing *zamal* reflects an important peculiarity about the anticipated effects of the plant. The priest smokes only when he is possessed by the spirit. His actions are then those of the spirit, who is often represented in the process of smoking *zamal* (see Plates). But smoking *zamal* is as natural for the gods as smoking cigarettes is for man. The possessed priest, consequently, must feel nothing and in no case must reveal any effects of the drug: this indifference is the *sign* of possession. By demonstrating that he is not affected by a drug accessible only to the gods, the priest shows that he has entered their universe. He can thus act as they do, or can at least act as an intermediary between gods and men.

The ritual use of *zamal* as a test, analogous to the ordeal of walking on hot coal, or performing the knife dance, extremely limits its secular use. It does happen that some young men finish the "ciga" begun by the priest, but, in the Indian community, the sacred role of the plant and the awe accompanying it, constrain its widespread use. On the other hand, the sacred role of the plant in communication with the spirits, a role it shares with other plants, has given it an important place in home gardens and in the pharmacopoeia.

(b) *Traditional secular uses.* Planted in home gardens or in sugar cane fields, *zamal* served a therapeutic function, magical as well as pharmaceutical. It scared off certain evil spirits and was also used in infusions prepared by the healers. The rigorous laws made the healers cautious in their choice of herbs and *zamal* has now been replaced by less dangerous plants in the preparation of medicinal infusions.

Boiled roots were used to reduce infants' vomiting, and an infusion of the leaves was used to rid one of fever, but these uses also have now practically disappeared. Several roots of *zamal* are still occasionally planted in a field, particularly where squash is grown to rid the area of parasitic insects.

In veterinary medicine, it is quite common to pulverize *zamal* leaves in the drinking water of chickens to prevent contagious and infectious diseases. *Zamal* is also used for the aggressive properties it is supposed to impart: the leaves are pounded and mixed into the food of dogs to make them vicious; fighting cocks are sometimes given tiny balls to eat, made of a mixture of minced onions and *zamal* leaves to make them combative.

Human consumption of the plant, outside of religious ceremonies, seems always to have been somewhat limited. Known by all, experimented with by many adolescents in the fields, it has never posed a major problem. Two sociocultural trends seem to have coexisted for a long time, which are the bases of present-day forms of consumption of the plant: consumption by agricultural workers as opposed to consumption by the elite, and these two trends scarcely ever coincide.

It is still recalled that some old Indians, from the region of Calcutta, who smoked for pleasure, placed *zamal* in a small coconut filled with water. But this usage has disappeared. The majority of the Indians, of Tamil extraction, regard the drug with some reticence, while insisting that it would not present the same dangers for them that it would for other ethnic groups: "When the creole or Malagasy people smoke *zamal*, they become wicked, but not the Malbars, they are more level-headed." *Zamal* seems to have been used for a long time especially in certain shanty-towns.

Some individuals in the countryside, white or creoles of color, prepared *zamal* cigars. Mature, almost yellow, leaves were gathered and mixed with tobacco leaves. The mixture was then washed in water in which citron had been boiled. A mixture of honey and alcohol was then poured copiously over the leaves, and they were placed in a press to dry out for a month. The dry mixture was then pounded and smoked in ordinary pipes. Cigarettes have tended to replace such preparations.

On the other hand, some Réunion writers were influenced by Baudelaire, Théophile Gautier, and Maurice Magre. Impressed by the Indian ceremonies in which the plant played a significant role in communication with the supernatural, they formed small groups which added the poetic exaltation of *zamal* to the use of the plant as a drug. Several literary works resulted (M. A. Leblond, *Sortilèges* [Charms]; J. Albany [1951, 1970] *Zamal*), glorifying *zamal* in the poetic-mystical manner of French poets. *Zamal* became both the symbol and the means of rejection of the most rigid forms of Western thought, mixed with an Indian point of view that valued its mystics. This current of thought seems to have lasted until around 1950, and to partly underly present ideological trends.

II. APPEARANCE OF NEW MODES OF CONSUMPTION

Réunion has seen considerable social changes in the period since the 1950s. Having become a French department, it has received an unprecedented influx of money that produced a new middle class, supported by public works and the tertiary sector.

At the same time, secondary education has broadly expanded, while the urban population has grown more rapidly than that of the country areas, giving rise to the peri-urban proliferation of shanty-towns. High wages created economic and social problems leading some employers to hire manual laborers from outside the island (from the Comores), thus creating a doubly marginal sub-proletariat. During this period also, continental French from all geographical and social levels have been coming to Réunion in increasing numbers, along with their families. And flights between the island and Mauritius have multiplied.

Zamal cannot be considered apart from these changes. In many respects the new society has created a milieu much more favorable to use of the plant than was the preceding one. Discreetly at first, and then more and more overtly, new modes of use have begun to appear. Here again, the two principal trends can be found, the sub-proletarian and the elitist.

The former has mainly attracted the workers from the Comores, enclaved in densely populated communities in shanty-towns outside of Port and the capital, Saint-Denis. They have ties with the vendors from Mauritius and collaborate with them in the collection of cannabis from the countryside; part of the cannabis crop is clandestinely exported to Mauritius. The cigarette seems to be the principal mode of use in this group, and most of the users are male, but precise data on the extent of use are lacking.

The other trend is the indirect result of the extremely rapid social mobility by means of education, affecting a large portion of Réunion's youth. Following an ideology reminiscent of that of the late nineteenth-century poets, groups of continental youth, and students from the lycées, began to smoke on the beach or outside the schools. They have had no difficulty in procuring the drug which grows quite freely in many places. These young people have been joined by musicians from dance orchestras, prostitutes, and marginal individuals, both continental and creole. There is great variation in the methods of use. Many young people are only occasional users; others tend to form groups of habitual users.

The authorities have decided to deal quietly in regard to legal trials and sanctions. They feel, and rightly so, that the phenomenon does not present a social menace, and that any exaggeration of the conflict would lead to results quite opposed to those that might be desired.

Clinical observations of the phenomenon are also rare. The psychiatric hospital has received groups of youthful smokers on only two occasions. The first group, committed by the police in 1971, consisted of young people who met in a house to smoke *zamal* cigarettes. They had been initiated by members of a travelling Mauritian orchestra and were harvesting *zamal* themselves in fields on the eastern part of the island. The decision of the psychiatrists was to not admit them to the hospital and only to exercise some surveillance over them. The group quickly quit smoking.

In 1973, another group presented a more serious problem. Several boys and girls between seventeen and twenty years old had formed a community for two years, led by a woman from France, an artist with a strong personality. She was hospitalized for a psychotic episode, and the entire group joined her soon afterward. After an investigation by the police, they were all still smoking numerous cigarettes daily. Following brief hospitalization, they were all sent home under surveillance.

These two cases serve to illustrate the new pattern, which in its general aspects is similar to that which has been observed elsewhere in the world with regard to marihuana. It is clearly opposed to the traditional island pattern, as well as to that of the urban sub-proletariat. Moreover, it seems that the reactions of society are relatively moderate because of the weak lines of communications between the two groups of users. The separation which is elsewhere apparent between social classes, and which drug usage continues to bring into question, is emphasized in Réunion by a more radical separation, to the extent that the sub-proletarian class of Comores does not participate at all in the same activities as the other members of society. At the same time, ritual uses have regressed to the point of being purely symbolic.

Thus, the relationship between man and the plant has evolved in close correlation with relationships between different groups of men. In a society in which division into ethnic and cultural groups is less significant than class structure, the use of cannabis moves from forms profoundly marked by the cultural antecedents of particular ethnic groups to forms characteristic of social classes and age groups. This realignment is closely related to that in other countries under metropolitan influences. The specific aspects of Réunion society alter these generalizations in a relatively slight manner aside from the almost absolute barrier separating the Comores from the rest of the population.

It would be erroneous to consider cannabis as an isolated phenomenon in Réunion. Furthermore, interesting as it may be to observe as a cultural phenomenon, it must be emphasized that cannabis is completely overshadowed by the formidable problem of alcoholism.

The contrast between cannabis societies and alcohol societies, emphasized throughout this volume, shows up quite clearly here. In Réunion alcoholism is more widespread than in most countries of the world. The real cultural choice between alcohol and cannabis has yet to be explained, in a country where both are easily accessible and neither is costly. The relationship between this choice and the influence of legislation, which in Réunion favors alcohol, must be carefully studied.

REFERENCES

ALBANY, J.
   1951   *Zamal*. Paris: Bellenand.
   1970   "Vavangue." Unpublished manuscript, Paris.
CHAUDENSON, R.
   1973   *Le lexique du parler créole de la Réunion*, two volumes. In press.
MEERLSMAN, R. P.
   [1895?]   "Histoire de la Paroisse de St-Gilles-les-Hauts." Unpublished manuscript.

Social Aspects of the Use of Cannabis in India

KHWAJA A. HASAN

ABSTRACT

Cannabis in India is used in three forms — *ganja*, *bhang*, and *charas*. *Bhang* is obtained from the dried leaves of *Cannabis sativa* or *Cannabis indica*. The oleo-resinous exudate of the plants is called *charas* and the flowering tops are called *ganja*. *Ganja* and *charas* are mixed with tobacco and smoked in clay pipes; *bhang* is eaten orally in the form of small balls or used as a beverage called *thandai*. While alcohol is generally looked down upon in Hindu society as it is tabooed to the *Brahman* and *Bhagats* (devotees), the use of cannabis is socially sanctioned and is associated with religio-social ceremonies of the Hindu god, *Shiva*. Cannabis is offered to *Shiva* on *Shivaratri* day in temples as "food of god." This paper examines what role cannabis plays in the social life of the people, particularly in villages, and whether freedom to obtain and use these drugs results in addiction as a massive problem.

ETHNOHISTORICAL ASPECTS

The use of intoxicating drinks and drugs is known to have existed in ancient India. Aryan settlers are believed to have used a drink called *somarasa*, the juice of a mysterious plant called *soma*. The *Grihya* and *Dharamsutras* do not mention anything about *soma* but the *Srautasutras*, which describe the religious practices of the Aryans, do mention the sacrifices connected with the drinking of *somarasa*. Some substitutes of *soma* are also suggested by the *Srautasutras*. For example, a beverage called *masara* is mentioned as a substitute for *somarasa*.

Masara was prepared from germinated rice or germinated barley, fried grains, and certain roots, herbs, and spices known under the generic name *nagnahu*, which mainly served as yeast (Gopal 1959: 166–167). It is also mentioned in the *Srautasutras* that *masara* was used in the preparation of *sura* which was a common liquor of the Sutra period and was

For Plate, see p. xiii, between pp. 266–267.

offered to deities. However, *Dharamsutras*, the literature dealing with the interaction between religion, family, and society, condemns drinking of *sura* and prescribes severe punishment for a Brahman who drinks it. It is recommended in this literature that a Brahman who drinks *sura* should be branded on his forehead with the sign of a *sura* pot and condemned to exile (*Ibid.*). Thus it seems likely that the use of liquor was confined to the so-called lower castes.

The Buddhist Age in India began in the sixth century before Christ, and Buddhism gradually supplanted Brahmanism as a national religion. Buddhism prohibited the use of intoxicants to its followers (Report 1955: 4). However, Brahmanism was revived in the tenth century of our era. Modern day Hinduism, therefore, is the result of cumulative influence of post-Vedic times (Mackenzie 1913: 120). Historically, the consumption of alcoholic drinks and hemp drugs is reported to be in use up to the 8th or 9th century A.D., i.e., prior to the advent of Muslims into the country (Mitra 1955: 234). Opium was brought to India by the pre-Islamic Arab traders during 570–632 A.D. (Terry 1931: 242–251). During the medieval period the habit of drinking developed considerably. This may be attributed in part to the example set by the kings and their courtiers. However, not all the medieval kings indulged in drinking. It is reported that King Allauddin Khilji in the year 1310 had imposed a total prohibition on the capital city of Delhi, and Aurangzeb, a king in the Moghal dynasty who was a staunch follower of Islam, abstained from drinking (Report, *op.cit.*). One wonders what the situation was regarding the use or abuse of hemp drugs and opium during the medieval period.

The British introduced the system of excise taxation in India for the first time in the history of the country. The East India Company and its successor, the then Government of India, enacted laws in the year 1790 in consonance with the policy that was followed in the United Kingdom. The Royal Commission of 1893 to inquire into the prevalence of the opium habit, and another commission appointed by the Government of India two years later, collected a mass of information on the prevalence and effects of these drugs (both opium and hemp). In 1907 an agreement to reduce the export of opium to China was reached, which was stopped completely in 1913–1914 (Report, *op.cit.*).

Legislative measures against the production, possession, and sale of intoxicating drinks and drugs were also taken in India. For example, in 1910 an act, known as the United Provinces Excise Act IV, was passed by the legislature of that province which under article 17 (1) includes the following measures:

(a) No excisable article shall be manufactured,
(b) No hemp plant shall be cultivated,
(c) No portion of hemp plant, from which any intoxicating drug can be manufactured, shall be collected,
(d) No liquor shall be bottled for sale,
(e) No person shall use, keep or have in his possession any materials, distilling utensils, implements or apparatus whatsoever, for the purpose of manufacturing any excisable article other than toddy; except under the authority and subject to the terms and conditions of license granted in that behalf by the Collector.

Thus, the British did not impose prohibition of intoxicating drinks and drugs in India. Instead, they introduced a system of licensing the manufacture of alcoholic beverages and the production and sale of narcotic drugs. They also followed a policy of restricting consumption by raising taxes from time to time. The production of opium in India was curtailed drastically through governmental control. For example, in 1910 about one million acres of land was planted to poppies. This was curtailed to one-fifth of a million acres in 1948 and to about 75,000 acres in 1958 (*Times of India*, New Delhi, May 24, 1959, Sunday Magazine Section).

In the post-independence period, the concept of the Welfare State was promoted in India and the followers of Mahatma Gandhi demanded a system of prohibition throughout the nation. Several states introduced prohibition. In some states "wet" and "dry" districts were declared while in some other areas "wet" and "dry" days of the week were introduced. This gave a fillip to illicit distillation, smuggling and even to resorting to the use of denatured spirits. The system of control on the production and sale of hemp resulted in smuggling of *ganja* from Nepal. Newspaper reports reveal that new methods are continually adopted in the smuggling business. In January of 1972, about 100 deaths were reported from methanol poisoning in the Capital City of Delhi (*Overseas Hindustan Times*, New Delhi, dated January 29, 1972, p. 1).

ALCOHOL AND CANNABIS: DIFFERENCES IN CULTURAL ORIENTATION

While our knowledge of ethnohistorical aspects of the use of alcohol and drugs in India is by no means complete, the above account throws some light on how present day sociocultural norms are derived from the past and on differences in the use or non-use of different intoxicants at present. This paper is an attempt to discuss differences in the cultural goals and orientation toward the use or non-use of different intoxicants in Hindu society. These differences are based on an individual's membership in a *varna* and caste, or other groupings such as the "holy" as against the "ordinary," or are related to the nature of interaction between members of a kinship group as against others. While the objective of this paper is to discuss mainly the use of cannabis in India, reference to the use of alcohol is inevitable since the use or non-use of these two groups of intoxicants represents differing cultural values in Hindu society.

Consumption of alcohol in villages in India is confined to the use of *daroo* or *sharaab* (wine), *tharra* (country-made liquor), *taari* (toddy — the juice of fan palm, date palm and coconut trees), and denatured spirits. Among the hemp drugs in common use are *ganja*, *bhang*, and *charas*. *Bhang* is obtained from the dried leaves of hemp plants. The oleo-resinous exudate is called *charas* and the flowering tops are called *ganja*. While the use of hemp drugs seems to have social sanction among Hindu castes, alcoholic beverages do not find a place of honor or even proper conduct. This does not mean that there is no use of alcohol among Hindus. It only indicates a differential in cultural and religious orientation toward these two groups of intoxicants. Alcohol in any form is absolutely prohibited to the Brahman, the highest *varna* in the Hindu caste system. The prohibition of alcohol goes back to the Vedic periods. Among the twice-born castes, the *Kshatriya* are known to use alcohol and meat as mentioned by Carstairs (1954). The Kayasthas of north India also use alcoholic beverages. However, even in these castes, individuals who drink alcohol try to give up wine and meat with the coming of old age and begin to devote themselves to religion — a cultural goal to die "pure" and pious (Hasan 1967).

Among the *Shudra* and the untouchable castes, the use of alcohol is not prohibited. It is in this group of castes that we find that some alcoholic beverages are used quite commonly. In a study of a village inhabited predominantly by the so-called lower castes near the City of Lucknow, in 1959–1960, I found that out of 62 respondents among Hindu castes, 45 (75%) did not object to using wine and country liquor, while 41 (66.1%) did not object to using denatured spirits (methyl alcohol), while 42 (67.7%) did not object to using toddy. However, 54 respondents out of 62 (87.1%) did not object to using one or more forms of hemp drugs. Table 1 gives the exact number of respondents by caste showing no objection to using one or more of the intoxicants.

The figures from Table 1 reveal that more people in the village used hemp drugs than alcohol. This difference is due to the religious and cultural sanctioning of hemp drugs, while alcohol is seen differently. For example, a person who wants to become a *Bhagat* (devotee) must pledge before his *guru* (religious preceptor) that he will not consume liquor, meat, onion, garlic, etc., nor will he have sexual intercourse (even with his own wife) after becoming a devotee. However, hemp drugs are not forbidden to him. *Bhagats* and holy men (saints) are, therefore, free to use these drugs while they are forbidden to take alcohol (Hasan 1971). Since Brahmans are accorded the highest status in Hindu society, their practices, (fasting, vegetarianism, ablution) and avoidances (teetotalism) are valued and respected, and *Bhagats* of other castes adopt many of these practices to bring themselves closer to the supernatural. Many lower-caste individuals, generally those over 40 years old, become *Bhagats* and must, therefore, give up alcohol although they can continue to use hemp drugs.

The use of *ganja*, *bhang*, and *charas* is associated with religio-social ceremonies among the Hindus. It is believed that the god *Shiva* (also known as *Shankar*) was very fond of hemp drugs; and these drugs are still offered to *Shiva* on *Shivaratri* day in temples as being "foods of the god." It was due to this religious association that Brahmans and *Bhagats* did not abstain from using these drugs while they abhorred alcoholic drinks.

The festival of Shivaratri is observed on the fourteenth day of the dark half of the month *Phalgun* (February-March). People celebrate by expressing happiness as they believe that *Shiva* was married on this day.

Table 1. Number of respondents (caste-wise) showing no objection to using one or more forms of intoxicants in Chinaura (1959–1960)

		(total)	Wine	Country liquor	Denaturated spirit	Toddy	Hemp drugs
1.	Ahir	12	4	4	2	3	8
2.	Lodh	10	7	7	7	7	9
3.	Pasi	14	12	12	12	12	12
4.	Chamar	12	12	12	12	12	12
5.	Dhobi	4	4	4	4	4	4
6.	Kumhar	2	1	1	Nil	Nil	2
7.	Marau	1	Nil	Nil	Nil	Nil	1
8.	Nau	1	1	1	1	1	1
9.	Bhujwa	1	1	1	1	1	1
10.	Kayastha	1	1	1	Nil	Nil	1
11.	Teli	1	1	1	1	1	1
12.	Lohar	1	Nil	Nil	Nil	Nil	1
13.	Kurmi	1	Nil	Nil	Nil	Nil	Nil
14.	Dom	1	1	1	1	1	1
15.	Muslim	18	Nil	Nil	Nil	Nil	Nil
Total Hindu Caste		62	45	45	41	42	54

Shiva is considered to be both the Creator and Destroyer of men, and is a god to be feared. In Hindu mythology, it was *Shiva* who swallowed the poison that came out of the churning of the sea, which otherwise would have destroyed mankind. Thus, people also observe a fast on this day to honor *Shiva*.

It is not clearly known why Hindus associate hemp drugs with *Shiva*. According to Underhill (1921: 66, 70), the plant *soma* was identified with the moon and so was *Shiva*. The *Satapatha brahmana* mention the importance of offerings to the spirits of the dead on the new moon days, for the moon comes to earth on this day and *soma*, the food of the gods and the departed, is unobtainable on that day, therefore the spirits will be without food unless the worshipper provides it (*Ibid.*: 112). Some scholars believe that *soma*, the mysterious plant, is cannabis (O'Flaherty 1971: 128), however, the idea has been strongly opposed by Wasson (1971: 10). In this book, *Soma: divine mushroom of immortality*, Wasson argues that *Rg Veda* placed *soma* only on the high mountains, whereas hemp grows everywhere; and that the virtue of *soma* lay in the stalks, whereas the leaves and the resin of cannabis are used as intoxicants, while the stalks of hemp are woody (*Ibid.:* 16). Wasson's scholarly analysis of numerous verses from *Rg Veda* and ethnohistorical and ethnobotanical data advance very convincing arguments for identifying *soma* as the mushroom, fly-agaric *(Amanita muscaria)*.

BHANG AND *THANDA*

In villages as well as cities *ganja* is usually mixed with tobacco and smoked in a funnel-shaped clay pipe (Plate 1). *Charas* is also used in the same manner. However, *bhang* is eaten in the form of small balls or used as a beverage. The famous decoction prepared from *bhang* is called *thandai*. In cities, *bhang* may also be added to the milk of the indigenous ice cream, called *gulfi*. A slang term for *gulfi* mixed with *bhang* in north India is *hari gulfi* (green ice cream).

Preparing *thandai* is a time-consuming process. A number of dry fruits, condiments, and spices are used in its preparation. Almonds, pistachio, rose petals, black pepper, aniseed, and cloves are ground on the toothed stone grinding plate (*silauti*); water is added so that a thinly ground paste is obtained. This paste is dissolved in milk and then *bhang* is added to the mixture. Some people add asafoetida also because of its medical properties. A few spoons of sugar or jaggery (boiled brown sugar) are added finally and then the decoction is ready for consumption.

It is generally believed that *thandai* (literal meaning: cold drink) makes the body of the user cool and comfortable. It is obvious that the drink has good nutritional value for it contains many protective foods. Almonds are fairly rich in proteins and fats which have a high calorie value. The drink, *thandai*, therefore, serves as a supplement to a diet poor in proteins and the condiments supply mineral salts. During the hot summer months from March to October people perspire heavily, the consequent loss of salt is compensated by its intake in food as well as in decoctions like *thandai*. Finally, dehydration is also offset, at least partially, by the consumption of *thandai*.

The preparation of *thandai* and the social atmosphere it creates has great significance. Members of the same family, caste or a circle of friends from the village or the neighborhood gather in the parlor of a friend. Different ingredients of the drink are collected and ground on the toothed stone grinding plate. The whole process takes an hour or so. While preparing the drink, individuals talk about friends, family members, prices of goods and services and a host of other problems. However, members of the *Shudra* and the untouchable castes do not join the *thandai* parties of the twice-born castes. They generally have their own parties.

Raw *bhang* in the form of small balls is also eaten in the villages and cities. *Bhang* eating is usually accompanied by eating any kind of sweets — jaggery, or sweetmeats. It is said that the intensity of intoxication is greatly enhanced by combining *bhang* with sweets. Both *ganja* and *bhang* are easily obtainable in small quantities from licensed dealers. These items are relatively cheap for small quantities can be purchased by spending a few *paises* for a single dose.

GANJA AND CHARAS

Ganja and *charas* also play an important role in the social life of the people in villages as well as cities. *Charas* may be mixed with tobacco and sometimes cigarettes of this mixture may be prepared by the user. No commercial cigarettes of this mixture are found or sold in India. *Ganja* is smoked in a funnel-shaped clay pipe called *chilam*. Almost anybody except the untouchables (sweeper caste) can join the group and enjoy a few puffs. The base part of the bowl portion of the funnel-shaped clay pipe is first covered with a small charred clay filter. Then the mixture of *ganja* and tobacco is placed on this filter. A small ring, the size of the bowl of the funnel-shaped clay pipe, of rope fiber called *baand*, is first burnt separately and then quickly placed on top of the smoking material. The pipe is now ready for smoking. Usually four or five persons gather around a pipe. One person starts taking puffs slowly. After igniting the fire material by taking small puffs he finally takes a really big puff and immediately passes the pipe to the person sitting next to him. Thus, in reality it is the last big puff which is inhaled fully by the smoker, the earlier smaller puffs are merely to ignite the fire; the smoke of those smaller puffs goes to the mouth and is released but not inhaled. In this way, the smoking pipe takes one or at the most two rounds and is enjoyed by several persons.

The smoking of *ganja* or even of ordinary tobacco may bring members of different castes or ordinary individuals and *Bhagats* together over a common pipe. However, ritual purity of the pipe is always preserved for the clay pipe is never touched by the lips of the smoker. The tubular part of the *chilam* at its bottom is held in the right hand and the left hand also supports it. The passage between the index finger and the thumb of the right hand is used in taking puffs from the pipe. Since nobody touches the pipe with his lips, the ritual purity of the pipe is maintained.

The first man before taking his first puff offers the smoke to *Shankar* (another name of *Shiva*) by saying in a high pitched voice, "*Jai Shankar, Kata Lage na Kankar.*" In so doing, he fortifies himself as well as others in the smoking party with the knowledge that the great god Creator-Destroyer relishes the smoke and prays that the smoke will not give trouble to their throats. Again, while they sit in squatting position on a *chabootra* (raised platform) in front of one person's house or gather in an open space while the host prepares the *chilam*, they talk about social problems, weather, crops, prices, marriage negotiations and so forth. Such gatherings may take place any time during the day except early morning. After a smoke they again go back to work. Thus such smoking parties are like "coffee breaks" in the American culture.

DRINKS, DRUGS, AND HINDU SOCIAL ORGANIZATION

Vegetarianism, fasting, observing proper ablution practices, and teetotalism are highly valued in Hindu society for these are associated with Brahmans, the highest *varna* in the Hindu caste system. The members of lower castes adopt these practices when they become *Bhagats* (devotees) under the influence of a holy man. In the village Chinaura many individuals over 40 years of age and some younger individuals became *Bhagats* (devotees). One who becomes a *Bhagat* is given respect for superior knowledge and wisdom and ties with *Shiva*. Members of both sexes could become *Bhagats*. A *Bhagat* can be recognized from his or her outward appearance as he or she wears a *kanthi*, a necklace of small wooden beads. Since ordinarily individuals over 40 years of age become *Bhagats*, the latter usually are senior citizens as average longevity in India is considerably lower than in industrial societies.

Becoming a *Bhagat* does not necessarily mean that one is required to use hemp drugs, although one must not use alcohol, meat, onion, garlic, and must abandon sexual activity. I found only one *Bhagat* in Chinaura who did not even smoke tobacco. This man belonged to the Ahir caste (milk producing caste), and was also chairman of the *gaon sabha* (village assembly). However, generally *Bhagats* were seen smoking and using hemp drugs, although with the exception of a few individuals, regular and excessive use was not noted.

In this village, I also found an example of how members of lower castes or even untouchables can get higher individual status by becoming *Bhagats* and by using hemp drugs. A man belonging to a sweeper caste (untouchable) worked as an employee of the Railways in the city. His duties included cleaning toilets in the railroad cars and at the Railway Station in the city. He learnt the use of *ganja, bhang, and charas* under the influence of some holy man. Later he left his well-paid job and became a *Bhagat;* he returned to the village and indulged excessively in smoking *ganja*. Even members of higher rank Shudra castes like Pasi, Chamar, and Bhujwa joined his smoking parties. Normally, Pasis, Chamars, and Bhujwa would not sit with a member of the sweeper caste and smoke through a common *chilam*. Leaving a well-paid job did not lower his prestige; in fact, this enhanced his status for this meant renunciation of the material world. After becoming a *Bhagat*, he started working as a *naut* (exorcist and medicine man) in the village.

The two basic elements of Hindu social organization are kinship and caste and the use of alcohol or cannabis has an interesting relationship with the nature of social interaction that can take place over a smoking pipe or a bottle of alcohol. While to members of Shudra castes, alcohol may serve as a unifying force, it may be responsible for isolating an individual in other castes. For example, Brahmans and orthodox Vaish families denounce the use of alcohol and those who drink are looked down upon. On the other hand, marriage parties or *biradari panchayats* (caste assemblies) are occasions on which drinking among the members of the same caste of the Shudra group are common. Among the Pasi, Chamar, Dhobi, Dom, and many other low caste groups, usually toddy is offered to guests at feasts. If an individual is "outcasted" by the caste assembly for violating any of the rules, some cash fine is imposed upon him and he is supposed to give a feast to the members of the caste. The number of individuals to whom the feast is to be given, is specified by the *chowdry* (Chairman of the caste assembly); this may range from one hundred to two hundred individuals. Outcasting means total isolation of the individual and his family from the caste. No one will smoke from the hubble-bubble of a person who has been outcasted nor will water be accepted at his hands. If an outcasted member agrees to give a feast to the *biradari* (caste) in which toddy or some other alcoholic beverages are served, he can be taken back at the very meeting of the assembly in which the feast is given.

Drinking among the kinship groups is ordinarily permissible. Male and female members of the same family among the Pasi, Chamar, Dhobi, Dom, and many other castes, can sit and drink together. But a woman may feel shy to drink in the presence of her son-in-law and she may sit separately to drink. Similarly, the housewife may feel shy to drink in the presence of her father-in-law. Drinking among kinship groups is usual at festivals or during harvest or when a close relative comes to stay. Drinks may also be offered to the would-be-in-laws at the time of negotiations for marriage. Drinking outside one's kinship or caste groups is rare in the village unless one goes to the toddy shop or a bar.

EFFECTS OF CANNABIS

The use of cannabis has generally been described to have threefold effects on human beings: (1) physiological changes, (2) neuro-psychiatric manifestations, and (3) sociological aspects of chronic use (Goodman and Gilman 1955: 170–174). Cannabis is used both orally and smoked by the Hindus of north India. We do not know the physiological effects of the consumption of *thandai* nor the effects that eating *bhang* may have on the body. However, it is important to note that smoking *ganja* in its cultural context involves taking only one big puff at a single smoking party. There is certainly a need to conduct physiological studies of the use of cannabis in these forms.

Reports of sociological effects of the use of cannabis suggest effects on the personality associated with prolonged use: loss of desire to work, loss of motivation, and loss of judgment and intellectual functions. Chopra *et al.* (1942) have studied sociological, psychiatric, and criminological aspects of the use of *Cannabis sativa* in India. The inquiries they conducted in various jails and mental centers revealed that in many cases even a single dose of *ganja* or *charas* smoke was reponsible for a heinous crime.

It would be interesting to know how many users of the drug did not commit crimes and how many criminals committed crimes of similar nature without having used the drug.

Although it is true that the use of hemp drugs is not looked down upon among Hindu castes, there is no evidence of physical dependence. People use these drugs sometimes as a means of recreation but usually there is no desire to continue usage nor is there any tendency to increase the dosage. Only occasions of festivity and ceremonial functions are meant for using these drugs in most cases. The number of regular users is negligible. In Chinaura, with a population of 1190 at the time of study, not more than four individuals were found to be regular users.

REFERENCES

CARSTAIRS, G. MORRIS
    1954 Daru and bhang: cultural factors in the choice of intoxicant. *Quarterly Journal Studies on Alcohol* 15:220–237.

CHOPRA, R. N., G. S. CHOPRA, I. C. CHOPRA
    1942 Cannabis sativa in relation to mental diseases and crime in India. *Indian Journal of Medical Research* 30:155–171.

GOODMAN, L. S., A. GILMAN
    1955 *The pharmacological basis of therapeutics.* New York: Macmillan.

GOPAL, R.
    1959 *India of Vedic Kalpsutras.* Delhi: National Publishing House.

HASAN, K. A.
    1967 *The cultural frontier of health in village India.* Bombay: Manaktalas Company.
    1971 The Hindu dietary practices and culinary rituals in a north Indian village: an ethnomedical and structural analysis. *Ethnomedicine* 1:43–70.

INDIA
    1910 The United Provinces Excise Act IV, as modified up to 1923.

INDIA PLANNING COMMISSION
    1955 *Report of the Prohibition Enquiry Committee.* Delhi: The Manager of Publications.

MACKENZIE, D. L.
    1913 *Indian myth and legend.* London: Gresham.

MITRA, S. K.
    1955 *Social welfare in India.* New Delhi: Publication Division, Ministry of Information and Broadcasting, Government of India.

O'FLAHERTY, W. D.
    1971 "The post-Vedic history of soma plant," in *Soma: divine mushroom of immortality.* Edited by R. G. Wasson. New York: Harcourt Brace Jovanovich.

Overseas Hindustan Times
  1972   New Delhi, January 29th, p. 1.
TERRY, C. E.
  1931   "Drug addiction," in *Encyclopedia of the social sciences*. Edited by E. R. Seligman and A. Johnson, volume five. New York: Macmillan.
Times of India
  1959   New Delhi, Sunday Magazine Section, May 24th.
UNDERHILL, M. M.
  1921   *The religious life of India*. London: Oxford University Press.
WASSON, R. G.
  1971   *Soma: divine mushroom of immortality*. New York: Harcourt Brace Jovanovich.

Cannabis in Nepal: An Overview

JAMES FISHER

ABSTRACT

Cannabis has been grown in Nepal, in both wild and cultivated varieties, for an extremely long time; but its uses, and attitudes toward them, have begun to change in recent years.

Traditionally, Hindu yogis (more often than not pilgrims from India) have used cannabis as an aid to meditation, and male devotees use it as a symbol of fellowship in their frequent *bhajans*. It is also used for a wide variety of *Ayurvedic* medicinal purposes, both human and veterinary. Finally, it is used by older people of many castes to while away the time when they are too old to work in the fields and, until recently only secretly, by younger people in search of fun.

The advent of the hippie era brought increased cultivation, greatly inflated prices, and large-scale smuggling into the provinces of northern India. Over an approximately eight-year period the attitudes of young, middle-class, urban Nepalis changed to the extent that smoking *gānjā* (marihuana) or *charas* (hashish) came to be regarded as a novel, acceptable, and pleasurable mark of sophistication.

All dealers' licenses were revoked on July 16, 1973, and at present it is illegal to buy, sell, or cultivate (but not to use) cannabis. Three factors contributed to this government crackdown: (1) Nepalese alarm that their own youth were being corrupted by cannabis; (2) United Nations pressure to join other "respectable" nations in outlawing cannabis; and (3) U. S. pressure for narcotic control. Despite the loss of tax revenues by the government (approximately $100,000) and profits by farmers and dealers, there has been little critical response to the new restrictions.

Despite Nepal's high public profile in the popular press as a pharmaceutical paradise, no research of the detailed and systematic kind reported elsewhere in this volume has been done there. The notes that follow therefore represent only a brief and necessarily sketchy overview of the variety of cannabis uses, and attitudes toward them, in Nepal. The botanical

I gratefully acknowledge Dr. Khem Bahadur Bista, Mr. J. Gabriel Campbell, and Mr. Michael Stern for their assistance in collecting some of the data reported and for their helpful criticism of an earlier draft of this paper.

details of cannabis cultivation and preparation are virtually all identical with those described elsewhere in the Indian sub-continent. These will not be chronicled here, since they are already adequately covered in works such as the Indian Hemp Commission Report (1894) and Chopra and Chopra (1957) as well as in the article by Hasan in the present volume.

Few regions of the world compress so much ecological and cultural diversity into such a small physical space as Nepal. From the southern border — a flat, tropical, alluvial plain called the Terai, barely above sea level — to the permanent snow and ice of Mt. Everest (29,028 ft.) and the other Himalayan giants of the northern border, is a distance of barely 100 miles. The Terai is inhabited by various tribal groups as well as by high and low caste Hindus speaking Hindi and related dialects, and cultural equivalence on both sides of the unnatural border with India is readily apparent. Along the northern border live Tibetan-speaking Buddhists who speak, look, and act very much like their counterparts just over the border in the Tibet Autonomous Region of the People's Republic of China. Between these two extremes, in the great hilly heartland of Nepal, live both Aryan and Mongoloid peoples whose indigenous culture is mixed with influences from the north and from the south.

Despite this diversity, cannabis is found in most parts of the country, and it is only in the extreme north that cannabis is not grown at all. It is widely found, in cultivated and uncultivated varieties, in the middle hills; in the Terai it does not grow wild, but it is extensively cultivated there. It is commonly believed that the higher the altitude, the better the cannabis, and one dealer in Kathmandu claims that the highest quality cannabis is grown at seven or eight thousand feet. However that may be, the price of cannabis products in Kathmandu is the same regardless of the altitude of origin. I have seen cannabis growing above 10,000 feet in northwest Nepal, but the upper limits of its cultivation are not precisely known. Nevertheless, most of the cannabis grown in Nepal comes from the Terai, where agriculture is much more productive generally than in the highlands. According to government revenue records, the bulk of excise taxes on cannabis are collected in the Terai, and the five districts which produce the most cannabis are all in the Terai: Bara, Parsa, Siraha, Dhanusa, and Mahatari.

The near ubiquity of cannabis in Nepal notwithstanding, no one knows how long it has grown there or from whence it came. Geographical evidence suggests it came via India rather than directly from China, which may have been its ultimate origin (Li, this volume), since cannabis is not found along the Tibetan marches but is grown in the areas of north India bordering Nepal. Cannabis may have come to Nepal millennia ago, or perhaps it was carried into Nepal during one or more of the migration waves from India beginning in the 12th century. These migrants passed eastward through the mountains, and cannabis is found more extensively in the west than in the east. In many areas of the western hills cannabis grows all over the vast terraced hillsides as far as the eye can see. According to local humor it is very convenient to travel in west Nepal, where cannabis grows so prolifically there is no need to bother carrying a supply of cigarettes.

The uses of cannabis, and attitudes toward them, vary considerably in different cultural and ecological zones. Although cannabis is found and used in most parts of the country, the percentage of people in any given locality who use it for psychotropic purposes tends to be quite small, although it is in wide use as cattle fodder and fiber, especially in the hills. Users tend to be male rather than female and older rather than younger, but the vagaries of specific local situations make generalizations about caste avoidance or use of cannabis difficult to formulate. There is no association of use of cannabis by Brahmins and of alcohol by Chhetris (a caste reputedly of Rajput origin) along the lines reported by Carstairs (1954) for Rajasthan. In Nepal the highest as well as the lowest castes use cannabis, and Nepal, like the Indian subcontinent generally, illustrates the fact that cannabis use in traditional societies is not restricted to groups at the lower and disadvantaged range of the hierarchy.

One of the most pervasive traditional uses of cannabis in Nepal is not strictly Nepalese at all but largely Indian. Because of its traditional association with Shiva, the Himalayas attract many pilgrims from India, including *sādhus*, or Hindu mendicant holy men, who visit, among many other places, the Shivite shrines and temple of Pashupatināth. Of course Nepal produces its share of these *sādhus* also, but they are all followers of one or the other Indian ascetic traditions. Many of these itinerant holy men use cannabis extensively for a variety of reasons. They use it as an aid to meditation, claiming that it helps them overlook the discomforts of living in conditions alien to them — such as cold weather — so that they can concentrate on higher matters.

Shiva is frequently depicted with a bowl filled with herbs under his arm as one of the emblems of the mendicant, and there is a traditional association between Shiva and cannabis. For Shivites, smoking cannabis is a way of offering it to Shiva. But in interviews with *sādhus* at Pashupatināth, the holiest Hindu shrine in Kathmandu, it became apparent that cannabis use is by no means confined to members of Shivite sects. On the contrary, those *sādhus* who used cannabis belonged to a wide spectrum of Hindu sects. It is the combination of the general austerity of asceticism, the unaccustomed climatic rigor, and religious beliefs which produce conditions in which the use of cannabis is almost a professional technique.

One extreme example of ritual use is that of unusually austere *sādhus* called *aghoris*. Under the influence of cannabis, *aghoris* indulge in such ritual practices as eating excrement, urine, and the flesh of corpses. Professor Bharati (1965) reports that cannabis functions as a deinhibiting agent in certain esoteric Tantric rituals. Hinduism is in many ways a puritanical religion, and cannabis helps to psychologically shore up adherents who partake of these somewhat exotic practices — dietary in the case of the *aghoris* and sexual in the case of Tantric rituals.

The use of cannabis by *sādhus* is culturally constituted since they have renounced the world and whatever proscriptions against its use may exist for their more worldly brethren. It is public knowledge that these ascetics use cannabis, and it is an act of merit for a layman to donate cannabis to a *sādhu*. Thus in addition to those areas where it is grown for essentially commercial reasons, countless households have a few plants growing nearby so that they will have something to offer to the occasional itinerant *sādhu* who passes by.

A second category of cannabis users consists of male devotees to sing at *bhajans*, Hindu devotional meetings often associated with *bhakti* sects. These *bhajans* are not necessarily associated with Shiva,[1] since although the Himalayas have literary associations with Shiva, the ordinary Hindu layman worships Shiva as one among many other deities. These *bhajans* often take place in auspicious locations such as in, around, or near temples and *satals* (pilgrimage shelters), but they are also held in private houses.

At *bhajans*, the *gānjā* (marihuana) is passed around in a *chilam* (clay pipe) among the singers and musicians sitting on the floor. To partake of the *chilam* is not in any sense obligatory, but is clearly a way of symbolically stating the fact of devotional fellowship. As with *sādhus* it promotes good *bhakti*.

In Kathmandu, at least half a dozen more or less public *bhajans* take place every night and by and large the same people attend repeatedly. These men might be farmers or business men during the day, but they come at night to share the fellowship of the singing of hymns, usually in Hindi, although their own language is either Newari, a Tibeto-Burman language, or Nepali in the case of Brahmins or Chhetris. Participants in *bhajans* apparently can belong to a number of castes of various rank,

---

[1] Bhim Sen, Ganesh, Machendranath, Vishnu, and Saraswati are only a few of the deities worshipped in Kathmandu *bhajans*.

although sharing the *chilam* would preclude the lowest castes. Women sometimes participate in *bhajans* but rarely if ever smoke the *chilam*.

As with the *sādhus*, this devotional use of cannabis is publicly known, but *bhajan* singers are not in any sense highly regarded because they use cannabis, however exemplary they may be as devotees. On the contrary, there is if anything a tendency to regard any layman *ganjari* (one who uses *gānjā* excessively) as slightly reprehensible, although not seriously objectionable.

The third traditional use is not ritual or social but medicinal. Indigenous medical systems, most conspicuously *Ayurvedic*, use cannabis extensively to treat a variety of ailments in both humans and animals. It is an ingredient in compounds used to treat diarrhea, cholera, tetanus, rheumatism, and insomnia, among many other maladies. It is also employed as a cough suppressant, digestive aid, stimulus to whet the appetite, soporific, aphrodisiac, and antimalarial agent for hill people who move to the Terai. Cannabis is never prescribed alone but always in a mixture with other herbs or ingredients. A compound used in the treatment of diarrhea and cholera, for example, contains some fifteen different ingredients including dried ginger, black pepper, nut grass, sea salt, black salt, opium, cannabis, and the ashes of a clam shell. In these preparations cannabis is first washed in a cloth with water seven times to remove impurities.

Cannabis even functions as a tranquilizer for children. It is sometimes mixed with sweets and given to children to help them sleep or keep them quiet while, for example, a mother works in the fields. By giving her child a small amount of *gānjā* in forms such as *agnikumar* or *jatikari*, she keeps him less active and less likely to get into trouble while she is occupied in other ways. *Ayurvedic* practitioners believe that too much cannabis, like too much alcohol, can have deleterious effects and that overindulgence can result in madness, weight loss, and decreased semen.

Finally, cannabis is used by older people of many castes simply to while away the time when they are too old to work in the fields anymore. They use it to ease their aches and pains as they sit around during the day when there is little else that they can do.

The situation among the Tibeto-Burman speaking Magars of Dolpā District in the mountains of northwest Nepal, half way between Mustang and Jumla, is different in several respects from that described above. There cannabis is used neither ritually nor socially nor medicinally. Although it is extensively cultivated, it is never used as an intoxicant. The seeds are extricated from the rest of the plant and then pressed into a dough-like pulp. This moist, doughy substance is kneaded at the top of a slanted washboard-type surface so that the oil is squeezed out and drains to the bottom of the board where it is collected. This substance is used for cooking, and is the main source of cooking oil in this area of Nepal. Without it preparation of food would be impossible. This use contrasts with the intoxicant uses described in so many other parts of the world and with its use as a grain in China.

Although they are well aware of the euphoric qualities of the plant consumed in other forms, these Dolpā Magars never smoke *gānjā* or *charas* (hashish),[2] and the cooking oil has no hallucinatory effect; they have no compunctions about using alcohol for similar purposes and do so frequently. The low caste blacksmith/carpenters (*kami*) in the area do smoke *gānjā* and *charas*, and avoidance of this low caste behavior accounts for the Magars' abstinence.

Cannabis is used in some areas on popular and festive occasions by those who do not otherwise indulge themselves. Such occasions include Shiva Ratri, when enormous numbers of pilgrims who give cannabis *prasad* (gifts) to *sādhus*, come to Kathmandu from India. Another occasion is Krishna Astarmi (Krishna's birthday), when school children (particularly boys) smoke *gānjā* or *charas* or drink *bhang*. This use is not only public but, in at least one locality near Kathmandu, is actually sponsored by the local school itself.

All these uses have existed in the context of a society which had long since learned to accommodate, regulate and restrict them within traditional and secure limits. This situation was profoundly altered in the mid-1960's when the "hippie" invasion began. With the discovery that marihuana and hashish (not to mention hard drugs) were openly and very inexpensively available, a small resident colony of international world travellers became quickly established in Kathmandu. The price of *charas* quickly skyrocketed from about $15 per kilogram (retail) to about $70 per kilogram. Smuggling across the border into India increased, and it has been estimated that in recent years more marihuana was exported than consumed in Nepal (Rana 1973).

His Majesty's Government had begun to regulate by law and license the cultivation, sale, and export/import of cannabis (and other intoxicants) with the promulgation of the Intoxicants Act of 1961 and the Intoxicants Rules in 1962. This legislation, with its various amendments over the years, established a system of excise and sales taxes on the sale and commercial cultivation of cannabis, for which licenses were then required. Typically, a farmer would apply to grow cannabis on, say, one

---

[2] Elswhere in west Nepal, in the Jumla area, for instance, high and low Hindu castes smoke cannabis in addition to using it for cooking oil.

bigha (about one and 5/8 acres) of land for a license fee which by 1967 had been raised to $450. He would then exceed the licensed limit and earn large untaxed profits; to combat this tax evasion the tax rate was lowered to $350 per *bigha*. In addition, the 30 odd shops in Kathmandu who catered to the "hippie" clientele each had to pay a tax of Rs. 2,000.

At the same time, the attitudes of young, middle-class Kathmandu Nepalese began to change. Whereas cannabis use had been largely confined to older people (at *bhajans*, it is the older men, not the youngsters, who puff on the *chilam*), it now came to be regarded as a novel, pleasurable, and acceptable way to have fun with one's friends. For a few Nepalese, it became a mark of sophistication to use cannabis openly, unlike previous times when boys would sneak a few puffs in much the same furtive way that their American counterparts used to try corn silk cigarettes behind the barn.

Although Asian models have vaguely influenced Western marihuana use, in the mid-1960's these ideas returned to the Himalayas in a totally mutated form which had nothing to do with the traditional uses outlined above. Although Westerners may admire *sādhus* and *bhajan* singers, they are in fact involved in a totally different system which threatened to overwhelm the orderly regulatory mechanisms which tradition had established.

The beginning of the end of this era came on July 16, 1973, when His Majesty's Government revoked all licenses to cultivate, buy, and sell marihuana. It is now illegal to traffic in cannabis although it is still not illegal to possess or use it. What is owned can be used until the supply is gone. A comprehensive new law expected to be passed by the National Panchayat in 1974 will allow cultivation for the traditional uses mentioned earlier but will ban all other uses of cannabis or any other drug His Majesty's Government considers potentially harmful.

Three factors have contributed to this governmental crackdown. The first is Nepalese middle-class alarm that their own youth were being corrupted, through "hippie" influences, by cannabis. Where they had previously regarded cannabis abuse as a foreign problem, they now began to see some of their own young people turning into "hippies," and this development disturbed them. What in earlier and simpler times could be called "innocent excess" (Atkinson 1882; reprinted 1973) had become a threat.

The second source of pressure was exerted by the United States government as part of its world-wide effort to control the growth and traffic of so-called narcotic drugs. The United States government is more concerned about heroin than marihuana but regarded it as convenient to persuade the Nepal government to ban both.

The third factor is pressure from the United Nations to outlaw cannabis. The International Narcotics Control Board takes an extremely hard view of cannabis and regards it as a grave and insidious danger in the same league with heroin; the 1972 report heaps scorn on Nepal for not cooperating fully with its suggestions. For a small country like Nepal, United Nations' opinion and approval mean a great deal, but it is ironic that Nepal has, largely in response to the pressure of more "advanced" Western nations, abandoned a system — governmental control of production and distribution — toward which many Western nations are now belatedly striving. It is a further irony that the cannabis trade in Kathmandu, which arose in response to Western demand, has now been liquidated largely in response to a different kind of Western demand.

There have been several consequences of this governmental intervention. In the first place, the government now loses revenues of $100,000 from the sale of licenses. In addition, the farmers and middlemen and retail traders lose their profits. Although some of them surreptitiously sell off their previously acquired stocks, few plan to stay in the now illegal business. For them it is just a business in which, as in any business, it is unwise to take excessive risks. In any event, the prices in these clandestine transactions have not changed under the new policy, probably because most sales were made to casual buyers who will not buy if it is not readily available; thus demand has decreased with supply. Dealers do not necessarily use cannabis themselves, and as one of them put it, "you don't have to like it to sell it."

The Kathmandu dealers are able to shift their resources into other fields, such as handicrafts. But perhaps those most hurt by the ban are hill farmers in the west for whom cannabis was a small but crucial cash crop.

All these losses notwithstanding, there has been little outcry against the new order, although individuals do complain privately. One *sādhu* complained that although he formerly had nearly lived on cannabis, now he is lucky if he gets a puff a day. "This place is as bad as Banaras," he said, where it has been illegal for a long time. Cannabis is certainly not impossible to find now; it simply takes more time and trouble to find a reliable source.

Dealers regard the new rules as unfair. They say that in Western countries many different kinds of high-quality alcoholic drinks are available, but not in Nepal except at exorbitant cost. Thus the new restrictions work against the interests of poor people, who do not have the money to buy alcohol but can afford cannabis.

One *sādhu* has the last word in his belief that divine retribution eventually rectifies whatever wrongs governments perpetrate. According to him it is obvious why Singha Durbar, the central government secretariat, burned down shortly after the decision to revoke all licenses was made. Lord Shiva was so infuriated with these restrictions against cannabis, which he regards as his special drug, that he fired up his third eye, focused it on the government secretariat, and obtained his revenge by burning the structure down to the ground.

REFERENCES

ATKINSON, EDWIN T.
    1882   "The Himalayan districts of the north western provinces of India," vol. X of *The Gazetteer N.W.P.*; reprinted 1973 under the title, *The Himalayan Gazetteer*.

BHARATI, A.
    1965   *The tantric tradition*. London: Rider & Co.

CARSTAIRS, G. M.
    1954   Daru and bhang: cultural factors in the choice of intoxicant. *Quarterly Journal for Studies on Alcohol* 15:220–237.

CHOPRA, I. C., R. N. CHOPRA
    1957   Use of cannabis drugs in India. *U.N. Bulletin on Narcotics* 9:4–29. January–March.

KAPLAN, JOHN
    1969   *Marijuana: report of the Indian Hemp Drugs Commission of 1893–1894*. Silver Springs, Maryland: Thomas Jefferson Publishing Company.

HIS MAJESTY'S GOVERNMENT OF NEPAL
    1961   *Intoxicants Act*.
    1962   *Intoxicants Rules*. Nepal Law Translation Series 16, Nepal Press Digest (Private) Ltd.

RANA, PRAKRITA, S.
    1973   "Consequences of ban on 'ganja' cultivation in Nepal," in *The rising Nepal*, December 15th, 4.

UNITED NATIONS
    1972   *Report of the International Narcotics Control Board for 1972*. New York.

The "Ganja *Vision*" in Jamaica

VERA RUBIN

ABSTRACT

Traditional multipurpose use of *ganja*, introduced to Jamaica in the mid-nineteenth century by indentured laborers from India, was diffused to the black working class and has become endemic in the past forty to fifty years.

Smoking *ganja*, although illegal, is prevalent among working-class males and the non-smoker is a deviant who may pose a threat to the peer group. Reactions to the first smoking experience are culturally recognized determinants that validate the status of non-smokers as well as smokers. The *ganja* vision, a culturally standardized phenomenon occurring generally at the time of the first smoking experience, confirms the role of the smoker. The phenomenon is compared to the institutionalized vision quest among American Indians of the plains. The vision phenomenon, a culturally patterned experience with standardized content, usually in the context of a *rite de passage*, thus differs from idiosyncratic "hallucinatory" experiences. Hallucinogenic reactions are neither generally sought nor experienced by working-class males in Jamaica.

Cannabis, one of the oldest multipurpose plants known to man, source of hemp as well as hashish, of medications as well as manufactures, has had a divergent ethnohistorical course over the millennia, in differing civilizations and societies. The available evidence on the diffusion of cannabis from its Asiatic origins, reveals marked sociocultural differences in primary uses of the plant — for manufacturing, magico-religious, medicinal and psychoactive purposes and even in the dietary — and in the context of its use.

Public attention has been focused on the psychoactive properties of cannabis, particularly in their manifestations in Western societies, obscuring the extraordinary versatility of the plant. Schultes believes that the earliest use was for fibers, probably followed by magico-religious and medical use. References to cannabis appear in the pharmaceutical and religious works of the early civilizations of China and India,[1] and *kan*, the root word, occurs in the Old Testament (Benetowa 1968).

Documentation is becoming available of the early multipurpose use of cannabis in Eastern Europe, diffused through trade routes from Asia (Benetowa 1936; Kabelik *et al.* 1954). Cultivation of cannabis in southern Russia, which eventually became the leading world manufacturer of hemp rope, goes back to the 7th century B.C. While manufactures were probably the primary commercial consideration, cannabis was also traditionally used in folk medicine for its analgesic and antibiotic effects. Hemp "porridge" was a common food in Eastern Europe, and soups and juices made of hemp seeds are reported to have been served in medieval monasteries. There is also archaeological evidence of their ancient use for ritual purposes. Hemp seeds have been found by the Soviet archaeologist S. I. Rudenko in Scythian funerary remains in the Altai, as had been reported by Herodotus.

The latter provides one of the earliest recorded accounts of apparent psychoactive use of cannabis: the vapor of the hemp seeds in the Scythian funeral rites is alleged to have induced trance (Emboden 1972). It has, however, been suggested this was a feature of shamanism and that the ecstatic "howling" reported by Herodotus was the "characteristic shouting by shamans" in trance (223).

Cannabis reached Western Europe, in due course, possibly following the Moorish invasion of Spain in the 8th century A.D. Judging from subsequent history, use of cannabis for manufactures became a significant factor in empire building. It was introduced to the New World by the Spanish in the 16th century and to the British colonies by the early settlers, in both cases intended primarily for textile manufactures.

The earliest introduction to Western Europe of the use of "hashish," i.e., the psychoactive use of cannabis, has been attributed to the soldiers returning from the Napoleonic campaign of 1798, in Egypt.[2] Little is known about its psychoactive use, however, until the discovery of the "hallucinogenic" effects of cannabis by the mid-19th century French

---

[1] The first recorded use is reported in a Chinese pharmacopoeia about 2737 B.C. (Grinspoon 1971). The earliest reference in sacred writings of India is found in the Atharva Veda (2000-1400 B.C.) where *bhanga* is mentioned as a "sacred grass" (Chopra 1969:216).
[2] Hashish may have been introduced by returning Crusaders, between the 11th and 13th centuries. Although the precise source and the various uses of cannabis during this period are matters of historical conjecture, the Crusader route may account for Rabelais' familiarity with the various properties of cannabis, fictionalized as "the plant Pantagruelion." As Grinspoon (1971) points out, Rabelais the physician appears to have recognized in the 16th century the only recently reported analgesic and antibacterial qualities of cannabis.

avant-garde writers who formed the Club des Hachichins.

The search for hallucinogenic experiences via hashish, however, apparently did not spread beyond the circle of literati in Paris, or beyond French borders, with the exception of the American writer, Fitzhugh Ludlow, whose influence on his readers was also minimal.

The major non-textile use of cannabis in the United States during the past century was as a medication, following a report in 1843 by W. B. O'Shaughnessy who had been in the public health service in India. Cannabis was listed in the U.S. pharmacopoeia in 1850 and was used in general practice until the passage of the Marihuana Tax Act of 1937. That period marks the rise of the campaign against the "evils" of marihuana in the United States stemming from its use by Mexican-American "laborers" in the southwest and by black jazz musicians in New Orleans.

The stigma attached to the use of marihuana by marginal groups in the U. S. is characteristic of other societies as well, reflecting attitudes of the "establishment," generally, to the lower classes. Cannabis provided a convenient rationale for explaining away social problems rooted in poverty and underdevelopment.

The middle-class white American "marihuana habit" is a more recent phenomenon. While the 19th century romantic literature apparently had little impact on hallucinogenic experimentation, outside of literary circles, interest in the U. S. in hallucinogenic experiences was sparked by the work of Aldous Huxley and curiosity about mescaline and nativistic peyote cults. The mid-1960's in the U.S. were also marked by experimentation with LSD, and as McGlothlin notes (this volume), marihuana use by middle-class youth followed rather than preceded such experimentation. The spread of the "marihuana habit" to middle-class groups in other societies probably derives from the United States rather than from indigenous use. The writer would argue, in fact, that the contemporary "marihuana habit" differs sufficiently from traditional cannabis use — in expectations, motivation, patterned responses and life styles of the users — to constitute a distinctive subculture.

Current concerns about the effects of cannabis (both scientific and popular) stress ineluctable mind-altering phenomena and the "amotivational syndrome." These are treated, ethnocentrically, as universal reactions to inherent pharmacological properties of the plant. And cannabis has been classified as a hallucinogen, along with LSD, mescaline and psilocybin (McGlothlin 1966).

For the majority of consumers in non-industrial societies, however, particularly in the laboring classes, cannabis remains a multipurpose plant, used in the dietary, as an herbal in the tradition of folk medicine, and both as energizer and as tranquilizer — as stimulant and sedative — as the situation requires. Cannabis has also been used in ritual, and is still used in India as an offering to the gods. There is considerable subcultural as well as cross-cultural variation in the motivations for use of cannabis, the related expectations and situationally conditioned reactions. Recent multidisciplinary research on the effects of long-term chronic use of cannabis in Jamaica, the West Indies,[3] corroborates the hypothesis of cultural conditioning of cannabis use and reactions.

Introduced to Jamaica in the mid-19th century by indentured laborers from India, *ganja* use was diffused to the black working class and has become endemic in the past forty to fifty years.[4] Jamaica, consequently, provides an advantageous natural setting for anthropological and clinical studies of the parameters and effects of long-term smoking. Anthropological research was carried out in rural and urban communities to examine patterns of working-class use and to select subjects (chronic smokers and controls) for the clinical studies.[5]

The anthropological studies, and comparison with the *Report* of the Indian Hemp Drugs Commission of 1893, led to the premise that a "*ganja* complex" had been introduced to Jamaica, along with the plant, by the indentured Indian cane cutters. This paper deals with one aspect of the *ganja* complex, as it was developed in Jamaica — the *ganja* vision, as a form of initiation rite to becoming a smoker.

Given the endemic nature of *ganja* use in the Jamaican working class, it was more difficult to locate demographically comparable controls than to find long-term chronic smokers willing to volunteer for the clinical studies.[6] Multipurpose *ganja* use in the working-class milieu, particularly

---

[3] The project was carried out by the Research Institute for the Study of Man, in collaboration with the University of the West Indies, under NIMH Contract No. HSM-42-70-97.

[4] Cannabis, for hemp production, was introduced to Jamaica at the end of the 18th century, but did not become a plantation crop, and was apparently not used for dietary, medicinal or psychoactive purposes before the migration of Indian indentured workers, starting in 1845. The first anti-*ganja* legislation in Jamaica was enacted in 1913, twenty-four years before the Marihuana Tax Act in the United States.

[5] Clinical studies were undertaken at the University Hospital by the Faculty of Medicine of the University of the West Indies.

[6] The clinical sample consisted of 60 working-class males (30 smokers and 30 non-smokers) ranging in age from 23 to 53 years, average age 34 years. All but 12 of the 60 had had an initial smoking experience, between the ages of 8 and 36 years. Smokers had their first experience earlier than controls: onset of regular use ranged between the ages of 9 and 25 years (average age 15 years). Duration of smoking ranged from 7 to 37 years, with a mean of 17.5 years.

Frequency ranged from 1 to 24 spliffs (*ganja* cigarettes) daily, with an average of 7. *Chilam* pipe smokers took from 1 to 24 pipeloads per week, with an average of 7

in rural areas, is a cultural regularity, used in the dietary and extensively in folk medicine. *Ganja* smoking is also a manifest — if somewhat secluded — practice, despite the stringent legislation against possession and use. Young boys are occasionally involved in obtaining small supplies of *ganja* for older family members or friends and have certainly witnessed their smoking, at home or in "the bush." Socialization to *ganja* smoking is commonly through a peer group. It is the rare working-class Jamaican male who has never had an initial experience of smoking cannabis as an informal *rite de passage* to "manship."

Whether or not the initiate becomes a regular smoker, however, is determined — both by himself and his peers — by his reactions to the first experience. Most of the non-smokers in the study reported neutral reactions, i.e., they experienced nothing. There were several cases of negative reactions, similar to the "novice anxiety" reactions reported in the literature — dizziness, auditory sensations, fear of madness. The first smoke was characteristically a few "draws" on a communal spliff or cigarette, pharmacologically insufficient to produce reactions such as those described by one control: "All the whole world of insects and animals I think I hear crying and howling." None of the controls reported a positive reaction, retrospectively phrased by the smokers as "it sweet me."

A positive initial experience validates regular smoking; a negative early experience generally validates non-smoking — that is, sanctioned deviance from peer group norms. This culturally-accepted screening mechanism provides peer recognition of the individual's innate "capacity" to qualify as either smoker or non-smoker, phrased as "he doesn't have the head for it." *Ganja* smoking is considered undesirable by the middle class and by those members of the working classes who aspire to higher status. Heavy *ganja* smokers, consequently, are found generally in the lower socio-economic strata — small farmers and fishermen with limited resources, laborers, and semi-skilled artisans. The screening process which validates non-smoking may thus be an aspect of anticipatory socialization to higher status — a device which secures the individual but does not endanger cohesion and solidarity among working-class people.

Controls as well as smokers were intensively queried about their reac-

---

weekly. Pipe smoking is less prevalent than spliff smoking as it is more easily detectable.

Based on the frequencies of spliff smoking, light use is defined as 1–4 spliffs per day; moderate use as 4–7 per day and heavy use as 8 or more daily.

Ganja samples submitted by the smokers contained Δ^9THC ranging from .7% to 10.3% (mean weight) with a mean of 2.96%. The potency of *ganja* smoked varies according to availability and regular smokers consume various grades as available.

tions to the first smoking experience. To underscore the validity of their culturally deviant status, non-smokers frequently commented that they had failed to see the "little old lady" — a vision experience only reported by regular smokers.

Sometimes I hear them say they see a little old lady come before them and dance and laugh and do all sort of things and it makes them feel like doing the same things.

The initial positive smoking experience is an informal *rite de passage* into the *ganja* subculture, associated with feelings of sociability, meditation, and relaxation and with the special occurrence of a formalized vision. Experiencing the vision definitively validates smoker status — "You can't tell some man that when you smoke herb you don't see old lady." The occurrence of this vision phenomenon, generally on the first *ganja* smoking experience, and its content, are culturally standardized. The major features of the vision appear in the following account:

I felt happy, man, I felt happy when I used it that first time. Now the first thing I saw (I was just going into a little doze) is a little woman about this length [three feet tall]. But stouter than a drum and all dressed in pure green. And she wheeled and wheeled and she wheeled, her face was all around, and she wheeled and she wheeled and I was there, admiring, admiring. And how I got to wake up, I saw she had a little rod, just about like this and she wheeled and came toward me and I opened my eyes. And I just woke up and didn't see her again. And the next morning I did my work as nice as ever. I tried it and it did good. So I say this thing must be good. I started to use it regular.

The "little lady" in the vision may be dressed in various colors, red, white, green; the pattern of the vision may vary somewhat, as in that of "little men," dressed in different colors, described in the following:

Gradually as I was growing up and I saw the others smoking and nothing happened to them, I got into it and I smoked it too. The first time I enjoyed myself because I saw some little men in red dancing before me. And I just took it and amused myself. And I considered that must be how everybody feels when they take it the first time. And I just enjoyed myself with the little men I see until I left. Just some short men, they had on red clothes and they danced. About ten of them, it was just a little group of them going on with some dancing before me. [They were] different, different colors — some looked white and some looked like black men and some looked like brown men. They were smiling like something 'sweet' them and I just humored the joke with them. They never spoke, they just danced until they disappeared. It didn't make me feel dizzy, for I was conscious. [It never gave you any "visions apart from that?"] No, after I smoked it the first time I smoked it again and I just felt normal as any other man.

The culturally standard vision of the "little dancing" person or creature, which characterizes the first *ganja* experience for some subjects, may be comparable to the vision quest for guardian spirits of the Plains Indians of North America. The vision, an institutionalized phenomenon among various Plains Indian societies, "designates a culturally prescribed dream, hallucination or any unusual auditory or visual stimulus which is interpreted as a communication from supernatural entities, and results in the recipient's acquisition of power, advice or ritual privileges" (Albers and Parker 1971:203). Both the quest for the vision and its content conformed to culturally prescribed systems of belief and to structural factors in Plains Indian societies: "The manifest content of the standardized visions was highly stereotyped and stylized with regard to their form, symbolic content and behavioral directives."[7]

Sociocultural interpretation of the phenomena of Plains Indian collective visions indicates that "... the vision functioned as an anticipatory socialization device, easing problems of role transition" and that "... in some social contexts the vision served to solidify the individual's identification and cohesion with societal organizations" (Albers and Parker 1971:205). It is in the latter context that we may draw some functional analogies between the *ganja* vision in Jamaica and those of the Plains Indians. The *ganja* vision confirms the role of the smoker and his transition into the *ganja* subculture, possibly also his transition to "manship," and solidifies his "identification and cohesion" with the peer group.

Recent research further indicates that there were structural and role limitations on both the Plains vision quest and its outcome. Among the Plains Indians, in cases where the vision served as a validation of status, "unsuccessful individuals" did not dream. This may be compared, structurally, to the absence of the *ganja* vision among the Jamaican experimenters who did not achieve the status of smokers. On the other hand, there is only limited comparability as to the structural requirement of further validation of status in Plains Indian society. Albers and Parker (1971) note that in cases where the vision was employed as a functional device to achieve new status the individual had to verify the credibility of his vision through socially recognized achievements. Further research would be necessary to determine whether there may be a comparable situation in *ganja* smoking sets in Jamaica.

Ten smokers in the Jamaican clinical sample reported in standardized form the personal experience of the initial vision, and second person "dem say" accounts were frequently related by other subjects, non-

---

[7] Reichel-Dolmatoff, describing a hallucinogenic cult in the Amazon, observes that the visions induced by hallucinogenic drugs are standardized and that younger members of the cult group "still do not have well-defined hallucinations" (Reichel-Dolmatoff 1970:173).

smokers as well as smokers. The phenomenon appears to represent a collective vision, or myth, related to initiation into the *ganja* subculture and perhaps to origins of *ganja* use in Jamaica. More intensive research would be required to determine how pervasive the vision experience is, whether it represents a "quest" that validates smoking and perhaps grants special status in the peer group, and whether special psychological traits characterize the individuals who experience the vision.

HALLUCINATIONS

Cultural variables undoubtedly condition hallucinogenic reactions to cannabis. The vivid accounts of hashish smoking by Baudelaire, Gautier, and their contemporaries, provided a backdrop for Western cultural expectations and social concerns. Gautier's fantastic description of his reactions to "the greenish paste" focused on the bizarre: "Hallucination, that strange guest had set up his dwelling place in me" (Solomon 1966: 168). Even in less baroque Western literature, as previously noted, cannabis has been classified as a hallucinogen, along with lysergic acid diethylamide (LSD), mescaline and psilocybin.

There is a significant psychological difference, however, between hallucinations and visions; hallucinations are usually idiosyncratic phenomena which may be triggered by personality and/or pharmacological factors; visions are culturally patterned experiences, usually in the context of a *rite de passage* or of a ritual. The quantity and potency of the initial "smoke" by Jamaican subjects would not warrant a pharmacological explanation of the phenomenon, and certainly not of the patterned cultural content of the vision.

Similar folk uses and reactions to other plants, not generally considered hallucinogens, have been reported. Tobacco, for example, *Nicotinana* spp. which has been used in folk medicine and magic by American Indians "from Canada to Patagonia," is also "a vehicle for ecstasy." Wilbert (1972:55) reports that among the Warao Indians of Venezuela the use of tobacco in this context is "conceptually and functionally indistinguishable from the 'true' hallucinogen." He observes that there is "an obvious cultural conditioning toward specific ecstatic experiences that have nothing to do with the chemical action of the tobacco plant itself" (80).

The complex of beliefs and behaviors surrounding *ganja* in Jamaica is structurally linked with use by the lower class, urban and rural. The peasant takes *ganja* for energy when he works in his fields, the fisherman to ward off fatigue at sea. *Ganja* makes you "feel to work" and staves off hunger during work, but when taken before the evening meal, it enhances the appetite. If he smokes before an evening dance, the farmer can "win a contest"; if he takes *ganja* before bedtime, he can sleep restfully and wake refreshed and energized to start his day's work. Taken in congenial group settings, it can evoke religious meditation; taken in solitude, it is said to aid in problem solving. The subjective "mind altering effects" are thus selectively and conditionally experienced. *Ganja* teas and tonics are also used extensively in the working class — by males and females, adults and children, both as prophylactic and medication for a wide range of ailments. The *ganja* syndrome is characterized by situational determinants that reinforce working-class use and condition the range of reactions experienced, including the initial vision.

Contrasts in reactions to cannabis are becoming apparent within Jamaica itself, as a subcultural phenomenon. Use has recently spread to the middle class; however, it is not as pervasive as in the working class and carries a different set of psychocultural expectations. These include concepts of enhancement of creativity, pleasure in listening to music, escape from boredom, return to a "child-like" state of absorption in details, search for the "ultimate experience" in sex. Smoking or ingesting small amounts of *ganja* is reported to induce "tremendous" hunger and to act as an "instant" aphrodisiac. Aphrodisiac qualities, however, are seldom mentioned spontaneously by working-class subjects.[8]

It is clear from the Jamaican data that "hallucinations are *not* an invariable consequence of marihuana use" (Fort 1970–1971:519). In the Jamaican working-class setting, hallucinogenic reactions are neither regularly sought nor generally experienced. The one exception to this is the initial vision of the "little lady" who dances and beckons the smoker, usually in a congenial manner. This culturally patterned experience appears to serve the function of "vision quest" (possibly the spirit of the plant) which legitimates smoking for the working-class initiate.

Contrasts in the "marihuana habit" of middle-class Jamaicans, and the *ganja* complex of working-class Jamaicans, reinforce the thesis that psychoactive reactions to cannabis are conditioned by the cultural formulation of both experience and behavior.

---

[8] Laboratory analysis of samples submitted by several middle-class users reveals only "traces" of THC, supporting the thesis of reactions conditioned by psychocultural expectations.

REFERENCES

ALBERS, PATRICIA, SEYMOUR PARKER
   1971   The plains vision experience: a study of power and privilege. *Southwestern Journal of Anthropology* 27 (3)(Autumn):203–233.

BENETOWA, SULA
   1936   *Le chanvre dans les croyances et les coutumes populaires.* Warszawa: Nakladen Towarzystwa Naukowego Warszawskiego.
   1968   "Tracing one word through different languages," in *The book of grass: an anthology of Indian hemp.* Edited by George Andrews and Simon Vinkenoog, 15–17. New York: Grove Press.

CHOPRA, GURBAKHSH SINGH
   1969   Man and marijuana. *The International Journal of the Addictions* 4 (2) (June):215–247.

EMBODEN, WILLIAM A., JR.
   1972   "Ritual use of Cannabis sativa L: a historical-ethnographic survey," in *Flesh of the gods; the ritual use of hallucinogens.* Edited by Peter T. Furst, 124–236. New York: Praeger.

FORT, JOEL
   1970–1971   Pot or not. *International Journal of Psychiatry* (9):517–521.

GRINSPOON, LESTER
   1971   *Marijuana reconsidered.* Cambridge, Mass.: Harvard University Press.

INDIAN HEMP DRUGS COMMISSION
   1893–1894   *Report of the Indian Hemp Drugs Commission, 1893.* (Reprinted, 1969; Silver Springs, Maryland: Thomas Jefferson Publishing Company.)

KABELIK, JAN, *editor*
   1954   "Hemp as medicine." Olomouc, Czechoslovakia: Hygienic Institute, Pharmaceutic Faculty, Palacky University. (Mimeographed.)

MC GLOTHLIN, WILLIAM H.
   1966   "Cannabis: a reference," in *The marihuana papers.* Edited by David Solomon, 455–472. New York: New American Library.

O'SHAUGHNESSY, W. B.
   1843   On the preparations of the Indian hemp, or gunjah (Cannabis indica); their effects on the animal system in health, and their utility in the treatment of tetanus and other convulsive diseases. *Provincial Medical Journal Retrospect of the Medical Sciences* 5:343–347.

REICHEL-DOLMATOFF, GERARDO
   1970   *Amazonian cosmos: the sexual and religious symbolism of the Tukano Indians.* Chicago: University of Chicago Press.

SOLOMON, DAVID, *editor*
   1966   *The marihuana papers.* New York: New American Library.

WILBERT, JOHANNES
   1972   "Tobacco and shamanistic ecstasy among the Warao Indians of Venezuela," in *Flesh of the gods: the ritual use of hallucinogens.* Edited by Peter T. Furst, 55–83. New York: Praeger.

Plates

	Page
Typification of *Cannabis sativa* L. by *William T. Stearn* (pp. 13–20)	ii/iii
Cannabis: An Example of Taxonomic Neglect by *Richard Evans Schultes, William M. Klein,* *Timothy Plowman,* and *Tom E. Lockwood* (pp. 21–38)	iv/viii
Ethnobotanical Aspects of Cannabis in Southeast Asia by *Marie Alexandrine Martin* (pp. 63–75)	ix
The Social and Cultural Context of Cannabis Use in Rwanda by *Helen Codere* (pp. 217–226)	x
Réunion: Cannabis in a Pluricultural and Polyethnic Society by *Jean Benoist* (pp. 227–234)	xi/xii
Social Aspects of the Use of Cannabis in India by *Khwaja A. Hasan* (pp. 235–246)	xiii
Sociocultural and Epidemiological Aspects of Hashish Use in Greece by *C. Stefanis, C. Ballas,* and *D. Madianou* (pp. 303–326)	xiv/xvi
Cannabis Usage in Pakistan: A Pilot Study of Long Term Effects on Social Status and Physical Health by *Munir A. Khan, Assad Abbas,* and *Knud Jensen* (pp. 345–354)	xvii/xix
Magico-Religious Use of Tobacco among South American Indians by *Johannes Wilbert* (pp. 439–461)	xxi/xxvii

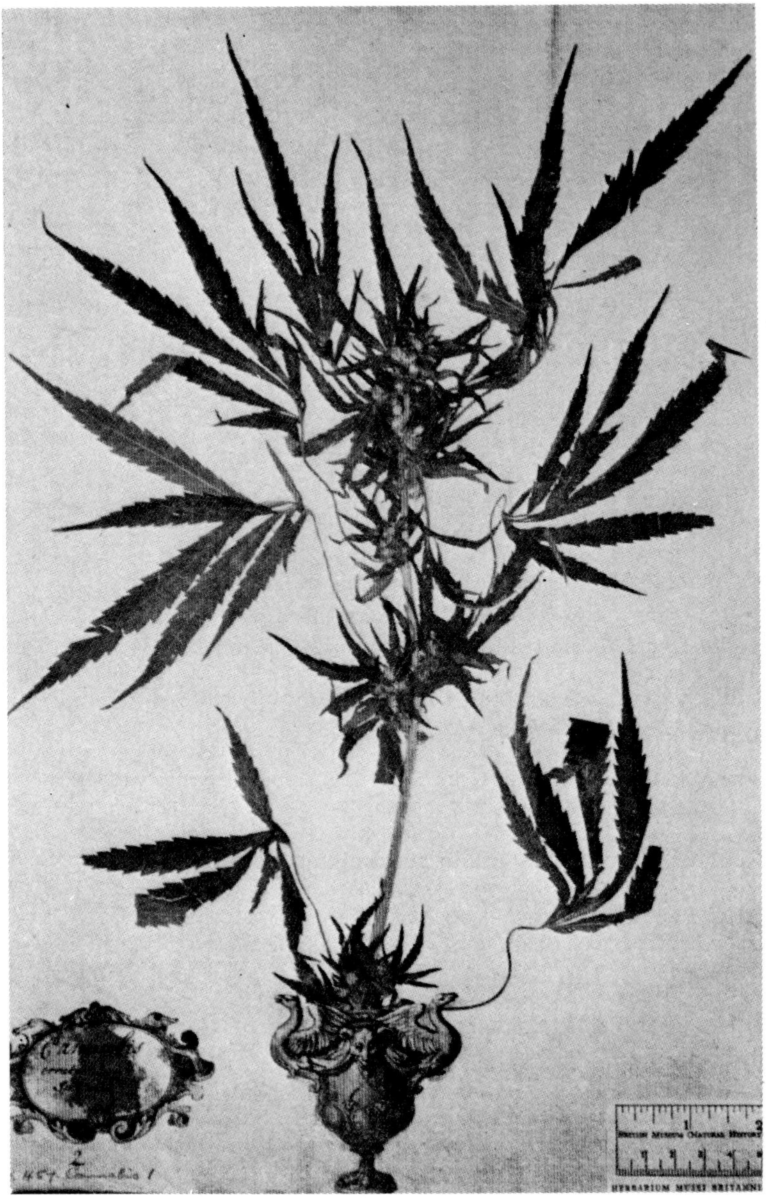

Plate 1. Pistillate specimen of Cannabis in the Clifford Herbarium at the British Museum (Natural History), London. This specimen has been taken as lectotype of the name *Cannabis sativa* L.

Courtesy: British Museum (Natural History)

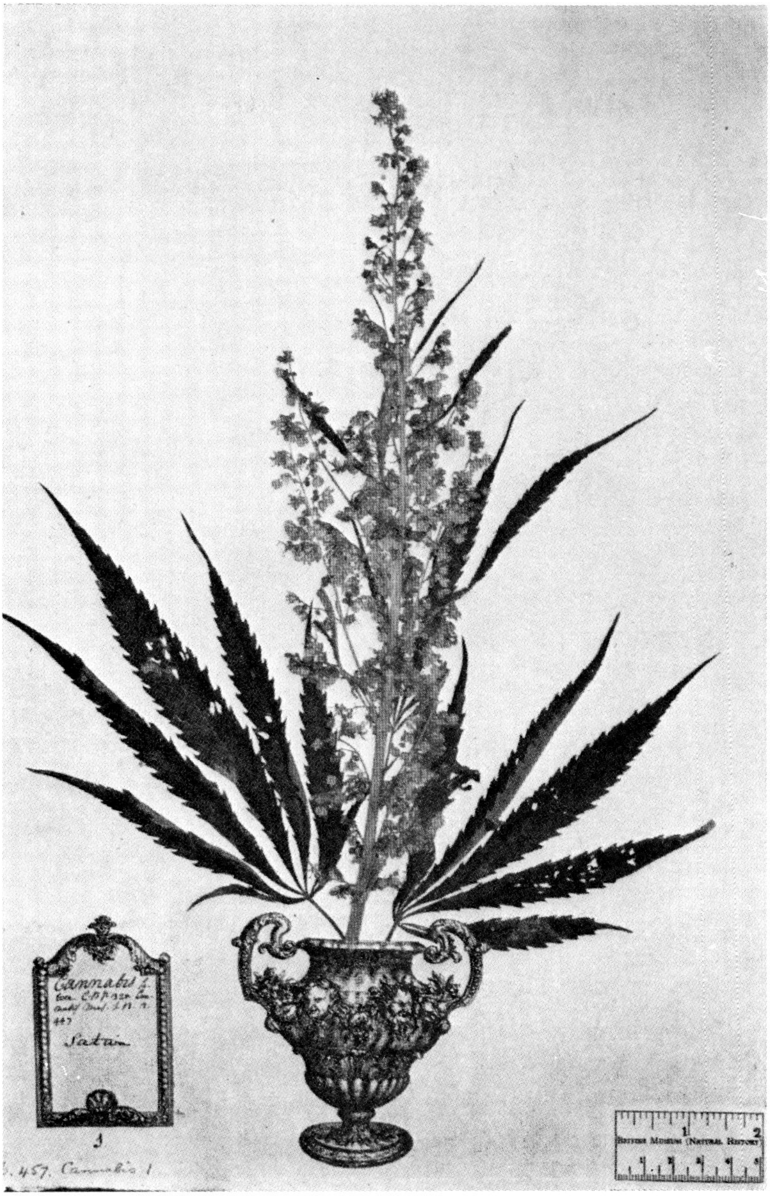

Plate 2. Staminate specimen of Cannabis in the Clifford Herbarium of the British Museum (Natural History), London.

Courtesy: British Museum (Natural History)

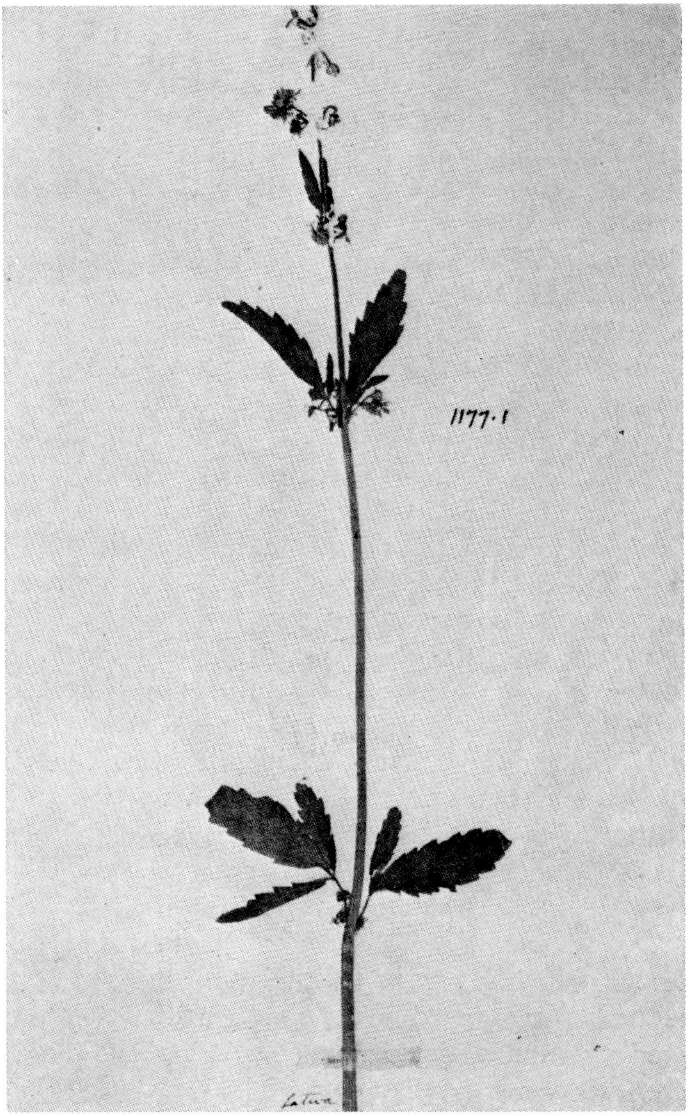

Plate 1. Specimen No. 1177.1 of Cannabis in the Linnean Herbarium
Courtesy: Linnean Society of London

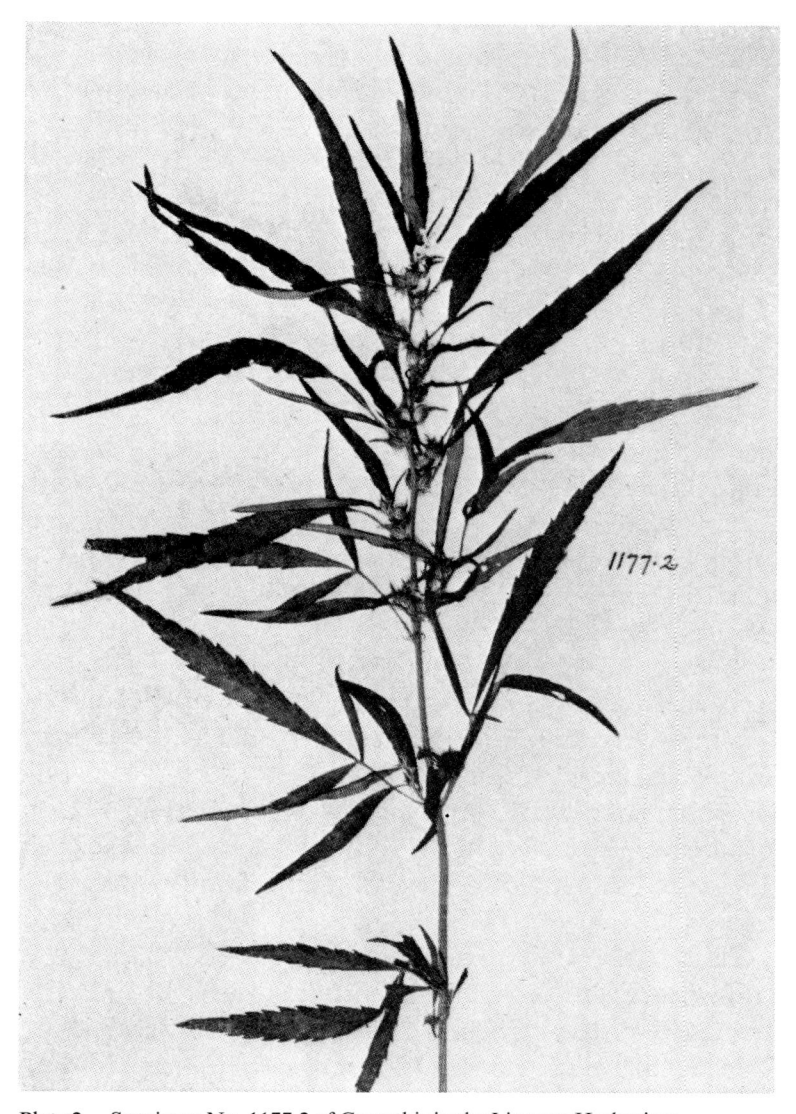

Plate 2. Specimen No. 1177.2 of Cannabis in the Linnean Herbarium
Courtesy: Linnean Society of London

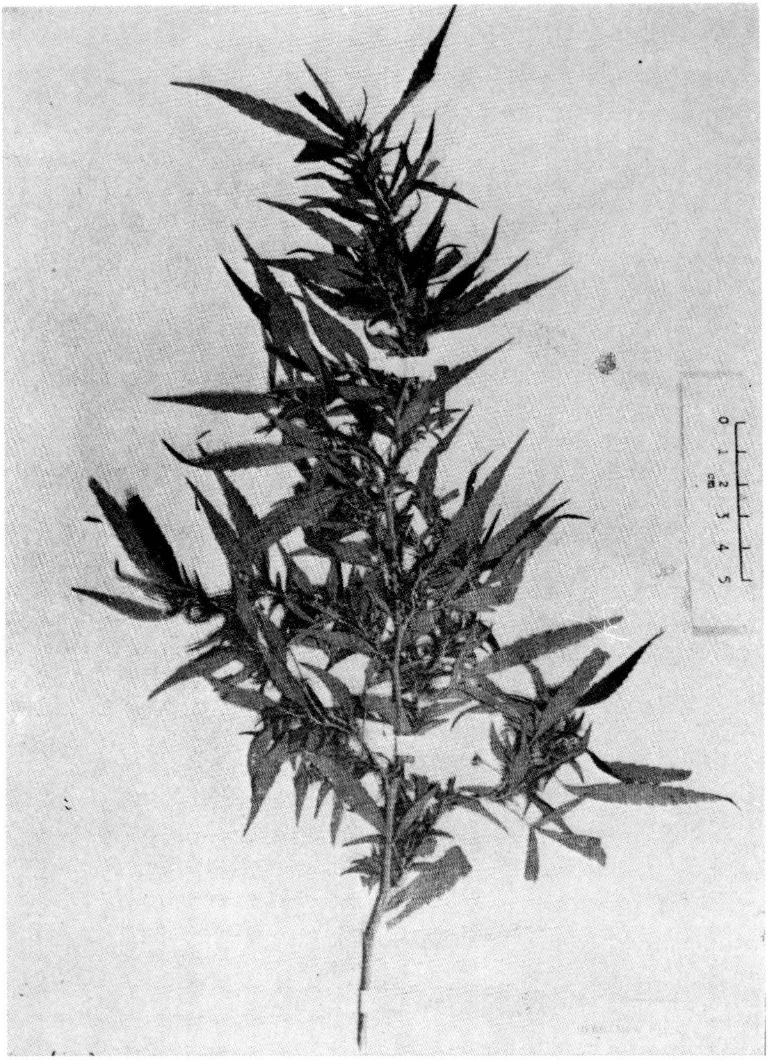

Plate 3. Type specimen of *Cannabis indica* Lam. in the Lamarck Herbarium, Muséum d'Histoire Naturelle, Paris

Courtesy: Muséum d'Histoire Naturelle

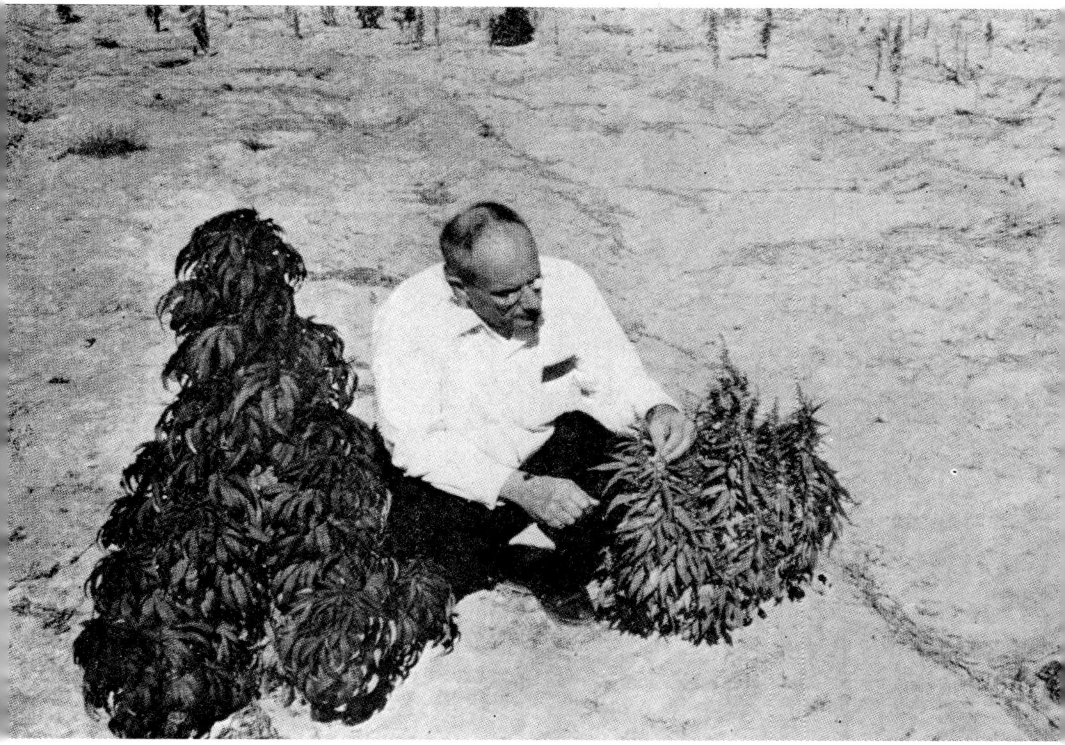

Plate 4. *Cannabis indica* (left: pistillate individual; right: staminate individual) in fields near Kandahar, Afghanistan. Pistillate plant: source of specimen *R. E. Schultes 26505* (Econ. Herb. Oakes Ames)

Photograph: R. E. Schultes

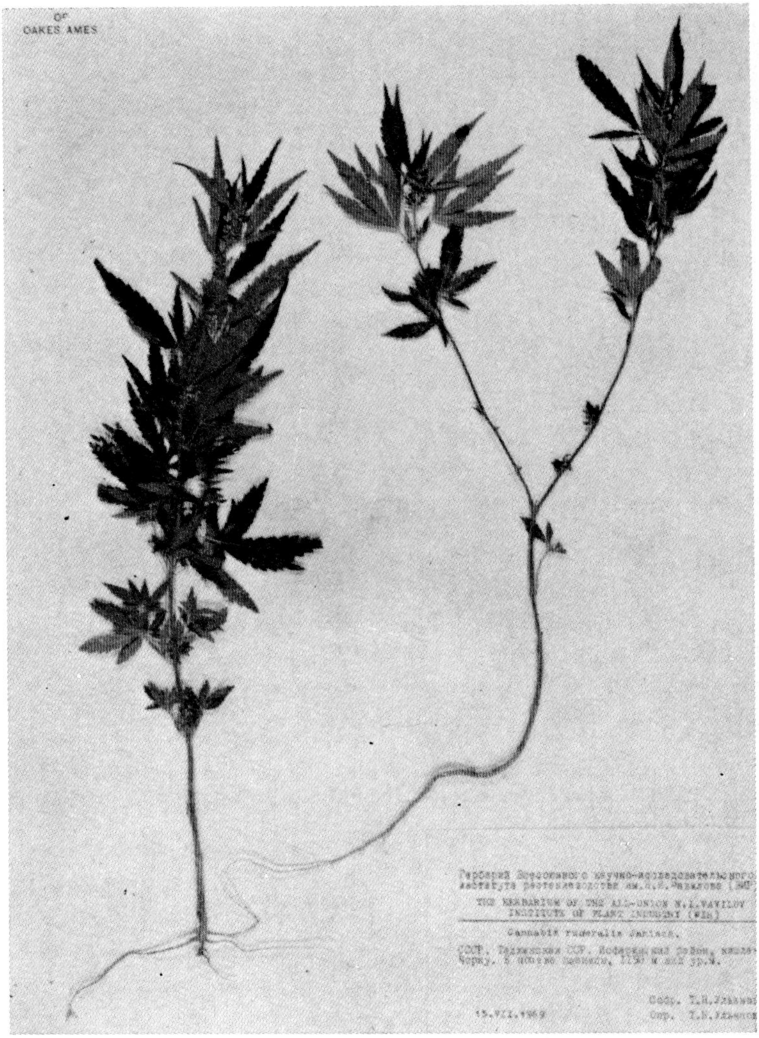

Plate 5. *Cannabis ruderalis* J. n. Specimen from the Herbarium of All-Union N. I. Vavilov Institute of Plant Industry (Wir). Soviet Union, Tadzjikskaia SSR. Isfarinski Raion, Kishlak Chorku. V Poseve Pshenitsy. Alt. 1150m. July 15, 1969. *T. N. Ul'ianova sine num.* (Econ. Herb. Oakes Ames)

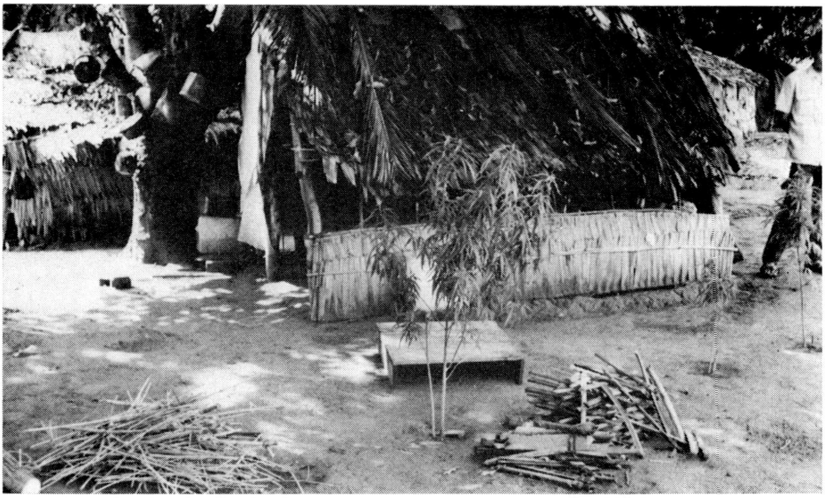

Plate 1.

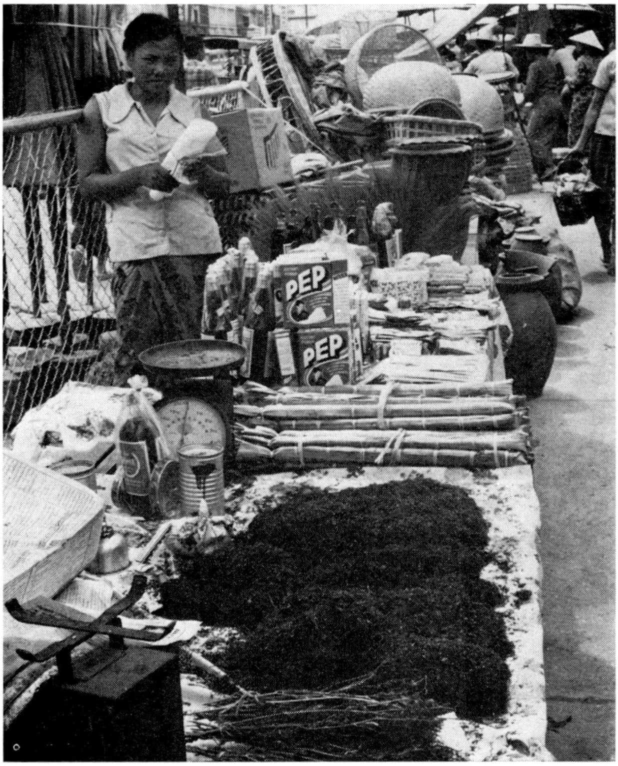

Plate 2.

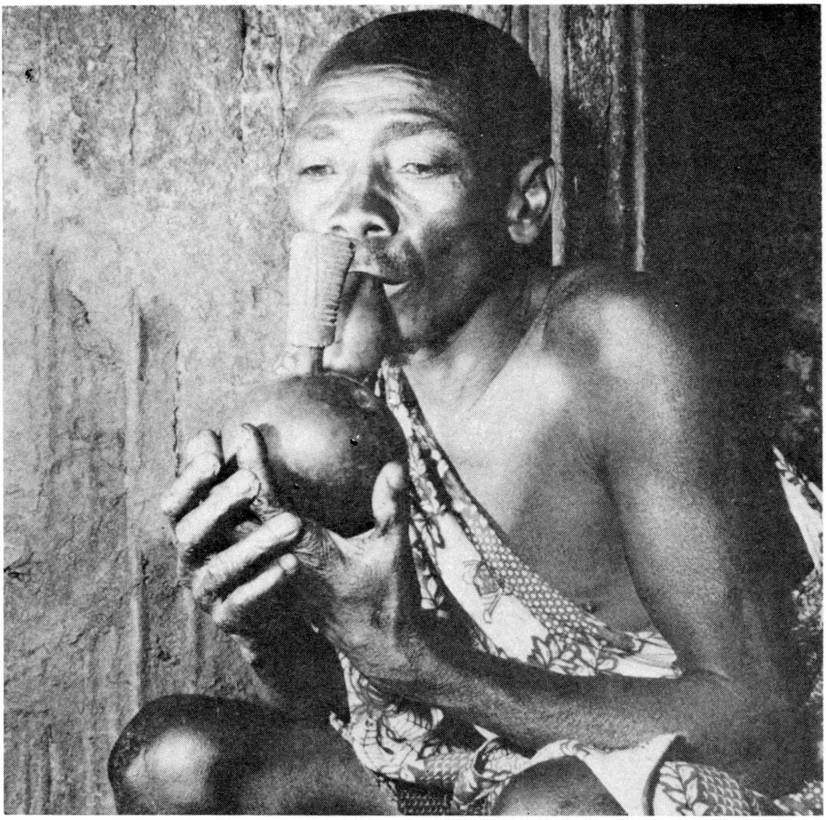

Plate 1.

Photograph: L'Institute pour la recherche
scientifique en Afrique centrale

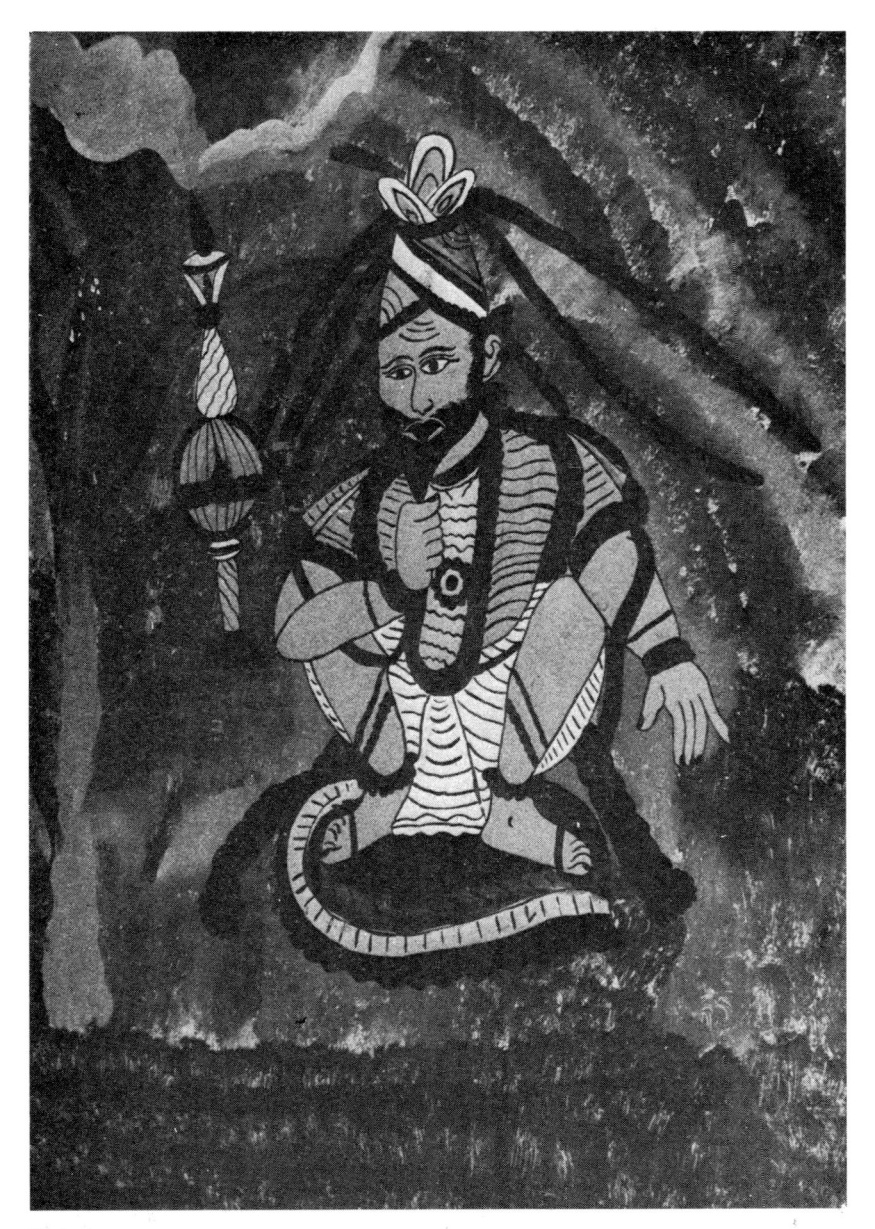

Plate 1.

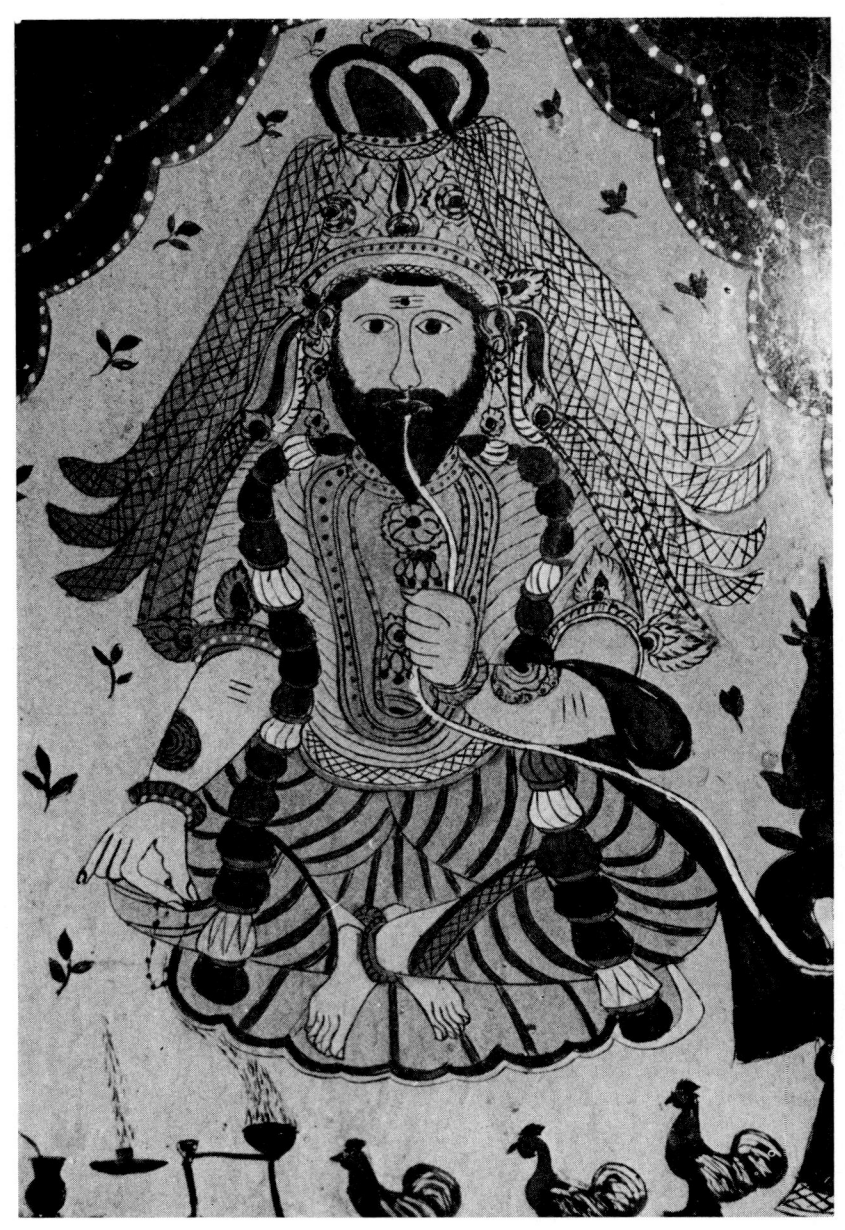

Plate 2.

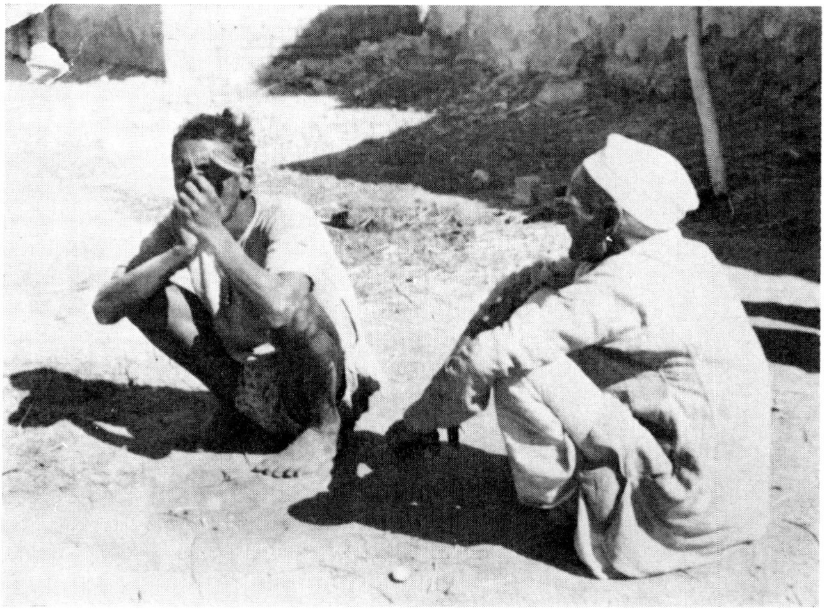

Plate 1. Smoking *ganja* in a funnel-shaped clay pipe

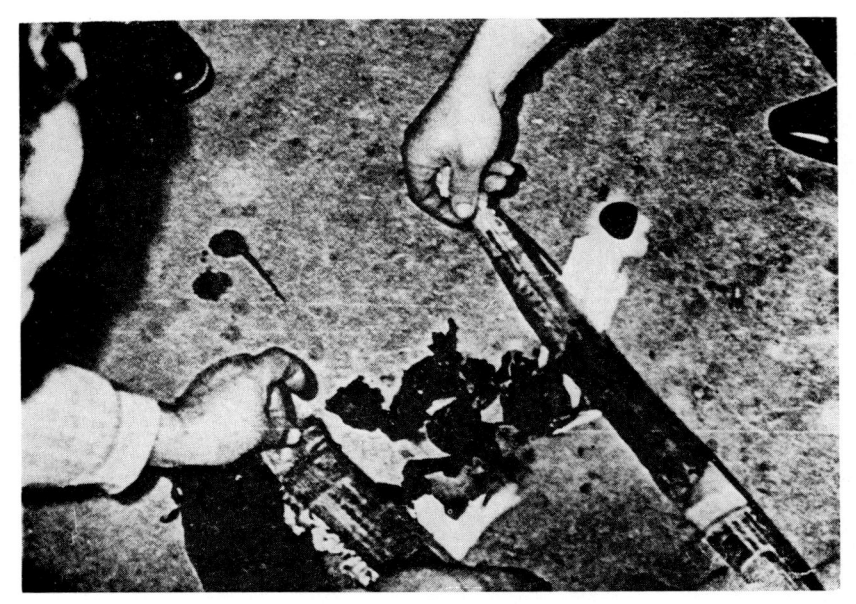

Plate 1. Preparation of hashish cakes (*tsikes*). Hashish powder, rolled in newspaper, is soaked in water and heated over a flame. This roll is then crushed to form a solid cake

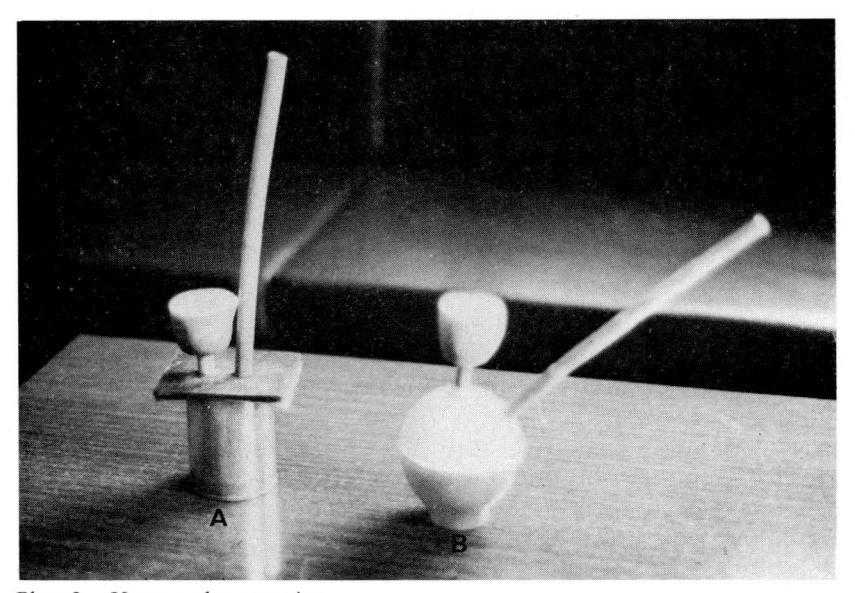

Plate 2. Homemade water pipes
A. Tin can with hollowed raw potato attached in which the mixture of hashish and tobacco is placed; and bamboo smoking pipe
B. Plastic piggy-bank replaces tin can

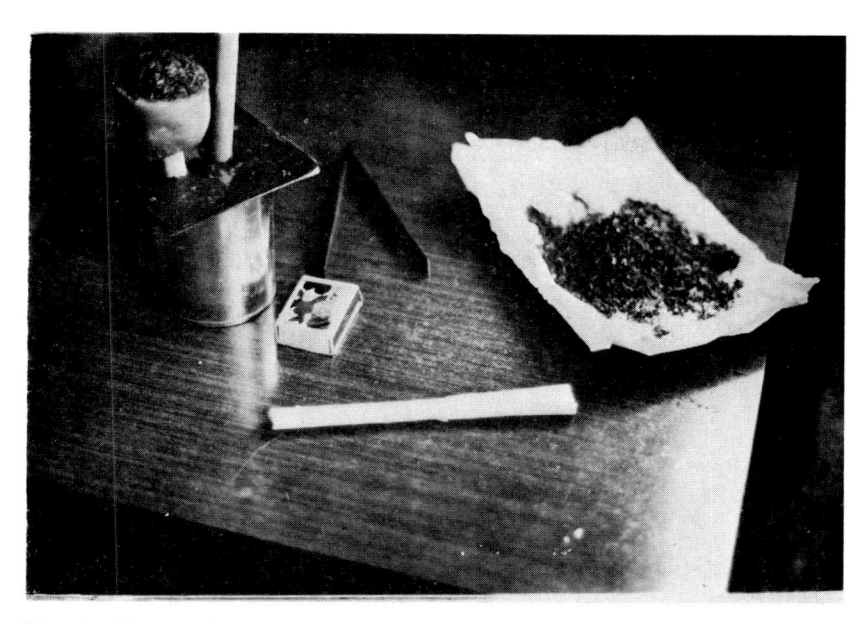

Plate 3. Homemade water pipe (*loulas*) with potato filled with the mixture of hashish and tobacco; and finished cigar (*tsigariliki*) with attached stiff paper pipe (*tzivana*)

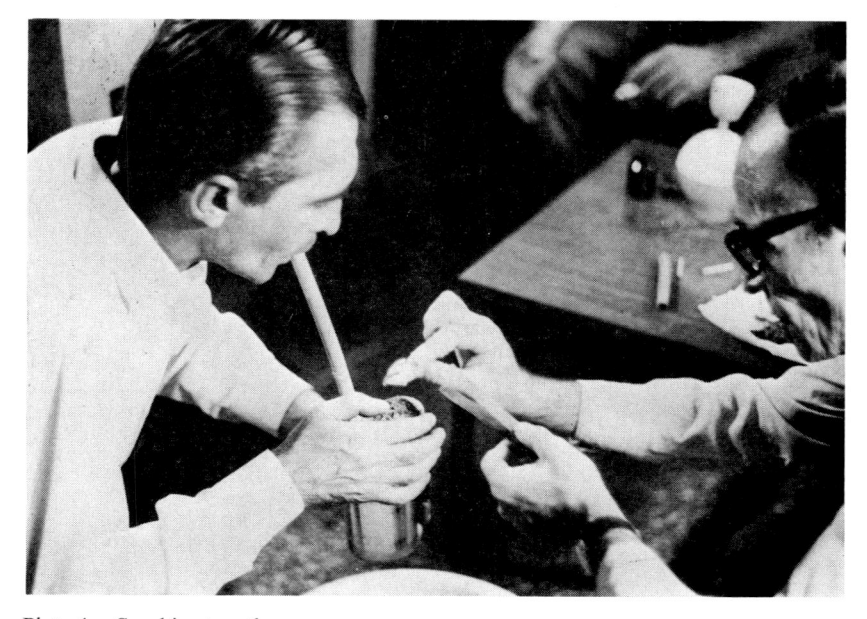

Plate 4. Smoking together

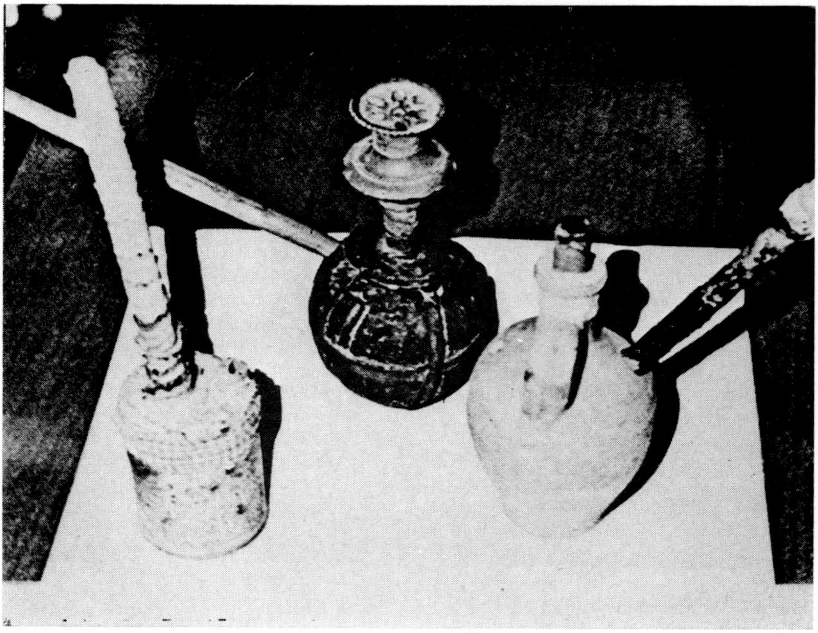

Plate 5. Smoking devices

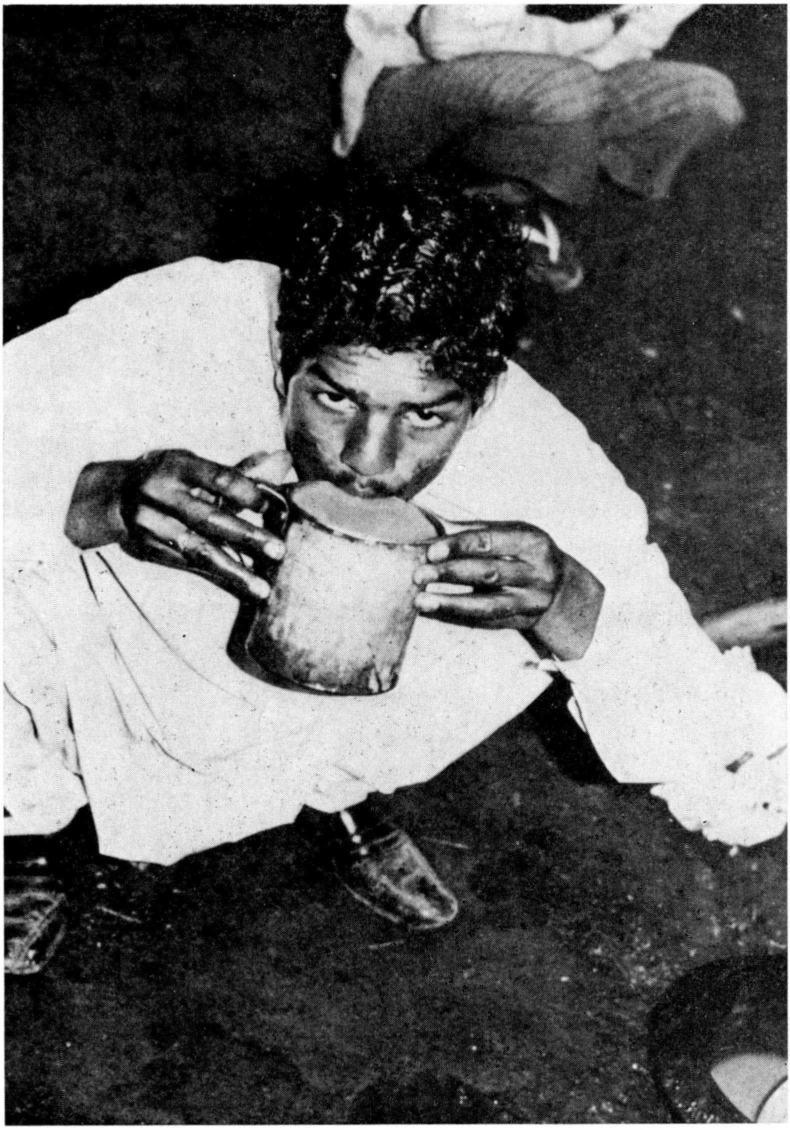

Plate 1. *Bhang* drinking

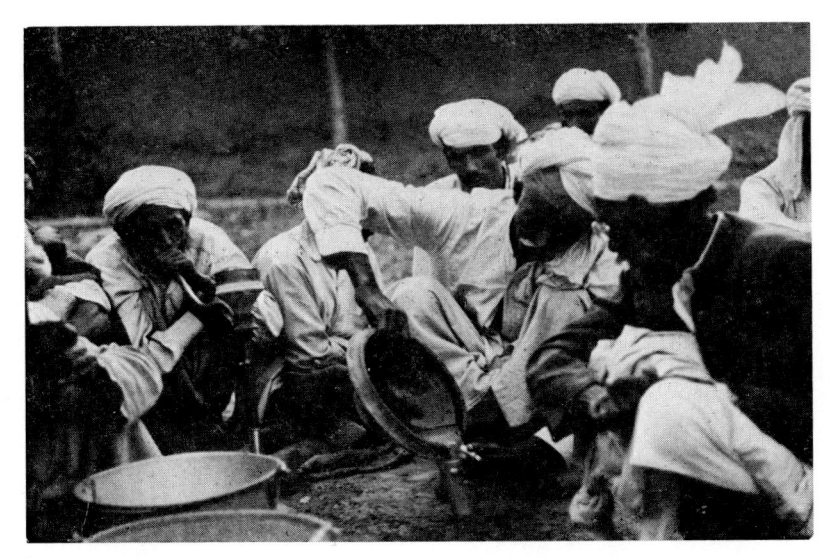

Plate 2. *Bhang* preparation

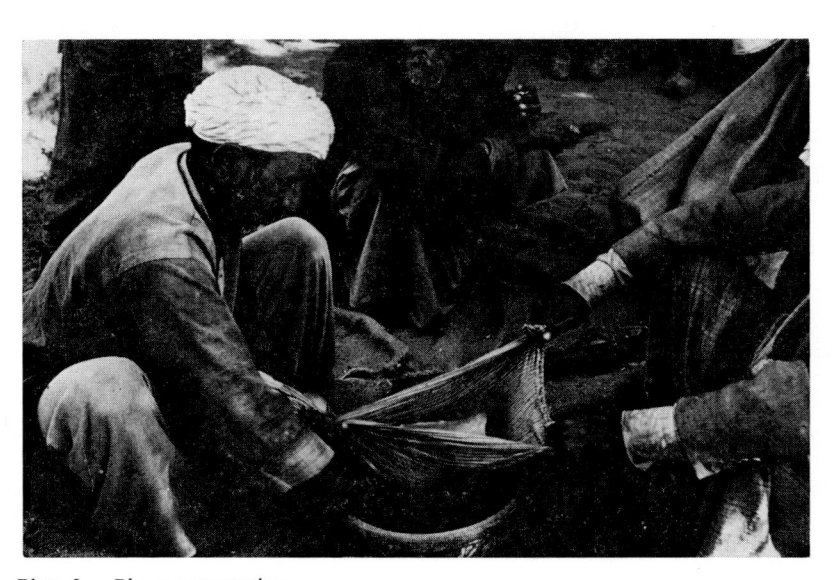

Plate 3. *Bhang* preparation

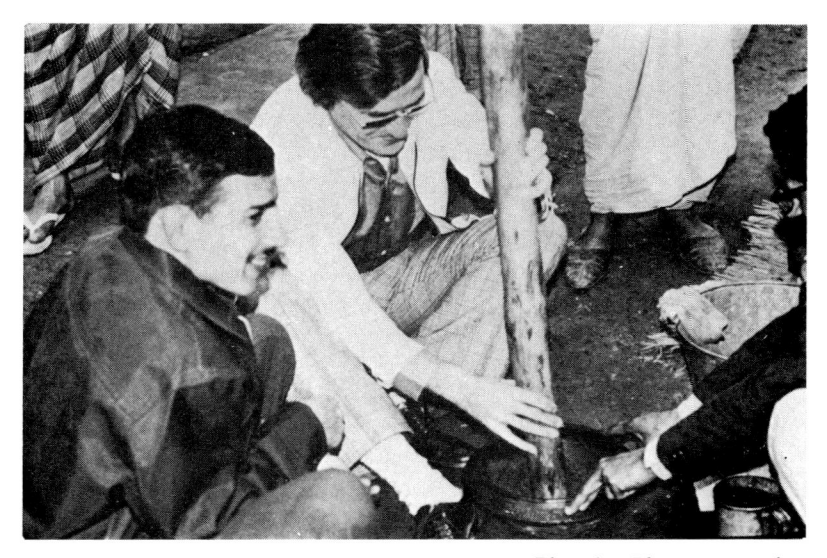

Plate 4. *Bhang* preparation

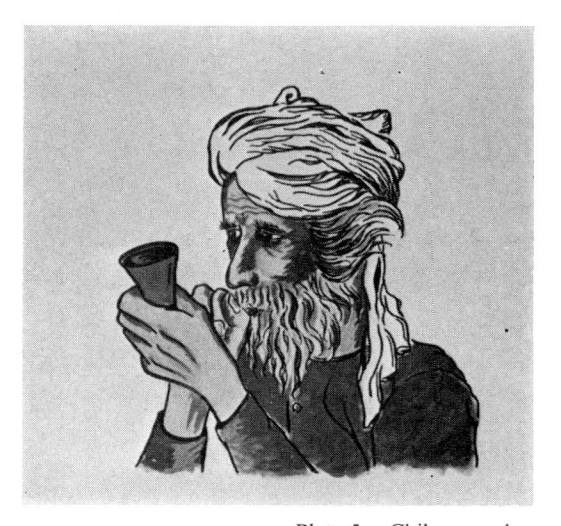

Plate 5. Chilam smoker

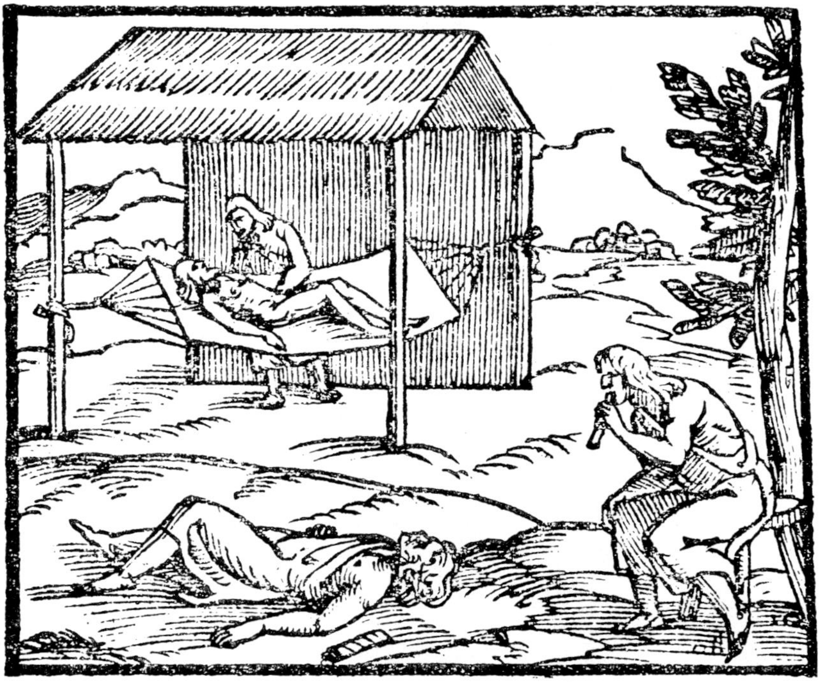

De cómo los médicos curan a los enfermos

Plate 1. Woodcut published by Benzoni (1565) showing Indians of Haiti smoking tobacco from a cigar or pipe. One smoker has dropped his cigar and lies on the ground intoxicated by the smoke he has consumed. A shaman cures a sick person in his hammock

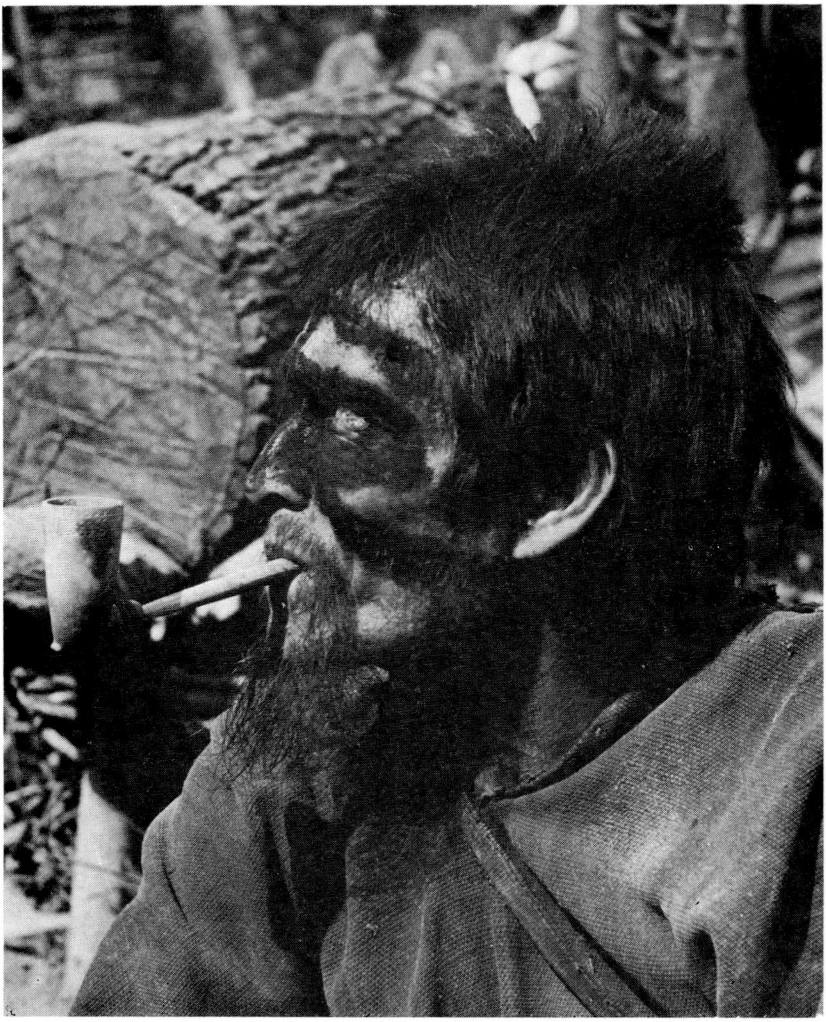

Plate 2. A Yupa Indian smoking the pipe. Courtesy Luis T. Laffer

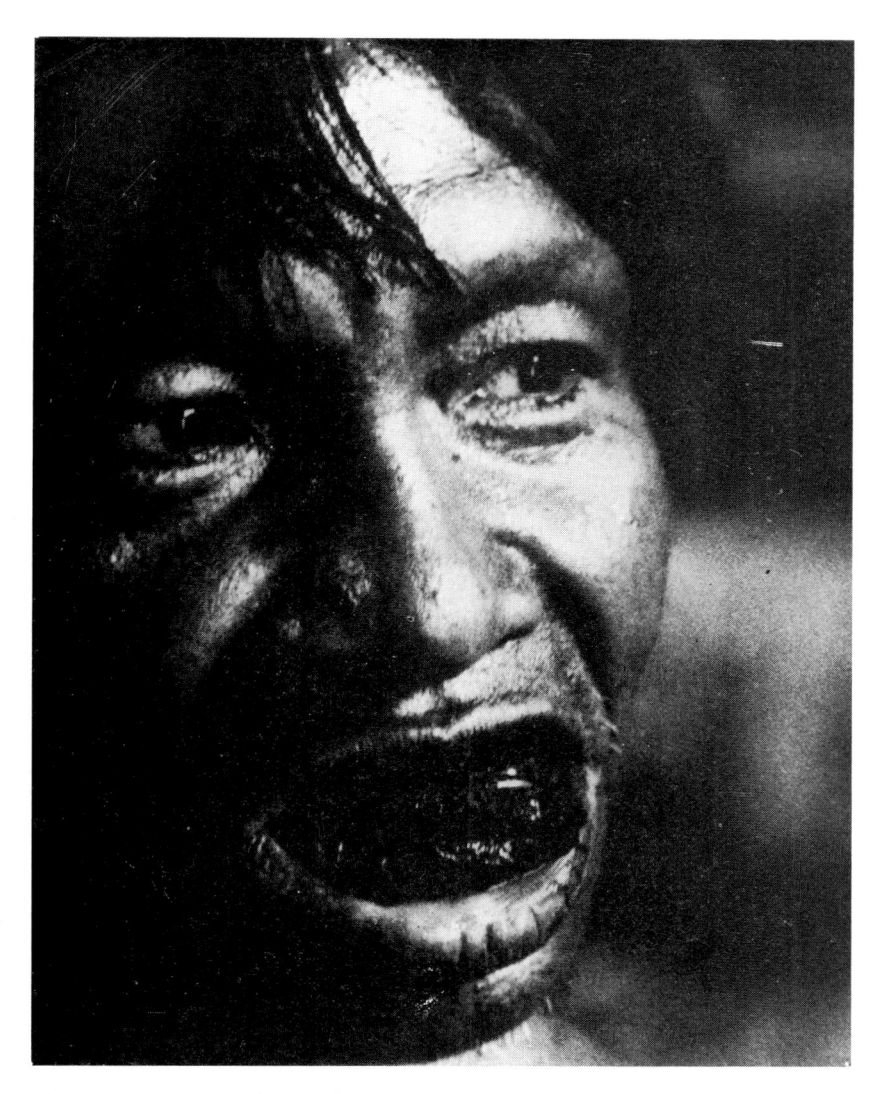

Plate 3. Yanoama Indian sucking on a wad of tobacco (Photograph courtesy Barbara Braendli)

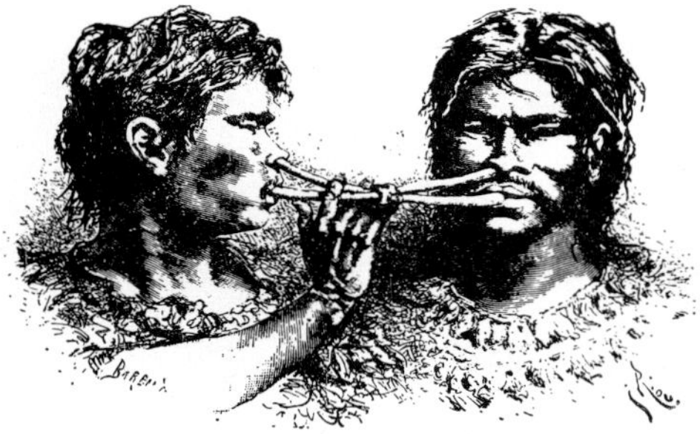

Plate 4. Witoto Indians taking snuff by blowing powder up into the nostrils of a partner (After J. Crévaux, *Voyages dans L'Amérique du Sud.* Paris 1883.)

FUMIGATION A LA CIGARETTE

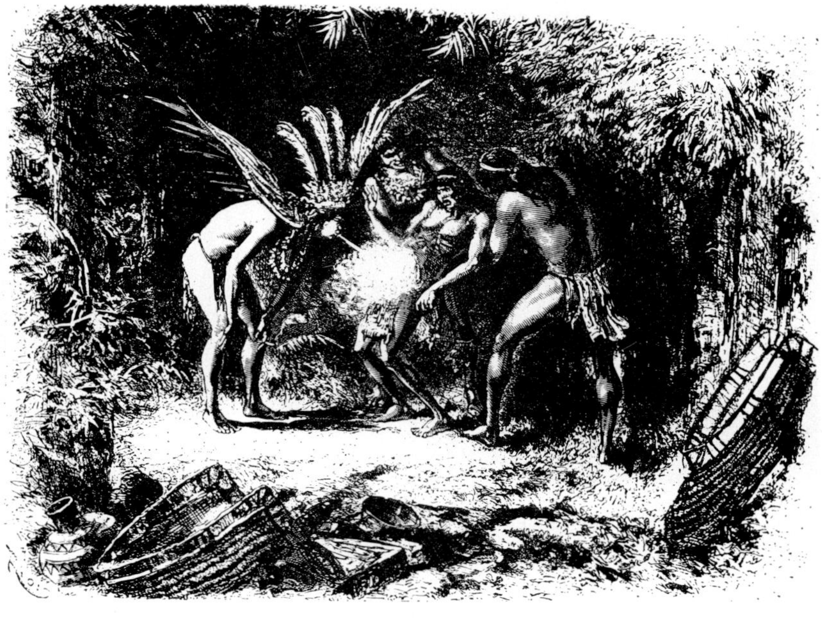

Plate 5. Roucouyenne Indian is treated by tobacco smoke blowing shaman (After J. Crévaux, *Voyages dans L'Amérique du Sud.* Paris 1883)

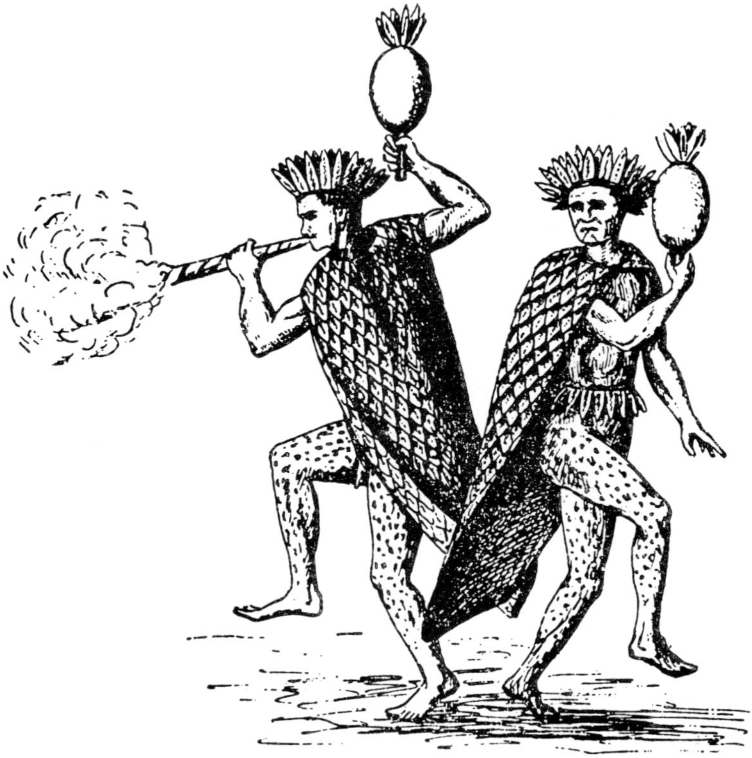

Plate 6. Tupinamba shamans wearing feather cloaks, smoking a cigar, and carrying rattles (After Métraux, 1928)

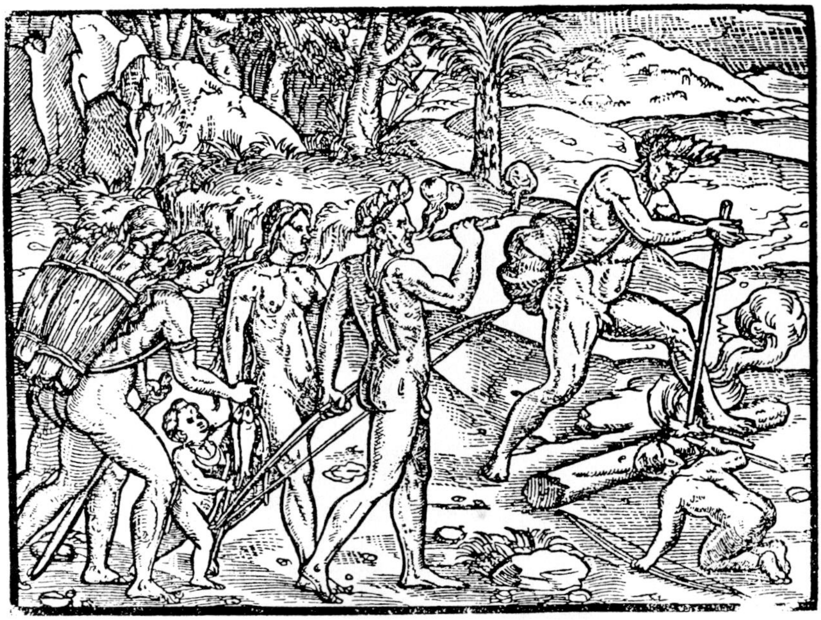

O fumador de tabaco e a fabricação do fogo (Thevet).

Plate 7. Woodcut published by André Thevet in *Les sigularitez de la France antartique*... Paris 1557, showing Tupinamba Indians smoking a cigar and making fire.

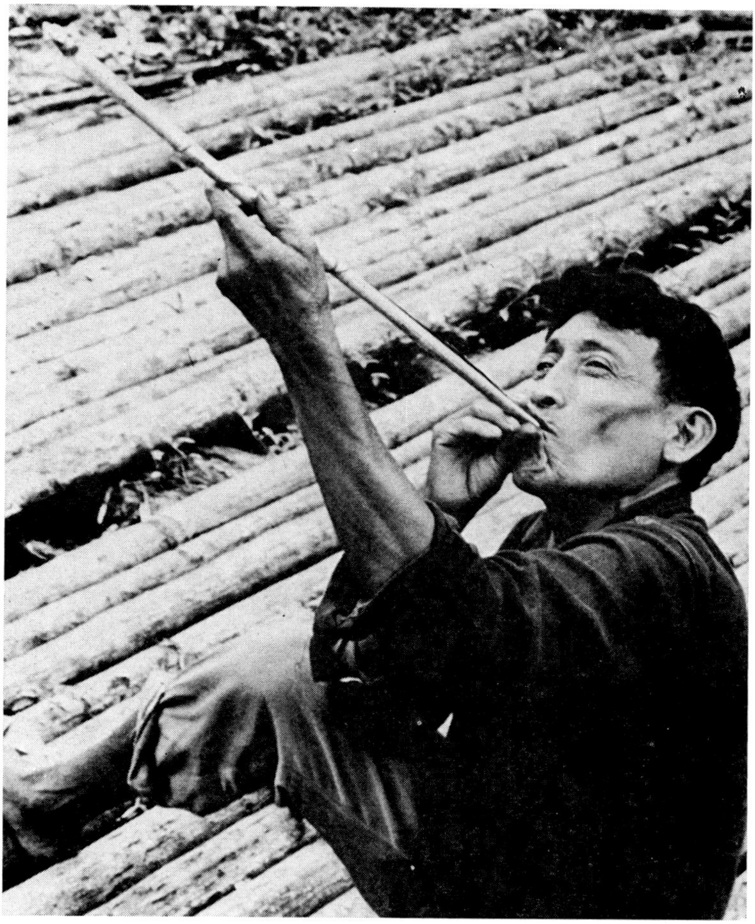

Plate 8. Priest-Shaman carrying out the feeding of the gods by holding the long cigar vertically and pointing it in the direction of the Supreme Spirits. (Photograph by Johannes Wilbert)

PART THREE

Medical, Pharmacological and Ethnometabolic Studies

Cannabis sativa *L. (Marihuana)*: *VI. Variations in Marihuana Preparations and Usage - Chemical and Pharmacological Consequences*

ALVIN B. SEGELMAN, R. DUANE SOFIA, and FLORENCE H. SEGELMAN

ABSTRACT

Relatively little is known regarding the drug effects of marihuana in man, *vis-à-vis* the different methods of preparing the plant material prior to actual use. A search of the scientific literature reveals cryptic references which lead one to believe that there may indeed be subtle as well as frank pharmacological differences in the marihuana induced effects in humans. These differences may depend on the sundry methods whereby various hemp products are prepared and used throughout the world.

Although marihuana is usually employed in this country by means of smoking the crushed and dried plant material, recent reports related to us from certain fringe groups of the drug subculture describe a heretofore unknown and novel method of marihuana preparation and use. Reputedly, the simultaneous ingestion of marihuana teas together with smoking cigarettes prepared from previously water-boiled marihuana plant material, results in increased psychotropic effects both in terms of intensity as well as duration. The known aspects of this ritual will be briefly described.

In our laboratories, using experimental conditions chosen to simulate the extemporaneous manner of preparation, it was found that the boiling water treatment of marihuana led to marihuana that was significantly enriched in cannabinoid substances, including delta-9-tetrahydrocannabinol which is considered to be the major psychoactive component of marihuana. This may explain, at least partly, the alleged claims made for the increased biological potency of marihuana so prepared. Furthermore, preliminary animal experiments indicate that marihuana teas may indeed exhibit biological activities. Finally, the potential health hazards inherent in this newly described practice, based on the fact that illicit marihuana is frequently misrepresented and adulterated with other drugs, will be discussed.

Supported by U.S. Public Health Service Research Grant RO1–DA–00328 (to Alvin B. Segelman) from the National Institute on Drug Abuse. We wish to thank Dr. Monique C. Braude, Executive Secretary, National Institute of Mental Health, Food and Drug Administration Psychotomimetic Agents Advisory Committee, for helpful advice and for furnishing cannabinoids and marihuana plant material for certain studies.

INTRODUCTION

The Indian hemp plant, botanically known as *Cannabis sativa* L., has long been known to man as a source of numerous preparations possessing intoxicating properties (Bouquet 1950). It is presently debatable as to whether or not *Cannabis* is a monotypic genus (viz., represented by the single species *sativa*). Schultes (1970a) and Quimby *et al.* (1973) have dealt with this subject in some detail. For the purpose of the present discussion, hemp will be considered to be synonymous with *Cannabis sativa* L. The plant itself, probably native to central Asia, is now distributed throughout most temperate and tropical regions of the world where it is either cultivated or grows wild as an herbaceous annual weed. Cannabis is usually dioecious, that is, having the female and male flowers borne on separate plants. Although it was previously believed that the male plants were biologically inactive in terms of intoxicating properties, recent evidence has demonstrated that both female and male plants contain psychoactive constituents (Fetterman *et al.* 1971; Small and Beckstead 1973).

Hashish of the Middle East and *charas* or *churrus* of the Indian peninsula represent the resinous secretion that spontaneously exudes from especially the flowering tops of the female plants. *Ganja* of India is prepared by collecting the tops of the female hemp plants; *bhang* refers to the product of the entire hemp plant or various mixtures of the leaves, stems and flowering tops. Marihuana, the product most often encountered in North America, is similar to *bhang*. *Hashish* is generally considered the most potent in terms of intoxicating properties, followed by *ganja* and *bhang* in order of decreasing potency. Nearly all these hemp preparations may be used alone or incorporated into various commodities suitable for eating, drinking, smoking and even snuffing (Bouquet 1950; 1951).

CHEMISTRY AND PHARMACOLOGY

The chemistry and pharmacology of cannabis have been extensively reviewed and need not be discussed in detail here (Wolstenholme and Knight 1965; Mechoulam and Gaoni 1967; Joyce and Curry 1970; Gershon 1970; Mechoulam 1970a; Braude *et al.* 1971; Hollister 1971; Neumeyer and Shagoury 1971; U. S. DHEW 1971; Cotton 1971; Singer 1971; Mills and Brawley 1972; Nahas 1973; and U. S. DHEW 1972). Nevertheless, it will be useful to introduce certain relevant chemical and pharmacological data. From a chemical point of view, cannabis is unique in containing a large number of different but closely related fat-soluble compounds collectively referred to as cannabinoids (Figure 1) (Mechoulam and Gaoni 1967), that have thus far not been found elsewhere in nature. The majority of the cannabinoids have been isolated and identified only since 1964, when Gaoni and Mechoulam (1964) characterized the compound (−) *trans*-Δ^9-tetrahydrocannabinol[1] (Δ^9-THC) and identified it as the major psychoactive constituent of hashish.

Figure 1. Some selected cannabinoids

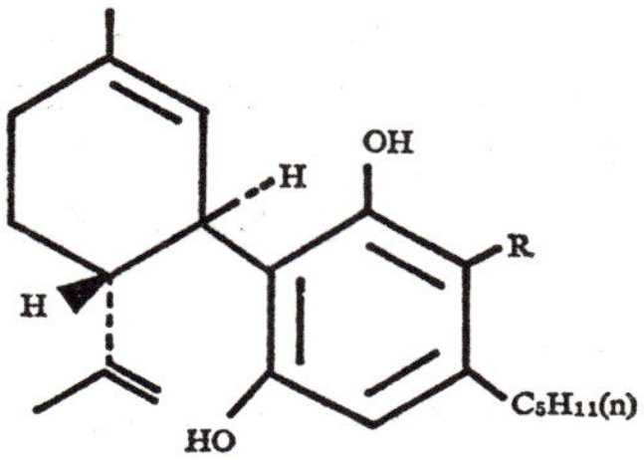

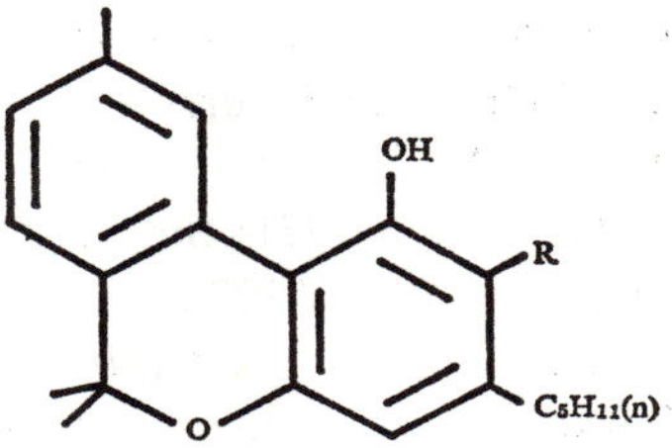

I, R=H, Cannabidiol (CBD)
II, R=COOH, Cannabidiolic Acid (CBDA)

III, R=H, Cannabinol (CBN)
IV, R=COOH, Cannabinolic Acid (CBNA)

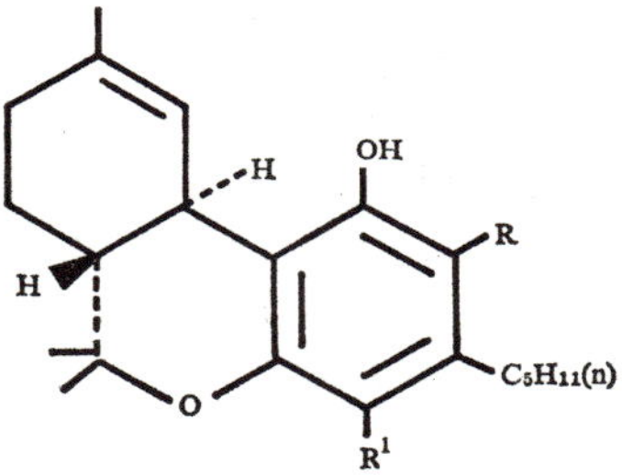

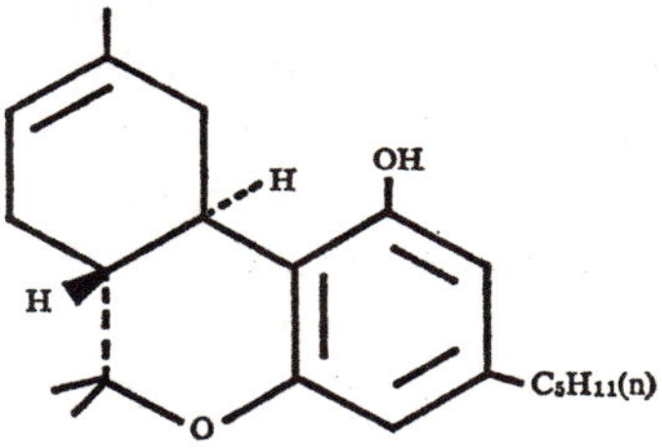

V, R=R¹=H, Δ^9-Tetrahydrocannabinol (Δ^9-THC)
VI, R=COOH, R¹=H, Δ^9-Tetrahydrocannabinolic Acid A
VII, R=H, R¹=COOH, Δ^9-Tetrahydrocannabinolic Acid B

VIII, Δ^8-Tetrahydrocannabinol (Δ^8-THC)

Note: The Δ^9-THC acids are not biologically active *per se*, but are converted (decarboxylated) by heating (smoking) to furnish the psychoactive Δ^9-THC.

It is now generally accepted that Δ^9-THC is one of the principal cannabinoid constituents and the major psychoactive component present in most hemp preparations (Isbell *et al.* 1967; Mechoulam *et al.*

---

[1] We prefer to designate the cannabinoids according to the dibenzopyran numbering as used by Chemical Abstracts. Thus, Δ^9-THC is equivalent to Δ^1-THC of a different numbering system commonly used. For a full discussion, see pp. 209–212 in (Joyce and Curry 1970).

1970a). A second minor cannabinoid, (–)-*trans*– Δ^8-tetrahydrocannabinol (Δ^8-THC), has also been found to exhibit psychoactive properties (Grunfeld and Edery 1969; Hively *et al.* 1966) while the remaining cannabinoids have been shown to be lacking in observable psychopharmacological effects (Edery *et al.* 1971). Large quantities of both Δ^9-THC and Δ^8-THC have been synthesized and are available for research purposes. This is also the case for cannabis plant material and "crude" extracts therefrom (Scigliano and Waller 1970). However, pharmacological experiments in animals and humans have been carried out using Δ^9-THC (Joyce and Curry 1970; Gershon 1970; Mechoulam 1970a; Braude *et al.* 1971; Hollister 1971; Neumeyer and Shagoury 1971; U. S. DHEW 1971; Cotten 1971; Singer 1971; Mills and Brawley 1972; Nahas 1973; and U.S. DHEW 1972).

It has been demonstrated that approximately 50 percent of the Δ^9-THC content of marihuana cigarettes was delivered unchanged via the smoke to the lungs of the users, providing that the entire cigarettes, including the butts, were smoked (Manno *et al.* 1970). The Δ^9-THC is apparently rapidly absorbed from the lungs and subsequently produces typical pharmacological effects. Although it has been reported that the ratios of the cannabinoids found in marihuana smoke approximate the ratios of the natural cannabinoids in the plant (Truitt 1971), relatively little is known concerning the chemistry and pharmacology of the smoke from cannabis preparations (Fentiman *et al.* 1973). Might there perhaps be present one or more components of the smoke which are biologically active *per se* or which in some other way modify the biological effects of the psychoactive Δ^9-THC?

Isbell and co-workers have reported that the absorption of Δ^9-THC is approximately three times less effective by mouth than when smoked (Isbell *et al.* 1967).[2] When considering the variety of hemp preparations containing cannabis or hashish which are intended to be taken by mouth, the question arises: are there present in these preparations heretofore undiscovered biologically active substances which could contribute to the overall perceived effects in humans? This important question has not been resolved to date.

In 1843 O'Shaughnessy described the preparation of the hemp confection known as *majoon*, "Four ounces of *sidhee* [*bhang*] and an equal quantity of *ghee* (clarified butter) are placed in an earthen or well-tinned vessel, a pint of water added, and the whole warmed over a char-

---

[2] In fact, the absorbtion of Δ^9-THC may be up to six times less effective by mouth than when smoked as pointed out by Kiplinger and Manno (1971).

coal fire. The mixture is constantly stirred until the water all boils away... the mixture is then removed from the fire, squeezed through cloth while hot – by which an oleaginous solution of the active principals and coloring matter of the hemp is obtained – and the leaves, fibres, etc., remaining on the cloth are thrown away. The green oily solution soon concretes into a buttery mass, and is then well washed by the hand with soft water so long as the water becomes colored. The coloring matter and an extractive substance are thus removed, and a very pale green mass of the consistency of simple ointment remains. The washings are thrown away; Ameer [the proprietor of a place for hemp users in Calcutta] says that these *washings are intoxicating and produce constriction of the throat, great pain and very disagreeable and dangerous symptoms* [italics ours]." (344–345) Is this perhaps one of the earliest indications that cannabis contains water-soluble biologically active substances? We shall return to this interesting concept later. Incidentally, the *majoon* described above appears to be similar to the arabic confection *dawamesc* which the French physician Jacques-Joseph Moreau used to study the effects of hemp in humans (Nahas 1973).

Schultes' remarks concerning peyote cactus intoxication could apply as well to hemp: "The very real – and often overlooked – differences between peyote intoxication and mescaline intoxication must be constantly borne in mind. Amongst aboriginal users, it is the dried head of the cactus, with its *total* [italics ours] alkaloid content, that is ingested; mescaline injected is employed only experimentally and then produces the effects of one of the alkaloids without the physiological interaction of the others that are present in the crude plant material. As a consequence, descriptions of the visual hallucinations found in psychological writings should not necessarily be too closely evaluated with the visual effects experienced by Indian peyotists" (Schultes 1970b: 33). The points that we are trying to emphasize are (i) the Δ^9-THC content of a particular cannabis preparation may not be a reliable index of psychoactive activity, (ii) possible pharmacological interactions between different hemp constituents, perhaps leading to subtle differences in perceived effects, cannot be and indeed should not be excluded at the present time.

STABILITY AND VARIATIONS IN POTENCY

In 1970, during the course of a program designed to assess the chemical constituents of hemp preparations, we obtained for study a 43-year-old sample of an alcoholic cannabis fluidextract (Kubena *et al.* 1972). This preparation had formerly been official in the *United States Pharmacopoeia* (*Pharmacopoeia* 1926). Using gas-liquid chromatography, it was shown that the fluidextract contained 0.4% Δ^9-THC, 0.1% cannabidiol and 0.04% cannabinol. Furthermore, we found that this preparation, even after the extended storage period of 43 years, still contained sufficient biological activity to induce the characteristic ataxia in dogs, following oral administration of the fluidextract to animals according to USP X (*Ibid.*).

These observations were totally unexpected because it had generally been assumed that cannabis preparations rapidly lost their potency with time (Bradbury 1899; Hamilton 1915; Eckler and Miller 1917; and Hamilton 1918). For example, Hooper (1894: 49) reported, "Ganjas always lose their strength when kept for some time, and many dealers in India obtain new supplies annually, and always consider the drug worthless after being kept three years." The *Dispensatory* later stated, "It is recognized in India that ganja rapidly deteriorates on keeping, that which is one year old being not more than one-quarter as potent as the fresh drug, while two-year-old ganja is practically inert and is required by the Indian government to be burned in the presence of excise officers." (Wood *et al.* 1926:278).

These conclusions have, in fact, extended to contemporary times (Trease and Evans 1966; Wallis 1967). But experimental data of greater significance resulted from further biological testing of the fluidextract. After the alcohol had been removed from the fluidextract, the residue was reconstituted in an inert vehicle, propylene glycol. Aliquots of the reconstituted mixture, calibrated to contain various amounts of Δ^9-THC, were tested in an operant conditioning lever-pressing procedure, based on alternative responses of food approach and shock avoidance (Kubena and Barry 1972).

In this procedure, rats were trained to make one response following injection of Δ^9-THC (4mg/Kg) and the alternative response after injection of the vehicle alone. Previous experiments with various drugs, including cannabinol, cannabidiol, morphine, cocaine, atropine, scopolamine, ethyl alcohol, chlorpromazine, chlordiazepoxide, pentobarbital, mescaline, LSD-25 and dimethyltryptamine showed that this bioassay was highly specific to Δ^9-THC. Hence, this procedure can serve to furnish valuable information regarding specific measurements of the subjective states induced by Δ^9-THC. Accordingly, psychoactive drugs can be shown to be similar or different, presumably on the basis of the induced perceptual states (Kubena and Barry 1969).

The data in Table 1 shows the results of this bioassay and clearly

Table 1. The effect of prolonged boiling water treatment on the Δ^9-THC content of marihuana

Marihuana material	Δ^9-THC, Percent	
	Calculated	Found
Untreated marihuana	1.86[a]	1.90
Boiling water treated marihuana	2.65[b]	2.56

[a] Determined from the supplier's assay results.
[b] Calculated by assuming that a total of 1.86g of Δ^9-THC remained unchanged in the 70g of dried, boiling water treated marihuana derived from 100 g of starting untreated marihuana plant material.

indicates that the marihuana fluidextract was approximately three times more potent when compared with equivalent amounts of pure Δ^9-THC. Unfortunately, the small amount of fluidextract available at the time precluded further studies to discover the phytoconstituents responsible for the observed increase in biological activity.

Presently there is an ever-increasing body of evidence which points to the fact that there may be heretofore uncharacterized biologically active constituents present in hemp. For example, contrary to previously published data (Persaud and Ellington 1967, 1968; Geber and Schramm 1969a, 1969b) which showed teratogenic effects in animals following injections of crude marihuana extracts, Borgen and co-workers (1971) were unable to reproduce these undesirable effects in rats, using pure Δ^9-THC. These investigators concluded, "It is quite possible that Δ^9-THC is indeed not teratogenic in the rat, but instead, another substance in the plant which occurred in the extracts was responsible for the defects observed previously. This other substance may be another of the cannabinoids known to exist in marihuana, or some other as yet unidentified compound" (485).

In a separate study, Karniol and Carlini (1972) found that the results from testing two different marihuana extracts indicated that they were approximately three to five times more active in rabbits, rats and mice when compared with the results obtained with Δ^9-THC. Very recently, Galanter et al. (1973) reported that marihuana, calibrated to contain known doses of Δ^9-THC, and pure Δ^9-THC were not absolutely equivalent when smoked. In another investigation, an *in vivo* study (Poddar and Ghosh 1972) was made of the comparative effects following the administration of a cannabis extract and Δ^9-THC on the activities of two rat liver enzymes, tryptophan pyrrolase and tyrosineα-ketoglutarate. Both the cannabis extract and the Δ^9-THC increased the two enzyme activities, but it was found that the cannabis extract elicited a greater response than did equivalent amounts of Δ^9-THC. In preliminary experiments Gill and collaborators (1970) presented evidence for the presence in cannabis of water soluble substances having pharmacological activities. It has also been reported (Klein et al. 1971) that a semi-purified alkaloid fraction derived from Cannabis sativa showed pharmacological activity (viz. – decreased motor activity) in mice.

The significance of the above examples as applied to humans, in terms of biological activities other than those attributed to Δ^9-THC alone, remains to be established.

NOVEL METHODS OF USE

We have recently received reports (Segelman and Sofia 1973) indicating that certain fringe groups of the drug subculture in this country are preparing and using marihuana according to a novel procedure. Briefly described, these individuals prepare and utilize marihuana as follows: the marihuana is first mixed with enough water to completely cover the plant material and is subsequently boiled for periods of time ranging from one to several hours. Additional amounts of fresh water are added from time to time in order to keep the plant material covered with liquid and thus prevent possible charring. The mixture is then allowed to cool and is passed through a cheesecloth filter. The filtrate (viz.–marihuana tea) is set aside and stored in a refrigerator because it has been found that the tea is prone to mold growth when kept at ambient temperatures. The boiled marihuana material remaining on the filter is removed, manually expressed free of entrapped liquid which is added to the reserved tea and finally spread out and allowed to spontaneously air-dry.

In some instances the damp marihuana is dried in household ovens, while certain more enterprising groups use hot-air hair dryers. The resulting dried marihuana is used to prepare cigarettes in the usual manner, with no adjustment being made in the approximate weight of plant material for individual cigarettes. These cigarettes are smoked normally except for the following variation: just prior to smoking, the reserved marihauna tea is consumed at once. We have presently no data regarding the amounts of tea ingested. Individuals employing the described procedure claim that the subsequent effects of the smoked marihuana are perceived to be significantly more profound, both in terms of intensity and duration, than are the effects experienced by smoking marihuana according to more conventional methods. We have not determined with certainty to what extent the described practice is carried out. However, essentially similar practices have been related by reliable sources from certain areas of the eastern United States, including New Jersey, Delaware, Pennsylvania, and Massachusetts.

We decided it would be worthwhile to study this problem under controlled laboratory conditions for the following reasons: first, it was of interest to assess the stability of the cannabinoids under the conditions of prolonged boiling. Reasonable stability of the compound Δ^9-THC could only be assumed on the basis of the long history of hemp products taken in the form of infusions or confections of various kinds involving heating during some stage of their preparation (Bouquet 1950, 1951). Of course, as mentioned earlier, it was known that approximately 50 percent of the cannabinoids survived the heat of combustion generated during smoking (Manno *et al.* 1970), but no stability studies had been done on the cannabinoids under boiling water conditions. Second, it was important to determine whether or not the marihuana tea showed pharmacological activity.

In order to stimulate the boiling water treatment of marihuana as described above, the following procedure was employed: a total of 100 g of marihuana [analyzed for Δ^9-THC, 1.86% (84% as the acid); Δ^8-THC, 0.03%; CTD, 0.19%; CBN, not quantitable] previously slurried with 1500 ml of distilled water was continuously refluxed for five hours using a Clevenger apparatus designed to collect volatile oils lighter than water. No precautions were taken to exclude light or air. Following refluxing, the slurry less the volatile oil was allowed to cool to room temperature and was suction filtered. The marihuana on the filter was washed with hot water and the wash filtrates were combined with the initial filtrate. This combined solution (*viz.*- marihuana tea) was frozen and lyophilized to give 30 g of a dark brown residue that was set aside for pharmacological testing. The remaining damp marihuana was allowed to air-dry for five days and was found to weigh 70 g. Thus, 30 percent of the dry weight of the original marihuana was removed by the boiling water treatment. The cannabinoid profiles of the boiling water treated marihuana and the untreated (non-boiled) marihuana were determined by gas-liquid chromatography (Figure 2a and 2b; see pages 282-285).

The data in Table 2 shows that the boiling water treated marihuana contained 1.4 times more Δ^9-THC than was found in the untreated marihuana. Under the conditions of the experiment, the biologically inactive Δ^9-THC-acid was quantitatively decarboxylated to furnish the psychoactive Δ^9-THC (Figure 3a and 3b). This was not unexpected since it was known (Mechoulam 1970b) that the cannabinoid acids smoothly decarboxylate at temperatures approaching 103°. The finding that was

Table 2. Responses[a] of rats to treatment with Δ^9-THC compared with the 43-year-old marihuana fluidextract

Δ^9-THC mg/Kg	Δ^9-THC	Marihuana fluidextract (0.4% Δ^9-THC)
16.0	100	–
4.0	93	–
2.0	77	–
1.0	33	91
0.5	0	45
0.25	–	9
0	8	–
ED_{50} (mg/Kg)	1.40	0.51
95% Confidence limits	0.93–2.12	0.32–0.80

[a] Percentage Δ^9-THC response (approach for half the animals, avoidance for the others) in tests with several doses and the 43-year-old marihuana fluidextract containing this compound by rats trained to make differential responses to 4 mg/Kg and the non-drug control conditions (0mg/Kg). See Kubena and Barry (1972).

surprising was that the cannabinoids present in the original untreated marihuana proved to be stable when subjected to the relatively drastic conditions of prolonged boiling. In fact, if one compares the gas-liquid chromatography analyses of the boiling water treated marihuana and the untreated marihuana (Figure 2a and 2b), it is quite clear that they differ quantitatively and not qualitatively. We (Kubena et al. 1972) and others (De Zeeuw et al. 1972) have shown that many of the cannabinoids appear to be relatively stable when they are present in crude cannabis preparations. In such cases, the complex mixture of phytoconstituents apparently retards the decomposition of the cannabinoids, and this phenomenon may also explain the stability of the cannabinoids remaining in the boiled marihuana plant material.

Thus, the reputed claims made for the increased biological potency of the boiling water treated marihuana can be explained, in part, as follows: the boiling water treatment of marihuana removes water soluble materials equivalent to 30 percent of the weight of the starting plant material, thus leading to marihuana correspondingly enriched in water-insoluble compounds, including Δ^9-THC, one of the major psychoactive compounds present in the plant. Obviously, those persons who smoke the same approximate weight of this boiled material as the untreated marihuana, would experience more profound drug effects.

We next turn our attention to the lyophilized aqueous extract (hereafter referred to as marihuana tea). Measurable amounts of Δ^9-THC or any other cannabinoids were shown to be absent from this material. It was

Table 3. The effect of Δ^9-THC and marihuana tea on hexobarbital sleeping time in mice[a]

Test compound	I.P dose mg/kg	N	Sleeping time in minutes (Mean ± S.E.)	Percent increase
Propylene glycol vehicle	–	16	49 ± 4	–
Δ^9-THC	5.0	8	49 ± 2	0
	10.0	8	100 ± 7[b]	104
	20.0	8	105 ± 12[b]	114
Distilled H_2O vehicle	–	16	41 ± 2	–
Marihuana tea	12.5	8	44 ± 4	7
	25.0	8	58 ± 5[b]	41
	50.0	8	59 ± 3[b]	44
	100.0	8	81 ± 8[b]	98

[a] Thirty minutes following administration of the test drugs or their vehicle each mouse was given an injection of hexobarbital sodium (125 mg/kg, I.P.). Sleeping time for each animal was measured by the time in minutes from the loss to regaining of the righting reflex observed for at least ten seconds after the animal was placed on its back.
[b] $p \leqslant 0.05$ when compared with its respective vehicle-treated control group.

decided to compare the effects of the marihuana tea with Δ^9-THC on hexobarbital sleeping time and alteration of painful stimuli, two pharmacological parameters known to be affected by Δ^9-THC (Garriott et al. 1968; Sofia and Barry 1972). Table 3 shows the results of each treatment condition on the hexobarbital-induced anesthesia in mice. A potentiation effect was observed in those mice pre-treated with either 10.0 or 20.0 mg of Δ^9-THC. Varying the pre-treatment dose of the marihuana tea produced significant prolongation of hexobarbital sleeping time following the three highest doses.

Table 4 summarizes the data obtained in the hot plate test system with each treatment group. All doses of Δ^9-THC produced a significant increase in mean reaction time to the noxious stimulus (viz.- heat) except those animals given 0.3 mg/kg. The three highest doses of the marihuana tea showed analgesic effectiveness, but were much less potent (viz.- ED 50 values approximately 1/200th that of Δ^9-THC) than Δ^9-THC.

On the basis of these results, work is underway directed toward isolation of the constituent(s) responsible for the observed activities. Moreover, the reputed claims that the effects of smoked marihuana can be augmented by consumption of marihuana teas has led us to initiate experiments in mice which will determine the extent of any interactions of the marihuana tea with Δ^9-THC. Also, experiments are being planned

Table 4. The effect of Δ^9-THC and marihuana tea in the hot plate analgesic test[a] in mice

Test compound	I.P. doses mg/kg	Control reaction time[b]	Drug reaction time[b]	% Increase in mean reaction time	# *Analgesic*[c] # Tested
Propylene glycol vehicle	–	7.8 ± 0.7	7.7 ± 0.6	0.0	0/8
Δ^9-THC	0.3	8.3 ± 0.6	10.0 ± 1.5	20.7	3/8
	0.625	7.4 ± 0.5	11.6 ± 1.5[d]	57.3	4/8
	1.25	7.6 ± 0.4	11.0 ± 1.0[d]	45.2	5/8
	2.5	7.5 ± 0.6	11.7 ± 1.1[d]	56.2	5/8
	5.0	7.6 ± 0.7	12.7 ± 2.1[d]	68.7	5/8
	10.0	7.4 ± 0.6	16.8 ± 1.1[d]	126.2	7/8
Distilled water vehicle	–	7.9 ± 0.2	7.9 ± 0.5	0.0	0/8
Marihuana tea	100.0	8.1 ± 0.7	8.9 ± 0.9	11.0	2/8
	200.0	7.0 ± 0.5	9.6 ± 0.5[d]	37.0	4/8
	300.0	8.0 ± 0.6	12.4 ± 1.7[d]	54.7	6/8
	400.0	7.5 ± 0.6	12.0 ± 1.0[d]	60.6	7/8

[a] This method for assessing analgesic activity was based on the reaction time of mice to lick their forepaws and/or jump after exposure to a copper surface hot plate heated and maintained at 54 to 56°C. A control reaction time (measured to the nearest 0.1 second) was obtained 24 hours prior to any test for drug effect. Only those mice with a control reaction time of ten seconds or less were used. On the test day, mice were administered the test drugs or their vehicles and thirty minutes later each mouse in a group re-exposed to the hot plate surface and the reaction time once again recorded.
[b] These data represent the mean ± S. E. for 8 mice in a group.
[c] The number of mice per group showing a 40% or greater increase in their pre-drug reaction time. These data are used to calculate the ED_{50} value (95% confidence limits); for Δ^9-THC, 1.3 (0.5–3.1) and the marihuana tea 216.0 (135.0–346.0).
[d] $p \leqslant 0.05$ when compared with its respective pre-drug control reaction time.

which will test the marihuana tea in the operant conditioning lever-pressing procedure described earlier (Kubena and Barry 1972), using rats trained to make one response following injection of Δ^9-THC and the alternative response after injection of the vehicle alone.

For the moment, we would call immediate attention to possible serious consequences which may result from consumption of marihuana teas. Because drugs are often misrepresented in the illicit marketplace, it is not unusual to find contraband marihuana adulterated with various non-cannabis substances. For example, during one particular three-month period in 1970, it was reported by a government agency that nearly 20 percent of the seized samples alleged to be marihuana instead proved to be another substance (Johnson and Gunn 1972), including tobacco, phencyclidine (PCP), catnip, parsley, lysergic acid diethylamide (LSD), oregano, tea, opium, alfalfa, wild carrot, chamomile, thyme, stramonium and stramonium preparations. Consider a street sample of marihuana impregnated with significant amounts of LSD. Although LSD is not biologically active when smoked, dangerous effects could result from ingesting teas prepared from LSD-containing marihuana. It may not be unreasonable to assume that marihuana may be adulterated with various drugs which, when smoked are inactive but which, when ingested in the form of teas may induce a variety of undesirable physiological effects in the user.

Finally, we should mention those items known as "drug cookbooks" and "underground formularies." These usually represent booklets containing compilations of research reports taken from the scientific literature as well as hearsay formulations – their purpose to provide "do-it-yourself" instructions for the laity who wish to prepare psychoactive materials. In some cases the information is useless (*viz.*–"powdered bananidine extract prepared from the scraped inside of banana peels" and claimed to have psychedelic properties). On the other hand, some of the formulations may conceivably lead to the preparation of toxic products, particularly in the hands of the scientifically uninformed. For example, the following excerpt from one such "drug handbook" (Barbour 1967:63–64) describes the preparation of a cannabis extract as follows: "(a) obtain 200 gm of dry cannabis and grind all of it to a very fine powder. Use a screen and pestle first, and then a pepper or coffee grinder. (b) Soak the powdered cannabis in enough 90% ethanol so that the level of the ethanol is 1 in. above the powder. Soak with periodic stirring for 2 days. (c) Filter the ethanolic solution, store in a corked flask, and label it 'solution #1.' (d) Again soak the cannabis sample in 90% ethanol, but in a percolator. The percolator must be on a hot-plate rather than on an open flame. (The vapors of ethanol are extremely flammable.) (e) Percolate, adding more ethanol as necessary, for at least two hours. (f) Pour off the ethanol solution and filter. (g) Mix this solution with solution #1 and evaporate off the ethanol until about 25 ml remains. Makes 4 full doses."

Assuming that the cannabis plant material in this particular case contains one percent by weight of Δ^9-THC and allowing for complete extraction, the final product will contain a formidable quantity of Δ^9-THC, that is, 500 mg per dose or 2000 mg per 25 ml final product. Of course, the more potent the plant material used, the greater would be the actual amount of Δ^9-THC consumed. Nahas (1973) has reviewed two reported cases of apparent acute hemp toxicity. One case (Heyndrickx

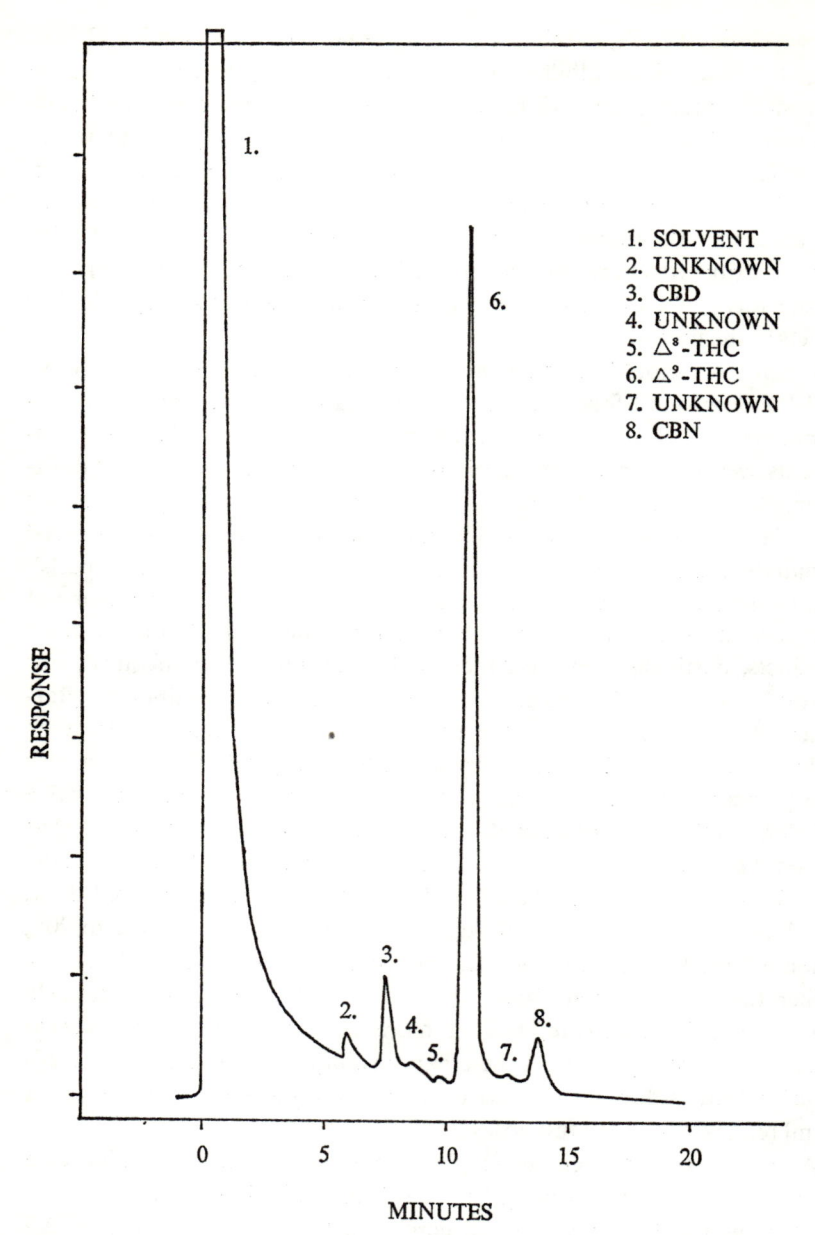

1. SOLVENT
2. UNKNOWN
3. CBD
4. UNKNOWN
5. Δ^8-THC
6. Δ^9-THC
7. UNKNOWN
8. CBN

Figure 2. Gas-liquid chromatography analyses

a. Boiling water treated marihuana.

b. Untreated marihuana (see next page).

The analagous peaks (*viz.* – boiling water treated marihuana/untreated marihuana) are in the approximate ratio of 1.4 to 1.0, thus showing enrichment of the cannabinoids in the boiling water treated marihuana.

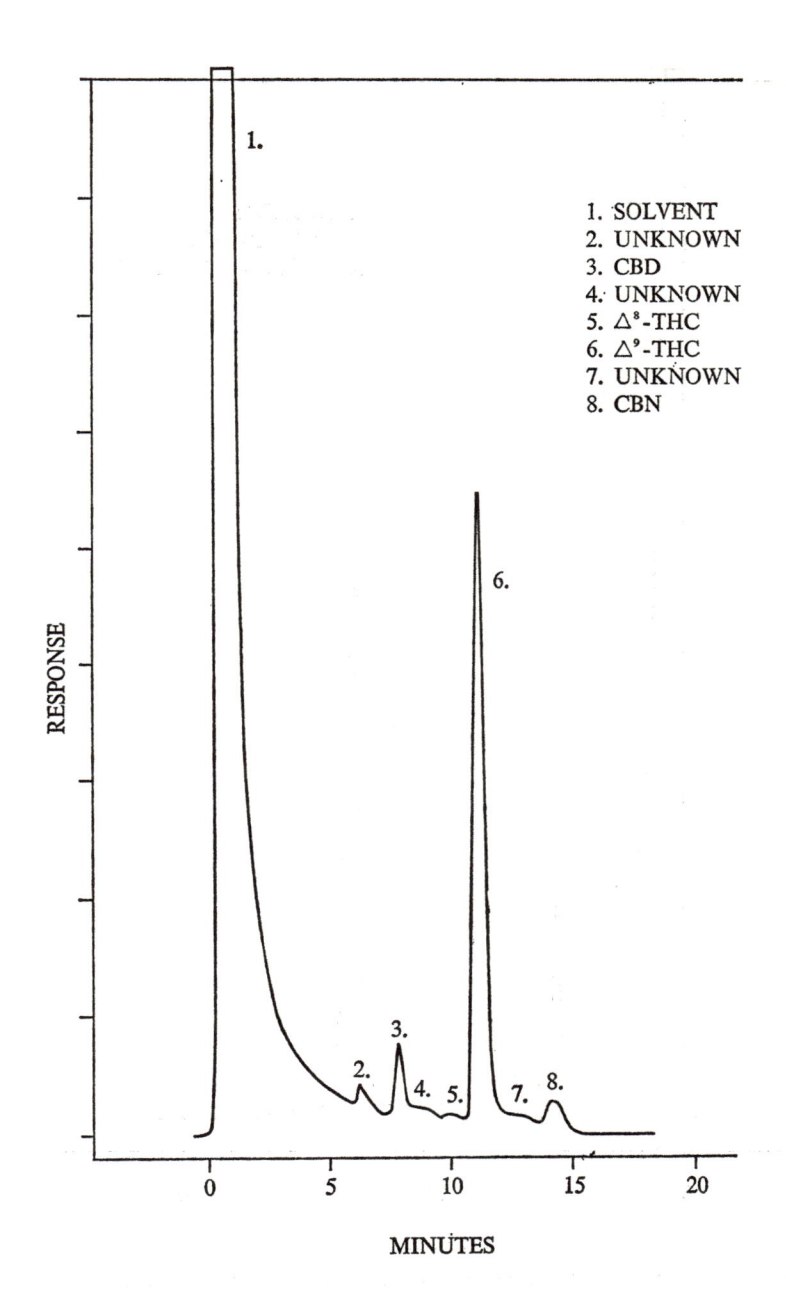

1. SOLVENT
2. UNKNOWN
3. CBD
4. UNKNOWN
5. Δ^8-THC
6. Δ^9-THC
7. UNKNOWN
8. CBN

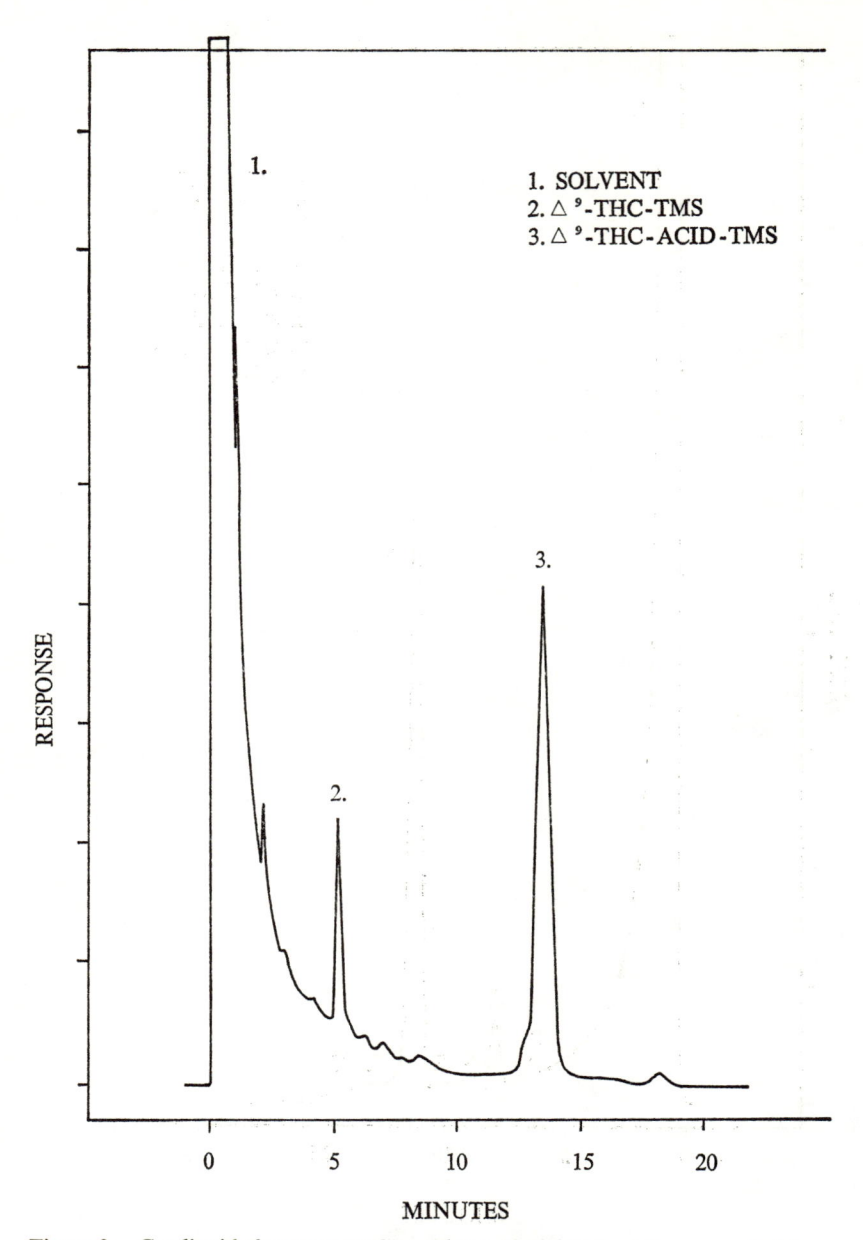

Figure 3. Gas-liquid chromatography analyses of silylated marihuana materials
a. Untreated marihuana showing that the total Δ^9-THC content comprised 84% Δ^9-THC-acid and 16% Δ^9-THC.
b. Boiling water treated marihuana showing the absence of the Δ^9-THC-acid-TMS peak, indicating that the Δ^9-THC-acid was quantitatively decarboxylated to furnish Δ^9-THC as a result of the boiling water treatment (see next page).

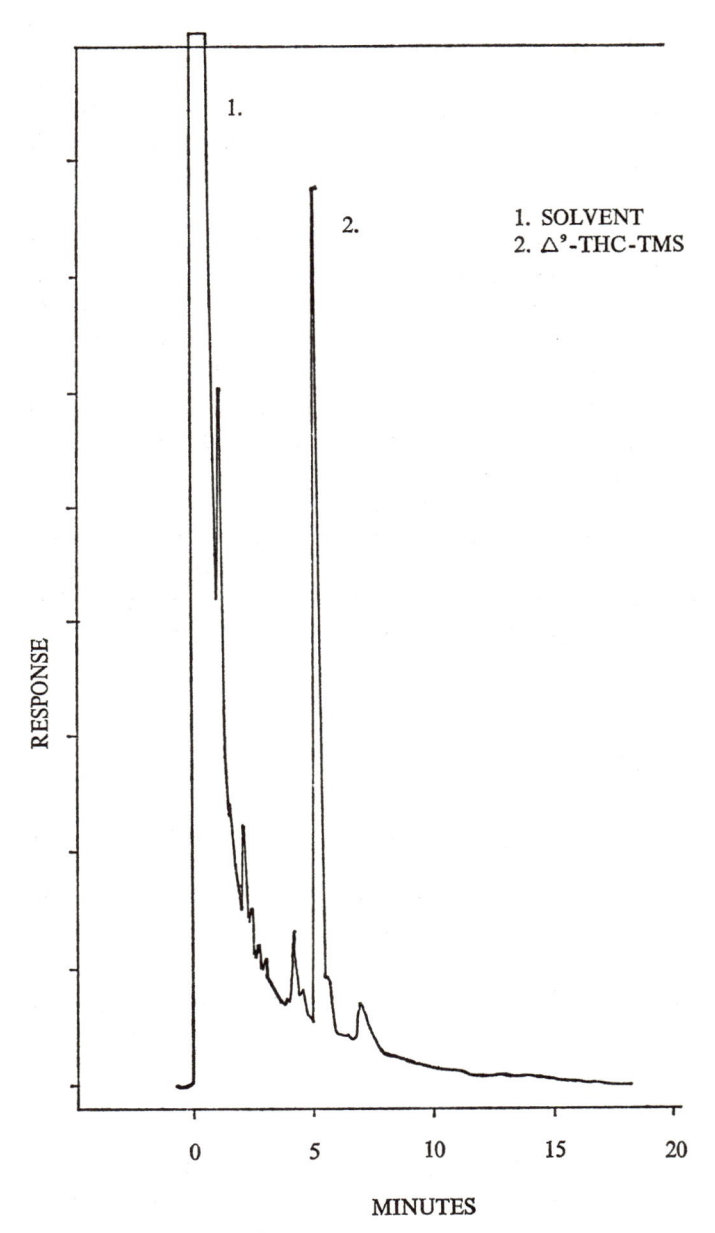

Cannabis sativa L.: Chemical and Pharmacological Consequences

1. SOLVENT
2. Δ⁹-THC-TMS

RESPONSE

MINUTES

The silylation step is carried out to prepare the trimethylsilyl (TMS) derivates of the cannabinoids. This is necessary in order to be able to distinguish the Δ⁹-THC-acid (as the Δ⁹-THC-acid-TMS derivative which is heat-stable) from the Δ⁹-THC (as the Δ⁹-THC-TMS derivative) when both cannabinoids are present in the same sample. Otherwise, the Δ⁹-THC-acid rapidly decomposes (decarboxylates) on the hot chromatography column to form Δ⁹-THC.

et al. 1970) resulted in the death of a 23-year-old student while the other (Gourves *et al.* 1971) led to a coma of four days duration in a young French soldier who had attempted suicide by smoking high doses of hashish. On the basis of the amounts of hashish claimed to be lethal, Nahas calculated that the lethal I.V. dose of Δ^9-THC for a 70 kg man would be approximately 200 mg. We are aware of the death of a young college student that was apparently associated with the consumption of large quantities of concentrated alcoholic extracts prepared from cannabis (Wille and Warren 1973). There is also evidence (Hays 1973; Anonymous 1972) for the appearance in the illicit market of increasing quantities of preparations referred to as "liquid hash" or "liquid hashish," some having high Δ^9-THC contents alleged to range from 20 to 56 percent. These preparations appear to represent concentrated alcoholic extracts prepared from marihuana and hashish.

It is speculative, of course, but one cannot help but wonder concerning some possible consequences if cannabis were given legal status and consequently made more or less freely available. Would society need to deal with various and sundry hemp preparations, some perhaps exhibiting socially unacceptable effects – or toxic effects heretofore not yet realized?

CONCLUDING REMARKS

In 1969 at a conference dealing with cannabis, Mechoulam and co-workers reported, "It is not yet known whether other natural cannabinoids, which are inactive *per se*, influence the activity of Δ^1-THC. There are grounds to believe that this may indeed be the case. Habitués believe that hashish samples of different origin show more than quantitative differences. Thus Afghanistan hashish is supposed to cause euphoria exclusively while Lebanese hashish may on occasion induce depression. We do not know any data which support or disprove such claims." (1970b:104–105). At the same conference, Joyce stated, "before we can attach too much importance to so-called pure substances, we must show that the pure substances are identical to the crude substances, and at present this is not proved." (Joyce 1970:155–156). These thoughts are no more or no less appropriate today than they were a few years ago.

If one reflects on the fact that various types of hemp preparations – *bhang*, *ganja* and *hashish* serving as prototypes – may be eaten, drunk, smoked and snuffed, then some questions arise.

For example, although it is generally agreed that Δ^9-THC is the major psychoactive substance present in hemp, might there not be also present in various hemp products – based on the particular modes of preparation and methods of use – other cannabis constituents exclusive of cannabinoids which also contribute to the pharmacological effects in man? Is it reasonable to suppose that over the centuries, by trial and error, man has learned to use certain hemp preparations while excluding others, based on *a priori* knowledge that desirable or otherwise advantageous drug effects will result from the use of the particular preparation which he has chosen to use?

Continued and imaginative interdisciplinary studies are needed to provide insights into these very important queries.

REFERENCES

ANONYMOUS
    1972   *PharmChem Newsletter* 1 (7). Palo Alto, California: PharmChem Laboratories.

BARBOUR, R. G., *editor*
    1967   *Synthesis and extractions of organic psychedelics*. USA: BarNel Enterprises.

BORGEN, L. A., W. M. DAVIS., H. B. PACE
    1971   Effects of synthetic Δ^9-tetrahydrocannabinol on pregnancy and offspring in the rat. *Toxicology and Applied Pharmacology* 20:480–486.

BOUQUET, R. J.
    1950   Cannabis. *Bulletin on Narcotics* 2:14–30.
    1951   Cannabis. *Bulletin on Narcotics* 3:22–45.

BRADBURY, J. B.
    1899   Some points connected with sleep, sleeplessness, and hypnotics. *Lancet* I:139–144.

BRAUDE, M. C., R. MANSAERT, E. B. TRUITT, JR.
    1971   Some pharmacologic correlates to marihuana use. *Seminars in Drug Treatment* 1:229–246.

COTTEN, M. DE V., *editor*
    1971   Marihuana and its surrogates. *Pharmacological Review* 23 (4):263–380.

DE ZEEUW, R. A., TH. M. MALINGRÉ, F. W. H. M. MERKUS
    1972 Δ^1-Tetrahydrocannabinolic acid, an important component in the evaluation of cannabis products. *Journal of Pharmacy and Pharmacology* 24:1–6.

ECKLER, C. R., F. A. MILLER
    1917   On the deterioration of crude Indian cannabis. *Journal of the American Pharmaceutical Association* 6:872–875.

EDERY, H., *et al.*
    1971   Structural requirements for cannabinoid activity. *Annals of the New York Academy of Sciences* 191:40–50.

FENTIMAN, A. F., JR., R. L. FOLTZ, G. W. KINZER
  1973 Identification of noncannabinoid phenols in marihuana smoke condensate using chemical ionization mass spectrometry. *Analytical Chemistry* 45:580–583.
FETTERMAN, P. S., *et al.*
  1971 Mississippi-grown *Cannabis sativa* L.: preliminary observation on chemical definition of phenotype and variations in tetrahydrocannabinol content *versus* age, sex, and plant part. *Journal of Pharmaceutical Sciences* 60:1246–1249.
GALANTER, M., *et al.*
  1973 Δ^9-Transtetrahydrocannabinol and natural marihuana — a controlled comparison. *Archives of General Psychiatry* 28:278–281.
GAONI, Y., R. MECHOULAM
  1964 Isolation, structure and partial synthesis of an active constituent of hashish. *Journal of the American Chemical Society* 86:1646–1647.
GARRIOTT, J. C., *et al.*
  1968 Pharmacologic properties of some cannabis related compounds. *Archives Internationales de Pharmacodynamie et de Therapie* 171:425–434.
GEBER, W. F., L. C. SCHRAMM
  1969a Teratogenicity of marijuana extracts as influenced by plant origin and seasonal variation. *Archives Internationales de Pharmacodynamie et de Therapie* 177:224–230.
  1969b Effect of marijuana extract on fetal hamsters and rabbits. *Toxicology and Applied Pharmacology* 14:276–282.
GERSHON, S.
  1970 On the pharmacology of marihuana, *Behavioral Neuropsychiatry* 1: 9–18.
GILL, E. W., W. D. M. PATON, R. G. PERTWEE
  1970 Preliminary experiments on the chemistry and pharmacology of cannabis. *Nature* 228:134–136.
GOURVES, J., *et al.*
  1971 Case of coma due to Cannabis sativa. *Presse Medicale* 79:1389–1390.
GRUNFELD, Y., H. EDERY
  1969 Psychopharmacological activity of the active constituents of hashish and some related cannabinoids. *Psychopharmacologia* 14:200–210.
HAMILTON, H. C.
  1915 Cannabis sativa: is the medicinal value found only in the Indian grown drug? *Journal of the American Pharmaceutical Association* 4:448–451.
  1918 The stability of Cannabis sativa and its extracts. *Journal of the American Pharmaceutical Association* 7:333–336.
HAYS, D.
  1973 'Liquid hash' worries cops as outside drug law. *The Star-Ledger*, Newark, New Jersey, Tuesday, May 15.
HEYNDRICKX, A., C. SCHEIRIS, P. SCHEPENS
  1970 Toxicological study of a fatal intoxication in man due to cannabis smoking. *Journal de Pharmacologie Belgique* 24:371–376.
HIVELY, R. L., W. A. MOSHER., F. W. HOFFMANN
  1966 Isolation of trans-Δ^6-tetrahydrocannabinol from marijuana. *Journal of the American Chemical Society* 88:1832–1833.

HOLLISTER, L. E.
   1971   Marihuana in man: three years later. *Science* 172 (3878):21–28.
HOOPER, D.
   1894   Extract of Indian hemp. *Yearbook of Pharmacy Comprising Abstracts* 484–489.
ISBELL, H., *et al.*
   1967   Effects of delta-9-tetrahydrocannabinol in man. *Psychopharmacologia* 11:184–188.
JOHNSON, D. W., J. W. GUNN
   1972   Dangerous drugs: adulterants diluents, and deception in street samples. *Journal of Forensic Sciences* 17:629–639.
JOYCE, C. R. B.
   1970   "Discussion," in *The botany and chemistry of cannabis*. Edited by C. R. B. Joyce and S. H. Curry. London: J. & A. Churchill.
JOYCE, C. R. B., S. H. CURRY, *editors*
   1970   *The botany and chemistry of cannabis*. London: J. & A. Churchill.
KARNIOL, I. G., E. A. CARLINI
   1972   The content of (—)Δ^9-*trans*-tetrahydrocannabinol (Δ^9-THC) does not explain all biological activity of some Brazilian marihuana samples. *Journal of Pharmacy and Pharmacology* 24:833–835.
KIPLINGER, G. F., J. E. MANNO
   1971   Dose-response relationships to cannabis in human subjects. *Pharmacological Reviews* 23:339–347.
KLEIN, F. K., H. RAPOPORT, H. W. ELLIOTT
   1971   Cannabis alkaloids. *Nature* 232:258–259.
KUBENA, R. K., H. BARRY, III
   1969   Two procedures for training differential responses in alcohol and non-drug conditions. *Journal of Pharmaceutical Sciences* 58:99–101.
   1972   Stimulus characteristics of marihuana constituents. *Nature* 235:397–398.
KUBENA, R. K., *et al.*
   1972   Biological and chemical evaluation of a 43-year-old sample of *Cannabis* fluidextract. *Journal of Pharmaceutical Sciences* 61:144–145.
MANNO, J. E., *et al.*
   1970   Comparative effects of smoking marihuana or placebo on human motor and mental performance. *Clinical Pharmacology and Therapeutics* 11:808–815.
MECHOULAM, R.
   1970a Marihuana chemistry. *Science* 168 (936):1159–1166.
   1970b "Discussion," in *The botany and chemistry of cannabis*. Edited by C. R. B. Joyce and S. H. Curry. London: J. & A. Churchill.
MECOULAM, R., Y. GAONI
   1967   Recent advances in the chemistry of hashish. *Fortschritte der Chemie Organischer Naturstoffe* 25:175-213
MECHOULAM, R., *et al.*
   1970a Chemical basis of hashish activity. *Science* 169 (3945):611–612.
MECHOULAM, R., *et al.*
   1970b "Some aspects of cannabinoid chemistry." In *The botany and chemistry*

of cannabis. Edited by C. R. B. Joyce and S. H. Curry. London: J. & A. Churchill.

MILLS, L. A., P. BRAWLEY
1972 The psychopharmacology of "Cannabis sativa": a review. *Agents Actions* 2:201–215.

NAHAS, G. G.
1973 *Marihuana-deceptive weed.* New York. Raven Press.

NEUMEYER, J. L., R. A. SHAGOURY
1971 Chemistry and pharmacology of marijuana. *Journal of Pharmaceutical Sciences* 60:1433–1457.

O'SHAUGHNESSY, W. B.
1843 On the preparations of the Indian hemp, or gunjah (Cannabis indica); their effects on the animal system in health, and their utility in the treatment of tetanus and other convulsive diseases. *Provincial Medical Journal Retrospect of the Medical Sciences* 5:343–347.

PERSAUD, T. V. N., A. C. ELLINGTON
1967 Cannabis in early pregnancy. *Lancet* II:1306.
1968 Teratogenic activity of Cannabis resin. *Lancet* II:406–407.

Pharmacopoeia of the United States of America
1926 10th Decennial rev. Philadelphia: J. B. Lippincott.

PODDAR, M. K., J. J. GHOSH
1972 Effects of cannabis extract, Δ^9-tetrahydrocannabinol and lysergic acid diethylamide on rat liver enzymes. *Biochemical Pharmacology* 21:3301–3303.

QUIMBY, M. W., et al.
1973 Mississippi-grown marihuana — *Cannabis sativa.* Cultivation and observed morphological variations. *Economic Botany* 27:117–127.

SCHULTES, R. E.
1970a "Random thoughts and queries on the botany of Cannabis," in *The botany and chemistry of cannabis.* Edited by C. R. B. Joyce and S. H. Curry. London: J. &. A Churchill.
1970b The plant kingdom and hallucinogens (part III). *Bulletin on Narcotics* 22:25–53.

SCIGLIANO, J. A., C. W. WALLER
1970 "The marihuana programme of the centre for studies of narcotic drug abuse, N. I. M. H.," in *The botany and chemistry of marihuana.* Edited by C. R. B. Joyce and S. H. Curry. London: J. & A. Churchill.

SEGELMAN, A. B., R. D. SOFIA
1973 *Cannabis sativa* L. (Marijuana). IV. Chemical basis for increased potency related to a novel method of use. *Journal of Pharmaceutical Sciences*, in press.

SINGER, A. J., *editor*
1971 Marijuana: chemistry, pharmacology, and patterns of social use. *Annals of the New York Academy of Sciences* 191:1–269.

SMALL, E., H. D. BECKSTEAD
1973 Common cannabinoid phenotypes in 350 stocks of *Cannabis. Lloydia* 36:144–165.

SOFIA, R. D., H. BARRY, III
1972 The influence of SKF-525A on the analgesic actions of Δ^1-tetrahydrocannabinol. *Federation Proceedings* 31:506.
TREASE, G. E., W. C. EVANS
1966 *A textbook of pharmacognosy*, 9th ed. London: Tindall & Cassell.
TRUITT, E. B., JR.
1971 Biological dispositions of tetrahydrocannabinols. *Pharmacological Review* 23:273-278.
U.S. DEPARTMENT OF HEALTH, EDUCATION AND WELFARE. NATIONAL INSTITUTE OF MENTAL HEALTH.
1971 *Marihuana and health: a report to the congress from the secretary.* Washington: U.S. Government Printing Office.
1972 *Marihuana and health: second annual report to congress from the secretary.* Washington: U.S. Government Printing Office.
WALLIS, T. E.
1967 *Textbook of pharmacognosy*, 5th ed. London: J. & A. Churchill.
WILLE, L., E. WARREN
1973 Marijuana abuse: teen death may arm researchers with facts. *The Star-Ledger*, Newark, New Jersey, Wednesday, January 10.
WOLSTENHOLME, E. W., J. KNIGHT, *editors*
1965 *Hashish: its chemistry and pharmacology.* Boston: Little, Brown & Company.
WOOD, H. C., JR., *et al.*, *editors*
1926 *The dispensatory of the United States of America*, 21st ed. Philadelphia: J. B. Lippincott.

Social and Medical Aspects of the Use of Cannabis in Brazil

ALVARO RUBIM DE PINHO

ABSTRACT

Cannabis seeds were brought to Brazil by African slaves, mainly from Angola by the first half of the fifteenth century. Cultivation was concentrated in the northeast areas of sugar cane plantations and cannabis was used for curing, religious rites, divination and mystic hallucinations. Marihuana use has spread among fishermen and longshoremen in the coastal cities and became known as the "opium of the poor." A study of prisoners revealed a high incidence of marihuana use.

Various studies include the findings that acute effects of smoking are conditioned by the plant material and the nutritional status and personality of the user, among other factors. The influence of regular smoking (one to three per night) was not evident in the work or ethical conduct of professional drivers. Clinical examinations of fifteen heavy smokers did not reveal any pathology.

In a study of 728 patients at the psychiatric hospital in Bahia, it was found that the role of marihuana was not a significant factor. Both constitutional and pharmacological factors should be considered. Acute schizophrenic psychoses occurred in some young people who were involved in youth movements and were known to have used marihuana. Complete and rapid remission of the psychoses occurred. It becomes difficult to delimit the etiological role of cannabis, in view of multiple pharmacodependencies among certain users and the diametrically opposed views of the mental consequences of chronic cannabis use taken by psychiatrists who diagnose acute reactions accordingly.

It is not certain if cannabis already existed in Brazil when the first Portuguese discoverers arrived. It is certain, however, that by the first half of the fifteenth century, cannabis seeds were brought by African slaves. A charter of Don João III, King of Portugal, dated in 1549, authorized the owner of each sugar plantation to buy up to 1200 African slaves. The planting of sugar cane was localized, in the northeast, the same region in which, through the centuries, the largest plantation of cannabis and a great number of smokers in the rural areas were concentrated.

The majority of the slaves imported at this time came from Angola and nearly all the traditional synonyms for marihuana in Brazil (*maconha, diamba, liamba, moconha*) had their origin in the Angolan language. Another name, seldom used now, is very significant as to origin: *fumo d'Angola* [smoke of Angola].

Describing the habits of the population in the sugar plantations in the northeast during the colonial period, Freyre (1937) noted that the owners allowed the slaves to plant cannabis amidst the sugar cane. And, while the whites smoked cigars and tobacco, the Negroes smoked marihuana, and in it found dreams and stupefication. Freyre affirms that during the periodic intervals of activity on the plantations, such a pastime avoided the risks of slave laziness, thus contributing to the stability of the workers.

The opposite occurred on the coffee plantations in the southeast, where the slave work load was heavier and the discipline more intense. In this area, it appears that the use of cannabis was uncommon and, moreover, was not tolerated. A popular saying remains in the region: *Maconha em pito faz negro sem vergonha* [Marihuana cigarettes make a shameless negro].

Either because cannabis already existed in Brazil or it was immediately introduced on contact, there are indications that smoking marihuana was observed among the Indians even during the Colonial period. And in the north, including the Amazon, whose rural population developed with less participation of Negroes, marihuana smokers are also found in certain communities.

There are records of the utilization of cannabis in popular religious rites in the interior zone of the northeast. The predominant sect there is the *Catimbó*, of Indian origin, with private and public ceremonies, in which spirits are received and sick people cured. Religious syncretism in *Catimbó* includes the cult of African deities and the use of plants presumed to be of value for medical treatment and magical practices. Among them, marihuana is judged capable of inducing divination, revelation of secrets and mystic hallucinations. Such influences came directly from the Angolan groups, who formed the *candomblé de caboclo*, on the northeast coast, *macumba* in Rio de Janeiro and *umbandismo* in the southern region. In these cults, alcohol use is frequent and marihuana does not fail to appear. This does not occur in the *candomblé nagô*, in Bahia. In this sect, derived from the Sudanese Negroes, there is less receptivity to syncretism: alcohol and marihuana do not appear in the rituals and are, in general, considered undesirable and condemned as vices.

Proclamations from the 19th century on impeded the use of marihuana in urban centers, including Rio de Janeiro, capital of the Empire, where imprisonment was the penalty for offenders. The prohibitions of the nation's capital, however, did not reach the planters and smokers of the provinces and were not accompanied by police vigilance.

The most extensive plantations were always maintained in the northeast, particularly in the state of Alagoas, for sale in the capital cities of the region and, also, in those of the south. Some smokers in the rural zone had small plots of cultivation next to their own houses, exclusively for personal use, a fact that is still not uncommon.

According to the observations of Doria in 1915 (1958) some preconceptions and superstitions were tied to the cultivation of the plant. When it began to branch, the terminal bud was cut to foster the development of the plant. This process was called *capacão*, a popular synonym for castration. It was not to be done by women, especially during menstruation, under the sanction of acquiring masculine qualities. While cutting the bud, whistling and speaking obscenities were to be avoided (habitual practices among agricultural workers in the region). Harvesting should be restricted from feminine influences.

Preparations of cannabis in teas and brews were always exceptional in Brazil. It is reported that they were indicated, in the rural milieu, for therapeutic purposes: for toothache and menstrual colic. It is possible that, in such cases, there is some anodyne effect.

Smoking in clay pipes, known as *maricas*, seems to have been the preference of the slaves. This has continued in some places, of evident Angolan influence, especially among the inhabitants along the banks of the São Francisco River.

Descriptions of the past century and the beginning of this one, emphasize the northeastern custom of group meetings for the *queima da herva* [burning of the grass]. On Saturday nights and on holidays, the smokers got together, generally in the house of the oldest member, and seated around a table, passed the *maricas* from one to another. Similarly, *jangadeiros* [raft fishermen] and canoemen in the same boat at sea or on the São Francisco River, adopted an identical system of "assemblies." It is doubtful that these traditional meetings for collective smoking still occur in such populations; at least, it can be affirmed that they are no longer frequent.

Smoking in the form of cigarettes became, in this century, the dominant form of marihuana use among peasants and probably the only form seen in the urban populations.

In the period from 1915 to 1930, several doctors from the northeast related their observations on the use of marihuana, which was no longer restricted to the rural areas. While it was a traditional habit in the country encompassing population groups from certain localities, the use of cannabis took another form in the coastal cities. Still another name was added to the extensive terminology – "opium of the poor" – faithfully expressing the economic level of the smokers. The greatest frequency of use was among fishermen, longshoremen, and agricultural workers, but the use was also spread among prostitutes and vagabonds. The presence of the vice reached a significant level in the penitentiaries and in some military barracks.

For the same period and subsequent years, there are newspaper articles revealing the clandestine trade that was established, transporting marihuana from the northeast by sea to the large capitals of the south. Rio de Janeiro became the largest importer, but cargoes for distribution in São Paulo were also unloaded in the port of Santos. The correlation between cannabis and social marginality was established in all these cities. To the newspaper articles were added pronouncements by doctors, warning against the criminal effects of marihuana. During the war, information from the health and police authorities (Farias 1958) expressed a concern about the migration of dealers to Bahia, where North American sailors were seen as buyers capable of paying high prices. It was referred to as a secret fact that some foreigners of an elevated economic level in Brazil were also consumers of marihuana, in sharp contrast to the sociocultural level of the great majority of the users.

In the decade of the 1950's, it was noted that some eccentric writers and artists were secretly habitual smokers of marihuana. In 1957 and 1958 (Pires da Veiga and de Pinho 1962), we examined the subjective symptoms of acute intoxication. Although we had the declared support of the police authorities for the research, and we assured the subjects of confidentiality, it was not possible for us, in Bahia, to obtain the collaboration of any of the intellectuals who were supposed users. This was probably a consequence of their respect for social pressures. The investigation was made partly in the prisons and partly in our private clinic, interviewing only known criminals or marihuana users without criminal records but who were adopting irregular family and professional lifestyles very like the *marginais* (people who are in a marginal state with regard to the rest of the society).

In a prison of 321 convicts (de Pinho 1962) all, without exception, had already tried marihuana, although there were only 36 habitual smokers. The correlation of cannabis users and criminals who had committed crimes against property was two times higher than that of criminals who had committed crimes against persons. Such findings were discovered when we sought to correlate alcoholism with the type of criminal offense. This fact confirmed findings among non-prosecuted offenders: the incidence of marihuana use was high among the thieves of the city. Nearly always, there were corresponding childhood antecedents of family disorganization and moral abandonment besides poverty and dependence on other intoxicants.

Comparison of the age of first use of marihuana between smokers never prosecuted and those in prison is interesting. Among those in prison, the habit began much later, while among the former it began, generally, during childhood or adolescence. Re-evaluation of the material permitted us to conclude that for those who had been prosecuted, the prison frequently functioned as an environment conducive to the habit.

A study (Pires da Veiga and de Pinho 1962) of 50 marihuana users at this time revealed that the effects of intoxication were conditioned by multiple factors: the authenticity of the cannabis (much is adulterated by the dealers) and its varieties; the age of the plant; the method of smoking; the rhythm of consuming cigarettes; the personality and nutritional condition of the user. Also, tranquility, comfort and liberty appeared as very important factors, proportionate to the noisier euphoric stimulations. There were individual preferences with regard to the surroundings however, in general, the beaches appear to be the locales. Collective smoking in small groups was the preferred setting for nearly everyone.

In 1969 and 1970, the habit was appreciably diffused, at least in the regions of greatest demographic density. The commercial trade of marihuana had multiplied in the large cities and along the highways. In Bahia, we observed its increased incidence in a well-defined group: that of professional drivers. They were almost all men of the lower middle class with stable families, consuming one to three cigarettes a night. They smoked alone, at home, without the tumult of intoxication. The influence of this habit was not evident in their work or ethical conduct.

During this period an increase in very diverse social aspects occurred with regard to the use of cannabis in Brazil. In the larger population centers, there was a great diffusion of fortuitous or habitual use among middle- and upper-class adolescents. This started merely with recognizably maladjusted youth, assimilated more or less transitionally to the hippie communties. Later, it appeared in clubs, bars, public festivals and even in dances at private residences. In spite of legal prohibitions, the trade is easily carried on. Vendors of cigarettes, tobacco and ice-cream, cashiers at restaurants and bars and employees of the schools are frequently middlemen for the sale of marihuana. Low-class brothels, patronized by *marginais*, continue to permit the storage and sale of marihuana. But, in the larger cities, the plazas and the beaches of the residential neighborhoods — the most elegant and those of the middle class — also have their special places for this trade. The majority of buyers are young, at the pre-university level. In the universities, appreciable differences are noted according to the course of study. Diverse observers concur that the students of the arts, communications, and human sciences seem to adopt the habit more than the candidates in medicine, engineering and other technical professions. Nearly always, the attitude of older people is that of rejection of the use of marihuana, and at times even terror of its use. But young people, even those who do not adhere to the habit, take a relatively permissive position with regard to its use.

In one of the studies carried out in the decade of the 1950's (de Pinho 1962), on the basis of material from the *marginais* and prisoners, our attention was drawn to the frequency with which dependency on other intoxicants was recorded in the histories of chronic marihuana users. And the fact gained significance on comparison with the backgrounds of alcoholics who in general are dependent only on alcohol. What is observed at present among young Brazilians who become habitual cannabis users is that once the continual use of marihuana is established, there follow in progression experiences with other intoxicants, established simultaneously or successively and other dependencies, especially that of amphetamines. According to the police authorities, the chronic user of only marihuana is rare or, if they exist in great numbers, they do not become known or arrested. The offenders in prison, including the adolescents, are, nearly always, multidependents.

With regard to the comparison with alcoholism, it is worthwhile to record two interrelated facts. Contrary to tradition, the present adolescents of the upper and middle classes reveal an appreciable disinterest in alcoholic beverages. On the other hand, parents do not show the anxiety formerly observed with regard to the possibility of alcoholism among their children. This contrasts with their accentuated fear in relation to marihuana and other intoxicants.

It is important to appreciate the problem as it refers to medical aspects. Clinical and laboratory examinations in 1969 (de Pinho 1969) of 15 heavy smokers did not reveal any bodily disturbance related to chronic intoxications. There was even some coincidence, in several of our observations, with an excellent state of nutrition, perhaps comprehensible, if one takes into account the appetite that acute intoxication customarily provokes.

Brazilian psychiatrists are divided with regard to the means of evaluating the mental consequences of chronic use of cannabis, reaching radically opposed positions: those that underestimate and those that exaggerate the possibility of the occurrence of mental consequences. Such a debate is not relevant to the frequent theme of ethical decadence, which ought not to be attributed to the pharmacological action of the intoxicant, but to a set of social and economic conditions habitually associated with the situation. The divergence grows, however, in importance in the relationship between the chronic use of marihuana and psychoses.

This difference of attitudes cancels out an appreciation of the statistical data, since the acute psychopathological pictures occurring in chronic marihuana users are diagnosed by some as toxic psychoses and by others as schizophrenias. And the etiopathogenic role of cannabis becomes even more difficult to delimit in view of the constant coincidence with other pharmacodependencies.

In 1957 (de Pinho 1962), we made an inquiry at the public psychiatric hospital of Bahia, obtaining responses from 728 patients that we deem reliable. Among this group, there were 327 schizophrenics and 44 patients diagnosed as psychopathic personalities. Of the total, there were eight individuals with backgrounds of marihuana use. Among these eight, only four had been admitted in psychosis: one with the Korsakoff syndrome, one with general paralysis and two with well defined schizophrenia. Therefore, we considered, that the role of marihuana in these cases was not significant.

Keeping in mind the dissemination of marihuana in recent years, especially among young people, it is understandable that, at the present time, a much larger number of the patients hospitalized reveal a background of marihuana use. It is, however, worth noting that the psychoses observed in marihuana users without a history of other dependencies have, in common, a schizophreniform physiognomy, never presented in our casuistry, and other traditionally known syndromes of exogenous reaction.

Our personal observation conforms fully to the taxonomy proposed by Lucena (1961) on relating the psychoses of cannabis users at least as they are presented in our milieu: a) precipitation of a previously unapparent schizophrenic process; b) intensification of the symptomatology already characterized before, especially, proportionate to the exacerbation of delirious production; c) rise of symptomatic schizophrenic complexes, with benign evolution.

In each of these possibilities, it is evident that there should be supposed the participation of an endogenous factor (the constitution) and an exogenous factor (the intoxicant). In all the cases, it is necessary to recognize the essentiality of predisposition, but there is no reason to deny the additional performance of cannabis.

Analyzing the etiopathogenic complex in a wider multidimensional perspective, we think, however, that psychogenic factors can be included, whether they contribute toward the precipitation of psychosis, or whether they provide the content for psychopathological production. It is important to bear in mind, also, the change of life plans and the loss of social roles.

Between 1968 and 1971, political modifications were reflected in youth movements, interrupting certain social programs, avoiding collective manifestations and impeding the exercise of some leadership roles. Our casuistry at the time included acute schizophrenic psychoses occurring in some of these young people who were known to have used marihuana more or less continuously. Complete and rapid remission of the psychoses was demonstrated. Such cases behaved thus like "psychogenic reactions in an altered sphere," in the sense of Kurt Schneider. A predisposed constitution and the intoxication to precipitate the traumatic events repeat themselves, meanwhile, in all the characteristics of the symptomatic model of schizophreniform.

In 1971, an Antitoxicant Law was passed in Brazil which prohibits the private planting, cultivation, harvesting and exploitation of all varieties of toxic plants. In spite of the formal enforcement of this law and the strongly repressive measures that it prescribes, it does not appear to have caused until now any appreciable change in the system of marihuana trade, in its diffusion or in its medical repercussions. Police activity seems more oriented toward the dealers and users of lower social levels who, in general, present asocial behavior and reactions of various types. Families of the middle- and upper-classes are anxious about conflicts between children and parents, and marihuana is frequently the theme of these conflicts. Among parents, there is a tendency to attribute to cannabis the slowness of young people in assuming their identities and responsibilities. The younger generation, while it includes many individuals with deviant behavior, including dependence on drugs, has a much greater proportion of those who harmoniously overcome the problems of age and launch themselves in the adequate fulfillment of their social roles. Many among these have had an occasional marihuana experience, they do not seem to have any biases against it, but are pessimistic with regard to the productivity of those who use it continually.

In Brazil, there are those who think that the juvenile vogue of smoking marihuana is beginning to decline. There are those who judge that there is less talk of the subject in certain areas, because acceptance by the communities is consolidating. It is too early to confirm or deny either of these two possibilities, as well as the consequences that will result from one or the other.

SUMMARY

In Brazil, where the use of cannabis has existed since the Colonial period, it was first a habit of the slaves. Its use was later consolidated in certain population groups in the rural zones. In this century, it spread to the small cities of the coast and, later, to the metropolises. In the urban areas it has lasted for decades, particularly among the criminals and *marginais* which led, always, to the image of asociability and danger attributed to the users.

In recent times, occasional or habitual use appeared extremely common among middle- and upper-class youth in the urban nuclei. The young people who established the habit followed it by other intoxicants, especially amphetamines.

Upper-class adults transferred to marihuana the fears they formerly had about alcohol, while the young people, even the non-users of marihuana, appear to have a permissive attitude with regard to cannabis.

In recent years our attention has turned to the relationship between chronic use of marihuana and psychosis. It is beyond doubt that marihuana exacerbates the delirious production of the schizophrenics. But we have also observed benign schizophrenic syndromes in cannabis users. The analysis of such cases in a multidimensional perspective suggests the interrelationship of the constitutional and the toxic factors, but also of psychogenic factors, including the relationships with social situations.

REFERENCES

DE PINHO, ALVARO RUBIM
    1962   Problemas sociopsicológicas do maconhismo. *Neurobiologia* 25:9–19.
    1969   *Communicão ao IX Congresso da Sociedade de Neurologia, Psiquiatria e Higiene Mental do Brasil*. Rio de Janeiro.

DORIA, RODRIGUES
    1958   "Os fumadores de maconha: efeitos e males do vício. (Memoria presented to the II Pan American Scientific Congress, Washington D.C. December 27, 1915)," in *Maconha*, 1-14. Rio de Janeiro: Ministério da Saúde.

FARIAS, ROBERVAL C.
1958 "Relatorio apresentade aos Srs. Membros da Comissão Nacional de Fiscalizacão de Entorpecentes. Inspecão realizada de 7 a 19 de Novembro de 1943 nos Estados do Bahia, Sergipe e Alagoas, visando o problema do comérico e uso da maconha," in *Maconha*, 105–113. Rio de Janeiro: Ministério da Saúde.

FREYRE, GILBERTO
1937 *Nordeste*. Rio de Janeiro: Jose Olímpio Editôra.

LUCENA, JOSÉ
1961 "La symptomatologia du cannabisme," in *The Third World Congress of Psychiatry*. Vol. I. 401–406. Toronto: University of Toronto Press.

PIRES DA VEIGA, E., ALVARO RUBIM DE PINHO
1962 Contribuicão ao estudo do maconhismo na Bahia. *Neurobiologia* 25: 38–68.

Sociocultural and Epidemiological Aspects of Hashish Use in Greece

C. STEFANIS, C. BALLAS, and D. MADIANOU

ABSTRACT

The first section of this paper traces the history of cannabis as it relates to ancient Greece, Byzantium, the Greek-speaking populations under Ottoman domination, and modern Greece. While it is clear that ancient Greeks were aware of the use of the plant by neighboring peoples, there is no evidence to indicate that they utilized it in any way or that hashish was incorporated into the Greek cultural inventory before the mid-nineteenth century. Socioeconomic conditions and geographical centrality are posited as key factors which led to the introduction of hashish to modern Greece, first in the island of Syros and then to other port cities. A second section deals with demographic and epidemiological data on current hashish use and compares the total hashish using population to the general Greek population and to a sample of subjects in a clinical study in Athens on chronic effects of hashish use.

This paper has two objectives: first, to present the principal historical and cultural reasons why Greeks did not incorporate hashish smoking into their cultural inventory until the middle of the nineteenth century and the reasons which led to its adoption by one section of the Greek population, a section best considered as a cultural subgroup; and second, to present the results of a study of the sociocultural and epidemiological characteristics of this subgroup, utilizing data from the archives of the Greek narcotics control authorities. The goal of this latter study was to determine the representativeness of the total hashish smoking population of Greece in terms of the general Greek population and to what extent the experimental sample from our earlier clinical studies[1] is representative of the total Greek hashish using population.

[1] From 1971 to 1974, the Psychiatric Clinic of the University of Athens was engaged in an extensive and systematic investigation of the physical, psychiatric and psychological effects of chronic cannabis use. This work was supported by the National Institute of Mental Health (United States) by means of a subcontract with the Interna-

For Plates, see pp. xiv–xvi, between pp. 266–267.

HISTORICAL BACKGROUND

Cannabis in Europe

Presently available facts convince us that cannabis was not long in moving from the highlands of Central Asia to the European mainland. Reiniger (1967) describes the presence of cannabis seeds and hulls among remnants of herbs in a pot found in a tomb of the third century B.C. discovered near Wilmersdorf, Germany. These are the only known facts from antiquity. Other published sources supporting the archaeological findings do not exist. It is well known that no reference to cannabis is made either in the Egyptian papyri or in the New Testament.

The first reference revealing the use of cannabis in Europe appears in Herodotus (*Book IV*) about 450 B.C. The Greek historian mentions that the Scyths not only cultivated cannabis several centuries before Christ but used it also as an euphoriant, "they threw cannabis seeds on red-hot stones and become drunk by inhaling the smoke." It seems certain that the Scyths, as mentioned by Papadopoulos (1959), were using not only the seeds, which are devoid of euphoriant properties, but also the tufts of the female plant. Herodotus further mentions that cannabis grew wild in Thrace but was also cultivated for its fiber which was used for weaving.

The widespread use of cannabis in Western Europe, at least for commercial purposes, during the pre-Roman period is well documented by the following characteristic references: Athenaeus (A.D. 170–230) mentioned that the tyrant of Syracuse, Hieron II, who lived between 270–215 B.C., obtained cannabis from the valley of the Rhône in order to manufacture rope for his navy. Pliny the Elder (A.D. 23–79) notes that the sails and canvas of the Roman galleys were made from cannabis fiber.

It has not yet been established how cannabis reached Europe from Asia. Did it first arrive through Russia to northern Europe or from the Middle East through the Mediterranean ports and the Aenos peninsula to

---

tional Association for Psychiatric Research. The mass of data obtained from an experimental subsample of hashish users and a control subsample are now being processed and only preliminary results have been reported thus far (*Report on chronic hashish use in Greece*, published by the National Institute n.d.). In order to better evaluate the data obtained in these clinical studies, a parallel investigation of the historical and cultural background of cannabis use in Greece was pursued. The results of this investigation are reported in this paper. These data, in turn, have stimulated an ongoing socioanthropological study of contemporary patterns of cannabis use in Greece.

southeastern Europe? Both routes are probable. The possibility should not be overlooked, however, that cannabis may have been cultivated in northern Europe at the same time as it was in Asia, a view supported by Hartwich (1911). Nevertheless, the derivation of the word cannabis favors the view that the Middle East area was the main avenue of cannabis traffic from Asia to Europe. It is probable that the word cannabis derives its origin from the Assyrian words *qunubu* and *qunabu* which signify "a way to produce smoke."

Cannabis and Ancient Greece

There is no evidence that cannabis was used by ancient Greeks for commercial, ritual, or euphoriant purposes. Herodotus, a profound observer of their mores and customs, mentions as noteworthy that "some other people" [the Scyths] were using cannabis. There is no reference indicating that *nectar*, the "sweet drink" of the Olympian gods, contained cannabis as did *soma*, the favorite drink of the God Indra, which was offered to mortals so they might find happiness. Furthermore, there is no evidence to indicate that cannabis was used at the Aesculapian shrines or at the Oracles. The plants principally used at these sites to modify consciousness were the *solanoids*, i.e. *hyoscyanus albus, datura stramonium,* and *mandragora*. It has been maintained that the prophetic delirium of Pythia was due to the inhalation of cannabis, but no evidence exists to corroborate this hypothesis (Ballas 1968).

The principal sources on ancient Greece which would be likely to refer to cannabis, should it have been used in ancient Greece at all, make no mention of the substance. It is significant that Theophrastus (372–287 B.C.) the famous master of the Peripatetic School, who described in great detail the plants known at the time on Grecian soil, makes no mention of cannabis. The restriction of cannabis to neighboring populations of Greece and the lack of its dissemination to the Greeks even during the first post-Christian period, is documented by a reference made by Plutarch (A.D. 46–127). In his work *On rivers' and mountains' names* (1615) he mentions, some four hundred years after Herodotus, that the people of Thrace used a herb similar to oregano, the tops of which they threw into the fire after meals and, inhaling their smoke, became drunk and fell into deep sleep. Cannabis is described in detail by Dioscorides (A.D. 59–79), a Greek doctor of the Roman army, whose *Materia medica* remained standard for centuries. Dioscorides wrote that cannabis has two varieties, "wild" and "domestic." The domestic variety produced a tall plant; the stems were used for making strong rope and the seeds were used pharmaceutically. He recommended the seeds for curbing sexual desire and the fluid extract for earaches. According to Papadopoulos (1959), the plant that Dioscorides described as "wild" was not cannabis at all since Dioscorides mentioned that it had red flowers.

Galen (A.D. 131–201), the famous Greek doctor of Pergamum, whose medical discoveries remained unchallenged until the sixteenth century, emphasized the euphoriant qualities of cannabis. He also observed that abuse or overdose of cannabis causes sterility (Galen 1821–1833:XII) and that "The seeds produce stomach trouble, headache and a disturbance of the body 'humours'. However, some people use them with other 'tragimata', beverages that are taken after dinner to produce pleasure" (Galen 1821–1833:V).

Cannabis is also mentioned by Pausanias, the geographer and traveller who lived in the second century A.D. His *Description of Greece* (1966) remains an invaluable source of information on the topography and legends of ancient Greece. The reference he makes to cannabis, however, does not provide evidence for or against its use by the Greeks during the Roman period. Reiniger (1962) misquotes him when he claims that Pausanias mentions that cannabis was cultivated in Elis in northwestern Peloponnesus. The pertinent reference in Pausanias runs as follows: "The land of Elis is fruitful, being especially suited to the growth of fine flax. Now while hemp and flax, both the ordinary and the fine variety, are sown by those whose soil is suited to grow it, the threads from which the Seres make the dresses are not produced from bark, but in a different way...." (Pausanias 1966).

The Byzantine Empire

The Byzantine Empire constituted a state combining Hellenic culture, Greek language, Christian religious beliefs, and Roman political traditions. Within its boundaries it encompassed several ethnic groups: Greeks, Latins, Syrians, Armenians, peoples of Mesopotamia, and even North Africans. It has been categorized primarily as an Orthodox-Christian state and only secondly as a Greek state.

The Greek inhabitants of the Byzantine Empire had come into contact with Moslem Arabs many centuries before the conquest of Byzantium by the Turks. Since the seventh century A.D., the Arabs had captured many provinces from Byzantium, including Alexandria and Jerusalem. Crete and Cyprus were only recaptured by the Byzantines after lengthy wars. The close geographical and social contact of Arabs and Byzantines enabled the former to become acquainted with the Greek language and to familiarize themselves with Greek culture. The influence of this relationship was such that the Arabs gradually adopted Greek as an international language of communication with other nations.

The Moslem Turks, who replaced the Arabs in occupying the outer rim of Byzantine provinces and who by A.D. 1250 had expanded their domination to a much larger part of the Byzantine Empire, continued this tradition and also adopted Greek as their diplomatic *lingua franca*. It is not surprising, therefore, that Mohammed II, the conqueror of Constantinople, spoke Greek to perfection. The cultural influence of Hellenism in the Moslem world before the total conquest of Byzantium was matched to some degree by Moslem influence on Byzantine cultural patterns. There is no evidence, however, to indicate that Byzantine Greeks, conquered first by Arabs and then by Turks, acquired the use of narcotics, either opium or hashish.

From the above, we can conclude that cannabis was not used by the Greeks during the classical era or the Roman period. For these times, it was described by historians and chroniclers as a somewhat exotic plant used by non-Greek nations, i.e. Thracians and Scyths. We can also extend this conclusion for the Greeks of the Byzantine period. Not because of any source material to verify it but because of the lack of written evidence to the contrary. It appears certain that cannabis, in contrast to alcohol, was never introduced into the cultural life of Byzantium. It is clear that it was neither used for ritual nor medicinal purposes and its possible use as an euphoriant does not appear consistent with the austere Christian atmosphere of the Byzantine period.

Period of the Ottoman Occupation

The fall of Constantinople in 1453 was followed by the official dissolution of Byzantium. Within two centuries the occupation of the entire Greek polity, with the exception of the Ionian Islands, was completed. A large number of the Greeks escaped to western countries; many were lost during the persecutions and slaughters that followed each new conquest, especially the conquest of the capital city of Constantinople. The largest part of the Greek population, however, survived and remained under Ottoman rule.

The cultural survival of this population was due largely to the policies inaugurated by Mohammed the Conqueror after the fall of Constantinople. Almost immediately following the conquest, he granted substantial religious and administrative privileges to the Christians, recognized the Patriarchate and allowed the organization of autonomous community life. These policies, which had incalculable consequences for the survival of Hellenism, were demonstrably dictated by the need to secure financial support from Christian subjects, primarily for the maintenance of the army since at that time the fledgling empire relied entirely on the strength of the Ottoman armed forces. Mohammed could have easily destroyed or "islamized" the occupied Christian-Greek population, but this was an option never seriously considered (Paparigopoulos 1932).

The political consideration that privileges to Christian subjects would widen the gap between the Eastern and Western Church contributed heavily to the issuance of these benevolent policies. Tolerance toward Christian subjects, which persisted throughout the four centuries of Ottoman occupation, allowed the subjugated Hellenes to organize themselves into separate legal communities of an autonomous nature, to enjoy a certain degree of freedom of movement and to worship more or less freely. As a consequence, they were able to preserve their customs, their religious and educational institutions and even their national and cultural identity. There were Greeks, the "Phanariotes," who were in such favor that they were able to occupy the highest posts in the Ottoman civil service. For about two centuries before the War of Independence of 1821, these individuals almost continuously held three of the highest Ottoman positions: Great Interpreter of the Court (equivalent to Minister of Foreign Affairs), Dragoman of the Navy and the Ruler of the Lands along the Danube. On the other hand, hardships, persecutions, and attempts to islamize the population (e.g. janissaries, *paidomazoma*) were not absent during the Ottoman occupation. Revolutionary movements, attempts to overthrow Ottoman domination and to restore freedom and Greek national life, were also continuous. It is noteworthy that of the Greek favorites of the Court, Rulers of Danubian Lands, Great Interpreters, and the like, thirty-eight were beheaded or slain "because they did not want to serve their masters as much as the subjugated Greek Nation" (Koukou 1971).

All available, unbiased sources (Pentzopoulos 1962) indicate that the Christian population and particularly the Greeks did not assimilate into Moslem society and throughout the occupation they kept alive their religious and national consciousness. The fact that a thorough search of the literature covering the period of the Turkish occupation does not even reveal suggestive references to the use of hashish by the occupied Greeks, must be placed within the context of their communal and cultural autonomy. The basic euphoriant for the Greeks continued to be alcohol. Absolutely no reference to hashish exists in the Greek demotic songs which were disseminated throughout the Ottoman Empire and contain a wealth of information about Greek mores and folk customs. No historian or traveller of that period mentions the use of hashish by the Greek, or Christian population under the Turkish occupation (Simopoulos 1973).

What was the relation of the Turks to hashish? Hashish smoking was undoubtedly widespread among the Moslems of the Ottoman Empire. It appears, however, that its use was not as prevalent among Turks as among the Moslem inhabitants of Arabic origin. A painting in Nicolas de Nicolay's book, reproduced by Stringaris (1964), depicts a group of Turkish soldiers in the streets of Constantinople, around 1500, inebriated by hashish. A very typical epic poem, the "Benk u Bôde," by the Turkish poet Mohammed Ebn Soleiman Foruli from Bagdad (Gelpke 1966) written in the middle of the sixteenth century, deals in allegorical form, with the dialectical battle between wine and hashish. Under the guise of a fencing match between alcohol and hashish, this most interesting poem describes with surprising accuracy the euphoriant properties of these two substances as well as their consequences. Significantly, Foruli's poetry ranks the two substances on the basis of social criteria. (This was also emphasized by Brunel [1955].) Foruli considers wine the drink of the rich and the powerful (he likens it to a Sheikh, a guest of the Sultan), "while hashish," he says, "is the friend of the poor, the Dervishes and the men of knowledge, i.e., of all those who are not blessed with earthly goods and social power." This description gives us further illumination: that in spite of Quranic prohibition, the Turks, or at least those of the higher social classes, by the sixteenth century had already begun to adopt the habits of the conquered population and were indulging in alcohol.

The distribution of hashish, alcohol, and opium use among the population of occupied Constantinople was reported by Eulogio Efendi (Stringaris 1964), the Turkish historian of the seventeenth century. He relates that during his days in Constantinople there were more than 1000 beer shops, 104 wine distributors, and only 60 "tekés," i.e. hashish smoking places. The view that hashish was disseminated mainly by Dervish sects (a Dervish religious school even existed in Athens under Turkish rule and its building may still be seen in Monastiraki) and among the poor Turks is supported also by other sources. Kerim (1930) mentions that hashish was widely known in Syria, Asia Minor, Constantinople, and especially Prusa and in the area of Smyrna. In all these places, Greeks, although in separate communities, lived in symbiosis with the

Turks. However, no evidence exists indicating that Greeks adopted hashish use, which they considered antithetical to their own mores and customs.

Hashish in Greece after the Liberation

When the modern Greek nation was founded in 1830 after the 1821 War of Independence, only one geographical section of the area then inhabited by Greeks was included in the new state. In total area, it encompassed 47,516 square kilometers with a population of 753,000. In 1870, with the annexation of the Ionian Islands, the Greek land mass increased to 50,221 square kilometers and the population to 1,457,000. By 1920, with the annexation of Macedonia, Epirus (in 1912), and West Thrace, Greece had expanded to 127,000 square kilometers with a population of 5,016,889. By 1928, after the arrival in 1922 of the displaced Greeks from Turkish Asia Minor, the population had swelled to 6,204,684 and with the annexation of the Dodecanesus in 1947, its geographical expanse had been enlarged to its present size of 131,944 square kilometers. The present population of Greece, as of the census of 1971, amounts to 8,768,641. In 150 years there was a tenfold increase in population and a tripling of its physical size. Perhaps more significantly, Greeks living outside the boundaries of the state had been brought within the polity and, as a consequence, the total Greek population acquired greater homogeneity in language, religion, and national identity (Sandis 1973). The economic base of the nation, at least to the end of the last century, was predominantly agricultural. It is significant that in 1853 only three cities existed with a population of over 10,000: Hermoupolis, capital of the island of Syros; Athens; and Patras, the port of western Peloponnesus (Tsaousis 1971).

It appears that hashish was not traditionally used as a folk medicine in Greece. Dionysos Pyrros, a Thessalian who studied medicine in Italy and had a vast knowledge of folk remedies, does not mention hashish in his *Doctors' textbook* which was printed in 1832. However, "Cannabis semen — Cannabis sativa" is mentioned in the first official *Greek pharmacopoeia* issued in 1837 based on a Bavarian text. It reads as follows: "a yearly plant, indigenous in the East but also growing in Europe when planted." It can be argued that this indicates that the introduction of cannabis into Greek therapeutics was influenced by Western European medicine. "Cannabis semen — Cannabis sativa" is also mentioned by the first Professor of Pharmacology at the University of Athens, N.

Kostis, in his 1855 *Handbook of pharmacology:* "a plant, indigenous in the East and especially in Persia, but cultivated in many areas of Europe and Greece...." He classifies this plant in his section on "Pharmaca Mucilaginosa" but not in the narcotics category. Cannabis is first mentioned as a narcotic in 1875 by Th. Afendoulis in his *Pharmacology,* described as follows:

Herrba siva Summitates floribuendae Cannabis indicae, a plant, indigenous in India and cultivated there as well as in Egypt, recently also in Greece in the areas of Argolis and Navpaktos in the Peloponnesus. In medicine as well as in everyday life, flowering tops of the female plant are used by Indian, Egyptian and Arab peoples.

This author also refers to the use of cannabis derivatives by Easterners and Egyptians in the diet.

All pertinent sources refer to hashish as definitely appearing in Greece after 1850. Introduced from the East, its starting point was the island of Syros in the Cyclades (Kouretas 1937; Papadopoulos 1959; Stringaris 1964). An analysis of the demographic, social, and cultural status of this island, therefore, is of considerable interest.

Until 1790 the population of Syros was 4,000, the majority Catholic (as a result of the Venetian occupation) and Greek-speaking. As a result of the War of Independence in 1821 and the persecution of the inhabitants of other Aegean islands (Chios, Psara, Crete, Rhodes) by the Turks, a large number of displaced Greek Orthodox people flooded into Syros. These refugees were instrumental in establishing the town of Hermoupolis around the harbor while the older stratum of Catholic inhabitants remained in Ano Hora, the old village in the hills above the new town. The development of Hermoupolis was meteoric. Within a very short period of time it grew into the leading port of the nation, to such a degree that English businessmen of the day were identifying Syros as Greece. These developments came at a time when the bulk of the Greek bourgeoisie (important merchants and wealthy professionals) was living outside of Greece in such places as Constantinople, Austria, Rumania, or Russia.

An urban-commercial society, with the first beginnings of industry, was formed in Hermoupolis. By 1828, it was the largest city of Greece with a population of 14,167 drawn from various parts of the nation. The majority were from Chios and other islands of the Aegean, later followed by Greeks from Asia Minor; the new inhabitants concentrated on new commercial enterprises and related industry. Hermoupolis quickly gained fame as an important port of call, a necessary stopover between

East and West, between North Asia and the Black Sea. Until 1880 it maintained its national leadership in commerce and industry; the first Greek shipyards and factories were established in Hermoupolis. As a result, this city developed the first urban proletariat of Greece, the first labor syndicates, and experienced the first strikes and labor unrests. As social counterpoint to this laboring class, a strong bourgeois class emerged and flourished. In its social activities, lifestyle, and habits this latter group had close resemblance to the Western European bourgeoisie of the time.

The older Catholic stratum of Syros was initially contained in the area known as the Kastro, in the hills above the city. These Catholic Greeks retained a traditional style of life based on agriculture and were culturally alienated from the urban life of the port city. Nevertheless, from 1890 and on, given the growing demands of new enterprises, they began to be drawn into the urban labor pool. In spite of the antipathy between the Catholic inhabitants of Kastro and the rich Greek Orthodox newcomers of the port (numerous clashes have been recorded), the Catholics were eventually forced to seek wage work as longshoremen, shipyard hands, and in the tanning factories of Hermoupolis, coming to the port to work by day and returning to their village by night — the first Greek example of migration for úrban work without physical abandonment of the village. Although the needs of the port and of the flourishing factories and commerce lured workers from all of Greece, the first true proletariat was recruited from Kastro.

These workers, over time, developed a distinctive social form with a characteristic cultural style. Syros became the meeting place of Eastern, primarily Arabian, and Western European influences. In Hermoupolis, laborers were exposed to both as ships and crews from Europe, Egypt, and the Middle East made it a regular port of call. Among other elements of culture, Syros was introduced to Western European music, which was quickly adopted by the upper class, and to Arabic and Middle Eastern musical forms (Vamvakaris 1973). As important, however, the refugees from the Peloponnesus, mainland Greece, and from Pontos brought along with them the tradition of Greek demotic songs.

The blending of these elements created a variant type of folk culture, tangentially related to that of the middle class but clearly differentiated. Within this multi-cultural context a music form developed with overt oriental characteristics and influence; the basic instruments were the *bouzouki* and the *baglamas* which bear resemblance to the mandolin and guitar. This new music developed in Syros but was soon transplanted to Piraeus, the seaport of Athens, from there to be spread to working people in all the harbors of mainland Greece. After World War II, this music acquired significant dimensions and diffused rapidly throughout the Greek lower class. From 1950 on, it could be considered as the national music of the country. Popularly known as *rebetiko* music, it is socially akin to American blues and jazz (Vamvakaris 1973).

From 1870, due to economic developments in continental Greece, Piraeus began to compete commercially with Syros. By 1880 it had gained ascendancy, and with the opening of the Corinth Canal in 1893 the decline of Hermoupolis commenced. At this point the labor force gravitated away from Syros toward Athens and Piraeus. We would maintain that the roots of hashish use in Greece are to be found in the Syros type of sociocultural setting. During the cultural florescence of this island, similar social, economic, and cultural events took place in Smyrna, an important port city of Turkish Asia Minor that had a basically Greek population which dominated local trade and industry. In view of close similarities between the development of Smyrna and Syros, the use of hashish by the inhabitants of the former place cannot be dismissed. In fact, this view is strongly supported by the fact that there was a considerable number of known hashish users among the Asia Minor Greeks repatriated in 1922.

It is not coincidental that all sources place the appearance of the first cases of hashish smoking on the mainland around 1870–1880, that is, at the time that socioeconomic conditions, comparable to those experienced by Syros, were developing in Piraeus. Stringaris (1964) reports that hashish appeared on the Greek scene during this decade, Kouretas (1937) places its use by prisoners around 1885, Petropoulos (1971) mentions that it was introduced by the prisoners of Smyrna, Mysiri, and Prusa as the "weed of the poor," *hashish-el-foukara*. Indeed it was the poor of Piraeus and its surrounding neighborhoods that constituted the bulk of the hashish smoking population of the region.

It appears from a report of the mayor of Orchomenus in Peloponnesus, requested by the government, that the cultivation of hashish was introduced in Greece about 1875 by immigrants from Egypt, Cyprus, and other eastern areas and by the last decades of the nineteenth century it was being openly and systematically cultivated for local use and export. Excerpts of this official statement follow:

Ten years ago the cultivation of hashish was disseminated to Orchomenus from the surrounding boroughs of Mantinea. Cultivation tests in these boroughs were made previously by Egyptians, Cypriots and other immigrants from the East, who had come to Greece and taught the cultivation and processing of this product.... As soon as the cultivation of this product was started in the borough of Orchomenus, great agricultural activity was observed among the people .... Hashish by the leaf costs 50–80–90–100 lepta (100 lepta = one drachma) per oka (one oka = 2.82 lbs), the price depending upon quality and demand, while the price of the powder varies from 10 to 20 drachmas per oka. Abroad the price is triple or quadruple (*On hashish: a report by the Mayor of Orchomenus in Montinea* 1887).

Papadopoulos (1959) estimates that before 1915 about 26,000 acres in Greece were put to hashish cultivation.

From the onset, and up until the 1960s, hashish use in Greece was limited to the working class, widely used by longshoremen, boatmen, sailors, porters, skinners and slaughterers, as well as by cart drivers (Stringaris 1964) and later by truckdrivers, who still utilize the substance. Examples of hashish smoking and implements are shown in Plates 1–5. Significantly, the spread of hashish use is correlated with the development and dissemination of *rebetiko* music (Petropoulos 1971). The use of hashish constituted an essential element in the behavior and personality of *rebetiko* musicians and singers and the evidence indicates that the development of this musical genre and the proliferation of its practitioners is intimately linked to the dynamics of the hashish cult in Greece (Stringaris 1964).

Stringaris also reports that the first admissions to the newly established mental hospital "Dromokaiteion," of hashish users, diagnosed as mentally disturbed, were in 1885. Our own investigation of the hospital's files casts doubt on this assertion: the first admissions of mentally disturbed hashish users appear to have been in 1912, while admissions of morphine and cocaine addicts are recorded as starting in 1901. Up to 1937 the prevailing term for institutionalization due to hashish use was "hashish mania"; after that date the term is replaced by "hashish psychosis." Even up to 1941 there were some admissions utilizing this terminology. From 1943 to 1947, hashish users admitted to the Dromokaiteion mental hospital were diagnosed as having "mixed or other toxicomanias."

On March 27, 1890, following a decision of the Medical Council, the Department of Interior issued a circular prohibiting the importation, cultivation, and use of hashish as an imminent threat to society (*Excerpt of the 1890 report of the Health Council* 1892). Despite passage of this restrictive law, in force until 1920, hashish was regularly used in the *tekedes*, cafes frequented by hashish smokers, in the harbor area of Piraeus and in the center of Athens. The habitués of *tekedes* were mostly younger, jobless, tough guys who, as a rule, existed by underground activities and were usually at odds with the law and the authorities. Known quite widely in Greece as *manges* (Petropoulos 1971), they had their own code of honor, a paradoxically tender and touchy personality, and fiercely rejected the established social order.

In the 1920's hashish use flourished. The reasons were primarily twofold: Greek soldiers, returning home after the disastrous war in Asia Minor, brought back hashish smoking habits which they had adopted in Turkey; and about one and one-half million Greek refugees from the destroyed areas of Asia Minor were repatriated to Greece. Among this latter population were individuals who either smoked or knew about hashish. It is more than probable that the poor living conditions to which they were subjected after repatriation in such slum areas as Tavros, Assyrmatos, Kokkinia, and Drapetsona, contributed to an increase of hashish smoking and to the establishment of more *tekedes*. But the problem is more complex. The population that came from Asia Minor consisted primarily of war widows and children (Zabathas 1969) in need of immediate relief and support which was hardly available and certainly not forthcoming. Hygienic conditions were very poor and death rates exceptionally high. Given these conditions, this population by 1923 had shrunk by 45 percent; in some parts of Greece no children of refugee parents were born during an entire year. Such social and physical hardships might well have contributed to the further spread of hashish use among this large minority population. In the years that followed, hashish use persisted in spite of proscriptive legislation. The retail price was low making it accessible to the majority of the population (Vouyoucas 1971).

From 1932 until 1970, the narcotics laws of Greece became increasingly severe and passed through various stages. Up to the end of the civil war in 1950, these laws were not strictly enforced and hashish use flourished. After this date a gradual decrease in the illegal cultivation and use of hashish took place. The latest version of the law, which is enforced, can be summarized as follows: a drug addict has to be confirmed as such by designated officials of the government medical service. Such an addict is then considered sick and subject to "attenuating circumstances" in the court trial required by law. As an addict, he will be given a lighter sentence than the non-addict. Punitive and corrective measures that may be imposed by the courts include imprisonment from 1 to 10 years; fines ranging from 50,000 to 10,000,000 drachmas; deprivation of driver's license for at least two years and up to life; confiscation of private property where the drug was found; dishonorable discharge from the armed forces; and prohibition against foreign travel.

Finally, while the rate of hashish use among the lower class continues to fall, a rise in hashish use may be observed among the teenage and student population of the middle and higher classes.

STUDY OF THE HASHISH SMOKING POPULATION

As stated earlier, this section reports on the epidemiological and sociocultural profile of the entire reported hashish using population based on data generated from the official Greek narcotic archives. We compare this population to the general Greek population and then to our experimental sample, utilized in previous clinical studies, in order to assess its representativeness.

Data Sources

In order to reach these objectives, a search of the archives of the following three narcotic units was undertaken: (1) Athens Metropolitan Police, (2) Piraeus Metropolitan Police, and (3) Athens Suburban Constabulary. These three archives encompass information for all of Greece with the exception of the city of Patras and the island of Corfu. The records studied cover the period 1958–1973.

Methodology and Methodological Problems

The archival search was conducted by a psychiatrist and a social worker who systematically collected data in the headquarters of the three narcotic units for two to three hours per day over a period of five months. Each narcotic unit has devised its own system of record keeping so that any given drug abuser may have a record in two or even all three units. Adding to the complexity, the archives of each unit include different kinds of information and the range of information recorded by each unit may vary depending on the time period in which they were collected. Practically all records, however, contain the following data: (1) name and surname, (2) nickname, (3) parents' name, (4) place of birth, (5) date of birth, (6) place of residence, (7) occupation, and (8) other illegal activities.

Only the oldest files of one unit provide data such as starting age and events associated with initiation to hashish smoking. Some files include information about imprisonments, although most of these only include dates of arrest for drug abuse without mentioning if the user was released after identification or remanded for trial. In a number of cases, records list the characterization "drug abuser" without indicating the type of drug used. In such cases the researchers, who had established good working relations with the narcotic squads, discussed the question in detail with pertinent police officials. In a very few cases, where only ambiguous or very incomplete information was available, such files were excluded from the study.

After this process, all usable records (5,589) were compared and cross-referenced so that for every drug abuser one final card was generated, as complete and inclusive as possible. Of the 5,589 records 1,893 were duplicates, leaving 3,696 as the basic pool of information. Subjects were classified by drug used and identified as hashish users only if they were utilizing this substance exclusively. Out of the total of 3,696 drug users, 3,128 were males who used only hashish, 107 were female hashish users, 330 were heroin addicts, 52 used other drugs such as amphetamines, barbiturates, etc., and 186 were foreigners arrested in Greece.

Since the experimental sample of our previous studies included only males, women were excluded from the archival analysis. Individuals arrested in Greece but residing permanently abroad were also excluded. Out of 3,021 males classified as exclusive hashish users, 125 had incomplete records. Due to the lack of standard classification of socioeconomic status in Greece, categorization of subjects' status was empirically determined according to educational background, occupation, and place of residence. On this basis, five categories were generated: (1) high, (2) middle, (3) working, (4) illicit activities, dependent, etc., and (5) peasantry. With regard to place of birth and place of residence, subjects were allocated into nine geographical areas. The Department of Attika was separated from the rest of central Greece, as it includes the two major urban centers, Athens and Piraeus.

Results

As previously mentioned, we attempted: (A) to analyze, given all their limitations, the data from the police archives concerning the total hashish population of Greece; (B) to compare the characteristics of the hashish population to the general population based on the 1971 census; and (C) to compare the total hashish population to the experimental sample.

A. Over the past twenty years Greece has become an industrially developed country; the proportion of the agricultural population has shifted from 55 percent to 35 percent. This has been accompanied by the large-scale movement of people from rural to urban areas, primarily to Greater Athens including Piraeus, which now contains one-fourth of the entire population of Greece. The urbanization process appears to

Table 1. Distribution of the hashish users population according to place of birth and residence

c/n	Area	General population	Hashish population Place of birth Number	Hashish population Place of birth Percentage	Place of residence Number	Place of residence Percentage
I.	Department of Attika	2,797,849	1175	38.89	2323	76.89
I.1	Region of Athens	2,101,103	628	20.78	1378	45.61
I.a.	Borough of Tavros	15,795	12	0.39	77	2.54
I.2.	Region of Piraeus	439,138	395	13.07	633	20.95
I.3.	Rest of Department of Attika	257,608	152	5.03	235	7.77
II.	Rest of Central Greece	734,469	156	5.16	53	1.75
III.	Peloponnesus	986,912	531	17.57	146	4.83
IV.	Ionian Islands	184,443	74	2.44	11	0.36
V.	Epirus	310,334	38	3.77	9	0.29
VI.	Thessaly	659,913	114	1.25	57	1.88
VII.	Macedonia	710,352	192	6.35	128	4.23
VII.1.	Thessaloniki	345,799	88	2.91	76	2.51
VIII.	Thrace	329,582	40	1.32	18	0.59
IX.	Aegean Islands	417,813	188	6.22	41	1.35
X.	Crete	456,642	124	4.10	46	1.52
XI.	Asia Minor		216	7.14	—	—
XII.	Abroad		32	1.05	26	0.86
XIII.	Unknown		100	3.31	163	5.93

be even more significant for hashish users, as revealed by a comparison of places of birth and present residence of the total hashish population. In the region of Athens, for example, the locally born hashish using population is 50 percent less than the provincially born hashish using population which migrated to the urban center. A striking finding is that the incidence of hashish users in the borough of Tavros (Greater Athens) has increased in the last decade from 0.39 percent to 2.54 percent (see Table 1).

By contrast, the hashish using population of the provinces has been greatly reduced. For example, in the Peloponnesus the proportion of users has dropped from 17.57 percent to 4.83 percent; in Epirus from 3.77 percent to 0.29 percent (see Table 1). The question has yet to be resolved as to whether the movement of rural born hashish users into Athens means the gravitation of already socialized users to the center of hashish traffic or whether the urbanization process was instrumental in initiating the practice of hashish use.

The geographical distribution of the total hashish using population is shown in Table 2. Users tend to concentrate in certain areas but pri-

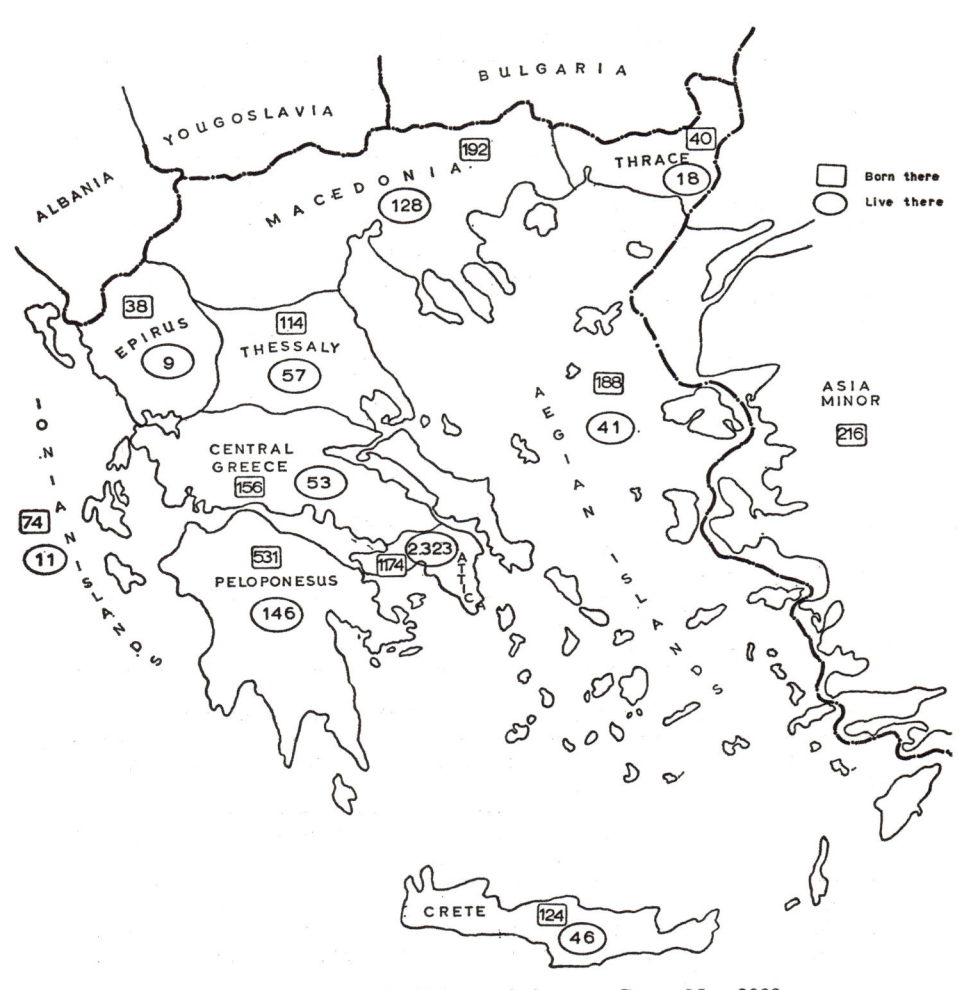

Table 2. Distribution of the total hashish population over Greece N = 2889

marily in the general area of Athens: the borough of Tavros has the highest incidence of hashish users 0.48 percent, compared to the region of Piraeus with an incidence of 0.14 percent, and Athens proper with 0.06 percent (see Table 3). Thessaloniki in Macedonia and Kalamata in the Peloponnesus have a relatively high incidence of hashish users, 0.02 percent and 0.14 percent, respectively. These latter figures can be attributed to the fact that the two provincial centers are port cities.

Analyzing the total hashish population by socioeconomic status reveals that hashish users are predominantly working class (61.60 percent). A high proportion are unemployed or are supported by underground activities

Table 3. Percentage incidence of hashish users in the general population

c/n	Area	General population	Hashish population Number	Percentage
I.	Department of Attika	2,797,849	2,323	0.082
I.1.	Region of Athens	2,101,103	1,378	0.065
I.1a.	Borough of Tavros	15,795	77	0.48
I.2.	Region of Piraeus	439,138	633	0.14
I.3.	Rest of Department of Attika	257,608	235	0.09
II.	Rest of Central Greece	734,469	53	0.007
III.	Peloponnesus	986,912	146	0.014
IV.	Ionian Islands	184,443	11	0.005
V.	Epirus	310,334	9	0.002
VI.	Thessaly	659,913	57	0.008
VII.	Macedonia	710,352	128	0.008
VII.1.	Thessaloniki	345,799	76	0.021
VIII.	Thrace	329,582	18	0.005
IX.	Aegean Islands	417,813	41	0.009
X.	Crete	456,642	46	0.010
XI.	Abroad at present	—	26	—
XII.	Unknown	—	163	—
	Total population of Greece (Census of 1971)	8,768,641	3,021	0.032

Table 4. Distribution of the hashish population to their socioeconomic status

c/n	Socioeconomic status	Total hashish population (N:2,628) Number	Percentage	Males (N:2,488) Number	Percentage	Females (N:107) Number	Percentage
1.	High	3	0.11	3	0.11	–	–
2.	Middle	335	12.74	326	12.94	9	8.18
3.	Working	1619	61.60	1599	63.50	20	18.18
4.	Unemployed, dependent, underground, etc.	562	21.38	452	17.95	77	70.00
5.	Peasantry	109	4.14	108	4.28	1	0.90

(21.38 percent). A smaller proportion (12.74 percent) belongs to the middle class. The peasantry (4.14 percent) and high class (0.11 percent) supply the smallest number of hashish users (see Table 4).

B. Eva Sandis, an American sociologist, who studied Nea Ionia, a refugee community in Attika (1973), found that occupational levels occupied by refugees from Asia Minor, migrants of rural Greece, and Athe-

Table 5. Job level of males by origins

Job level	Refugees percentage	Migrants percentage	Athenians percentage
Unskilled	7	5	1
Semi-skilled	27	40	33
Skilled	27	23	29
Petty proprietor	29	6	7
Lower white collar	4	10	12
Independent artisan	5	9	9
Middle white collar	1	7	9
Total percentage	100 ($N = 84$)	100 ($N = 123$)	100 ($N = 111$)

Table 6. Occupation and marital status of the two populations

	General population of Greece Number	Percentage	Total hashish population of Greece Number	Percentage	P
I. Occupational status	$N = 4,488,580$		$N = 2,628$		
Employed	4,268,639	95.10	2,066	78.62	<.001
Unemployed	219,941	4.9	562	21.38	<.001
II. Marital status	$N = 4,488,580$		$N = 795$		
Married	2,182,140	48.61	370	46.66	N.S
Divorced, separated, cohabiting	44,660	0.99	72	9.05	<.001
Widowed	483,200	10.76	0	—	<.001
Single	1,776,580	39.58	298	37.58	N.S
Not declared	2,000	0.06	—	—	—

nian respondents are lower for refugees than for migrants and Athenians (Table 5). Her findings are in accord with ours, since we found that the rate of unemployment among the hashish users (21.38 percent) was higher than that of the general population (4.9 percent). This difference is of significant importance ($P<0.001$) (Table 6).

Comparing the total hashish using population to the general population with regard to marital status, we find significant differences in the "divorced, separated and cohabiting " and the "widowed" categories ($P<0.001$) while no significant differences were found in the "married" and "single" categories (Table 6).

The two populations under consideration, males above the age of

16 years, show significant differences in age composition and education ($P<0.001$). Hashish users tend to be older, with a mean age of 44.46 years (S.D.=13.06) than the general population, mean age 41.32 years

Table 7. Comparison of personal characteristics of the two populations

	General population of Greece[a] ($N=3,334,185$)		Total hashish population of Greece ($N=2,896$)		
	Mean	S.D.	Mean	S.D.	P
Age	41.32	13.93	44.46	13.06	.001
Years of schooling	5.49	3.45	5.06	3.64	.001

[a] Male population above the age of 16 (census 1961)

Table 8. Age distribution of both populations

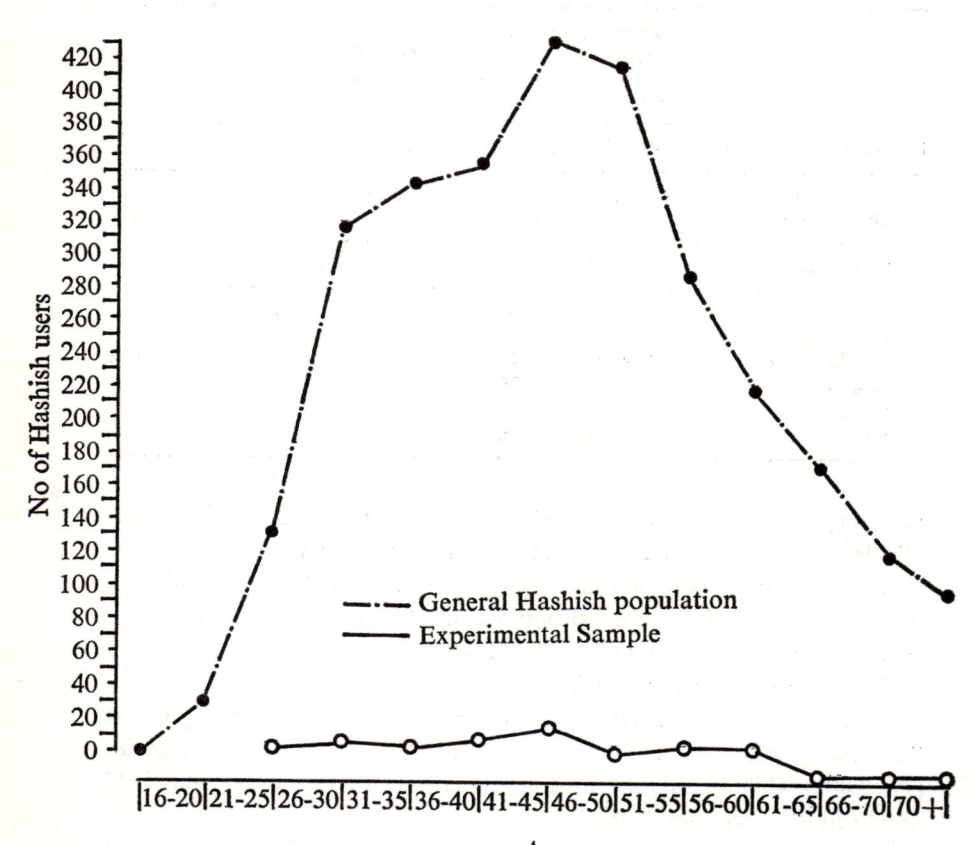

($S.D.=13.93$). Hashish users are also less educated, with a mean of 5.06 years of schooling ($S.D.=3.64$), than the general population, mean of 5.49 ($S.D.=3.45$) (Table 7).

C. A comparison of age in the total hashish population and our experimental sample indicates no significant difference between the two (Table 8). The total hashish population tends to be significantly more educated than the experimental sample ($P<0.01$). The mean years of schooling are 5.06 ($S.D. = 3.64$) for the total hashish population and 4.01 ($S.D. = 3.23$) for the experimental sample (Table 9). This difference is best explained by the fact that our experimental sample consisted primarily of lower working-class people.

As mentioned above, specifics on hashish smoking were available in the police archives for only a limited number of users (142 cases). Comparison of these data with those from our experimental sample focused on starting age of hashish smoking and years of use. The mean starting age for this accidental sample of the total hashish population is 23.52 ($S.D. = 7.05$) while that for the experimental sample is 18.05 ($S.D. = 4.32$), significant at $P<0.001$ level. No significant difference exists for years of use of hashish between the two populations (Table 10).

We may conclude that hashish users in Greece are derived primarily

Table 9. Comparison of personal characteristics of the total hashish population and experimental sample

	Total hashish population of Greece ($N = 2896$)		Experimental sample ($N = 58$)		Significance
	Mean	S.D.	Mean	S.D.	P
Age	44.46	13.06	42.74	11.26	N.S.
Years of schooling	5.06	3.64	4.01	3.23	.01

Table 10. Comparison of the hashish smoking data in the two populations

	Total hashish population of Greece ($N = 142$)		Experimental sample		P
	Mean	S.D.	Mean	S.D.	
Starting age	23.52	7.05	18.05	4.32	.001
Years of use	24.15	12.57	24.32	10.20	N.S.

from the working class and are differentiated from the general population with regard to age and education. On the other hand, our experimental sample is representative only of the lowest urban working class and is differentiated from the total hashish population of Greece by lower levels of education and earlier starting ages for the smoking of hashish. Differences between our experimental sample and the total hashish population may be attributed to the selection criteria imposed by clinical objectives which restricted admissions to the medical project to heavy chronic users only while the total hashish using population of Greece exhibits various degrees of use — from very occasional to heavy.

REFERENCES

AFENDOULIS, TH.
1875 *Pharmacology*.
[BALLAS, C. N.] Μπάλλαζ, Κ.Ν.
1968 Τό προφητικόυ παραλήρημα τῆς Πυθίας [The prophetic delirium of Pythia]. Athens: Soteropoulos.
BRUNEL, R.
1955 *Le monachisme errant dans l'Islam*. Paris.
[*Excerpt of the* 1890 *report*]
1892 Ἀπόσπασμα ἐκ τῆς ἐπί τῶν ἀποτελεσμάτων τῆς χρήσεως τοῦ χασίς ἐκθέσεως τοῦ Ἰατροσυνεδρίου (1890) [Excerpt of the 1890 report of the Health Council of Greece on the effects of hashish use]. *Greek Agriculture*, November: 525–529.
GALEN
1821–1833 *Opera omnia*, volume five, pages 349–350, in *Medicorum Graecorum opera quae exstant*. Edited by Karl Gottlob Kühn. Leipzig: Cnobloch.
1821–1833 *Opera omnia*, volume twelve, page 8, in *Medicorum Graecorum opera quae exstant*. Edited by Karl Gottlob Kühn. Leipzig: Cnobloch.
GELPKE, R.
1966 *Vom Rausch im Orient und Okzident*. Stuttgart.
Greek pharmacopoeia
1837 *Greek pharmacopoeia* (Athens Royal Press).
HARTWICH, CARL
1911 *Die menschlichen Genussmittel; ihre Herkunst, Verbreitung, Geschichte, Bestandteile, Anwendung und Wirkung*. Leipzig: Tauchnitz.
HERODOTUS
n.d. *Book IV*. Chapters 74–75.
KERIM, F.
1930 Les troubles psychiques dus à l' emploi du hashish. *L'Hygiène ment*.
KOSTIS, N.
1855 *Handbook of pharmacology*.

[KOUKOU, E.] Κούκου
1971 Ἡ διαμόρφωσις τῆς Ἑλληνικῆς κοινωνίας κατά τήν Τουρκοκρατίαν. [The development of Greek society during the Turkish occupation]. Athens: EKKE.
KOURETAS, D.
1937 "Drug-abusers in the army," in *Psychiatric topics in the army* (in Greek). Edited by D. Kouretas and F. Scouras. Thessaloniki.
NATIONAL INSTITUTE OF MENTAL HEALTH
n.d. *Report on chronic hashish use in Greece.* HSM 42-70-98.
On hashish
1887 Περί χασίς: "Ἔκθεσις τοῦ Δημάρχου Ὀρχομενοῦ τῆς Μαντινείας [On hashish: a report by the Mayor of Orchomenus in Mantinea]. *Greek Agriculture*, March: 110–114.
[PAPADOPOULOS, D. N.] Παπαδόπουλος, Δ.Ν.
1959 Κάνναβις [Cannabis]. Athens.
[PAPARIGOPOULOS, C.] Παπαρρηγόπουλος, Κ.
1932 Ἱστορία τοῦ Ἑλληνικοῦς Ἔθνους [History of the Greek nation]. Athens: Elephtheroudakis.
PAUSANIAS
1966 *Description of Greece.* London: Loeb Classical Library.
PENTZOPOULOS, D.
1962 *The Balkan exchange of minorities and its impact upon Greece.* Paris: Mouton.
[PETROPOULOS, E.] Πετρόπουλος, Ε.
1971 Ρεμπέτικα τραγούδια [Rebetika songs]. Athens: Chiotelis.
[PLUTARCH] Πλούταρχος
1615 Περί ποταμῶν καί ὀρῶν ἐπωνυμίας καί τῶν ἐν αὐτοῖς εὑρισκομένων: [On rivers' and mountains' names]. Tolasae: D. Bosc.
[PYRROS, D.] Πύρρος, Δ. (Θεσσαλός)
1832 Ἐγκόλπιον τῶν Ἰατρῶν [Doctors' textbook]. Navplion: Tobras.
REINIGER, W.
1962 "Historical notes," in *The marihuana papers.* Edited by D. Solomon. London: Panther.
1967 "Remnants from prehistoric times," in *The book of grass.* Edited by G. Andreus. New York: Grove.
SANDIS, E. E.
1973 *Refugees and economic migrants in greater Athens.* Athens: EKKE.
[SIMOPOULOS, K.] Σιμόπουλος, Κ.
1973 Ξένοι ταξειδιῶτες στήν Ἑλλάδα (1706–1800) [Foreign travellers in Greece: 1706–1800]. Athens: Simopoulos.
[STRINGARIS, M. G.] Στριγγάρης, Μ.Γ.
1964 Χασίς [Hashish]. Athens.
TSAOUSIS, D. G.
1971 *Structure of the neo-Hellenic society.* Gutenberg: Gutenberg Press.
[VAMVAKARIS, M.] Βαμβακάρης, Μ.
1973 Αὐτοβιογραφία [Autobiography]. Athens.

[VOUYOUCAS, C. N.] Βουγιούκας, Κ.Ν.
1971 Πρόληψις καί καταστολή τῆς χρήσεως ναρκωτικῶν οὐσιῶν διά μή θεραπευτικούς σκοπούς [Prevention and repression of the use of drugs for nontherapeutic purposes]. Thessaloniki.

[ZABATHAS, E.] Ζαμπαθᾶς, Ε.
1969 Οἱ ἐκ Μικρᾶς 'Ασίας 'Ελληνορθόδοξοι πρόσφυγες [The Greek-Orthodox migrants from Asia Minor]. Athens.

Marihuana and Genetic Studies in Colombia: The Problem in the City and in the Country

B. R. ELEJALDE

ABSTRACT

Colombia is a marihuana country. Cannabis is cultivated as a cash crop on a family basis and on plantations in the interior. Production has increased considerably within the past decade and is now an established export industry. Formerly used mainly by marginal unemployed groups, it has spread to the working class, students, and to the upper class. While marihuana smoking (principal form of use) was formerly rejected as socially undesirable, it is now considered acceptable in many circles.

Police statistics indicate high percentages of use by urban high school and university students. The high percentage may be due to sampling errors, but it is apparent that university students are continuing use started in the third to fifth forms of secondary school. Use in rural areas, previously limited by religious factors and the social custom of drinking, has shifted with the easy availability of marihuana and increase in the price of alcohol. Although the majority in the urban as well as rural areas are occasional users, the number of regular high frequency users is increasing in the rural areas, due to low salaries and unemployment. Marihuana is also used, on a limited scale, for the treatment of rheumatoid arthritis, asthma, and other clinical syndromes.

Several of our research findings are reported here. The number of abortions among marihuana users in the rural areas and in the urban low income population is higher than in the control groups, but the low levels of nutrition and other factors must be taken into consideration. The rate of congenital malformations is the same as that of non-marihuana users in control groups of the same social class. Chromosomal studies of regular marihuana users do not show any abnormality.

According to archaeological evidence, almost all the native tribes which still remain intact in Colombia have used hallucinogenic substances since long before the Spanish conquest. Coca, tobacco *(yague)*, and others have long been used by those pre-Columbian cultures for ritual, magical, medicinal and commercial purposes; or they have been used simply as a means of escape from the fatigue of work or to attain psychological states of euphoria. Use of such substances has been one of the features of the initiation of males into social life.

While it is not known exactly how long coca has been used in the native towns of Latin America, it is thought to have been used since long before the arrival of the Spanish.

In the San Agustín culture, Preuss (1931) found a head in relief at a site called La Estrella. The features of the face, at the level of the cheekbones, very similar to that found in other prehistoric statues *(Ibid.)*, have been interpreted by Pérez de Barradas (1941) as a representation of the act of chewing coca. Masculine figures found at the site depict individuals carrying a type of pouch or gourd which may have been used for depositing lime and tobacco, with which they mixed the coca (Lunardi 1935).

Other archaeological discoveries prove that coca has been used since the time of the Incan empire which passed it on to its descendants and neighbors. Nevertheless, no evidence of the use of marihuana has been found in any of these civilizations.

The history of marihuana in Colombia is especially interesting owing to the fact that for many years no publicity was given to the effects it produced on the human species. During this period from 1950 to 1955, marihuana was used only by persons of a low social class without any known occupation. But marihuana then spread rapidly, with a dramatic change after 1955 in the type of person who began taking it orally. Until then the majority of users of marihuana were arrested by the police and generally sent to jail with sentences varying from months to years. At that time punishment was mainly for the consumer and not the trafficker, who was not known.

During this period cultivation of marihuana was uncommon, and there were only a few small plots used by addicts who knew how to grow it. But the most common manner of obtaining it was from wild plants. These were found in various places in the country, including regions of natural vegetation within the cities themselves. Thus, it could be said that it was quite a common plant throughout the country.

With the spread of its use after 1955, small plots began to be converted into larger ones. And what previously had no economic significance began to be increasingly important because of its internal consumption. As a result, a small quantity of marihuana produced an appreciable amount of money.

Later, marihuana growing was carried out in a "family manner," that is to say, on land which the family cultivated. This was generally in places close to cities, where distribution to users was easy. As time passed and its effects became better known, marihuana was losing the myth of tragic consequences which had been attributed to it in previous years, and massive use started.

Colombian society was protected by high moral (principally religious) values which kept it within strict social rules that threatened violators with repudiation and punishment. However, the increase of information and access by a larger number of persons to the University as in other parts of the world created a rapid change in the last years of the 1950's.

Previously marihuana consumers were few in number and were severely punished. But with the change of attitudes, especially among the youth, the number of consumers was increasing steadily to the point where they became uncontrollable by the police. Given the limitations of the latter and the great increase of consumption and distribution, the result was that demand could not be met by wild plants. It was necessary to have recourse to its cultivation; this started with small areas near the cities which were easily detectable by the police. As a result, cultivation was initiated in rural areas and in greater amounts, making the enterprise a veritable commercial entity outside the law.

These phenomena (which took place starting from the beginning of the 1960's) and the increase in the number of consumers, created an immense network of producers who were growing it and middlemen. This network now extends throughout the Republic: not only in the large cities, but also in the country. It has been increased by exports to various countries of the world.

There are very few studies about the extent of the crops, dealers and consumers, and those which do exist only reflect some circumstances in the urban areas. In the country there are only a few indications of its trade and use.

The above phemonena led to an increase of production designed to increase local consumption and, basically, to infiltrate areas of the population where profits could be higher. After some time (1963–65), it began to be found that there were large crops of marihuana in very remote regions. Like those existing today they were principally devoted to export because of the demand in various countries of the world, mainly the United States. It increased business by making it profitable.

Along with the exporting there was wide internal distribution of marihuana. Previously its use had been limited to individuals without known occupations, many with social and psychic disorders or mental conditions of different kinds. It now began to be used by students, at first those of the lower class. Numbers increased and the use of marihuana spread to secondary schools. Here one noted an increase of marihuana starting with its use by small groups of the lower socioeconomic class. The drug's use by these groups of students was spreading and it began to penetrate the middle and upper social classes. This was due principally to the ease of obtaining it, as well as the abundance of literature publicizing the use of hallucinogenic drugs and marihuana. This was accompanied by the students' knowledge not only of the ease of obtaining it but also of the effects produced by the drug. Today a high percentage of students of the secondary schools of the large Colombian cities, varying according to the city, are occasional or frequent consumers of the drug.

Meanwhile, the lower socioeconomic classes, at the level of the worker, began to use the drug just like the middle and upper classes (principally the upper class). We can say that at this moment the highest centers of marihuana consumption in Colombia are students in all social classes, workers of the lower social class, and the upper class. All varieties of users exist in each of the groups.

From 1965 on, various amounts of marihuana began to be confiscated from cultivators and distributors. However, at that time deposits of it were not as large as those found in the last two or three years, produced for export to various countries of the world.

The purpose of this work is to present the various findings made about the types of marihuana distributed in Colombia, the manner in which they are distributed, the groups of population affected, the law's attitude concerning its use, and in addition, possible genetic effects produced by marihuana and its consequences for the species.

GROUPS OF POPULATION AFFECTED

As has been mentioned, the use of marihuana has been increasing in all groups of the population, principally among students and the lower and upper classes. The middle class still remains comparatively unaffected by the use of marihuana, although it is increasing every day. There are no clear statistics, nor have investigations been carried out of the different social strata which can provide fully accurate data. The few facts we know have been provided by the police and courts, who have partial statistics concerning individuals who have been found in possession, use or production of marihuana.

The use of marihuana by social class, according to these very partial and limited sources, is distributed as follows (Quiñones 1972):

Class Position	Percentage
Upper	22.7
Upper Middle	13.6
Middle Middle	54.5
Lower Middle	4.7
Lower	4.5

According to the statistics of the judicial authorities, the above data may be subdivided in the following manner: 66.1% were arrested for possessing marihuana; 11.6% were arrested for trafficking; 21.4% were arrested for consumption; no one was arrested for growing it; and only 1.9% for sponsoring the use of marihuana. These facts are especially significant, as only a fifth of the arrests were for consuming marihuana. As is obvious from the above data, no one was arrested between 1969 and 1972 for growing marihuana.

The use of marihuana is greater in large cities, and it is very difficult to find it in small towns which still uphold traditional cultural values.

The known age at which consumption started for various persons apprehended by the police may be subdivided as follows:

Age at Onset	Percentage	Age at Onset	Percentage
10	4.5%	16	22.7%
12	4.5%	18	4.5%
13	4.5%	19	18.2%
14	4.5%	28	4.5%
15	16.6%	36	4.5%

These statistics, though not a representative sample of the general population, are the only ones available to us.[1] They show a greater frequency of initiation into marihuana consumption during the ages corresponding to secondary school. As concerns the individual's position in the family it was found that .9% were only children, 12.5% the youngest child, 33% intermediate or middle children, 6.2% the oldest child, while no information is available for the remaining 47.4%.

Frequently, owing to the position of individuals arrested for using marihuana in the streets or distributing it openly, the crime is repeated. It is found that 6.2% reappear for the same crime, 26.8% reappear for another crime and 67% are not rearrested. This means a high percentage (26%) are arrested because of being involved in crimes other than using marihuana. This indicates that the legal finding and action on the use, consumption and production of marihuana occur only by chance, and the number of new dealers increases daily.

According to educational level they may be classified as follows: 59% of those arrested by the police for possessing marihuana finished their primary education; 27% completed secondary school; 8.9% had no

---

[1] It is important to note that the statistics presented refer only to a small sample of the population, that does not actually represent the numbers of consumers, as it only refers to cases detected by the police. These are very few in number compared to the immense use of marihuana in society.

education; and there is no information for 5.1%. This statistic also obviously contains errors, because as the cultural level increases it becomes more difficult for the police to arrest individuals using marihuana. For example, at the university level where probably the greatest consumption occurs, it nevertheless appears that no one is arrested by the police.

One of the most important findings concerning those arrested is that 0.9% displayed verbal aggressiveness; 77.7% were passive; 8% made an attempt at flight; 2.7% tried to bribe their way out; another 4.5% behaved in an "anti-social" manner; and there is no information for 6.2%.

Of the sentences received, 30.3% were acquitted; 1.8% were fined; 5.3% were placed on supervised probation; 4.5% were sent to a work school; 13% were sent for reeducation; the parents of 4.5% were notified; 3.6% were sent for help; 25.9% were placed under their parents' care; 1.8% under the care of other relatives; 6.2% were placed in institutions; 1.8% were pending; and no information is available for 1.3%.

The majority of individuals between 12 and 16 years of age were not punished for the use of marihuana; nevertheless, many of them were traffickers as well as users. It is important to mention that the law has been changed dramatically with regard to marihuana dealers since 1962. Trafficking is now only considered a misdemeanor, whereas it was previously cause for imprisonment.

The following data on individuals arrested under the effects of marihuana show how the social structure conceals the involvement of the different social classes: lower class, 49%; lower middle class, 20%; middle social class, 19%; upper middle social class, 1%. Eleven percent of those interviewed had no data concerning residence. No one belonging to the upper class was arrested, although it is known that they consume a large amount.

One of the few well controlled studies on the use of marihuana by students reveals that nearly 30% of the students in four main cities of Colombia (Bogotá, Medellín, Cali, Barranquilla) have used marihuana at least once. At first the use of marihuana was almost restricted to small groups of university students. Those who did so acted mainly out of curiosity. But then its use expanded until now 75% of university students have used marihuana on some occasion. The age at which they began to use it varies from 10 to 35, but 51% began between 15 and 17, corresponding to the third and fifth class of secondary school, thus localizing the problem at this level.

The difference in our population as compared to others is that in Colombia, university students use almost solely marihuana among the drugs which could be used. In the United States, according to Blumenfield *et al.* (1972) only 20% of the students interviewed used marihuana, and the rest other drugs.

It is important to mention that the use of alcohol is more moderate than would be expected in this student population: 43% of secondary school students partake occasionally of alcohol; 7% use alcohol regularly; and only 2% use it chronically and habitually.

One of the main problems in studying the incidence of use of marihuana in Colombia is to establish the occupations of those using it. According to police statistics (Quiñones 1972), 45.4% are students and 18.2% are persons whose job is unknown; the rest include various activities. However, these facts are somewhat remote from reality, since it is known that the number of regular adult users of marihuana is much higher; and yet these have not been detected.

Rural Areas

In rural areas the plant's use was long limited to only a few people. However, in recent years the number of persons using it has been increasing. At first they were emigrants from the cities to small towns. They began to implant not only the use, but also the cultivation of marihuana in rural communities. As the police were searching for these plants, crops were moved to more remote places, and its use in remote rural communities became more common. Nevertheless, there are no clear statistics providing concise information on its use.

The use of alcohol has been a cultural value of rural communities, where most men consumed alcohol on the weekends. With the increasing cost of alcohol and reduction of peasants' income the possibility of using marihuana has increased, particularly because it is grown locally. Furthermore, it is much cheaper and easier to obtain than alcohol, as it can easily be produced on one's own parcel of land.

It may be said that 90% of Colombian peasants use alcohol habitually and routinely about once a week, when it is generally consumed in abundant quantities.

One of the circumstances which has influenced the control of marihuana consumption in rural areas has been the retention of social values which, like religion, are static and have changed little.

In the last two years the migration of young North American tourists to Colombia has introduced the use of mushrooms and other types of hallucinogenic substances to the rural population and students of our cities. Many of the visitors come in search of these plants and have taught the natives not only how to find and recognize them, but also how to use them. This is why the use of hallucinogens is increasing in the Colombian Republic.

GENETIC STUDIES

The widespread use of marihuana and the need to study the possible teratogenic effects of new substances used by man have created special interest in knowing the possible genetic actions of this drug and its derivatives.

In 1965 Miras published his observations on rats taking an extract of cannabis in their diet: on the reduction of the growth rate and diarrhea. No congenital or hereditary abnormality was found. Since then some works have been published such as the one by Persaud and Ellington (1968). The latter describe the teratogenic effects of *Cannabis sativa* extract when administered daily in the 1st to 6th days of the gestation period, producing various deformities such as encephalocele, amelia, phakomelia *(facomelia)*, syndactyly and ventral hernia, but principally growth retardation and reabsorption of the ovum. These observations have been corroborated in part by Geber and Schramm (1969).

Recently, in a well-conducted experiment, Pace, Davis and Borgen (1972) studied the effects of tetrahydrocannabinol and marihuana extract, as well as the previous compounds marked with C^{14}. They found a complete absence of congenital defects in the animals studied with the two synthetics, cannabidiol and cannabinol.[2] According to the experiments conducted, they do not cross the placenta barrier by themselves, in quantities sufficient to affect the embryo. Studies carried out by others, Idanpaan-Heikkila *et al.* (1969) show that THC H^3 passes the placenta barrier with a maximum level of activity in the fetus in 30 minutes. From this we should be able to conclude, as do Pace, Davis and Borgen (1972), that marihuana is not teratogenic, at least in rats and hamsters.

Nevertheless, they found a reduction in the total weight of the litter and in the survival rate of the newborn. This last point, carefully studied, proved that the high rate of mortality of the newborn rats is due to the reduction of production of maternal milk, which disappeared when the rats were fed by "wet-nurses."

---

[2] Translator's note. The Spanish text refers to "the two synthetic cannabinodioles." Analysis of hashish has yielded "three types of related compounds: cannabidiol, cannabinol, and tetrahydrocannabinol (THC)." (Leech, Kenneth. 1973. *A practical guide to the drug scene*. London: SPCK, 42). The Spanish word appears to have contracted the first two of these compounds.

Another of the studies described in the publication by Pace, Davis and Borgen is the effect of THC on the maternal and fetal chromosomes of rats receiving different doses before and during gestation. They found no evidence of chromosomal abnormalities. This has been corroborated by studies carried out *in vitro* by Stenchever and Allen (1972), who put different amounts of tetrahydrocannabinol in a culture of human leucocytes, and found no structural or numerical abnormality in the metaphase studied. It is also described how amounts larger than 100 micrograms of tetrahydrocannabinol do not allow cell growth.

We have studied the rate of fertility, frequency of abortions, number of abnormal fetuses, and chromosome abnormalities in different groups of persons in the city of Medellín who smoke marihuana regularly.

1. Chromosome Studies

One group of 10 individuals (5 men and 5 women) have been consuming marihuana for periods varying between one and three years, for an average frequency of 1.3 times per week. They are all university students who are healthy from the medical point of view and have received no medical treatment of any kind for the last five years. None have consumed any hallucinogenic drug other than marihuana. Three of them have been exposed to very low doses of x-ray radiation (3.3 scans of the thorax), the most recent four years ago. All of them are psychologically normal individuals and have done well in their studies.

The chromosome study was made on peripheral blood following the normal methods (Moorhead *et al.* 1960), and no evidence of chromosome abnormalities was found in any of the 100 cells studied in each of the ten patients.

On the other hand, a study was made of a group of three students who, besides taking marihuana, have used LSD. An incidence was found of 30 gaps per one hundred complete metaphases (4600 chromosomes) studied and 15 breaks of chromatids with displacement.

Similar abnormalities were found in a couple which had only used LSD. We are able to deduce from this that the chromosome damage in the group which consumed both was probably caused by LSD, and not marihuana.

2. Studies on Reproductive Capacity and Fertility

The following groups were studied:

Six young couples of an average age of 26.5 years, each couple conceiving their first child which terminated in abortion before the first three months. They all used marihuana at least five times in the last two years, with an average of 7.8 times. Some of the wives smoked marihuana after knowing they were pregnant. The products of all the abortions were studied. No evidence of congenital deformities was found in any of the fetuses. One of the abortions was a shapeless mass, where only dead areas of placenta and membranes were seen. In chromosome studies carried out on cells originating from tissue cultures from the aborted fetuses no evidence was found of structural or numerical abnormalities of chromosomes. (There was one exception, where there was a large number of gaps and breaks in the chromatids. However, during the week when the latter conception occurred, the mother had had a bad attack of flu. She was treated with different drugs, principally aspirin and caffeine. This woman had been using tranquillizers of different types, particularly diazepam, for a number of years.)

Five young couples (average age 27.2) who used marihuana prior to the conception of the child (with a frequency varying from 1 to 15 times in the last twelve months before conception, with an average of 7.4 times) had perfectly normal pregnancies. The children (two male and three female) were normal, with no evidence of congenital deformities or hereditary illnesses. The chromosome study of these children showed no numerical or structural abnormality. Only one of the couples used marihuana in the first three months of pregnancy, through ignorance of her condition.

One group of fifty-one young couples, average age 28.4 years, used marihuana at least once during the five months prior to pregnancy, with an average of 4.7 times. The course of their pregnancy was followed and the products of the pregnancy examined.

These people belonged to the group with the largest incidence of spontaneous abortions in the city of Medellín. They were all from the upper middle and upper socioeconomic classes, and were of a high cultural level. They had an abortion rate which was 25.4% of the total number of spontaneous ones in the city. However, the abortion rate in this group was only 16.7%. Although the small size of this group does not allow us to draw any conclusions, it is important to note the significance of this observation. None of the children which did not abort had any kind of congenital deformity.

One group of fifteen couples was sent for genetic study after exhaustive gynecological-obstetrical studies for infertility, where no evidence was found of congenital deformities or detectable hereditary illnesses. Three of the women started to use marihuana after the end of the gynecological study and while still under genetic study, without telling the doctor. They became pregnant in the months following the end of the study, the latter not having shown any abnormality. Two of them gave birth to normal children in whom no abnormality could be identified. The third aborted when two and a half months pregnant, with a fetus which was behind schedule in its development, but without evidence of congenital deformities.

Like Pace, Davis and Borgen (1972), we are able to conclude that we have not detected any teratogenic effects: they came to this conclusion in rats and hamsters, and we in various human groups exposed to marihuana. Neither were we able to find chromosome abnormalities in users of the drug, nor in their offspring conceived after using cannabis.

Pace, Davis and Borgen used semi-synthetic alkaloids in their experiments and believe that the discrepancy between their results and others published in the literature on the subject may be due to the fact that the teratogenic substance present in marihuana is different from those they used. However, we studied couples who made more or less frequent use (normal for that social group) of the drug, all by means of inhalation, and no evidence can be found of any teratogenic effect.

In couples studied for infertility it is important to mention the great psychological tension they undergo because of their sense of reproductive frustration. One should also note the start of pregnancy after the use of marihuana, which both couples described as quite agreeable and as liberating them from their daily problems.

FACTORS WHICH HAVE INCREASED AND CONTROLLED THE USE OF MARIHUANA IN OUR COUNTRY

Colombia is a country where the different sociocultural groups correspond to geographic divisions. We can speak of the Atlantic Coast group, the Pacific Coast group, the Antioquia, Cundiboya (Cundinamarca-Boyacá) and Nariño groups. These groups are well defined and each has different cultural and social values. However, they also have common characteristics, such as religion and the importance of the family. In some areas, as on the Atlantic Coast, this is a polygamous matriarchal type of family, while in the central part of the Republic, Cundinamarca-Boyacá and Antioquia, it is a monogamous patriarchal type. One of the most important values is the attitude toward social realities. This is broadminded and overt on the Atlantic Coast, where a man may have two or three wives and conceive children by them with the full knowledge of the others. This situation of openness and clear knowledge of the men's extramarital relations and procreation of children outside marriage is looked upon without suspicion on the Coast. On the other hand, although the same phenomena occur in the Cundinamarca and Antioquia cultures (i.e., the men father children outside marriage by one or several women), it is not accepted by society and is kept hidden. Thus we should be able to classify the reaction to these cultural values on the Atlantic Coast as one of openness and sincerity. On the other hand, the Antioquia and Cundinamarca cultures in the center of the country have a hypocritical attitude to the situation.

This also expresses two distinct attitudes to the use of hallucinogenic substances (principally marihuana), in different parts of the country. Its use is high on the Atlantic Coast, though no accurate data exists. People of the Atlantic Coast are characterized by their excessive vivacity, love for parties and high consumption of alcohol. It is a society without high cultural or religious values, unaccustomed to steady work. The use of marihuana has been increasing and it is believed that 72% of the people between 18 and 24 have used it at least occasionally. Some use marihuana for rituals of the Afro-Cuban and Haitian types, for religious acts in which they claim to be following voodoo rites. Marihuana has been used for such pseudo-religious purposes in this part of the country. Its use has been extended to minors, who use it repeatedly. No great incidence of problems of any type has been found within the few medical centers existing in the region.

We can say that the use of marihuana on the Atlantic Coast exists at all social levels. Although it is not limited to any one level, it is found principally in the working class. Perhaps there may be a small group of people devoted to farming who still do not use marihuana to any great extent.

One may say that the lack of self-control and strict social values on the Atlantic Coast has caused its use to be more extensive and freer than in other parts of the country.

In the Cundiboya (Cundinamarca-Boyacá) and Antioquia cultures, moral values are stricter and religion has a stronger hold. This has resulted in a more restricted use of marihuana, as the Catholic Church has criticized it, maintaining the point of view that it is very harmful and belongs to the group of hallucinogenic substances. This has created a feeling of fear and respect, thus restricting the use of marihuana. Nevertheless, in the last five years the use of this drug has been increasing alarmingly. From the lower social strata, which were the first to use it, it has spread to students, and finally to the upper social strata of young people, who use it instead of alcohol.

On the Atlantic Coast the use of alcohol continues to be on the same scale as before. Its use is indiscriminate and generally associated with festive celebrations. On the other hand, the Cundiboya and Antioquia cultures have a tradition of weekend use of alcohol. The majority of the men meet in the town to imbibe. This also occurs in the cities, where the working class males meet on weekends to consume alcohol. The introduction of marihuana into these social groups has exchanged the use of one for the other, due principally to the high cost of alcohol and low cost of marihuana. They find they obtain similar results with marihuana as with alcohol, and at a lower cost.

In these last two cultures the use of marihuana is concealed and is not acknowledged or accepted socially, even though in practice the number using it is quite large.

The statistics given are based on the number of persons arrested for transporting or selling marihuana, but not on the number of users, which is much higher. The number of persons in universities who have used marihuana at least once is growing increasingly.

If we compare the use of marihuana and other drugs by university students, we find great differences in relation to the statistics of other countries, as very few people in our society use drugs other than marihuana. These observations are quite different from those made in the United States in the works of Millman and Wen Huey (1973) and Blumenfield and co-workers (1972). The latter show that besides marihuana, other drugs, such as darvon, LSD, mescaline, peyote, amphetamines, codeine, barbiturates and other compounds are used by college and university students. However, we have found nothing comparable to this among students surveyed in the city of Medellín, nor in the secondary colleges or university (Quiñones n.d.). The use of alcohol on a habitual basis among students is limited to small groups. This is true even though it may be said that 92% of students use alcohol at least sporadically after 15, and a small group of 7% do so habitually both in university and college (Quiñones 1972).

We believe that the factors influencing the increase of marihuana consumption have been mainly the publicity given to the pleasant sensations it produces, its actual use, and knowledge of the lack of harmful effects caused by it as compared with other drugs. The Catholic religion has also lost much influence, which is increasingly obvious at the different levels of society. This means that the religious sanctions which used to exist concerning the drug have fallen into disrepute, and very few people really believe in the problems pointed out by Catholic priests concerning the use of drugs.

The feeling of rebellion (mainly in youth) against established structures (mainly religion) has not only passively influenced its use, but also positively influenced marihuana use. The latter has become a demonstration of rebellion against structures they reject as being outmoded and against the people's interests. The increased use of marihuana has also been influenced by the ease with which it is obtained and its low cost compared to the use of alcohol. Alcohol is easier to acquire, but it costs more to obtain comparable results.

The statistiscs previously mentioned indicate that a larger number of students as well as individuals of the lower classes are marihuana users. Nevertheless these statistics are clearly vitiated because of the fact that no complete detection program has been carried out in the various social spheres where one would probably find a different incidence of the use of marihuana. It may be said that all individuals have been exposed to its use at least once.

Another factor contributing to the increased use of marihuana is the lack of control by authorities. This has been limited to the arrest of some distributors, but very rarely of large-scale producers. This has given rise to a state of impunity for growers and traffickers; they are rarely detected and very rarely punished or even imprisoned. Large quantities of marihuana are frequently found, ready for retail sale or export; nevertheless, the person implicated never appears and even less often does he receive any punishment.

Recently the Colombian Institute for Family Welfare sponsored a seminar on the study of hallucinogenic drugs and their use in Colombia. The Seminar's conclusion is simple: it shows the enormous lack of knowledge of the problem and the lack of policies for treatment. This applies principally to the use of marihuana, as other drugs are still not used to an extent which might be considered alarming.

The Government is interested in initiating campaigns to improve this situation. However, since previous campaigns in other fields have been ineffective, it makes one fear that there is little possibility of success in this one. Furthermore, the spread of scientific knowledge about the use of marihuana makes it increasingly difficult for exaggerated concepts to be accepted with any likelihood of curbing its use by young people.

Some such groups do exist. For example, "Unity against Marihuana" is made up of a few individuals trying to do something akin to Alcoholics Anonymous. It has been completely ineffective because of its reactionary nature. Those involved exaggerate marihuana's harmful conditions and by this very exaggeration have been completely discredited. They claim that marihuana produces an addiction leading to escalation to other drugs, as well as grave toxic reactions and sociological effects. They insist that individuals who smoke marihuana are especially dangerous and aggressive. This is contrary to the actual situation, for it has been shown that these individuals are passive *(Ibid.)* and less aggressive than normal persons, given the state of tranquility produced by the drug. The group also exaggerates the psychological effects of marihuana alleging that it is a grave hallucinogen and comparing it with LSD. Such reactionary and extreme claims turn out to be counterproductive: individuals who might have been influenced by such societies totally reject them. They regard the latter's effects as negative rather than positive.

BELIEFS

There are an endless number of popular beliefs about marihuana. There are those who believe that terrible harm is caused by marihuana, that it leads to antisocial behavior and causes a degeneration of the nervous system, turning the users into assassins and individuals with abnormal behavior. However, there are people, principally among the middle and lower classes, who attribute medicinal powers to marihuana. This belief was increased by a pseudoscientific use of marihuana in the form of liniments for application with ethyl alcohol, with curative powers against rheumatoid arthritis and asthma. There are those who continue to use it in this form, although it is now prohibited.

Other curative powers are attributed to marihuana mainly among herbalists who prepare infusions of different plants for cures of chronic illnesses.

RESEARCH

There are very few studies of marihuana in our country. They are limited to the few carried out by Dr. Richard Evans Schultes (in press) on the psychopharmacological drugs in the Colombian Amazon and in the country, and those by Dr. Alvaro Fernández Pérez on the botanical inventory of marihuana and other drugs in Colombia (personal communication). There has been research at the Universidad del Valle in Cali, by Drs. Argota and Guerra on the effects of marihuana on the level of cerebral amines (n.d.). They found that the psychopharmacological effects of marihuana are probably due to alterations of the subcortical amines in rats. They compared amounts of epinephrine, norepinephrine and cerotonine in four subcortical areas. By means of a tracheostomy they made the rats inhale marihuana smoke a number of times. The rats were then beheaded and their brains frozen, and an analysis was made of the above-mentioned substances. Considerable increases were found in the levels of norepinephrine and epinephrine in the hypothalamus and thalamus, and cerotonine in the grooved nucleus. The results obtained reinforce the possibility that the various effects of marihuana may be measured through the increases of the levels of these amines. An attempt has been made to carry out an epidemiological study of the general population. Most projects, however, suffer from grave defects and have up to now received no government support.

CONCLUSION

The use of marihuana has been increasing rapidly in all spheres of Colombian society. No study has been made of the size and implications of the problem, one that is aggravated by the profitable nature of the production, sale and export of marihuana.

In the studies we carried out we found no evidence of chromosome abnormalities in chronic smokers, nor has there been any increase in the number of abortions or abnormal children in couples who have consumed the drug.

There are still values in society which restrict the speed of the spread of the use of marihuana.

Although the legislation is strong, in practice it is weak and rarely applied, especially to large traffickers.

It is necessary to continue and initiate more extensive research to examine the long term effects of cannabis on different generations.

Marihuana, given its low cost in comparison with alcohol, is replacing the latter in its social function.

REFERENCES

ARGOTA, G., A. GUERRA
   n.d.   *Efectos de la marihuana sobre nivel de aminas cerebrales* [Effects of marihuana on the level of cerebral amines]. *Colombian Seminar on Pharmacology Proceedings* III:66.

BLUMENFIELD, M., et al.
   1972   Marihuana use in high school students. *Diseases of the Nervous System* 33:603.

FERNÁNDEZ PÉREZ, ALVARO
   n.d.   Personal communication.

GEBER, W. F., L. C. SCHRAMM
  1969   Effect of marihuana extract on the fetal hamsters and rabbits. *Toxicology and Applied Pharmacology* 12:276.
IDANPAAN-HEIKKILA, J., et al.
  1969   Placental transfer of tritiated-1-Delta 9 tetrahydrocannabinol. *New England Journal of Medicine* 281:330.
LUNARDI, FEDERICO
  1935   *La vida de las tumbas* [The life of the tombs]. Rio de Janeiro: Typ. do Journal do Comercio.
MILLMAN, D. H., M. A. WEN HUEY
  1973   Patterns of drug usage among university students: V. Heavy use of marihuana and alcohol by undergraduates. *American College Health Association Journal* 21:181.
MIRAS, C. J.
  1965   "Some aspects of cannabis action," in *Hashish: its chemistry and pharmacology*. Edited by G. E. W. Wolstenholme and Julie Knight, 37–47. London: J. & A. Churchill.
MOORHEAD, P. S., et al.
  1960   Chromosome preparations of leukocytes cultured from human peripheral blood. *Experimental Cell Research* 20:613.
PACE, H. B., W. DAVIS, L. A. BORGEN
  1972   Teratogenesis and marihuana. *Annals of the New York Academy of Sciences* 191:123.
PÉREZ DE BARRADAS, JOSÉ
  1941   *Arqueología y antropología precolombinas de tierra a dentra* [Precolumbian archaeology and anthropology of inland areas]. First edition. Bogota: National Publishing House.
PERSAUD, T. V. M., A. C. ELLINGTON
  1968   Teratogenic activity of cannabis resin. *Lancet* II:406.
PREUSS, K.
  1931   *Arte monumental prehistórico* [Prehistoric monumental art]. Translated by Walda Weldegg and Urbide Piedrahita. Bogota: Imprinta Nacional.
QUIÑONES, A.
  n.d.   *Campañas especiales estadísticas sobre consumo de alcohol.* [Special statistical campaigns on alcohol consumption]. National Police. Mimeographed copy.
  1972   *Policía nacional y la prevención y recuperación de toxicomanías* [The national police and the prevention and recovery of drug addicts]. First National Seminar on Drug Addiction. Bogota.
SCHULTES, R. E.
  i. p.   *El papel médico religioso de las plantas alucinogenas de la Amazonia y de los Andes* [The religious medical role of hallucinogenic plants of the Amazon and Andes]. *Proceedings of the Seminar on Improvement of the Colombian Man and Environment.*
STENCHEVER, M., M. ALLEN
  1972   The effect of delta-9-tetrahydrocannabinol on the chromosomes of human lymphocytes in vitra. *American Journal of Obstetrics and Gynecology* 114:819.

Cannabis Usage in Pakistan: A Pilot Study of Long Term Effects on Social Status and Physical Health

MUNIR A. KHAN, ASSAD ABBAS, and KNUD JENSEN

ABSTRACT

A detailed description is given of the various modes of consumption of cannabis, *bhang* as a drink and *charas* for smoking, in Pakistan, a society in which cannabis is socially accepted.

The study includes preliminary social and medical investigations of 70 healthy male subjects, all of whom had consumed cannabis for at least 20 years. These examinations showed no significant abnormalities and in no case was there evidence that the use of cannabis interfered with the subjects' ability to work. There was no suggestion that either tolerance to the drug or physical dependence on it occurred.

Observations made on subjects indicated that the drug tended to cause a slight fall in the blood pressure and an increase in the heart rate. Some transient dryness of the oral mucosa and a tendency to develop an irritant cough occurred after smoking.

Such extensive studies on a much larger scale are required on a population which is well adjusted and where cannabis is socially accepted, and where only cannabis is used.

INTRODUCTION

There is a vast literature on the subject of cannabis as a *drug*, although of uneven quality. A need was felt to study a society where cannabis use is accepted as a normal phenomenon similar to that of alcohol in Western countries. Only a few such studies have been performed by indigenous investigators having a thorough knowledge of the language and culture of the population. In addition, the long-term effects of cannabis have rarely been the object of study in a normal population.

The present paper describes an attempt to fill these gaps, as it reports a pilot study performed in Pakistan from January to March, 1973.

Pakistan is largely a rural country, with a population of approximately 55 million, is 803,420 sq. km. in extent, and the economy is mainly based on agriculture. Cannabis has been traditionally used for centuries. In

For Plates, see pp. xvii–xix, between pp. 266–267.

some parts of the country and in some sections of the community cannabis is used and, although not totally approved, is not socially prohibited. In contrast, alcohol is looked down upon, apart from a tiny minority of Westernized people. The use of cannabis is equally prevalent in both urban and rural areas and is virtually confined to adult males.

Our aim was to study the long-term effects of cannabis in a socially well-adjusted population in contrast to many previous investigations which were usually concerned with special subgroups. The inevitable conclusion of such studies is that the use of cannabis, mental illness and criminality are causally related. We feel, however, that it is unjustifiable to generalize from subgroups of deviants, hence the reason for this pilot study.

THE STUDY

There are vast regional and local differences in the habits and modes of cannabis consumption as well as the venues where cannabis is consumed. For this reason we selected two areas, one urban and one rural. Thirty-five subjects were selected from each area. Lahore, the urban area, is one of the oldest and largest cities in Pakistan and has a population of approximately 2.6 million inhabitants. We did not contact the subjects ourselves, as we thought that a direct approach might result in suspicion on their part. Instead, the subjects were contacted through a man who is active in community voluntary work. He is also esteemed by the local residents as a successful entrepreneur. The rural sample was drawn from nine villages near the city of Khanpur in the erstwhile state of Bahawalpur. The population of these villages ranged from 100 to 500 inhabitants.

In Lahore, 19 subjects were totally illiterate, 10 could barely read and write and 6 had had ten years of schooling. In the Khanpur area, 31 were totally illiterate, 3 could barely read and write, and only one had had ten years of schooling.

Fifteen of the subjects in Lahore were unmarried and 20 were married; 16 of the latter had an average of 5 children. In the Khanpur villages, 4 were unmarried and 31 married, 24 of these had an average of 6 children.

It is difficult to describe social class in the context of Pakistan economy. In Lahore most of our subjects belonged to the working class: 11 were skilled artisans, 14 were shopkeepers, 2 were laborers, 2 were clerks, 2 professional wrestlers, 1 was a beggar and 3 were well-to-do contractors. In Khanpur, 2 were beggars, 2 were laborers, 9 skilled artisans, 5 *mirasees* (traditional professional musicians who have a special social function in village life), 15 farm workers, 1 landowner and 1 restaurant owner.

METHODS

The only criterion for the selection of the subjects was that they must have been taking cannabis regularly for a minimum period of twenty years. They were not interviewed or checked for their physical, mental or social background before the selection. The urban sample was, therefore, taken from the old city of Lahore, which represents the traditional Pakistani way of living. Likewise, the rural sample was selected from the nine neighboring villages near the city of Khanpur.

Our assistant selected a group of thirty-five suitable subjects in Lahore who were asked to come in the morning without taking cannabis. The subjects were picked up by taxi in the morning at their homes, two at a time, and were remunerated in order to maintain interest in the study.

In Khanpur the subjects gathered at the Dera (landlord's house) of the village. The investigation was divided into the following three phases: before, during, and after the consumption of cannabis. Before the consumption of cannabis, each subject was medically examined and interviewed about his social background, work habits, history of cannabis use, etc. [Appendix I]. He was then offered either *charas* (which is smoked), or *bhang* (which is drunk) [Appendix II]. A questionnaire for assessment of subjective feelings was completed for both *charas* smokers and *bhang* drinkers [Appendix III]. For the *charas* smokers it was first completed half an hour after smoking (it takes about 5–7 minutes to smoke one cigarette), and for *bhang* drinkers it was first completed an hour after drinking (the glass is emptied at once). The questionnaire was filled in at hourly intervals for the next four hours. Blood pressure, pulse and general neurological examinations were carried out at the same time.

RESULTS

The modes of cannabis consumption were found to be different in urban and rural areas. In Lahore cannabis was taken in both forms, i.e., 7 out of 35 were only *charas* smokers but 28 used both *charas* and *bhang*. In Khanpur the villagers were almost exclusively *bhang* drinkers, with two exceptions who occasionally smoked *charas* as well. The average number of *charas* cigarettes smoked in Lahore was 14 a day. Each cigarette contains approximately between 1/2–1 gram of cannabis. In Khanpur where *bhang* was consumed, the average number of tumblers taken was 6. The amount of *bhang* varies per glass but, on an average 6 glasses would contain approximately 60 grams of dried leaves. There was also a seasonal variation in the consumption of *bhang;* in the summer when long cool drinks are popular the intake is higher. Drinking *bhang* usually took place before meals, while smoking *charas* was not related to any special time of the day.

The average age of the subjects in Lahore was 44 years, with a range of 29–75. The average age at which the subjects started smoking was 16 years with a range of 8–25 years. The average length of time they had been smoking was 28 years with a range of 21–57 years. The average age in Khanpur was 53 years, ranging from 32–80 years. The average starting age was 17 years with a range of 10–25 years, and the number of years they had been drinking was 35, the range being 20–65 years.

Respondents were asked about the history and present mode of consuming cannabis. The picture which emerged corresponded very closely to alcohol drinking. All our respondents from both areas commenced drinking or smoking cannabis in a very unself-conscious way, again rather like an average Westerner starting to drink alcohol. The reasons given were medical and social, but rather unspecific. Four of the subjects from Lahore and two from Khanpur had a previous history of alcohol or opium consumption. We must, however, point out that this is a regional variation and this picture would not be obtained in all parts of Pakistan. We found that in Lahore the respondents mainly used what are known as *uddas*[1] for drinking *bhang* in the company of their friends but smoked *charas* at work.

In the rural groups, the places known as Deras (the landlord's house) were found to be the focal point of social activities for villagers and were regarded as the centre of village political life. A certain group of people known as the *mirasees* [the musicians] were found to be the only group who were drinking *bhang* within the family.

All seventy subjects were given a full physical examination. No significant abnormalities could be detected and the previous medical histories were also negative. So was the family history. As can be seen from Appendix I, a lot of information was recorded but we have not discussed it here due to the lack of control groups. One very interesting medical point that emerged is that *bhang* drinkers, particularly from rural

---

[1] An *udda* is either a shop which specializes in selling cannabis, opiates, etc., or a meeting place attached to the local *mazar* [shrine].

areas, pointed out that they had never suffered from dysentery, which is very common in Pakistan.

In no case was loss of libido reported. All the subjects thought that there was no effect on sexual desire, but some (50%) felt that ejaculation was delayed. No impairment was reported by the subjects in work functions; in any case, all subjects led a normal active life. No one reported having to cease or curtail any occupational or other activity because of taking cannabis. Some subjects even remarked that their ability to concentrate was better after they had consumed cannabis. Again nothing very suggestive medically was discovered, except for the blood pressure and pulse. In all cases, the systolic pressure fell while the diastolic pressure rose and the pulse rate was increased. With regard to the systolic pressure, the pattern of change varied slightly in some cases. Nothing abnormal was found in the neurological examinations.

Other findings revealed that symptoms such as pupillary reactions (myosis), irritative cough, shortness of breath, dryness of mucosa of the mouth, etc., were present after smoking *charas*. Difficulty in breathing also occurred after *bhang* consumption and the blood pressure and pulse showed a similar pattern, after drinking and smoking. The other symptoms, however, were only present after smoking. Conjunctival injection was observed in both *charas* smokers and *bhang* drinkers but this complaint is common among Pakistanis due to various local conditions and we have, therefore, excluded this symptom.

In the third stage of the study, a questionnaire that was completed on the following day revealed that a hangover never occurs after *charas* or *bhang* as is seen with alcohol [Appendix IV].

DISCUSSION

The most significant point which emerged was that in a society such as Pakistan where cannabis consumption is socially accepted, habituation does not lead to any undesirable results. We have deliberately used the word habituation rather than addiction because we did not find either increased tolerance or withdrawal symptomatology, which are the essential prerequisites for addiction.

We are aware of the fact that our sample is not random; we feel, however, that it was the best that could be obtained for a pilot study under the given circumstances.

In the areas we have described, the use of cannabis is as prevalent as alcohol drinking in Western countries, and it seems to be a lesser problem than alcohol. Our study appears to show that cannabis does not produce any serious long-term effects.

There appears to be a growing fear of the ill effects of cannabis among the educated classes in Pakistan. This attitude is unquestionably borrowed from Western publications in this field. The older generation tends to see cannabis in a different perspective and is perturbed about the sporadic cases of drug addiction among the young generation.

CONCLUSION

As has been pointed out, this is a pilot study; however, we availed ourselves of cultural background information in making sure that the sample of subjects in our study was as representative as possible of the population at large and was not drawn from deviant groups.

It can be concluded that:
1. No signs were found of physical or mental damage after 20 years consumption of cannabis.
2. Cannabis use does not seem to lead to addiction or any conditions resembling alcoholism.
3. There were no findings of mental disease, criminal offences or social, working or family breakdowns in any of our subjects.
4. All subjects had myosis after cannabis consumption; the systolic blood pressure fell whereas the diastolic pressure rose and the pulse increased.

We feel strongly that this kind of study on a much larger scale is essential in order to answer a whole range of questions relating to the medical, cultural and social aspects of cannabis use.

APPENDIX I

QUESTIONNAIRE FOR THE *CHARAS* AND *BHANG* PILOT STUDY IN PAKISTAN

1. Name
2. Age
3. Profession
4. Monthly salary

5. Weight
   i. constant
   ii. gain
   iii. loss

6. Religion
7. Height
8. Ethnic group

9. Marital status:
   i. single
   ii. married

10. No. of children, if any:
11. No. of dependents in the family:
12. Educational status:
   i. illiterate
   ii. matriculate
   iii. graduate

13. Previous medical history
14. Family history
15. Present history
16. Narcotics used:
   i. *bhang*
   ii. *charas*
17. Other narcotics if any
18. The age at which *bhang* or *charas* started

19. Motivational reasons
20. Drinking or smoking habits
21. How often during the day
22. Working capacity
23. Drinking or smoking habits:
   i. in groups:
   ii. with family:
   iii. alone:

24. Sexual habits
25. *Physical examination:*
   General description of the physical appearance:
   i. pyknic
   ii. athletic
   iii. leptosome

26. Cranium
27. Cavum oris
28. Eyes:
   i. pupils
   ii. conjunctiva

29. Chest:
   i. respiratory modus
   ii. bronchitis

30. Blood pressure
31. Pulse:
   i. periphal vascular conditions:

32. Abdomen
33. Liver
34. Spleen
35. Kidney
36. Other U. organs

37. Extremities:
   i. UE motility
   ii. muscular tonus and strength
   iii. reflexes

38. LE:
   i. motility of joints
   ii. muscular tonus and strength
   iii. reflexes:
      a) patelar
      b) plantar

39. Sensory organs:
   i. smell
   ii. hearing
   iii. vibration

40. Sensitivity:
   i. cold
   ii. warm
   iii. stumpf   sharp

41. Pain
42. Tremor
43. Diadochinese
44. Romberg
45. FNF
Remarks

APPENDIX II

Charas

Charas is smoked; it is usually mixed with tobacco and is either smoked in a cigarette or is placed in a *chilam* pipe which is then lit and the *charas* inhaled deeply. *Charas* is the generally known form of hashish. These preparations are the unadulterated resins from the flowering tops of the cultivated female plants. The most desired substance resides in the microsopically small glandular hairs on the foliating leaves. Because of the pressure in the glands they burst and the resin flows out covering the small leaves in a sticky film. The extraction of the resin is simple, layers of the film are peeled off and pressed together making hard blocks which are then sold in the market.

Bhang

Bhang, on the other hand, is drunk. Dried cannabis leaves are steeped in water for about 15 minutes, then heated in water (not boiled). The water is discarded and the soaked leaves are washed and rinsed in running water for 15 to 20 minutes. The processed leaves are then crushed until a homogenized thick paste is obtained. This paste is then diluted in ordinary water, and in summer ice is added to it. Rich people mix it with almonds, sugar, cardamom, to make the drink more palatable. The drink is served in mugs and the quantity consumed is comparable to that of beer.

Bhang, the weakest of the three hemp products used in the Indo-Pakistan subcontinent, is made from the dried top leaves of the ripe uncultivated female plant which is green and has a potency nearly equivalent to that of marihuana.

APPENDIX III

QUESTIONNAIRE FOR THE ASSESSMENT OF SUBJECTIVE FEELINGS DURING AND AFTER INTOXICATION

1. Consciousness:
   i. normal
   ii. drowsy
   iii. somnolent
   iv. comatose

2. Hunger
3. Has he to pull himself together to feel normal
4. Time taken to reach the height of intoxication
5. Time taken until the effect of the drug has completely disappeared
6. Working capacity:
   i. increased
   ii. decreased
   iii. normal

7. Nausea
8. Aggressive
9. Irrelevant talk
10. Destructive
11. Mental state:
    a) Thought process
       i. acceleration
       ii. slow response
       iii. non-communicative
       iv. incoherence
       v. irrelevance
       vi. preservation
       vii. shouting
       viii. obsessional rumination
       ix. blocking
       x. ideas of reference
    b) Emotional response
       i. flattened
       ii. incongruous
       iii. depressed
       iv. excited
    c) Biological functions
       i. insomnia
       ii. loss of appetite
       iii. lack of energy
       iv. sexual desire
    d) Projection phenomena (delusions)
       i. persecutory
       ii. somatic
       iii. religious
       iv. magical
       v. grandiose
       vi. influence
       vii. misinterpretations
    e) Projection phenomena (hallucinations)
       i. auditory
       ii. visual
       iii. olfactory
       iv. tactile
       v. gustatory
    f) Cognitive disorders:
       i. derealization
       ii. depersonalization
       iii. specific body image disturbance
    g) Memory impairment:
       i. loss of recent memory
       ii. loss of past memory
    h) Clinical assessment of intelligence:
       i. below average
       ii. average
       iii. above average
    i) Present insight and judgement:
       i. adequate
       ii. fair
       iii. poor
       iv. very poor

Remarks

APPENDIX IV

HANGOVER SYMPTOMS ON THE CHECK LIST

Symptoms:

Vomiting
Loss of appetite
Heartburn
Lassitude
Continued thirst
Palpitation
Weakness of joints
Respiratory difficulties
Sleeplessness
Giddiness

Headache
Sweating
Disturbance of balance and gait
Pallor
Tremor
Nystagmus
General malaise
Anxiety
Depression

The Significance of Marihuana in a Small Agricultural Community in Jamaica

JOSEPH SCHAEFFER

ABSTRACT

A comprehensive field study, including videotape coverage and extensive laboratory research, was carried out in a small agricultural community in Jamaica, the West Indies. The research sought to explore whether cannabis altered the user's cognitive and psychological frame of reference in a specific socioeconomic and cultural context.

The findings indicate that 1) heavy cannabis smokers enact subtle alterations in daily agricultural activities directly related to cannabis-induced alterations in the stream of consciousness; 2) subjective (smoker) impressions of cannabis-induced alterations in specific tasks contrast with descriptions based on analysis of research records of those activities; 3) alterations associated with cannabis smoking seem to be appropriate to the users as members of the socioeconomic cultural system.

Multidisciplinary research procedures are suggested for further study of these findings.

INTRODUCTION

When smoked or ingested in sufficient quantity, psychoactive preparations of *Cannabis sativa* produce significant effects on the stream of consciousness.

These effects have been described in numerous reports and studies (Moreau de Tours 1845; Mayor's Committee 1944; Weil *et al.* 1968; Hollister *et al.* 1968; Manno *et al.* 1970; Goode 1970; Tart 1970; Grinspoon 1971). The effects of cannabis cited include: anxiousness followed by euphoria, a sense of well-being, and excitement; rapidly changing emotions; heightened sensory awareness; feelings of enhanced insight; fragmented thought; impaired short term memory; altered perception of time and space; altered sense of identity; increased desire for food; restlessness and hyperactivity followed by a relaxed, slightly drowsy state and sleep.

The intensity and duration of the effects depend to a degree on the potency, dosage and means of administration. Psychological set and setting are also factors in the subjective interpretation of effects (Goode 1970; Jones 1971).

Recent studies indicate that experienced users get moderately "high" from 2 to 20 mg tetrahydrocannabinol (THC, one of the primary psychoactive agents in cannabis) in smoked preparations and 5 to 40 mg THC in oral preparations (Isbell *et al.* 1967a, 1967b; Hollister 1969; Weil *et al.* 1968). Heavier doses, especially of ingested preparations, may produce intense anxiety, possibly leading to paranoia and depression, depersonalization, marked distortion in sensory perception, and hallucination (Mayor's Committee 1944). Usual effects begin almost immediately after the smoking of cannabis and last one to four hours depending upon the dose. They begin one-half to one hour after ingestion and persist for three to five hours (Mayor's Committee 1944; Isbell *et al.* 1967b; Hollister *et al.* 1968).

In attempts to elucidate the cannabis experience described by users, researchers have concentrated on studies of possible physiological, biochemical, and neurological effects. These studies are reviewed systematically in several summary reports (Canada 1970; Grinspoon 1971; USDHEW 1971; WHO 1971).

Viewed collectively these studies indicate that few cannabis-induced effects on either the stream of consciousness or the behavior stream are founded in effects on observable biochemical or physiological processes or in effects on external sensory mechanisms. We would expect, rather, that they are the result of a direct action of cannabis in the central nervous system.

An important conclusion from these studies is that psychoactive preparations of cannabis affect the primary centers of thought, perception, and emotion in the brain. The result is an altered stream of consciousness. A consequent modification of the "subjective grasp of experience" (Goode's phrase 1971) — of the "self," the body, and the material and social environment — is inevitable. To a lesser degree several essential qualities of behavior are modified as well. In other words, the users' frame of reference for thoughts, perceptions, feelings, and behavior is altered after cannabis use.

Since the subjective grasp of experience — with Goode (1971) let us call it the "subjective reality" — is altered after cannabis, we may assume that the relationship between that reality and an observer-defined "objective reality" may be altered as well.

These conclusions have critical implications for research in defined

Jane Schaeffer, my wife, and I had an opportunity to fulfill these requirements during recent research on cannabis use among inhabitants in a small community in Jamaica, West Indies, sponsored by the National Institute of Mental Health, Contract No. HSM–42–70–97.

THE RESEARCH COMMUNITY

The research was carried out during a one year field study in a small agricultural community, Valley, situated in hilly, shaley terrain in Jamaica's eastern Blue Mountain range. The research population includes 80 male and 85 female adults (over 14 years) and 82 male and 82 female children (14 and under) living in 85 households along a winding dirt road. The age distribution of the population is indicated on Table 1.

Most common living arrangements in the 85 households are summarized on Table 2. Forty-six percent of the households (34) include a man, a woman, and others. In 24 of these (32% of the total) the man and woman are married. Thirty-one percent of the households are denuded (headed by a single male or female)[1] and 19 percent are single person households.[2]

Information from each of the households concerning residents, land, dwellings, principal occupation, education, and religion is summarized on Table 3. Excluding information from single person households, we find an average of 5.7 persons per farm in Valley. If single persons are included in the sample the average per farm is 4.3. Zero to two-acre farms are prevalent but larger farms (5 to 7 acres) are not uncommon. Average education among adults is 4.2 years. Farmers with higher education usu-

---

[1] For the time being I have arbitrarily used Edith Clark's classification (1966:117). She distinguishes six types of residential groupings in Jamaica: "(A) simple family type households consisting of a man and woman with or without their children and possibly adopted children and non-kin persons; (B) extended family households, being an extension of simple family by the addition of other kin; (C) and (D) denuded family households, containing either a mother, or a father, living alone with his or her children. These might be either of the simple or the extended type; (E) single person households, and (F) sibling households. Type A is subdivided into two main groups: (I) a *primary* type containing children of the couple only and (II) a *secondary* type showing the presence of outside children. Thus II (a) shows households containing outside children of both the man and woman, II (b) those with outside children of the man, and II (c) with outside children of the woman.... Type II (d) households have adopted children only. Type III households are childless." Our term "common law" applies to relatively stable unions which have not been legally consummated.
[2] Many of these households are connected by historical family ties or by marriage or common-law relationships. The most important connections — those which are maintained and cherished over time — include exchanges of goods and services.

Table 1. Age and sex of valley inhabitants

Age	Number Male	Female
60 and over	24	27
22 – 59	40	46
15 – 21	16	12
7 – 14	41	46
0 – 6	41	36

Table 2. Household types in valley

Type household	Status	Number of households	Sub-totals	Percent of households
A (I) simple	married	11		
	common law	4		
A (IIb)	common law	1		
A (IIc)	married	1		
	common law	2		
A (III)	married	4		
	common law	1	24	28
B extended	married	13		
	common law	9	16	19
C denuded simple	male	3		
	female	3	6	7
D denuded extended	male	1		
	female	15	16	19
E single person	male	13		
	female	6	19	22
F sibling household		1	1	1
G combination		3	3	4
Total			85	100 %

populations. Certain alterations in the central nervous system associated with cannabis use are probably universal. Their interpretation and expression, however, are directly related to psychological, social, economic, and cultural variables. Consequently, their significance can only be understood if at least two research requirements are fulfilled: 1) cannabis use must be viewed in the natural (and not only the laboratory) setting; and 2) patterns associated with the use of cannabis must be considered in detail with contextual phenomena.

ally own more acreage and have larger incomes. Eighty-four percent of the households maintain religious affiliations.

The primary source of income is the crop market (see Table 4). Most common market crops are congo peas, carrots, coffee, and cocoa. Pimento and coffee are the most valuable crops financially. Average incomes vary with acreage under cultivation and type of marketing. Highest incomes result from the marketing of "own" crops plus the buying and selling (higgling) of "outside" crops. Most household incomes from marketing were under $ 300.00 in 1970. A few relatively large-scale farmers were able to gross nearly $ 1,000.00.

Farmers in Valley, as in many parts of Jamaica (see, for example, Comitas 1963) supplement market income with income from other occupations. Road construction and wage labor on neighboring farms are common alternatives to "own account" farming. As indicated in Table 3, several farmers have also perfected specialities as cooks, barbers, butchers, carpenters, painters, sawyers, shoemakers, tailors, etc.

Ease of access, to public areas and spring water, for example, has influenced most people to construct dwellings near a road or well-trodden path. Houses are usually situated on one-fourth acre to one-acre plots for which the owner has often paid a handsome price. A few fortunate families have constructed homes on corners of their own cultivated acreage.

Small business — three grocery and beer shops and two butcher shops — border the valley road; artisans and craftsmen work in their own dwellings. Two public buildings, the Baptist and Zionist churches, are at opposite ends of the mile-long main residential section.

As is the pattern in Jamaica, farm lands are strewn over the hills at varying distances. These lands stretch 5 miles to a southwest ridge. To the northwest they meet fields occupied by residents of an adjoining district one-half mile from the valley road; to the southeast they cover both sides of several land fingers along summer-dry stream beds. They border the lands of residents of a sister district, Richards Crossing, one mile to the south; to the east and northeast a winding road to the interior is a precise marker.

Approximately 70 percent of the available lands are under cultivation. Other lands are either in ruinate or pasture for livestock.[3] Of the cultivated lands, between 60 percent and 75 percent sustain mixed agriculture similar to farming (Conklin 1957). For example, on one plot, carrots,

---

[3] These lands are sloped between 10 and 40 degrees. The shaley soils (slightly acid in reaction and low in phosphate and potash) are far from ideal for farming.

Table 3. Summary information on households

Type	Total households	Av. size	Av. acres	Average education Male	Average education Female	Religion Type	Religion No.	Dwelling Cond.	Dwelling No.	Occupation* Male Type	Occupation* Male No.	Occupation* Female Type	Occupation* Female No.
A (Simple)	24	4.75	6.25	3.4	5.10	Bapt. Zion. Other	9 18 2	VP P F G VG E	2 8 8 5 0 1	cultivator cook baker butcher road work carpenter painter constable	15 1 1 1 1 1 1	market cook shopkpr. domestic account. relig. ass't.	12 3 2 5 1 2
B (Extended)	16	5.10	8.80	5.5 +1coll.	5.5 +1coll.	Bapt. Zion. Cath. Meth.	18 6 2 1	VP P F G VG E	0 5 2 3 4 2	cultivator carpenter minister factory van owner public work baker ass't.	12 2 1 1 1 1 1	market higgler teacher post mtr. shopkpr. minister's wife	4 1 1 1 1 1
C (Denuded Simple)	6	3.1	2.1	3.3	3.0	Bapt. Zion.	1 2	F P	3 3	cultivator market sell can. sawyer	3 1 1 1	cult. wage sell can.	1 1 1

D (Denuded Extended)	16	5.9	5.9	5.0	4.7	Bapt. 7 Zion. 3 Other 1	VP 2 P 0 F 5 G 5 VG 1 E 3	cult. market wage domestic tailor agric. peanut seller	1 5 2 2 2 2 1
E (Single Person)	19	1.0	1.78	3.4	4.5	Bapt. 5 Zion. 1	VP 5 P 5 F 5 G 1 VG 2 E 1	cultivator trucker factory farmhand wage labor	11 1 1 1 1
								higgler domestic	1 1
F (Sibling)	1	3.0	1.0	4.0		Bapt. 1	F 1	cultivator	1
G	3	11.0	6.9	5.3	5.3	Bapt. 1 Zion. 7 Other 2	G 1 P 2	cultivator butcher sell can. minister shoemaker labor	4 2 2 1 1 1
								market farmer daywork	1 1 2

Abbreviations under the title "dwelling" are: VP-very poor; P-poor; F-fair; G-good; VG-very good; E-excellent. sell can. is an abbreviation for sell *Cannabis sativa*.

* These are primary occupations.

Table 4. Average market income by size of farm

Acres	Coffee and Cocoa	Pimento	Other crops	Total income
0 – 2	$ 13.33	$ 5.30	$ 29.91	$ 48.54
2 – 4	18.05	9.36	184.80	212.21
4 – 6	18.57	56.81	230.29	305.67
6 – 10	35.35	52.68	253.68	341.71
10 – 15	84.38	37.24	491.98	613.60
15 +	105.09	251.33	862.92	1219.34

turnips, tomatoes, corn, congo peas, bananas, and plantains are intermixed. On another, climbing and sprawling vines of starch crops (sweet potato, cassava, and several types of yam) intermingle with sugar cane, coffee bushes, banana, breadfruit, jackfruit, avocado, citrus, pimento, cocoa trees, and several other vegetable, spice and non-food crops.

Cedar, cottonwood, tambrun, poinciana, and other trees fill the gullies. Bamboo usurps any available sunny land. Fruit bearing trees, (sugar plum, guava, otaheiti apple, and star apple) are desirable in the dwelling yard and are not uncommon on the hillside. Eleven mango tree variants grow in profusion. Several queenly guangos shelter the valley stream.

Cows, pigs, goats and fowl are the most common domesticated animals which roam the pastures and yards. Chickens are raised in pens and dogs stand guard at nearly every gate. Wild animals include pigeons, many small birds, cats, the mongoose, and rats.

Valley residents travel to neighboring and more distant districts along the road or connecting paths by foot, beast, daily bus, market truck, or private transport. Several Valley farmers own land in neighboring Crossing Ridge, school children make the daily trek to the Crossing primary school, and Valley residents visit relatives and friends occasionally in other not too distant communities. Churchville, a four-mile walk over the northeast hills, is the most important village center in the area. There one can find medical care, police authority, government services, and recreation.

The trucks and bus travel established routes to coastal towns and the capital. Many women ride these vehicles on the weekly two- to four-hour trip to market. Other Valley residents make arduous, distant journeys only rarely to visit relatives, attend funerals, or complete important business.

PATTERNS OF DISTRIBUTION AND USE

According to local historians, cannabis, known as *ganja* in Jamaica, was first introduced to Valley between 1910 and 1920 by traveling East Indians and by local farmers who made visits to coastal cities and the capital. Early use was limited to several individuals who cultivated their own small crops. Gradually, as its popularity increased, more farmers began cultivation for sale. By the 1940's, several dealers enjoyed considerable income from the distribution of *ganja* to practically every local household for tonics and tea mixtures and to a growing number of local smokers. Laws against cannabis enacted in 1913 (revised in 1940) did not seem to hamper trade.

Following a devastating hurricane in 1951 much of the cultivation ceased; the cannabis crop, along with most other crops, had been destroyed. The government introduced land development schemes which included visits to local fields by program officers who could recognize cannabis. The risk of discovery by the police seemed too great. Gradually, however, local residents began to cultivate cannabis. In the early 1960's a few dealers planted sizeable crops and contacted their former clientele.

According to recent interview data, by 1965, 80 percent or more of the residents were using cannabis in some form, in tea or tonic, or smoking. Today probably 75 percent of the adult residents smoke cannabis. Most women drink *ganja* tea and take rum tonic; 50 percent smoke it as well. Smokers consume varying quantities. Of the 40 discussed in this paper, 12 are heavy smokers, 8 are moderate smokers, 11 are light smokers, and 9 are very light smokers.[4] Most of these men began smoking *ganja* between the ages of 14 and 16. One teenager reported early use at age 12, while an older heavy smoker had his first smoking experience at age 25. The few women smokers began in their early twenties. Nearly all (both men and women) smoked tobacco cigarettes before cannabis.

Most men were introduced to cannabis smoking among older friends. Some were initiated into use during extended visits to the capital,[5] a few mention contact with Ras Tafarians during these visits.[6] Others began smoking when older family members or friends passed them the "weed" in the fields. These smokers often associate initiation with the acquisition

---

[4] A heavy user smokes 3 to 8 times a day (2 grams to 1 ounce). A moderate user smokes once a week to once a day (.5 grams to 2 grams). A light user smokes once a week to once a day. A very light user smokes less than once a week.
[5] Older smokers emphasize the importance of outside contacts in histories of use.
[6] Ras Tafarians are members of a Jamaican religious, race-conscious, "back to Africa" group in which cannabis is used heavily.

of their own farm plot. The women usually learned to smoke with their boyfriends or husbands, although some were introduced to cannabis by women smokers in the city.

Not long after initiation the smoker establishes a routine of use.[7] Variations in the routine are related to the purpose of use and the availability of *ganja*. Cultivation requirements, for example, affect men who like to smoke during arduous labor. When private cannabis crops end in January and household incomes decrease in April and May, smoking patterns change as well.

Dose averages vary among smokers. Some stop when they "first feel it affecting the brain." Others smoke standard amounts, e.g., one-half round (.5 to .6 grams) or one round (1 to 1.2 grams). Heavy users often smoke as much as they can get.

For many users dose is related to activity and the quality of the cannabis. "When you smoke in the field," one man suggested, "you don't smoke enough to block up (get very high)." Another said, "When you get the real thing a few draws (puffs) will do it." The duration of the effects is reported to be as short as one-half hour to as long as five or six hours (for the "strong stuff"). Most smokers report effects lasting two or three hours.

Not all smokers agree that the effects are in any way profound. Some say they feel "no different" after smoking. Others, however, report major changes in the stream of consciousness. All agree that effects can be consciously controlled.[8]

Reliable antidotes are available for the smoker who is affected too strongly: sugar-water mixed with lemon juice is the common remedy. If this should fail, the smoker can be bathed in lime juice. Symptoms requiring administration of the antidotes are dizziness, associated with a need to lie down, and "feelings of craziness." No heavy smoker mentioned a hangover from cannabis. Several moderate smokers mentioned thirst (sometimes hunger) as a frequent early-morning-after effect. One light user reported feeling physically weak after heavy use.

Withdrawal symptoms are uncommon when cannabis is not available to heavy users. A few, however, indicate some aggravation: one said, "I want it badly when I don't have it but I keep control of myself"; a second reported feeling "lonely" without cannabis. Several felt "angry

---

[7] Several men for whom first experience with cannabis was unpleasant (nausea and dizziness) declined a second trial. Their decision was supported by others who said, "His brains are too light so he can't use it."

[8] Several report using cannabis to "calm" themselves when they are particularly "vexed" (angry). That is, cannabis itself is used to control behavior.

and sad" or lifeless ("like I'm not living"). A long-time heavy smoker said, "The first day (without cannabis) is the worst day in my life; feel as though I might die; life mash up; no appetite; head hurt; feel like brains scatter." He reported feeling better on the second day and "fine" by the third.

The availability of cannabis in Valley is based on a fairly complex system of cultivation and distribution. Many users plant one to five "roots" for home use in some private spot. They sow the seeds in pans, trays, or secluded beds in February, March, or April, replant the suckers a few weeks later, and nurture the plants to maturity by September, October, or November. Their crops have often been consumed by January or February, and they then turn to local dealers.

Occasionally, a small-scale cultivator sells a limited surplus to local or distant dealers "to unload the crop quickly" for fear of the police and/or to make pocket money for Christmas. The extra "ganja money" is a vital addition to small market incomes. More stable local dealers stock-pile small quantities of cannabis during harvest seasons; when this is exhausted they travel to other districts to obtain supplies. Some connection with the police is necessary to succeed as a dealer over any extended time period. Protection costs money or cannabis, and loyal friendship, which is probably most important.

The benefits to the dealer are well worth the price of possible prosecution, a few years in prison. Mr. Fisher,[9] a local shopkeeper and the most successful dealer in Valley, has done very well indeed. He began handling bits of *ganja* in 1930; by 1935 he was selling 2 ounces (48 to 56 rounds) a week, and by 1955, 5 to 10 pounds a week in both small rounds and medium ($1/2$ to 1 ounce) packages. He is now satisfied to sell about 2 pounds a week since he is "getting old" and has already earned sufficient income to construct a good house and educate his children.

Most Valley smokers visit Mr. Fisher's yard to buy *ganja* several times a week during off-crop seasons. On special occasions or holidays he hires a teenager to vend it for him. If the Fisher cache is not of the highest quality, however, heavy smokers search for other dealers in nearby districts.

Several small-scale vendors appear in Valley from time to time. Two farmers who grow 200 to 500 plants yearly, supply rounds to local smokers until their crops have been sold to dealers. A female smoker has a friend who cultivates cannabis in a nearby village; she occasionally markets his crops by rounds in Valley.

---

[9] All names used are pseudonyms.

Large-scale cannabis cultivators are no longer common in the Valley area; several have died recently, and two are in prison. And only one extremely clever cultivator remains. In 1970, he planted 8000 roots on Crown land (interior land owned by the government). His major market targets are city dealers who drive to his home late in the evenings to purchase as much as 10 to 25 pounds of cannabis. He also supplies Mr. Fisher and other area dealers. Interestingly, he does not smoke *ganja* himself: "Nothing against it," he says, "it's just safer that way."

The price of cannabis varies with supply and demand and quality. Rounds have been selling for $ .20 for some time in Valley; an ounce costs $ 1.50 to $ 2.00; a pound sells for $ 24.00 to $ 40.00. Prices are highest between April and July and lowest between August and December.

"Kali" is though to be the best product, but few can define it precisely. One cultivator says that only 50 out of 5000 plants produce the rich, black, female buds called *kali*. Others insist that any "strong" female bud can be classified as *kali*. All agree, however, that its strength is greater than that of the normal leaves and buds of female plants. Male "bush" is used primarily for tea and tonic mixtures. On occasion, if the female plant is running low, it may be mixed with the male for smoking; the "weak and wasteful" male is rarely smoked alone.

Territorial patterns associated with smoking *ganja* in Valley are limited. Most solitary users smoke in their homes or yards, in their fields, in the yard or field of a trusted friend, or in a private area in the bush. For those who prefer to smoke in a group, the bush is the desired location. There they can relax together to enjoy "good and loving thoughts" in companionship. Safety from the police is the primary consideration and few users smoke in public.

Many Valley smokers and their relatives and friends fear the police. The fear is often based on personal accounts of police brutality, however, arrest itself is not shameful and prison terms are considered a "normal" part of life. Police surveillance techniques include search by helicopter, inspection of fields, observation in homes and shops, and questioning of "informers." Local officers know most smokers and/or growers and can crack down at will. Frequently, however, impending arrests are discovered in time and *ganja* crops and/or caches are destroyed. When arrests are carried out, legal loopholes may be available for those able to raise lawyers' fees.

General feelings concerning cannabis laws are negative. People say, "The government doesn't like us to get money so they try to stop *ganja*," or, "They (the government) know it's a good thing and they want to make money off it." Many associate the stringent laws with the power of the medical profession: "Doctors don't want us to have it because everyone would be healthy." Others believe the Bible ordains the use of cannabis and say that men have no right to impose laws against it.

Three informants felt that the laws should be stringent. The local minister and an elderly woman readily accepted news reports of violence related to the use of cannabis. The district dealer, on the other hand, associated "loose" laws with the free growth and sale of *ganja* and a decrease in his own business.

SUBJECTIVE EFFECTS OF CANNABIS

The prevalent subjective effects related to the use of cannabis by 25 Valley informants are summarized on Table 5. Most smokers associate the use of *ganja* with clear thinking, meditation and concentration,

Table 5. Reported effects of the smoking of cannabis*

Effects	Total resp.	No category mentioned	Positive resp.	No effect resp.	Negative resp.	Pos. & neg. at diff. times
Concentration	16	9	14	2		
Euphoria	15	10	15			
Reaction to others	13	12	8		1	4
Thinking	11	14	6	2	2	1
Sexual desire	11	14	9	1		1
Feel good	10	15	10			
Well-being	10	15	9		1	
Short and/or long-term memory	10	15	8 (both)	1	1 (short term)	
Agressive ("boldness in spirit")	8	17	6	2		
Work	21	4	13	3	1	4
Animation	13	12	8	2		3
Talking	10	15	8			2
Appetite	16	9	14	2		
Energy	9	16	9			
Strength	10	15	9		1	
Tiredness	15	10	11 (more tired)		1 (never tired)	3

* Responses of 25 informants are included in the chart. "Effects" are those mentioned by informants. During interviews we pressed for responses to questions concerning effects but did not suggest categories. Several interviews were given to each informant.

euphoria, feelings of well-being, positive feelings towards others, and self-assertion. A few express negative reactions with regard to one or another of these psychological effects. Such reactions are often reported to be related to dose, frequency of use, quality, or the "lightness of the brains."

Major effects emphasized by most smokers are related to patterns of work. Many report an increase in strength, energy, and/or rate of movement immediately after use, followed by relaxed feelings of steady power, and eventually fatigue. Many associate *ganja* with enjoyment of food and several warn of physical risks of use when food is scarce. Few smokers consciously experience any decrement in either short- or long-term memory. Of the 9 informants who mention memory, 7 indicate improvement, 1 finds no effect on memory, and 1 feels his short-term memory is "weakened." No smoker feels that *ganja* leads to violent behavior.

Several effects are mentioned by only a few informants: two speak of alterations in the time sense; two mention increased fear of sanctions against smoking; four enjoy a heightened perceptive capacity; six feel more confident; eight are more relaxed; and nine spend extended periods in daydreaming about daily activities and social relationships.

RESEARCH METHODS

Given the emphasis on the relationship between cannabis and work activity by Valley inhabitants, specific research was undertaken to determine cannabis-induced alterations in the stream of behavior during work activity. We employed several techniques including daily written observations and audiotape, videotape, and film coverage. We tested alterations in the stream of consciousness as subjects responded to prearranged signals with brief statements concerning their perceptions. To place the alterations in context we also carried out measurements of energy metabolism and nutrition and case studies of social-economic networks.

Following an introductory period of observation and interviewing in the community, a representative sample of 16 cannabis and non-cannabis smoking households was selected for intensive study. Procedures for covering daily activity in each sample household included interviews, extended observation, and tape review sessions. Research goals were explained, coverage techniques demonstrated and the permission and cooperation of all the subjects secured during the preliminary interviews.

In each household I observed the stream of activity of a central adult male informant throughout his waking hours for 14 consecutive days, listing all episodes in sequence (see Harris 1964); I noted all material items related to activity, and described encounters and the content of conversation. On selected days I carried videotape and photographic equipment to produce audiovisual records of representative sequences of activity (up to 120 minutes in length). When possible the sequence included complete activities. All behaviors of all informants in a given scene were framed at all times during coverage. At least three audiovisual records of each major activity were acquired for each cannabis smoker before, during, and after smoking.

Upon completion of audiovisual coverage in each household, tape viewing sessions were scheduled for the subjects and for their families and friends, when requested. On occasion videotape review was employed to stimulate responses concerning behavior in particular scenes.

Episodes of central female adults in each sample household were listed by Jane Schaeffer during the 14-day coverage periods. She briefly noted activities of other female adults and/or children, and maintained precise records of food intake. On selected days all foods consumed by household members were weighed before cooking, and the proportions of each food were weighed as they were distributed; waste food was also weighed. Foods consumed between meals were noted and weighed whenever possible.

Subjects in each household were taught to compile brief daily nutrition-activity booklets including statements concerning hourly activity, recipes for each meal, and estimates of food proportions given each household member. We checked these booklets during brief weekly visits throughout the field year.[10]

Medical studies of adults and children in sample households and selected other adults in the community were carried out to support the nutritional studies.[11]

Toward the end of the field research several nutritionists from Columbia University (Dr. Mary Bal, Dr. Orrea Pye, and Miss Judith Wylie) joined us in the field to conduct tests with a Kofrani-Michaelis respirometer and

---

[10] The USDA Handbook No. 8 was employed for analysis of nutritional data to establish baseline caloric and food composition values; these values were related to precise data for each informant to determine daily intake.

[11] Dr. Michael Ashcroft and Mrs. Eric Cruickshank from the University of the West Indies Hospital visited the community to administer medical history interviews, examine the subjects, and obtain venous blood samples and feces specimens. In the hospital laboratory hemoglobin and packed cell volumes were measured and a thin blood film examined. Serum albumin and globulin were estimated and VDRL tests performed. Stool specimens were examined for ova and parasites.

a Lloyd-Haldane gas analysis apparatus. We asked selected subjects to wear the seven pound Kofrani on their backs and to breathe into the attached respiration tube during normal activity before and after smoking cannabis. The volume of consumed air in liters was noted every 30 seconds and many of the tests were analyzed on the Lloyd apparatus. The activity tests were videotaped in their entirety.

The subjects were also involved in laboratory exercise studies (carried out with Dr. George Miller of the Epidemiological Research Unit at the University of the West Indies) in which they exercised on a cycle ergometer (Monark).[12]

Analytical procedures related to these field studies include an activity episode summary, an analysis of audiovisual records, energy metabolism studies, a nutritional survey, an exchange and social network summary, and analyses of special subject interviews.[13]

In the activity episode summary original lists are reduced to charts from which easy calculations concerning actors, time, place, activity, content of activity, social and exchange networks, food intake, energy expenditure, and physical context for activity can be made.

---

[12] Tests Ia and Ib (before and after cannabis) began at a cycle power load of 30 watts. This load was increased by 30 watts at three-minute intervals to the subject's maximal performance. In tests IIa and IIb subjects cycled 10 kilometers at a speed and in the manner of their choice against a flywheel load of one kilogram. Inspired ventilation, breathing frequency, heart rate, expired air composition, and pedal rate were monitored continuously during all tests. A second series of tests were carried out in the field situation with the Monark ergometer. I installed the machine in our yard to reduce the effects of a long journey to the city before testing and to facilitate increased numbers of tests on alternative days. Six subjects were presented with the task of riding a total of 50 kilometers on two successive days at the speed and in the manner of their choice against a flywheel load of one kilogram. Three subjects smoked one gram of cannabis before the test on day one and none on day two. The process was reversed with the other three subjects. Another six subjects were asked to complete the test only once. Three of these smoked cannabis before the test, and three had none. Pedal rate, distance, and time were monitored every 30 seconds during 14 of the 18 tests. In 4 tests they were monitored every 5 minutes. The exercise tests were analyzed to determine heart rate at specified oxygen consumptions, ventilation at specified oxygen consumptions, tidal volume (size of each breath), and maximum oxygen consumption achieved. Results indicate effects of smoking cannabis on oxygen consumption during exercise, on resting heart rate, on submaximal heart rate during exercise (heart rate up to the point of maximum work output), on submaximal ventilation, on tidal volume, on maximal exercise, and on oxygen intake.

[13] An exchange and social network summary was prepared from the daily activity episode summaries and the weekly interviews acquired in research households. It includes information on place of activities, persons met, purpose of meeting, nature of relationship, and exchanges of goods and services. Special subject interviews on cannabis and stream-of-consciousness tests were analyzed for specific classes of response. These were categorized and compared with those reported in the literature on subjective effects of cannabis.

We reviewed the entire corpus of visual/audiovisual records and selected comparable, clear sequences for analysis. Three assistants and I applied analytical operations to the sample sequences (outlined in Harris's *The nature of cultural things* 1964) to relate activity to effects in the environment and to determine the number and sequence of behaviors in various activities. We also applied techniques (Schaeffer 1970) to determine the organization and structure of behavior during work and social interaction. Patterns of behavior before and after smoking cannabis were then compared.

Another research assistant carried out microanalyses of rhythmicity in movement using several sample sequences from the videotapes. He marked onsets and endings of movements in each of six variable body parts to the one-tenth of a second for participants in the sequences, then compared rhythmic patterns in movement before, during, and after smoking cannabis.

Information gathered with the Kofrani-Michaelis[14] respirometer was analyzed on the Lloyd-Haldane apparatus to determine oxygen and carbondioxide content in expired air during activity before and after smoking cannabis.

RESEARCH FINDINGS ON CANNABIS SMOKING DURING AGRICULTURAL WORK: CASE STUDIES

Findings during daily coverage in sample research households can be clarified in four brief case studies. The first of these studies demonstrate effects of moderate use of cannabis on the rate and organization of movement and associated energy requirements during work: effects of heavy use are discussed in the second study and individual variations in effects are the subject of the final two very brief studies.

CASE STUDY I. Ethel and John Ellis (34 and 40 years old respectively) and their seven children occupy research household 01. They own 9 acres

---

[14] The Kofrani-Michaelis device consists of a dry gas meter for measuring the total volume of expired air during any type of activity. It is connected to an aliquoting device containing a 100-ml butyl rubber bag which continuously removes samples of each breath of expired air. Rubber bladders are employed to retain samples of the air for analysis. The Lloyd analyzer is constructed so that materials absorb first the oxygen and then the carbon dioxide in the air sample. The amount of each absorbed can be measured precisely to determine by extrapolation the energy used when the sample was collected.

of land purchased in bits and pieces since 1963. In 1970 Mr. Ellis worked 190 days in own account farming. He cultivated two $1/2$-acre carrot crops, $1/2$ acre of red peas, $1/2$ acre of congo peas, and maintained standing crops (coffee, cocoa, pimento, bananas, breadfruit, coconut, citrus, avocado, yams, etc.) on another 3 acres. The rest of his land lay in ruinate.

Mr. Ellis worked an additional 41 days on the road and 30 days as a wage laborer on neighboring farms. He also sold sno-cones during Christmas and other holidays and worked as a house painter when jobs were available. Mrs. Ellis marketed the household crops weekly throughout the year. All household members broke rock to sell to road construction crews.

The use of *ganja* in the Ellis household is limited by its cost and the risks of cultivation. Although Mr. Ellis holds certain negative ideas concerning the use of *ganja*, it is, nevertheless, a common household item. At certain times of the year (when his small crop is reaped between August and December) Mr. Ellis smokes as often as three times a day — once when he awakes at 6:30 AM, again before lunch at 11:30 AM, and finally before dinner between 3:00 and 5:00 PM. His usual dose is .8 grams. The *ganja* he prefers has a Delta 9-THC content of between 2.6 and 3.0.[15] He and his family also prepare tea and rum tonic mixtures from cannabis roots and green leaves to "keep away sickness."

Between January and August, when his own crop is gone, he smokes perhaps two or three times a week. During this period he shuns daily use, rationalizing that "If you smoke it too much, it spoils you, you become like a Rasta man, ignorant and violent."

During research with Mr. Ellis I observed him smoking *ganja* many times in the fields. He only indulged when alone or among trusted friends — never in public. The effects on his work patterns can be seen in a well documented example: on April 20, 1971, he forked by hand a piece of land in preparation for sowing carrots and turnips. Beginning at 8:15 AM he worked for 60 minutes without rest. Analyses of videotape segments indicate that he averaged 31 major episode movements per minute. He covered 393 square feet or 6.55 square feet per minute. At 9:15 he sat and smoked .91 grams of cannabis with a Delta 9-THC content of 3.0. He worked again at 9:25 AM and continued for 77 minutes until 10:42. He completed an average of 36 major episode movements per minute. He forked 200 square feet of 2.6 square feet per minute. (That is, he covered considerably less space with more major movements per time

---

[15] In all such statements the content refers to percent per amount smoked. We also have analyses of Delta-8, CNB, and CBD content of each cannabis sample mentioned in this article.

period after smoking. From 10:42 until 10:49 he rested and smoked one-fourth of a tobacco cigarette. Then between 10:49 and 11:52 (63 minutes) he worked steadily forking 290 square feet or 4.6 square feet per minute. At 11:52 Mr. Ellis smoked one-half cigarette, forked a bit more and relaxed into sleep for 85 minutes. Upon awakening at 1:45 PM he decided to stop work for the day.

A micro-analysis of his movements before, just after, and well after smoking during this work period indicates significant alterations in micro-rhythmicity. In six body parts analyzed separately there are, on the average, 30 percent fewer points of change per second (change from movement to stasis or stasis to movement) after smoking. The number of "configurations" of change in multiple body parts moving together is also strikingly lower after smoking.[16] These findings indicate that after smoking the internal organization of major movements is considerably less complex. We might have expected this finding given the increase in major movements after smoking.

The results of 12 Ellis tests carried out in the field with the Kofrani-Michaelis respirometer and the Lloyd-Haldane apparatus are summarized in Table 6. The data indicate that the number of kilocalories required to complete a task is altered significantly after smoking: for example, Mr. Ellis expends 31,500 kilocalories to weed one acre of cow grass. Before smoking he covers the same space while expending fewer kilocalories.

Table 6. Kofrani-Michaelis tests — Mr. Ellis

Activity	Average kilocalories before cannabis	Average kilocalories after cannabis
Plowing with fork	5724 per square*	7632 per square
Weeding small grass	11983 per acre	15437 per care
Weeding cow grass	27600 per acre	31500 per acre

* A square is 1/10th of an acre. The figures for squares and acres were extrapolated from precise measurements of expenditure in smaller space units.

Questions concerning the relationship between the effects of smoking cannabis on the organization of micro-movements and energy expenditure on the one hand, and food consumption on the other, now become salient.

[16] Body parts often change in concert — that is, the hand, arm, and leg change from movement to stasis at precisely the same moment. We borrow the term "configurations of change" from microanalysts of communicative behavior for these mutual changes.

Summary figures on consumption indicate that Mr. Ellis takes in 1,135,040 calories per year.[17] Monthly variations correlate with variations in total expenditure requirements (1,121,000 kilocalories per year). Weekly and daily figures indicate variations which are usually related to differences in day to day work patterns. Certain of these differences may result from acute and cumulative effects of smoking cannabis.

During the week of 1/18/71, for example, Mr. Ellis weeded his "middle year" congo pea crop. Daily work patterns are similar with regard to activity and space covered per unit of time. Energy expenditure was greater, however, on 1/20/71, the one day in the week on which Mr. Ellis smoked *ganja*. He smoked .6 grams at 8:25 AM and .5 grams at 10:48 AM: Delta 9-THC content was 2.25. Closer analysis shows that he covered the same number of square feet per minute (an average of 11.79 square feet per minute) on all four work days. The day on which cannabis was smoked (1/20/71), however, he expended an average of 1.1 more kilocalories per minute during field work.

A brief analysis of group field labor adds another dimension to a consideration of Ellis' *ganja* smoking pattern. On February 3, 1971, he and eleven other farmers plowed a field together with iron forks. Just after arriving, most men shared some of the *ganja* provided by the host farmer. For a short period (10 to 15 minutes) they "worked like demons," talking and laughing as they moved up the hill, forks pounding the earth in a close, straight line. Then, gradually, a quiet, dogged concentration replaced the gaiety. The sharply lineal work formation changed, as one, then another man dispersed to carry out his task in seeming solitude. The work pace, highly varied at first, became steady during the extended period of concentration and then slackened as evident fatigue set in. A farmer called for more "herb." Skliffs (*ganja* cigars) were rolled and passed and the acute effects began. Again, animation in social concert was followed by concentration, gradual dispersal, and fatigue. The process was repeated twice (a total of four times) during the day. Finally, after a filling lunch served in the field by the hosts' wife and a late afternoon hour of work, the party ended — the happy host satisfied with a "fine piece of forking."

As the behavioral patterns varied in concert among the men throughout the day, one had the impression of togetherness — of social cohesiveness. It was a cohesiveness based on similarities of behavioral patterns in sequence rather than focused social involvement. Ellis, himself, felt the

---

[17] The figures on calories and kilocalories were extrapolated from daily information on consumption and expenditure covering the first 180 days of 1971.

effects: "Relations with other people are better when I smoke," he said, "I don't interrupt nobody... I feel good about everybody."

CASE STUDY II. "Poppy" Silver (age 55 years) heads a second case study household. His companion of 12 years, Miss Amanda, their son, and one of Poppy's young nephews occupy a relatively well-built, well-kept house near the northwest end of the Valley. Poppy's lands include four acres inherited from his father, $1^1/_4$ acre he purchased in 1965, and a rented $^1/_2$ acre. Miss Amanda inherited another $1^3/_4$ acres from her mother. She rents 1 acre and reaps standing crops from several acres of ruinate family land.

Poppy farmed about an acre on his land in 1970. He rented out $2^1/_2$ acres — 1 acre to his first cousin, and $1^1/_2$ acres to a friend. Miss Amanda farmed $1^1/_2$ acres on her own with only occasional help from Poppy: she hired help or worked "partner" days.

Poppy is a specialist in other work activities: he is the most respected village sawyer, does carpentry on occasion, boils sugar in the only remaining private wet-sugar mill in the area, and cooks a fine curry goat for local holiday feasts.

As a heavy *ganja* smoker, Poppy is an interesting subject. He began smoking rather late in life (age 25) among friends and has been a daily user ever since. Occasionally during the past 30 years he has also cultivated and distributed *ganja*. He says he smokes 3, 4, or even 6 or 7 times daily (as much as an ounce a day), with a friend or two. He relates use to work and to intimate social involvements with several smokers. He likes *ganja* because he thinks better, concentrates deeply, enjoys relaxation, and has a feeling of well-being after smoking: his work spirit is enlivened, is stronger and more motivated in both work and play.

My observations concerning dose, frequency of use, and effects provide contrasts to Poppy's account. During the heavy use season, August to December, he smokes $^1/_2$ to 1 ounce daily in 3 to 8 sessions. Between January and August his use is more sporadic. The variations depend to some degree upon the availability of *ganja* and his financial status. *Ganja* becomes scarce toward and during early summer; as the congo pea crop slackens in January, and yams slow by April, income decreases as well. Variations are also related to activity patterns and cumulative effects. When Poppy works steadily for a time at weeding or sawing or when he works at carpentry among friends, he wishes to smoke frequently. Often after two heavy-use days, however, he is extremely tired and depressed; he rests to rejuvenate, usually without a smoke.

Figures on the effects of cannabis on work indicate that Poppy, like

Table 7. Kofrani-Michaelis tests — Mr. Silver*

Activity	Average kilocalories before cannabis		Average kilocalories after cannabis
Weeding bananas	10,923 per acre	1.57	17,107 per acre
Weeding with hoe	10,444 per acre	2.16	22,572 per acre
Plowing with fork	6,966 per acre		7,210 per acre

* To ensure the fact that the alterations were related to cannabis rather than fatigue or other possible factors, we compared many examples of behavior for each subject before and after use in various settings and at various times. All subjects smoked immediately before beginning work during several test days. On other days they began work without smoking. The cannabis patterns were evident no matter what the research schedule.

Mr. Ellis, alters the organization of movements after smoking. Energy expenditure and work patterns related to these alterations are affected as well (Table 7). In one Kofrani-Michaelis test in which he weeded small grass with a machete (first listing in Table 7), for example, Poppy covered 192 square feet in 12 minutes, while expending 48.12 kilocalories.

At this rate he would expend 10,923.24 kilocalories to weed one acre in 45.4 hours. In a comparable cannabis test he weeded 116 square feet in 11 minutes while expending 44.11 kilocalories. At this rate he could cover one acre in 71.1 hours, and would require 17,106.7 kilocalories.

A reduction of the Kofrani figures to percentages is informative. Poppy worked 1.56 times as long to weed an acre of bananas after smoking, and used 1.56 times as many kilocalories. When he weeded mixed grass with a hoe, he worked 2.29 times as long on an acre and required 2.16 times as many kilocalories. In both tests he was working alone.

Videotape analyses of several of Poppy's work sessions in agriculture indicate little variation in numbers of episode movements. His movements are, however, significantly more repetitive after smoking cannabis.

Poppy also smokes *ganja* during his non-agricultural activities. As a sawyer he exploits the extended period of concentration associated with cannabis by many workers to produce precise, repetitive movements essential to the task. During carpentry, a task usually carried out with other men, Poppy associates *ganja* use with social cohesiveness. Its effects are similar to those described on cooperation during field work. Just after smoking, animated movement commences followed by concentration on work, periods of immobility and staring, and eventual fatigue. On questioning during periods of quietness and staring, Poppy usually says "feeling good," "feel nice," "just all right."

The effects of cannabis on thought processes may be important in the sawing activity. Poppy learned to respond to a prearranged signal every 15 seconds while sawing with a brief statement concerning thought content. It appears that transcontextual ideas, interspersed among thoughts about the body, the tasks, or the immediate environmental context are significant after smoking. When Poppy saws after smoking *ganja*, 60 to 70 percent of his thoughts relate to the techniques of sawing, the saw itself, getting the job done, or his own body. Fifteen to 20 percent relate to things important in his daily life, e.g., his crops, a carpentry job, or meetings with other people. Abstractions concerning religion, worldly travel, and philosophical ideas occupy 5 to 10 percent of his thoughts. When he saws without *ganja*, his daily life (crops, etc.) assumes importance (60 to 65 percent of his thoughts). The immediate context (weather, trees) occupies 15 to 25 percent of his thoughts, 25 to 35 percent relate to the task at hand and few, if any, are abstract or philosophical.

CASE STUDY III. Two of the research households are single men households. A brief summary of each will serve as an appropriate background for several additional points concerning the effects of cannabis on work in Valley.

Elija Bickman is a 37 year old bachelor who regularly visits his long time lover and their children whom he supports by court decree. He owns 7 acres of inherited land, 3 of which he shares with his brother, Nathaniel. None of the land was under short-term crop cultivation in 1970. Standing crops covered $1^1/_2$ to 2 acres. These included 700 coffee, 100 cocoa, 300 banana, 10 breadfruit, 10 coconut, 4 citrus, 5 avocado, 1 ackee, "plenty" mango, a dozen other trees, and 400 yams. These crops must be weeded two or three times a year. Each weeding takes 90 hours (20–25 days) and requires 31,500 kilocalories.

In January, 1971, Elija received money from his sister in the United States to cultivate congo peas and carrots in anticipation of her return to Valley later in the year. Between January and June he prepared $3/_4$ acre for crops by weeding out cow grass, raking and burning debris, and building contours, for which he hired help several times. He also maintained a wage job as a handy man for a local shop owner during this period.

If the criterion is frequency, Elija is a moderate to heavy *ganja* smoker. He has smoked two to four times a day since he first tried *ganja* 18 years ago: he has "always liked it," he says, because it "make me feel happy, and whatever work I have to do I do it." He prefers to smoke alone during work and leisure time, primarily to remain unknown to the police.

In terms of quantity Elija is only a light to moderate smoker; his skliffs are small (.25 to .30 grams). He inhales deeply but quickly — much like a cigarette smoker in the United States, saying that "If you smoke a lot it ruin your body; it make you look meager; you spend money on weed (cannabis) and have no money to buy food." By titrating in this way, he is able to experience what he considers to be the "good effects" of cannabis frequently while avoiding undesirable effects, e.g., fatigue or hunger.

Our figures on work patterns, energy expenditure, consumption, and states of consciousness indicate that the effects of these smaller doses are insignificant. During seven weeding and forking days in the field, for example, Elija varied very little in either rate of movement or space covered before and after smoking. Summaries of variations in movements show an average minute to minute variation of .0519 before smoking; after smoking the variation is .0551. During weeding before smoking on one sample work day, Elija expended 313 kilocalories per hour; after smoking he expended 330 kilocalories per hour. Total space covered on two weeding days was practically equal (16.0 square feet per minute for 325 minutes on the non-smoking day and 15.4 square feet per minute for 300 minutes on the smoking day).

Comparisons of his thought content before and after smoking also indicate that the effects of small doses of cannabis in the natural setting are negligible (see Table 8).

To determine whether the minimal variations may have been due to the individual rather than the dose, we tested Elija under maximum dose conditions. On 6/10/71 we asked him to perform a repetitive task: then he smoked 1 gram of high quality cannabis (Delta 9-THC content: 2.5) and repeated the same task. The average variation in movements per minute before smoking was .0510. After smoking the average was .0661. During the first 40 minutes the average variation before smoking was

Table 8. Thought content before and after Cannabis

Thought content	Percentage of Response Before smoking	After .2g	After .1g
Philosophy, religion, procreation	0%	0%	4%
Other people, crops, food, the effects of the work	63%	54%	18%
The immediate environment context	13%	15%	20%
The work task itself, e.g., getting done, techniques of the task, effects of work on the body	24%	31%	58%

.0461. In the comparable time period after smoking it was .0794. Elija said he was "really red" from the *ganja*.

In the Kofrani-Michaelis tests he was given ample amounts of cannabis. Variations in kilocalorie expenditures and space covered before and after smoking are significant (see Table 9).

Table 9. Kofrani-Michaelis tests — Mr. Bickman

Activity	Average kilocalories before cannabis	Average Kilocalories after cannabis
Plowing with fork	6,865 per square	10,528 per square
Weeding bananas	14,110 per acre	21,073 per acre

CASE STUDY IV. Virgil Fisher (age 36), also a single man, is Valley's healthy warrior at 70 inches and 182.5 pounds. He has no land holdings and supports himself with day wages from road and field work. Generous friends and members of his family provide him with food and shelter as well.

Since Virgil's father is a local dealer, he has been familiar with *ganja* since childhood. By the time he was 14, he was "tiefing" some for his older friends and taking an occasional puff himself; he liked feeling the "bright spirit" once a day or so. Soon he became a regular smoker — one round a day (two or three smokes). By age 20, he was smoking two to three rounds or more (four to seven times a day). He maintained this pattern until *ganja* became scarce a few years ago. Between January and August in 1970 he consumed two rounds a day in morning, noon, and evening smoking sessions. During the heavy crop season he smoked "all the time — very hard."

Virgil associates three primary effects with cannabis: it helps him work faster; it gives him a big appetite; and it allows him to concentrate. He prefers smoking in solitude for two reasons: "Too many people start foolish argument (i.e. discussions) when they smoke," and "If you share with everybody you don't get enough for yourself." He does have one friend, however, Norman Hadley, a heavy user, with whom he smokes regularly. Hadley supports himself with savings from two years' wages as a ship hand on transatlantic freighters.

During research days in the field, along the road, and in the yard with Virgil, I was impressed with his ability to consume large amounts of cannabis without evident major effects. He did respond with brief periods of talking and laughter just after smoking and he did, on occasion, lapse into sleep two or three hours into the effects. Most of the time, however, he continued his day in the quiet, unobtrusive manner his Valley neighbors have come to expect.

Objective measures suggest interesting conclusions. The two example figures on Table 10 indicate that Virgil's reaction to cannabis with regard to kilocalories expended per unit of space is similar to that of other users.

Table 10. Kofrani-Michaelis tests — V. Fischer

Activity	Average kilocalories before cannabis	Average kilocalories after cannabis
Weeding small grass	20,137 per acre	22,760 per acre
Plowing with fork	4,983 per square	10,528 per square

Variations in movements per minute or in the organization of movements related to cannabis, however, are not evident. In two example comparable tests, the variation per minute is .0584 before smoking and .0601 after smoking — an insignificant difference.

It seems that Virgil either compensates to some degree in his behavior after smoking cannabis, thereby reducing the evident effects on the rate and organization of movement, or that, for some reason, he does not experience strong effects. The first suggestion is probably correct since expected alterations in efforts and associated energy requirements occur in his work after cannabis.

SUMMARY

To summarize tentative conclusions from these case studies: 1. Smoking cannabis is related to effective alterations in the rate and organization of movement and the expenditure of energy.

    a. Behavioral changes related to light or moderate use (defined by either dose or frequency) are not significant in agricultural pursuits over extended time periods.

    b. Behavioral changes related to heavy use are significant in agricultural pursuits over extended time periods.

    c. Alterations related to both moderate and heavy use are appropriate to social cohesiveness during work in group situations.

The four cases were chosen as examples of contrasting types in an attempt to emphasize the importance of understanding contextual phenomena, e.g., frequency, dosage and type of activity during use. As I proceed now to summaries of more inclusive data this emphasis remains crucial.

Data on agricultural pursuits and other activities among ten heavy users, eight moderate users, and twelve light users corroborate the data summarized in the above Conclusion. Total space covered or amount accomplished, in number of plants reaped, is usually reduced per unit of time after smoking. The number of movements per minute is often greater after smoking as is the total number of movements required to complete a given task.

In conjunction these findings may indicate that the user is more intense and concentrated after smoking — that he does a better weeding job, for example, because he enacts sufficient movements to root every weed. Alternatively, the extra movements per time and space unit may be related to cumulative inaccuracies resulting in the need for repetition. Several farmers watching themselves on videotapes commented on the completeness of their work, suggesting that the smoker supports the former view.

Data from the energy metabolism and exercise studies support the field observations. The comparative studies with the Kofrani-Michaelis respirometer and the Lloyd-Haldane apparatus covered 15 activities in 47 tests before, and 29 tests immediately after smoking, and 11 tests 2 to 4 hours after smoking cannabis. In addition, records of ventilation rate were acquired without gas analysis in 63 tests. The 12 subjects included our 4 case study subjects.

Results concerning energy expenditure during agricultural work indicate significant effects. The mean expenditure in a representative sample of heavy activity tests before smoking cannabis was 5.30 kilocalories per kilogram per hour, compared to 4.62 kilocalories per kilogram after smoking. The difference is significant at the 5 percent level. Tests of sitting showed no significant alterations before and after smoking cannabis. The findings, therefore, are probably not related to fundamental changes in metabolic rate but rather to the effort put forth by subjects.

Results from the laboratory exercise studies are as follows:
1. There was no evidence of any effect of smoking cannabis on the relationship between oxygen consumption and work done (i.e., metabolic function was not altered by cannabis).
2. Resting heart rate and sub-maximal heart rates during exercise were normal before smoking cannabis. After smoking both resting and sub-maximal heart rates were increased. Consequently, heart rates were high relative to the work load after smoking cannabis.
3. Sub-maximal ventilation was normal in all but one subject (.04 hyper-

ventilated) and was unaltered by cannabis. The tidal volume was reduced however, during exercise after smoking. The breathing frequency was increased.

4. Maximal ventilation and the maximal oxygen intake achieved were higher before smoking. That is, exercise performance appeared to have been reduced by smoking cannabis.

Results from the field ergometer studies concern movement rate and time of activity. Variations in pedal rate and distance per minute are, on the average, greater after smoking. Average speeds are not altered. In five of the six comparative cases the time required to complete the 50 kilometers was greater after smoking due to longer rest periods.

These energy-exercise results indicate that the primary effects of smoking cannabis are related to alterations in patterns of movement and associated energy requirements during work. Depending upon the task, greater numbers of movements and/or greater variations in numbers of movements per unit of time occur after smoking. These alterations are probably related to alterations in the tidal volume/breathing frequency relationship, especially under maximum work load conditions.[18] It is also remotely possible that the heart rate/stroke volume relationship is altered during work (exercise of any kind) after smoking cannabis and that, as a result, the maximum cardiac output is reduced. However, this could only be demonstrated by direct measurement.

POSSIBLE IMPLICATIONS

The implications of these findings for the total population are difficult to determine given the scope of the present research. Tentative suggestions based on limited results, however, are appropriate.

Men in our sample of 16 Valley households were found to expend an average of 1,116,725 kilocalories per year.[19] Average expenditures per month, week, and day vary in accordance with seasons and the exigencies of farming. Primary tasks requiring considerable kilocalories, e.g., weeding, contouring, and forking, must be completed in limited time periods between January and March, and for some farmers, in September and October. During other months, leisure time activity takes precedence and energy requirements for work decrease.

[18] Increased breathing frequency relative to ventilation achieved after smoking cannabis tends to induce a premature sensation of breathlessness. Maximum oxygen intake is reduced by low ventilation.

[19] These figures were summarized from daily information on consumption and expenditure for 15 men. The data cover the first 180 days in 1971.

Average figures on consumption indicate that men in the sample households are, in general, getting sufficient calories to meet expenditure requirements (1,110,554 calories per year). Both *ganja* smokers and non-smokers are adequately fed.

Average anthropometric values on height, weight, arm circumference, and triceps skinfold thicknesses for a sample of 31 male adults in the community (including men from the sample households) corroborate these findings. They are 66.6 inches, 141.7 pounds, 28.5 centimeters and 5.0 millimeters, respectively.[20] No significant differences appear when averages for heavy smokers and non-smokers are compared.

No superficial signs of specific nutritional deficiencies or of undernutrition were apparent in medical examinations of 31 male residents of Valley. With the exception of one case of hypertension, no serious disease was detected. Hemoglobin levels were adequate: seven protein values (albumin and globulin) fell within normal limits: intestinal parasites, when present, resulted in only slight infections. One may conclude that cannabis, no matter what the frequency or number of years of use, need not affect general physical health.[21]

With regard to energy expenditure related to the exploitation of land resources, the effects of smoking cannabis seem to be somewhat more significant. Members in the 85 Valley households hold a total of 406.5 acres. (The general distribution of these lands by household types can be seen on Table 3.) In ten of these households, lands are cultivated to capacity by men or women who expend the minimum number of kilocalories to exploit maximum land resources. None of the farmers in these households are heavy cannabis smokers; three are light to moderate smokers. Maximum land is exploited in six households with wage labor help; in one of these households the male adult is a heavy *ganja* smoker: he is also a dealer and is able to hire wage laborers to do most of his farming.

In 27 households available lands are partially uncultivated; in fifteen of these the potential farmer is old and/or infirm: two of the farmers are alcoholics who rarely work. Five are heavy ganja smokers; one of these never farms, four farm small acreage and do odd jobs.

In another 48 households adequate lands are unavailable. Men in seven

---

[20] Two points: 1) These figures are in striking similarity to those from other agricultural areas in Jamaica. 2) Figures on consumption for women and children indicate that the seeming health of the adult male farmers is gained at considerable nutritional expense to other household members.

[21] Our field study was part of a collaborative project of the Research Institute for the Study of Man and the University of the West Indies. Detailed psychological, neurological, and physiological studies were carried out on chronic smokers and non-smokers of cannabis. Results indicate no significant long-term effects of cannabis smoking.

of these households expend minimum possible kilocalories per task and experience great blocks of enforced leisure time. Several take odd jobs when possible; twenty-eight potential farmers are old and/or infirm; three of the women cannot maintain their acreage alone: two men are alcoholics; one farmer is also a butcher. Seven households are headed by heavy *ganja* smokers; four of these men prefer odd jobs to farming.

Since these statements are correlative, no firm conclusions concerning relationships between land exploitation patterns and smoking cannabis can be drawn at the present time. I do feel, however, that the data justifies a hypothesis and, possibly, further research. In Valley, heavy use of cannabis seems to alter the relationship between perception and action in such a way that the movement-energy-production pattern link in the agricultural system is altered. The results seems to be appropriate in the social-economic-cultural context. Briefly, a significant number of potential Valley farmers hold small acreage; due to slope degree and soil type some of this land is unsuitable for farming. Of the lands which can be cultivated, some must be left in ruinate for extended periods to avoid severe decline in crop yield. As a result, many farmers cannot farm. In a village in which the ethical code includes hard work and long hours in the fields, such farmers face a dilemma. They can leave the area to search for work elsewhere and some do. They can complete their field work quickly and maintain odd jobs in their spare time — a rare possibility due to the scarcity of such jobs. Or, they can work longer hours in the field and expend more kilocalories than would be necessary in the Valley context to adequately exploit available land. While doing so they can maintain a subjective impression of enhanced physical effort and capacity for work. The heavy use of cannabis during agricultural pursuits may be related to this alternative.

Lest this tentative conclusion be misunderstood as a suggestion that a direct and constant relationship exists between the heavy use of cannabis and decreased production, a word of caution is in order. The interpretation and exploitation of the effects of cannabis in Valley are systemic. They cannot be analyzed in proper perspective separately from the phenomena among which they occur and to which they are intricately related. Given another set of contextual phenomena one could expect different conclusions concerning their significance.

Two examples clarify this point. As mentioned above, the farmers with whom we worked, insist that cannabis-induced alterations in perception and action are associated with quality work. One weeds more completely or forks better, they say, after smoking cannabis. In Valley this improvement, if, indeed, it occurs with cannabis use, is achieved at an expense of time, space, and energy. Unfortunately, results are not worth the price. The terrain, soil, and climate are such that a partially clean weeding or chunk-dirt fork job are no less advantageous than clean weeding or fine-dirt forking. Crop yield and/or quality are about the same either way. One can well imagine a situation, however, in which alterations in focused energy and thought processes related to smoking cannabis may well pay off — a situation in which population pressures exist, available land is minimal, and soil, terrain, and climate are such that crop quality and yield are considerably increased by careful, concentrated farming.

Secondly, cannabis-induced alterations in perception and action may well be associated with increased production during work in other than farming activity. I am at present analyzing videotapes of cannabis users in sugar plantation areas in Jamaica.[22] I may find that cane loaders exploit rapid movements after smoking cannabis to accomplish more in, say, number of canes loaded per given time period.

CONCLUSIONS

An extensive literature indicates that psychoactive preparations of cannabis affect primary centers of thought, perception, and emotion. As a result the users' frame of reference when he is "high" for seeing, thinking, and acting in a psychological-social-economic-cultural context is altered.

An important problem related to this conclusion concerns the significance of cannabis-induced alterations to individual users as members of psychological-social-economic-cultural systems. A specific research question is implied by this problem: How are processes in relationships among individuals and between individuals and material elements in the environment altered when cannabis is in use? What are the consequences of these alterations in an ever broader systemic context?

Our specific concern in the present paper is the relationship between cannabis smoking and work in agriculture. Tentative results are based on analyses of detailed written observations, 200 segments of videotape, 150 tests with metabolic research equipment, laboratory exercise tests, and interviews.

Intensive data on 30 smokers indicates that the use of cannabis is related to effective alterations in the rate and organization of movement and the expenditure of energy during work. Most smokers enact more movements per minute — often with greater variation — and expend more

[22] These tapes were produced by Melanie Dreher, a member of the Research Institute for the Study of Man project, during recent field studies in Jamaica.

kilocalories per unit of space immediately after use. Between 20 and 40 minutes into the effects of cannabis the alterations decrease and patterns of behavior appear to be normal. Between 80 and 140 minutes after use, feelings of fatigue are often expressed in movements. Thereafter, the effects are no longer evident.

These effects depend to some degree on dosage, frequency, psychological set, and the situational context. The behavior stream is hardly altered when the dose is small. Infrequent use results in alterations seemingly irrelevant to the user's position in the larger socioeconomic context. Effects can be consciously reversed to some degree even after relatively heavy doses. They are greater, on the other hand, when the user wishes to exploit them. Varying elements in the environment mediate behavioral alterations. Weather, soil quality, and plant type, for example, must be considered in relation to the effects of cannabis.

The implications of these findings are difficult to determine without conclusive evidence based on analyses of a larger number of individuals and without extensive information on the social-economic-cultural context of use. Our hypothesis, however, is that cannabis use is subtly related to population, land, and economic pressures in Valley. To oversimplify: Land resources are relatively scarce. The topography is not conducive to cultivation. Average farms are small. Common agricultural products in the area do not bring high market profits. A population decrease has ended due to international pressures against migration and the difficulties of city life. Two results are particularly significant to our concern: (1) Valley inhabitants have a vested interest in decreasing total cultivated acreage and consolidating production. (2) Social cohesiveness among farmers is now more appropriate than rugged competition.

Both results may be related to cannabis smoking patterns. If relationships between cannabis use and alterations in patterns of movement and, consequently, energy expenditure during work discussed in this paper are substantiated, we may suggest a connection between heavy use and decreases in total cultivation in Valley. Preliminary analyses also indicate a connection between cannabis use, cohesion in social and exchange relationships, and cooperative effort during work and leisure time activity. A discussion of these analyses is in preparation.

SUGGESTIONS FOR FUTURE RESEARCH

In Valley we found that cannabis use is related to alterations in the stream of consciousness and in the stream of activity which, in turn, are probably related to alterations in the central nervous system. Though subtle, these alterations seem to be significant in the biological-social-economic-cultural system. To test these findings we suggest multi-disciplinary research. A team of anthropologists will carry out detailed studies in a research community at several levels of inclusiveness: 1. to determine the subjective interpretation of cannabis-induced alterations; 2. to determine cannabis-induced alterations in the stream of activity; 3. to determine the social-economic-cultural context for the use of cannabis; and 4. to determine the implications of use to the user as a member of a population in the defined social-economic-cultural context.

Concurrently, medical researchers, neurologists, and psychologists will carry out detailed studies with selected subjects; 1. to determine the relationship between cannabis use and physical health; 2. to determine alterations in psychological states after smoking cannabis and the relationship between those alterations and cannabis-induced alterations in perception and behavior during daily activity; and 3. to determine the relationship between the direct effects of cannabis in the central nervous system and alterations in the stream of consciousness and/or activity associated with cannabis.

Systems theory will permit the integration of findings and consequent statements concerning the relationship between the use of cannabis and 1. alterations in information processing and organization in the brain; 2. observable alterations in the stream of behavior at several levels of organization; and 3. alterations in the structure and organization of social-economic-cultural institutions in a research community.

REFERENCES

CANADA
    1970 *Interim report of the Commission of Inquiry into the Non-Medical Use of Drugs.* Ottawa: Information Canada.

COMITAS, L.
    1963 *Occupational multiplicity in rural Jamaica.* Washington: Proceedings of the American Ethnological Society.

CONKLIN, H. C.
    1957 *Hanunoo agriculture: a report on an integral system of shifting cultivation in the Philippines.* Rome: Food and Agriculture Organization of the United Nations.

GOODE, E.
    1970 *The marijuana smokers.* New York: Basic Books.
    1971 Ideological factors in the marijuana controversy. *Annals of the New York Academy of Sciences* 191:246–260.

GRINSPOON, L.
   1971   *Marihuana reconsidered.* Cambridge: Harvard University Press.
HARRIS, M.
   1964   *The nature of cultural things.* New York: Random House.
HOLLISTER, L. E.
   1969   Steroids and moods: correlations in schizophrenics and subjects treated with lysergic acid diethylamide (LSD), mescaline, tetrahydrocannabinol, and synhexyl. *Journal of Clinical Pharmacology* 9:24–29.
HOLLISTER, L. E., R. K. RICHARDS, H. K. GILLESPIE
   1968   Comparison of tetrahydrocannabinol and synhexyl in man. *Clinical Pharmacology and Therapeutics* 9:783–791.
ISBELL, H., C. W. GORODETSKY, D. R. JASINSKI, U. CLAUSSEN, F. VON SPULEK, F. KORTE
   1967a Effects of (-)-Delta-9-tetrahydrocannabinol in man. *Psychopharmacologia* 11:184–188. Berlin.
ISBELL, H., C. W. GORODETSKY, D. R. JASINSKI, U. CLAUSSEN, M. HAAGE, H. SIEPER, F. VON SPULEK
   1967b Studies on tetrahydrocannabinol. *Bulletin, Problems of Drug Dependence.* Washington: National Academy of Sciences, Division Medical Science, 4832–4846.
JONES, R. T.
   1971   Tetrahydrocannabinol and the marijuana-induced social "high," on the effects of the mind on marijuana. *Annals of the New York Academy of Sciences* 191:155–165.
MANNO, J., G. R. KIPLINGER, I. F. BENNETT, S. HAYNE, R. B. FORNEY
   1970   Comparative effects of smoking marihuana on motor and mental performance in humans. *Clinical Pharmacology and Therapeutics* 11(6):808–815.
MAYOR'S COMMITTEE ON MARIHUANA
   1944   *The marihuana problem in the City of New York: sociological, medical, psychological, and pharmacological studies.* Lancaster, Pennsylvania: Cattell Press.
MOREAU, J. J. (DE TOURS)
   1845   *Du haschisch et de l'alienation mentale.* Paris.
SCHAEFFER, J.
   1970   "Videotape techniques in anthropology: the collection and analysis of data." Unpublished Ph. D. dissertation. New York: Columbia University.
TART, C. T.
   1970   Marihuana intoxication, common experiences. *Nature* 226(5247): 701–704.
U. S. DEPARTMENT OF HEALTH, EDUCATION AND WELFARE, NATIONAL INSTITUTE OF MENTAL HEALTH
   1971   *Marihuana and health; a report to the Congress from the Secretary.* Washington: U.S. Government Printing Office.
WEIL, A. T., N. E. ZINBERG, J. M. NELSEN
   1968   Clinical and psychological effects of marihuana in man. *Science* 162: 1234–1242.
WORLD HEALTH ORGANIZATION
   1971   *The use of cannabis.* Report No. 478. Geneva: World Health Organization.

Chronic Cannabis Use in Costa Rica:
A Description of Research Objectives

W. E. CARTER and W. J. COGGINS

ABSTRACT

A report on the initial stages of research on chronic cannabis users in Costa Rica. Work on the project began in July, 1973, and is expected to terminate by September, 1975. It will involve in-depth studies of the sociocultural context of cannabis use, pulmonary and visual function studies, neuropsychological studies, and basic biomedical measurements. The format of the research will be explained in detail and preliminary findings discussed. Critical evaluation of the project's design will be welcomed.

In July of 1973, a two year study began on the effect of long-term cannabis use in Costa Rica. Sponsored and funded by the National Institute for Mental Health, the study is being coordinated by the University of Florida and facilitated by both the Costa Rican Ministry of Health and the Social Security Hospital (Hospital Méjico) of San José.

The goal of the research is to obtain in-depth material on the sociocultural context of long-term cannabis use, the effect of such use on interpersonal relations, job performance, motivation, aspirations, career development, and on the biology and psychology of the human organism. No studies are planned on acute effects. Rather, a final sample of approximately 40 heavy,[1] chronic users and 40 carefully matched non-users, will be selected and will be subjected to prolonged, controlled testing and observation in both the sociocultural and biomedical fields to measure the effects of chronic use. To facilitate close matching, initial work will encompass 240 individuals, 80 of whom will be long-term users, and 160 non-users.

Contract No. HSM–42–73–233 (ND).
[1] Heavy use is being defined as daily use, and chronic use as continuous use over at least a 10-year period.

Many ask why such a study should be carried out in Costa Rica. Perhaps the best answer is that, to date, no studies have been made of chronic cannabis use in any part of Latin America (if one excludes Jamaica from that geographical category), and that, during a feasibility study made in three Latin American countries, it was found that the Costa Rican health authorities were the most willing of all to host and support such research. During the past 10 years, cannabis use has spread rapidly through the middle and upper sectors of Costa Rican society, especially among the youth. Conservative estimates are that at least 25% of all university students use the drug, and that its use has become common in junior and senior high schools as well. This rapid diffusion of what was formerly a lower-class trait has greatly concerned Costa Rican authorities and has made them anxious to learn as much as they can both about use in their country and about possible implications for performance and health.

The sanitary code of Costa Rica specifies that all research on drugs be coordinated through the Ministry of Health and requires police and other law enforcement authorities to offer their full cooperation for such research. With the support of the Ministry, legal guarantees have been obtained for each of the researchers and subjects. Prosecution for cannabis production, sale, and possession continues unabated, however. This situation makes research a delicate matter.

Because of widespread police harassment, selection of both the experimental and control groups must be done with great care. To accomplish this, three social anthropologists are working in Costa Rica, gaining initial entry, establishing confidence by looking at non-threatening areas such as socialization of the young, and gradually establishing rapport through the technique of participant observation. These procedures are beginning to provide much contextual material on subject areas such as family, community, associations, and values. These areas are not irrelevant. Without them a full understanding of the function and meaning of cannabis in Costa Rican society will be impossible.

Fifteen months will be devoted to participant observation and interviewing in the natural context of communities and occupational groups. During this period of time, the anthropologists will concentrate on several basic objectives:

1. The collection of data as complete as possible on community life, patterns of interaction, life-crisis rituals, work patterns, daily, weekly and yearly cycles, religious symbols and rituals, economic life, and interaction with neighboring communities, social groups, and work groups.
2. General life history data for all individuals forming part of the original sam-

ple of 240, and in-depth life histories for those selected in the final sample of 80.
3. Genealogical studies of the final sample of 80.
4. The form and context of cannabis use, initiation of the user, self perception of the effect of cannabis, perception of the effect on the part of relatives and associates of the user, function of use, frequency, and dosage.
5. Collection of cannabis samples for laboratory analysis on a bi-monthly basis, in the form in which the drug is commonly consumed.
6. Analysis of market networks, with special emphasis on the role of cannabis in economic exchange. The impact that cannabis purchase makes on family budgets will be given special study, inasmuch as it may be associated with poorer nutrition, clothing, education, or housing for the entire family.
7. In-depth information on family interaction for those 80 individuals constituting the final sample.
8. Controlled comparison of interactional patterns of chronic users with those of carefully matched non-users.

One hypothesis of special interest to the anthropologists is that prolonged cannabis use may be associated with the a-motivational syndrome. Selection of only those cannabis users who are productive and successful could skew the sample by eliminating these who are at the lowest margin of society. In working with life history materials, the anthropologists will search for any contrasts which may exist between the subject and control group in terms of career ambitions as these change over the years. They will also collect information on the way a subject's family, friends, and employers perceive the effect of cannabis on his behavior and aspirations.

Because health, and therefore work habits and ambition, may be so directly affected by diet, during the second year of the research, nutritional studies are planned for all those forming part of the final sample. From the family of each subject and each control, data will be collected for four consecutive days. A daily register of foodstuffs will be compiled, using a combination of direct weighing and measurement of foods in the form in which they are consumed, and supplementing these measurements with information given by the housewife or maid responsible for preparing foods. Controlled comparison will then be made of nutritional patterns in the homes of chronic users and non-users.

Once an initial core of subjects and controls has been identified by the anthropologists, the physicians and psychologists attached to the team will begin medical, biological, and psychological studies. These will focus on the aspects of organ function which are of most concern as possible targets for the harmful effects of chronic cannabis use. The preliminary sample of all male, long-term cannabis users and 160 controls will receive a complete medical history and physical examination. The history will contain questions concerning tobacco, alcohol and other drug use, but will specifically omit questions concerning cannabis use. A medical-mental status and neurological examination will be included in this screening procedure. Finally, a battery of laboratory tests will be performed. These will include:

1. Blood count (hematocrit, hemoglobin, white blood cell count and differential, red blood cell count and red cell indices).
2. Erthrocyte sedimentation rate.
3. Urinalysis (pH, sugar, protein, acetone and specific gravity).
4. Stool — ova, parasite and occult blood.
5. Serological test for syphilis.
6. Two-hour post-prandial blood sugar after injection of 75 gms. of glucose.
7. Blood urea nitrogen.
8. Prothrombin time.
9. Alkaline phosphatase.
10. Serum bilirubin, direct and total.
11. SGOT and SGPT.
12. Serum protein electrophoresis.

Two of the objective and best documented effects of cannabis use are the enlargement of scleral blood vessels and the mild decrease of intraocular pressure. Subjective effects and color awareness are frequently reported, and pupil size has been reported to be both larger and smaller than normal in studies of the immediate effects of marihuana ingested by smoking. To better understand the effects of cannabis on vision, each individual in the original 240 sample will be given a routine test of visual acuity, refraction, slit lamp examination, applanation tonometry, routine funduscopic examination, and a test of color vision using Ishihara plates.

In setting up the final study group of 40 long-term cannabis users and 40 controls, subjects with chronic illness which can be attributed to causes other than cannabis will be excluded. Examples of such subjects will be those with tuberculosis, syphilis, alcoholism, severe infestation with intestinal parasites, or major visual abnormalities. Subjects with relatively minor illnesses or static deficits to which they have compensated well, such as old stable orthopedic deformities without serious locomotor impairment or work handicap, will not necessarily be excluded.

Since there has long been concern about the possible harm to brain function caused by cannabis, special care will be given to an evaluation of those areas measuring some aspect of brain function. Each individual in the original 240 sample will be given a standard "mental status examination" which neurologists and psychologists customarily perform. Individuals with neurological deficits which can be ascribed to other disease processes will be eliminated from the study.

The 80 individuals selected for the final sample, 40 of whom will be chronic cannabis users and 40 non-users, will be subjected to a series of special studies. These will focus on (1) visual function, and neurological response, (2) pulmonary function, (3) sleep electroencepholographic patterns.

The effect of chronic, heavy cannabis use on sight will be probed through a variety of tests, including:

1. Facility for dark adaptation, using the Goldman Weekers adaptometer. This measure gives information about the rate and extent of dark adaptation and the time at which the shift from the photopic to the schotopic system takes place. It is intended to test peripheral visual function.
2. Acuity, using two techniques.
a. Static visual acuity stressed by variation in illumination. Since functional acuity is related to illumination level, stepwise reduction in illumination may differentiate those subjects with sub-clinical impairment.
b. Dynamic acuity, using a target moving at standard rates across a field. Measure would be of the visual angular subtense of groups of letters moving across a field at varying rates. Previous studies indicate that hypoxic stress, for example, can be discriminated by this test.
3. Color balance, using an anomaloscope. The instrument presents a standard color with known hue and saturation. A variable spectral color is provided and the subject is instructed to make a match between this and the standard. The hue and saturation required for the match are an accurately established measure of color, balance and preception.
4. Pupillary response to stepwise reductions in light level, using the Goldman instrument with the addition of an infrared screening television camera and monitor to produce an image on the television screen enlarged sufficiently for photographing with Polaroid equipment for later measurement of pupillary size.

Measurement of the effect of cannabis use on pulmonary function will include the following:

1. Vital capacity.
2. Timed forced expiratory volume.
3. Maximum breathing capacity.
4. Arterial pH, p^{O_2} and p^{CO_2}.
5. Diffusing capacity (CO).
6. Maximum mid-expiratory flow rate.
7. Lung closing volume.

Sleep electroencephalography has demonstrated characteristic shifts in sleep level patterns caused by certain hypnotics and tranquilizers as well as by certain psychiatric disturbances. Previous studies have shown suggestive changes in sleep EEG patterns of short-term cannabis users, but no detailed studies of long-term users have been reported. The sleep EEG may itself serve as a bioassay method for pharmocologic compounds having CNS effects. Because of the many external stimuli which affect sleep patterns in normal man, assessment of changes which can be attributed to a drug effect require control of external stimuli and familiarization of the subjects with the experimental setting. For this reason, each of the chronic users and the matched controls will have eight consecutive nights of EEG recording as outpatients at the Hospital Méjico. The resulting data will be subjected to both visual scanning and computer analysis and will be interfaced with the social, behavioral and other medical data on the sample population.

Supplementing the insights coming from the sleep EEG's will be a battery of neuropsychological tests, designed to detect early evidence of brain damage. Seven of the tests will be essentially culture-free to the extent that they will require a minimum of linguistic or verbal instruction for understanding and response. These will primarily assess attentional, motor and/or somesthetic skills. All seven tests have been widely used in the assessment of brain functions in humans. Five tests will be specifically addressed to delayed memory retrieval (verbal and non-verbal) and intellectual cognitive skills.

All tests will be standardized on a separate subject sample in Costa Rica in the pre-test phase in order to reduce cultural sources of variation or error variance in performance. A tentative selection of these tests has been made contingent upon subsequent developments in Costa Rica. It includes the following:

1. Culture Fair Intelligence Test.[2]

The Culture Fair Intelligence Test, developed by Raymond B. Cattell for use with children and adults, was designed as a measure of general intelligence. In an attempt to make the instrument "culture fair" (i.e. minimally contaminated by differences in culture patterns of motivation, achievement, social status, etc.), Cattell employed nonsense material, presumably universally unfamiliar, as well as some common place material. The test, while heavily concentrated on perception, taps categories such as progressions, analogies and abstract reasoning. A visual mode of stimulus presentation is used with a multiple choice response mode. In general, the major reviews of the instrument raise some doubt as to its universal applicability. However, it has come closer to meeting such standards than any other test which has attempted to cut across cultures. Furthermore, it does appear to be a reasonably good measure of general intelligence. In lieu of a test designed specifically to measure general intelligence within a particular culture, Cattell's test would appear to be an appropriate instrument to employ. Split-half and test-retest reliability coefficients exceed 80 in most samples, and the vitality coefficients exceed 80 in most samples, and the vitality coefficients (i.e. as a measure of general intelligence) have ranged from .56 to .85 with the

[2] R. B. Cattell, Theory of fluid and crystallized intelligence: a critical experiment. *Journal of Educational Psychology*. 1963. 54:1–22.; R. B. Cattell, *Abilities, their structure, growth, and action*. New York: Houghton-Miffin, 1971.

Stanford-Binet, .73 with the Otis Group Intelligence Test, and .84 with the Wechsler-Bellevue.

2. Finger Oscillation Test.[3]

This test constitutes a measure of fine manual ability. The subject is required to depress rapidly a key for 10 seconds using his index finger. A Veeder-Root counter records the frequency with which the key is depressed during the time interval. Four 10-second trials per hand are administered. Scores are summed and averaged over trials for each hand. Difference scores between hands are used to determine the degree of manual laterality.[4]

3. Small Parts Manual Dexterity Test.[5]

This test measures the more refined aspects of motor ability, involving a precise coordination of finger and hand movements, as well as control of arm movements. The subject is required to use a tweezer to pick up small pins, place them in holes, pick up small metal collars and place them over the pins. Scores are computed on the number of pins that are inserted *and* capped during a three-minute interval with each hand. The subject starts with his preferred hand and is allowed to practice before the timed trial begins. The difference score between hands is also used to compute the degree of manual laterality.[6]

4. Halstead Tactual Performance Test.[7]

This task, as modified and administered in the Satz Neuropsychology Laboratory at the University of Florida, is designed to test unilateral tactile learning and central nervous system integrity. It provides a direct measure of the presence or absence of transfer capabilities from the dominant to the nondominant cerebral hemisphere. By eliminating all visual and auditory cues, the patient is required to pick up a specified number of wooden geometric shapes and place them in a formboard in a 15-second interval, using first the preferred hand and then the non-preferred hand. Evidence of the transfer of learning from the dominant cerebral hemisphere to the nondominant cerebral hemisphere is demonstrated by a significant reduction in the time required to perform the task with the non-preferred hand.

5. Finger Localization Test.[8]

This task is composed of three parts which combined measure the subject's ability to integrate and report sensory stimulation. Part I measures unilateral

[3] R. M. Reitan, Certain differential effects of lateralized brain lesions on the Trial-Making Test. *Journal of Nervous and Mental Disorders.* 1959. 129:257–262.
[4] P. Satz, K. Achenbach, and E. Fennell, Correlations between assessed manual laterality and predicted speech laterality in a normal population. *Neuropsychologia*, 1967, 5:295–310.
[5] J. E. Crawford, and D. M. Crawford, *Small Parts Dexterity Test.* 1959. New York: The Psychological Corporation.
[6] Satz, *et al.*, 1967.
[7] R. M. Reitan, *Manual for administration of neuropsychological test batteries for adults and children.* 1964. Indianapolis, Neuropsychological Laboratory, Indiana University Medical Center.
[8] A. L. Benton, Development of finger localization capacity in school children. *Child Development*, 1956. 225–230.

and bilateral differentiation between digits which should be complete in the absence of cortical dysfunction. The fingers of each hand are numbered one through five, beginning with the thumb: stimulation by touching the finger in question with the tip of a pen or pencil, out of the subject's range of vision, is reported by number. Part II requires the subject to identify the finger stimulated by pointing to the same finger represented on a diagram of each hand, Part III requires the subject to identify a letter of the alphabet which is traced on his finger tip. Scores are reported in terms of errors on each part of the task and are combined for total errors in terms of right and left sides.

6. Satz Block Rotation Test.[9]

This is a general screening exam for cortical dysfunction. In Part I the subject is required to rotate designs using a stimulus design composed of two to four red and white blocks. The orientation of the stimulus design is always horizontal and vertical, with the required rotation being a 90 degree turn to the left and to the right. Part I is composed of 16 trials, with the first trial used for demonstration, so that only 15 trials are scored. Part II is composed of one demonstration trial and 7 test trials which are scored. In Part II the stimulus design is always presented at a 45 degree angle to the subject, so that the subject must perform a 90 degree rotation from the 45 degree presentation, both to the left and to the right. Errors are recorded in terms of general, angulation, duplication and time (each trial has a 65 second time limit). These are computed with the subject's age and performance IQ to render a multivariate Z score which demonstrates the presence or absence of cortical dysfunction (Discriminant Function Analysis).

7. Raven's Progressive Matrices.[10]

The task consists of designs which the subject is required to complete using multiple choice options of the design part which best fits. No verbal responses are required. Answers may (1) complete a pattern, (2) complete an analogy, (3) systematically alter a pattern, (4) introduce systematic permutations, or (5) systematically resolve figures into parts. Scores are reported in terms of the number of items correctly solved and may be converted to percentile ranks.

8. Facial Recognition Memory Test (University of Florida modified version, 1971).

The subject is presented with 12 photographs of unfamiliar men and women, which he is asked to study for 45 seconds. At the end of this time period, the photograph is removed and an interpolative task of approximately one and one-half minutes is presented. The subject is then presented with a photograph of 25 pictures of unfamiliar men and women and asked to identify the 12 which appeared in the first photograph. This is a measure of non-verbal memory (short term). Scores are reported in terms of number of photos correctly identified.

---

[9] P. Satz, A block rotation task: the application of multivariate and decision theory analysis for the prediction of organic brain disorder. *Psychological Monographs.* 1966. 80(21): 1–29.
[10] J. C. Raven, *Progressive matrices.* 1960. New York: The Psychological Corporation.

9. Verbal Memory Task.

This will be an analog of the Wechsler Memory Scale,[11] as modified and administered in the Satz Neuropsychology Lab. Two short paragraphs of a narrative nature will be devised by the consulting psychologist in San Jose using material that is culturally homogeneous for the population to be examined. The subject will hear the paragraphs (one at a time) in colloquial Spanish and will be asked to relate to the examiner the content of the passage immediately upon hearing it for the first time. Scores will be based on the number of phrases correctly remembered or approximated for each of the two paragraphs. After a 90-minute delay, the subject will again be asked to repeat to the examiner the content of the two paragraphs which he heard earlier. Thus, two scores will be obtained: one for immediate short-term verbal memory and one for delayed short-term memmory.

10. Visual Reaction Times.[12]

The aim of this task is to measure the duration of attention on the part of the subject. He is required to press a button as soon as a neon lamp in front of him is switched on. A trial period of 10 stimuli will be given, during which the subject will be urged to press the button as rapidly as possible. No further encouragement will be given in the course of the test. The task itself consists of 50 consecutive stimuli presented at irregular intervals, varying between 2 and 5 seconds, without a preceding warning signal. The subject's time until response will be recorded by means of a 1/100 second chronograph, summating automatically the values of the answers. The mean of the 50 trials will denote the reaction time of the subject.

11. Continuous Choice Reaction.[13]

This task is also aimed at measuring the subject's vigilance. He is instructed to press a button, which is held in the subject's hand, each time one particular combination of designs appears on the projection screen in front of him. He is instructed to make no response to any other combinations of designs which are projected. A total of 500 combinations will be presented to the subject, with 170 possibilities for a correct response. There is a 1.5 second time interval between each projection. An error is recorded when the subject presses the button for an incorrect combination but fails to do so within the 1.5 second inter-trial interval. The score for each subject consists of the sum of errors and omissions.

Biomedical and psychological studies, as described above, will not begin for several more months. Data gathering by the social anthropologists has just begun. The first few weeks in the field have produced only superficial impressions on cannabis use in Costa Rica. They have, however, suggested a series of fascinating questions.

---

[11] J. Wechsler, *Wechsler Memory Scale*. 1945. New York: The Psychological Corporation.
[12] E. De Renzi, and P. Faglioni, The comparative efficiency of intelligence and vigilance tests in detecting hemispheric damage. *Cortex*, 1965. 1(4):410–433.
[13] *Ibid.*, 1965.

There seems little doubt that cannabis is widely diffused in the country. It seems to have begun as a lower class phenomenon and quite recently spread into the rest of society. Costa Rica seems to be a major source for distribution throughout the Western hemisphere, and the obtaining of detailed information on the productive and distributional systems seems well within the realm of possibility. Informants report an enormous variance in potency among different types of marihuana peddled on the streets of San Jose. Families of users are often divided, with some individuals abstaining and others using the drug heavily over a long period of time. Even among users, there seems to be no universal pattern. Some use cannabis only during their leisure hours; others for selected work tasks, while still others use it any time it becomes available.

In many ways the Costa Rican situation parallels that found in the U.S. more closely than does that reported from the recent Jamaican study. Cannabis is actively suppressed in Costa Rica today, and the price of the commodity fluctuates wildly in response to the degree of oppression. While the drug is widely diffused, this diffusion still seems to be limited to a minority of the population.

To be successful, the project must overcome continuous obstacles. If it succeeds, it promises to give us important additional insight into the effects of long-term heavy use on sociocultural, biological, and psychological development. Such insight would be a significant step forward.

PART FOUR

Traditional Usage of Other Psychoactive Plants

Man, Culture and Hallucinogens: An Overview

MARLENE DOBKIN DE RIOS

ABSTRACT

This paper, a summary of a monograph prepared for the National Commission on Marihuana and Drug Abuse, on the non-Western use of hallucinatory agents, assembles data on a dozen societies of the world where plant hallucinogens have been central to religious and healing activity. The societies have been chosen with regard to their placement along an evolutionary continuum, as well as the adequacy of available data on drug use. The paper delineates themes common to many drug-using societies, especially insofar as cultural variables such as belief systems, values, expectations and attitudes contribute to the structuring of one of the most subjective experiences available to scientific inquiry.

In recent decades, there has been a resurgent interest in hallucinogenic drugs. In particular, scholars have seen a need to reexamine the anthropological record in order to assess the global significance of drug-induced hallucinatory phenomena. Unlike their scientific colleagues interested in hallucinatory phenomena, anthropologists are less able to design research experiments to measure the effects of cultural variables on drug-induced altered states of consciousness due to the very nature of the fieldwork method. Although engrossed in a natural laboratory study where primitive and peasant peoples of the world utilize plants to induce visionary experience for specific cultural goals, the anthropologist nonetheless can still contribute to a general theory of hallucinations.

This paper will address itself to several topics: first, the important role of cultural variables such as belief systems, attitudes, expectations and values in structuring the patterning of drug-induced hallucinatory experience; second, some common themes linked to traditional societies that use plant hallucinogens. These pandemic themes emerged from a recent report prepared for the National Comission on Marihuana and

Drug Abuse on the non-Western use of hallucinatory agents (Dobkin de Rios 1973a). Finally, in order to obtain a more predictable index of collective visionary experience in diverse societies where plant hallucinogens are used, a model of drug effects is developed to take into account the importance of antecedent cultural variables, first discussed by Wallace (1959).

CULTURAL PATTERNING OF HALLUCINATORY EXPERIENCE

To those involved in studies of drug-induced hallucinations in a Western clinical setting, the idea that hallucinations are culturally patterned may appear to be something of an anomaly. Certainly, even a casual perusal of published drug effects in Western middle-class patients indicates a most idiosyncratic series of reports (cf. Ebin 1961; Aaronson and Osmond 1970). Yet, individuals who are reared in a society where hallucinatory drugs have been used traditionally, enter a drug experience with certain expectations about the content and form of drug-induced visionary experience: this is especially so when specific beliefs are held and the individual's experience is programmed by a skillful shaman or priest.

In this section, I would like to summarize my research on hallucinogenic use in traditional society, as well as my field research in the Peruvian coast, and in the Amazon city of Iquitos where a transitional Indian group used an hallucinogen, *ayahuasca* (containing various *Banisteriopsis* species) in folk healing. I will also focus on a few studies that validate the hypothesis that culture is a determinant of the stereotyping of hallucinatory visons. These expected drug visions have been found among a diverse number of the world's people who have used plants for their unusual properties, as a way to identify the source of bewitchment in illness; to see special divinities; to learn the ways of the animals they hunt; to divine the future; and in general, to place oneself in communication with the supernatural.

The following societies will be discussed to illustrate the production of stereotypic visions among individuals who use hallucinatory plants for cultural goal-oriented behavior: the Siberian reindeer herders, the Shagana-Tsonga of the Transvaal, the Amahuaca of the northwest Amazon, the Mestizos of the north coast of Peru, and the Peruvian rain forest transitional Indians.

Many more can be added to the list, while still others can only be guessed at, because the use of hallucinogens often leaves only a faint tremor in the archeological record (Dobkin de Rios 1973b, 1974). As Blum (1969) has shown in an attempt to utilize the Human Relations Area File (with a sample of 247 societies coded for easy retrieval of pertinent drug information), data on hallucinogenic drugs were both inadequate when available and frequently distorted or unclear. Cultural bias on the part of the Western observer who was often sensitive only to the mind-altering substances of alcohol and tobacco (Janiger and Dobkin de Rios 1973) has led to a real problem in cross-cultural analysis. It is only in recent years that these problems are being overcome, as a series of publications focusing in depth on drug use in traditional non-Western societies are being published (Castaneda 1968, 1971, 1972; Fernandez 1972; Emboden 1972; Dobkin de Rios 1972a, b, c; Furst 1972; Heim and Wasson 1958; Harner 1968, 1973). Moreover, anthropologists are beginning to get their feet wet, so to speak, by trying the plant hallucinogens that their informants speak of, and reporting their own experiences in contrast to those of their subjects (Dobkin de Rios 1972a; Harner 1968). Others like Castaneda have become apprentices to drug-dispensing shamans in a long-term, truly heroic attempt to obtain the insiders' view.

Case Studies of Cultural Patterning of Plant Hallucinatory Phenomena

Looking at a pastoral people first, the Siberian reindeer herdsmen of the Eurasian continent, we find reports of the cultural patterning of visionary experience due to the ingestion of the colorful mushroom, fly agaric (*Amanita muscaria*). Although Russian contact in 1589 drastically altered traditional culture and literally wiped out the use of the fly agaric mushroom (by replacing it with cheap and readily available vodka), some reports have come down, as early as the seventeenth century, which describe the last remains of drug use among these nomadic peoples. R. Gordon Wasson and his wife have written an important book (1957), *Russia, mushrooms and history,* in which they reproduce many of the early reports on the fly agaric. Some of these are summarized below (*Ibid.*: 233–338).

Visionary effects include the production of macropsia or micropsia, which entails seeing objects very large or quite small. Koryak shamans used the plants to communicate with malevolent beings, called *nimvits*. After consuming the plant, the shaman falls into a trance, at which time he enters another world and arranges meetings with dead kinsmen who give him instructions. Another group, the Chukchee, report a series of plant spirits who reside within the plant and tell the ingestor what to do.

The visions are seen to personify the mushroom and the mushroom men who appear are numbered according to the number of plants eaten. The shaman is taken by the arm and accompanied on a voyage through the world, filled with real and unreal forces. These creatures, reported by Bogaras, follow intricate paths and visit places where the dead reside (cited in Wasson and Wasson 1957:276).

The Yurak Samoyed, too, see man-like creatures appear before them when they ingest the fly agaric mushroom. The creatures run quickly along a path set by the sun and the intoxicated person follows closely behind them. To quote one author, Lehtisalo, "along the way the spirits of the fly agaric tell the shaman what he wants to know, e.g., the possibilities of curing a sick person. When they come out into the light again, there is a pole with seven holes and cords. After the magician ties up the spirits, the intoxication leaves him and he awakens. Now he sits down, takes in his hand the symbol of the Pillar of the World, the four-sided staff with seven slanting crosses cut into each side and he sings of what he has seen" (Wasson and Wasson 1957:280).

Moving to the African continent, we find the Shagana-Tsonga of the northern Transvaal, who use a plant hallucinogen, *Datura Fatuosa* to achieve a religious experience during female initiation at puberty. A student of mine, Johnston (1973) has written about a girl's puberty rite in which the plant is administered to young women ceremonially, in order to ensure communication with an ancestor god who grants fertility. Johnston has pointed out how the utilization of the *Datura* plant in the puberty school is culturally patterned in the direction of fertility, and represents an attempt to ensure the attainment of this primary goal. Stereotypic visions as well as auditory hallucinations are important to the young women. Hearing ancestral voices while under the effects of the drug is a cultural goal highlighted during symbolic ceremonial activity.

During the ritual, an initiate lies in a quasi-foetal position on a palm-leaf mat at first, during a dance which simulates childbirth. This is the part of the life cycle emphasized by the puberty school in preparing initiates for marriage. A series of ritual activities ensue prior to the ingestion of the plant which Johnston argues is done to condition the attitudes, expectancies and motivations of the initiates toward achieving certain culturally-valued goals — namely, the fertility god. The plant is administered to the initiates and the female leader officiating suggests to the girls that they will hear the voice of the ancestor god. Drumming and special music follows, while each initiate in turn is wrapped in a multi-colored blanket on the mat. Chanting continues, and the initiates report seeing *mavalavala* — bluish-green colored patterns, which are said to be fantasy journeys. Johnston likens this to a common house snake found in the area, believed to be a reincarnation of the ancestors. This vision is believed to hasten the hearing of the ancestral voices which assure the initiates of fertility.

Turning now to the cultural patterning of drug visions in Peru, I would like to cite two studies of mine, one among a Mestizo agricultural group in the north coast, and another among a transitional Indian group in the Peruvian Amazon city of Iquitos (Dobkin de Rios 1968a, b, 1970a, b, 1972a, c, 1973b). In both areas, plant hallucinogens are used in folk healing. In the north coast of Peru, a mescaline cactus (*Trichocereus pachanoi*), along with various *Datura* plants are used. In the tropical rain forest, *ayahuasca* (various *Banisteriopsis* species) is made into a drink used to heal illness. The plants are not viewed as curative agents, *per se*, in both areas, but rather as important divinatory and revelatory aids. Both coastal and rain forest healers use the mescaline and harmine substances to diagnose the cause of illness set within a magical framework of disease etiology. In the coastal region, healers use the hallucinogenic drink made from the cactus to obtain visions of which remedies, herbs, or pharmaceutical medicines they should prescribe for their patients. Coastal healers report that ritual polished stones, present on their healing table (*mesa*) can assume forms of plants and animal familiars to do their bidding in retribution against the cause of evil responsible for their client's illness. In the rain forest, the plants are used mainly to reveal the agent or person responsible for bewitching the patient before any therapeutic action can be taken.

Cultural stereotypic visions are most complete for the *ayahuasca* materials. Informants report a series of stereotypic visions with great frequency and jungle creatures such as boa constrictors and viperous snakes are said to appear before a man or woman while under the effects of *ayahuasca*. Although some people claim that the plant did not cause any visionary effects, most spoke of river and forest animals that filled their mind's eye. Often, the person responsible for bewitching them would appear in front of them. Others reported a panorama of activity in which a person would express his innermost thoughts toward the patient, such as sexual desire, vengeance or hate. At times, reports appeared of a person manufacturing a medicine which he slipped into a drink at a party, or threw across a doorstep late at night. In all cases, however, these patterned visions had to be interpreted by an experienced *ayahuasca* healer, so that he could lay the blame for the cause of illness definitely at the foot of some evildoer or maleficent spirit. The healer was not believed able to deflect the evil magic or neutralize its effects until it was clearly established what or who was responsible for its origin.

A frequent occurrence would be the appearance of a friend or acquaintance, or perhaps a relative, who might laugh sardonically at the patient. At times, only part of a body would appear in the vision and would later be identified by the healer. Part of the effectiveness of the healer was his omnipotence and the generally held belief that he would be able to return the evil to its sender and cure the person of the powerful magic that was responsible for this illness.

A particularly important stereotypic vision concerned the boa:

... A commonly reported vision is that a very large snake enters the circle around which a person is seated in the jungle or else enters a room where one is taking ayahuasca. If the patient is not frightened by this creature, the snake begins to teach the person his song... A frightening vision is often described in which a boa enters the patient's mouth. Often identified as the *Yacumama* of folklore, these boa constrictors are, in everyday life, enough to cause horror to the most stout-hearted person. Although poisonless, such a creature measures over 25 feet long and one foot wide. Its force is prodigious and people say it can eat animals of great size. If a person is able to remain cool and not panic, this is a sign that he will be cured. As the boa enters one's body, it is a further omen to the man or woman with such expectations that he will be protected by the ayahuasca spirit. (Dobkin de Rios 1972a:120.)

Another rain forest group, the Amahuaca, is reported in a personal narrative of some beauty by a man who was captured by the Indians and eventually became an *ayahuasca*-using shaman (Cordova-Rios 1971). Describing the widespread use of the plant hallucinogen among these semi-nomadic, horticultural and hunting people, Cordova-Rios indicates how cultural antecedent variables played an important role in Amahuaca drug visions. He points out that the Indians used the plant for culturally-specified goals, namely, to obtain insight into the habits and peculiarities of the animals they hunt as well as to facilitate inter-group relations and aid them in achieving political harmony. Poetically, Cordova-Rios gives us a chant used to evoke stereotypic visions, which shows how the Amahuaca used *ayahuasca* "to acquire the stealth of the boa, the sight of the hawk, the acute hearing of the deer, the endurance of the tapir, the strength of the jaguar, and the knowledge and tranquility of the moon" (1971:81).

This brief summary points out that various cultures which have utilized hallucinogenic plants often expect and indeed report hallucinatory visions that have definite cultural tuition, and that these visions, it must be once again stressed, are patterned and stereotypic. One might even state that a study of hallucinogenic use in Western society where so-called idiosyncratic reports occur, would turn up some kind of patterning from multitudinous reports. Grof (1972) has made a first step in this direction in his analysis of LSD intoxication among over 2,000 patients he treated.

Given the occurrence of cultural determinants of the patterning of visionary experience, it is interesting to examine a series of common themes among such drug-using societies.

COMMON THEMES LINKED TO HALLUCINOGENIC PLANT USE IN TRADITIONAL SOCIETY[1]

It is quite possible that the reasons similar themes have emerged among a dozen societies of the world may be due to coincidence. Possibly, diffusion may be at work. A third explanation is that the biological parameters of psychotropic drugs affect man's central nervous system in a similar fashion. This may set the stage for similarities in cultural elaboration of a finite number of symbols.[2] Physiological factors such as increased pulse rate and tachycardia may find their way into a mythopoetic theme of aerial voyage or floating through the air. However, I would choose not to take the simple biochemical reductionist route. Fernandez' (1972: 239) discussion of man's behavior as either instrumental or expressive is pertinent here. While instrumental behavior may change nature, the latter is a reflection of man's inner states which are projected outward onto nature.

Still another explanation is possible and comes from the work of Castaneda. He argues that we are indeed victimized by our culture (in this case the scientific paradigm of what is reality) and in fact, there are other ways of perceiving the world. Perhaps, one might argue, we should be paying more attention to the content of belief systems rather than their structure, in that beliefs concerning paranormal phenomena in Western culture are only just beginning to be amenable to technologically-sophisticated analysis. For example, many would agree that acupuncture achieves healing results, although we have no acceptable explanation within the scientific paradigm for how it operates. Discussions of hallucinogenic drug use as a threshold to paranormal phenomena are beginning to receive serious treatment in the literature (Grof 1972, cited in Long 1973). The years ahead may find verification that indeed primitive man had the inside track in some areas whose present validity is subject to doubt.

[1] Drawing upon my report on the non-Western use of hallucinatory agents, in this section I would like to summarize common themes. The reader is referred to the original document for detailed information and bibliographic references.
[2] A Jungian analysis of archetypes and hallucinogens is beyond the scope of this paper.

A. *Perception of Time and Hallucinogenic Drug Use*

As Eliade (1957:170) has written, one of the major characteristics of the sacred realm in traditional religions deals with man's experiencing of time. Perhaps the circularity and reversible elements of time, in which an eternal mythical present exists which primitive man periodically reintegrated into his religious rites, has been influenced by the use of plant hallucinogens in various societies. One of the foremost characteristics of such drug use entails the perception of time, which slows up almost to an imperceptible flow, or else is experienced indescribably fast (Ludwig 1969:13–14).

B. *Animals and Hallucinogenic Drug Use*

Animals seem to have played a vital role in teaching or revealing to man the properties of plant hallucinogens. Evidence is growing that animals indeed seek out psychotropic experiences (Ron Siegel, U.C.L.A., personal communication). Several societies who use plant hallucinogens have reported learning about drug plants from deer, reindeer or wild boars in their environment. Despite the apparent non-adaptive aspects of such animal behavior, this behavior is widespread. The observation by man of psychotropic drug use in animals is interesting to examine and may point out the antiquity of drug use in human society, since hunters and gatherers may have been the ones to observe animal plant use most carefully and imitate this behavior.

C. *Music and Hallucinogenic Drug Use*

A recurrent theme is the important role of music as an accompaniment to hallucinogenic drug sessions. In some reports, we find that healers or sorcerers claim that their musical productions evoke certain stereotypic visions.

Sometimes the music (i.e., singing, whistling, drumming, etc.) may be viewed as necessary to attain certain cultural goals such as seeing the person responsible for bewitchment, aiding in curing, foreseeing the future, etcetera. Fred Katz, an ethnomusicologist, and I analyzed tropical rain forest music from *ayahuasca* sessions (1971) and found that music can play a crucial role in bridging ordinary and non-ordinary realms of consciousness. The production of acute anxiety often accompanies access to these non-ordinary realms. Since the physiological effects of hallucinogenic plants tend to alter basic structures of perception, music, in a manner of speaking, replaces part of the structure and operates as what we have called a "jungle jim" of the unconscious, providing a series of pathways and banisters implicit in the unconscious structure of music itself (cf. Katz and Dobkin de Rios 1974).

D. *Spiritual Animation of Hallucinogenic Plants*

A common theme linked to hallucinogenic plant use deals with animated spirits of hallucinogenic plants. At times, these spirit animators are seen to be small — miniscule in size. Or else, they may be giant-like. Such visionary experience in psychiatric literature has been given the term micropsia or macropsia. Barber (1970) argues that the near universal reporting of small or very large figures in the wake of LSD-like experience can be related to a physiological phenomena where pupillary activity is altered in complex ways. Thus, we find reports of the *yagé* men, small people of the mushroom, tiny *hekula* spirits, etc. Hallucinogenic substances also seem to enhance visual effects by changing retinal image, permitting the appearance of geometric forms and patterns almost universally reported in the wake of use of LSD-like substances. In effect, these perceptions are the physiological structures in one's own visual system, including lattices, cones, cylinders and other geometrics, now suddenly amenable to observation under the effects of the drug (*Ibid.*:32).

E. *Animal Familiars and Plant Hallucinogens*

Shamanic transformations into animal familiars, aided by potions of hallucinogenic derivation, are common themes in drug-using societies, particularly in the New World. Pitt-Rivers has discussed some Central American beliefs in such spirit familiars and shamanic transformations (1972) which are quite generalizable to the drug experience (Dobkin de Rios 1973a). Where these beliefs exist, we find the shaman certain that he can control and beckon a series of familiars for his own personal use in curing or bewitching. It is possible that themes of shamanic transformation may be related to drug reports when one image often remains in the mind's eye while a second is superimposed upon it. The first then fades away. Such an illusion of man-animal transformation may have given rise to this common theme. The relationship of the shaman to his animal familiar(s) may indicate a mirror into the shaman's psychic need, to have some ontological security to permit him to control the world in which he lives. The shaman's unconscious feelings and needs may have been projected outward to the forces of nature to enable him to believe that his world is understandable and chartered and that he will not founder on its shoals. In this context, belief in spirit helpers stereotypically found in hallucinogenic visions enables man to put on a good face and go about the business of hunting, staying alive, curing illness and incapacitating one's enemies.

F. *Cultural Evolution and Plant Hallucinogens*

We can plot differences in hallucinogenic drug use from simple hunting and gathering societies to those of greater social stratification and complexity. With stratified societies, drug use seems to have been eliminated or in name, at least, removed from widespread use — usurped by specialized segments who controlled drug use as part of their sumptuary laws. Unauthorized drug use under these circumstances may have become a crime against the commonwealth (Harner 1970, personal communication). It may be that man's belief in his ability to bewitch an enemy and cause his death, the heritage of the power of the plant, could be dangerous to members of stratified society. In a state-level society, if a peasant shaman were permitted to continue using drug plants where beliefs existed that he could bewitch a state administrator, legitimate power may have been viewed as in jeopardy. Once usurpation of hallucinogens by higher ranking segments of society occur, we find the quick demise of drug knowledge predictable once cultural change in the form of conquest, colonialism, etc., occurs. Esoteric knowledge may not diffuse to the folk level again from whence it surely originated. It is possible that historical reports of drug use tend to be most complete at societal levels where hallucinogenic plants are in general use rather than among larger, more complex societies where only special castes may have employed the drug for communal or private ends. This problem of elite use of drugs occurred in my study of the Maya (1973b) where the very nature of hieratic structure may have been responsible for our lack of knowledge about Maya drug use until an analysis of their art became the vehicle to speculate on such use.

G. *Paranormal Phenomena and Plant Hallucinogens*

Although a near-universal theme linked to hallucinogenic plant use concerns the power of these plants to bestow divinatory success, there is little within the scientific paradigm to explain this often reported phenomenon. Grof claims to have isolated a brain wave pattern in LSD intoxication that operates as a threshold state to paranormal phenomena (cited in Long 1972); the years ahead should see further investigation of this area. Although there is no specific data on this point, the anthropological record does provide an interesting mainspring for analysis, since one of the principal reasons that shamans use hallucinogenic plants is to predict the future.

H. *Sexual Abstinence, Preparatory Diets, and Plant Hallucinogens*

Sexual activity may be discouraged in drug-using societies in order to canalize libidinal energy toward interior states of contemplation. Perhaps discharge of such sexual energy is viewed as detracting from the drug experience itself. As far as diets are concerned, various drug-using societies are concerned about food ingested prior to hallucinogenic experiences, perhaps in an effort to heighten the effects of the drug. The main effect of both sexual restraint and particular diets and food taboos, at another level, however, seems to be to shroud the actual experience in an aura of the unusual, the special, the non-ordinary. Thus, when the initiate or shaman comes to the experience, his expectations of entry into distinctive realms of consciousness is high, and he is, in effect, psychologically as well as physically prepared to encounter the experiences shortly to unfold.

Comments

Although the above makes no pretense to be an exhaustive list of hallucinogenic themes, it should serve to make generally clear to the anthropologist interested in recording hallucinogenic drug use in non-Western society certain themes that might be pursued.

AN ANTHROPOLOGICAL SCHEMA OF DRUG-INDUCED HALLUCINATIONS

As many writers since mid-century have pointed out, the ingestion of a plant hallucinogen is, in itself, hardly responsible for the ensuing drug effect. Since early reliable studies of hallucinogens, we know that the actual drug effects are mediated by setting and set, as well as a host of additional factors such as belief systems and values connected to the plant's use. Following Barber's formulation (1970:8), these antecedent variables interact with the consequent relations of the drug. It is only by subsuming the antecedent-consequent relations under general principles which relate to previously established antecedent-consequent relations that one can attempt to predict new or not-yet-verified relations and obtain a useful theory of drug effects.

Certainly, social psychiatrists have, among others, attempted to develop theories of drug-induced hallucinations, taking into account these interacting variables. The anthropologist, however, working in a natural laboratory where hallucinogens are used ritually by shamans, can neither control nor adequately measure dependent variables such as somatic effects, reduced intellectual-motor proficiency, changes in visual perception and other consequent effects. It is in the realm of antecedent variables, a somewhat overlooked area in contemporary theory building, that the anthropologist can indeed contribute. For one thing, as pointed out recently (Dobkin de Rios 1972b), the anthropologist can focus on the corpus of beliefs surrounding the groups' use of hallucinogens, the cognitive system dealing with the belief in the drug's efficacy and utilization of visionary content (especially when such plants are used for healing, witchcraft or religious activity), as well as the shared expectations of members of the community who expect to see certain visions and report them with frequency.

One of the main problems of anthropological theory building in this area of study is the lack of a shared paradigm. Harris (1968) points out that until recently, there was a lack of nomothetic approach in anthropology. In particular, he has lambasted idealistic as opposed to materialistic approaches to the study of man. While a phenomenological approach would view each event as unique, perhaps a cultural materialistic approach should be the umbrella under which theory is to be built in this area. Certainly, the verification in recent years of the hypothesis that culture is a determinant of the patterning of drug-induced visionary experience is an important step in this direction. Even Castaneda's fascinating studies of his apprenticeship to a drug-using Mexican shaman (1968, 1971, 1972) bring forth belief systems (e.g., the ally, the militaristic nature of shamanism) which have near-universal applicability. Anthropologists, whatever their theoretical approach, however, tend to acknowledge the superorganic nature of culture, whereby individuals recruited to a society by dint of birth are socialized in the total life ways of that group and from the beginning of language learning and even earlier acquire social characteristics. In the realm of drug-induced altered states of consciousness, we would be hard put indeed to explain the replication of stereotypic visions without such an overriding paradigm.

The lack of shared paradigm aside, a concatenation schema which looks at the interaction of antecedent and consequent variables can be presented as follows:

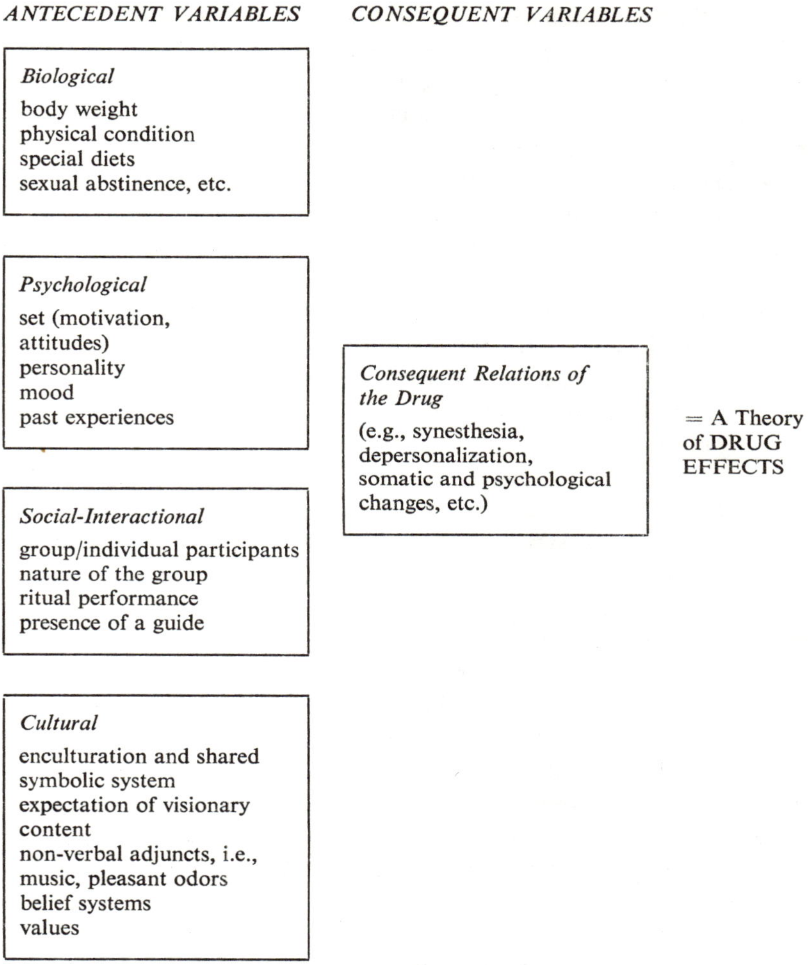

Man, Culture and Hallucinogens: An Overview

ANTECEDENT VARIABLES *CONSEQUENT VARIABLES*

Biological
body weight
physical condition
special diets
sexual abstinence, etc.

Psychological
set (motivation, attitudes)
personality
mood
past experiences

Consequent Relations of the Drug
(e.g., synesthesia, depersonalization, somatic and psychological changes, etc.)

= A Theory of DRUG EFFECTS

Social-Interactional
group/individual participants
nature of the group
ritual performance
presence of a guide

Cultural
enculturation and shared symbolic system
expectation of visionary content
non-verbal adjuncts, i.e., music, pleasant odors
belief systems
values

Figure 1. An anthropological schema of drug-induced hallucinations

Comments

Turning first to antecedent variables, I have set off four general areas, namely the biological, psychological, social-interactional and cultural as a purely heuristic device. Beginning with biological factors such as body weight, physical condition, etc., most shamans conducting drug sessions pay particular attention to these factors prior to drug ingestion. In addition, in many parts of the non-Western world, special diets and sexual abstinence accompany drug ingestion as mentioned above. Psychological factors generally subsumed under the term "set," including personality factors, mood, past experience, attitudes, etc., have been amply discussed in the psychiatric literature. Anthropologists working in field situations have only been able to comment on this in a superficial way due to the fact that they are outsiders. This is not to fault the anthropologist under such circumstances, since far too often, he is present at a drug session by the gracious consent of a shaman, who will stand for little meddling with his ritual activity.

The structure of the group, how this will effect the potentiation of the drug, the relationships of the members present and their role interactions, the ritual performance itself and the presence of a guide skilled in the use of the drug are important factors to consider in any attempt to predict drug effects. Shared enculturation in belief systems is another major area of concern, in that shared cognitive domains are important to the successful guiding of an experience (at least in non-Western cultures).

A shared symbolic system is indeed crucial to permit the guiding of individuals through a particular drug experience in order to achieve culturally-valued goals. Particular expectations of visionary experience are often the *raison d'etre* for non-Western drug experiences and prior socialization in this area is crucial to shamanic success. Non-verbal accompaniments to drug experience are widely utilized in non-Western societies to expand and fully exploit the drug experience. In particular, apart from pleasant odors which accompany many drug sessions, the vital role of music is worth re-emphasizing. The values and belief systems connected to the use of hallucinogens, finally, play an important role in evoking stereotypic visions which are used by different cultures for specific ends.

To be able to predict drug effects in man, we must consider the importance of the antecedent variables. With the "rediscovery" of hallucinogens in post-Industrial society, far too often such antecedent variables have been lost sight of, nonetheless, as anthropological studies of hallucinatory behavior have shown, sociocultural variables play an extraordinarily important role in structuring the form and content of hallucinatory experience. Perhaps the student of hallucinatory behavior might be best advised to pay particular attention to antecedent variables, even when the lack of cultural traditions and expectations are involved, in order to obtain a theory which predicts not only Western man's response to drug-induced altered states of consciousness, but rather, one which takes into account a more generalizable entity, namely all of mankind.

REFERENCES

AARONSON, BERNARD, HUMPHREY OSMOND
 1970 *Psychedelics: the use and implications of hallucinogenic drugs.* New York: Doubleday.

BARBER, THEODORE X.
 1970 *LSD, marihuana, yoga and hypnosis.* Chicago: Aldine.

BLUM, RICHARD, et al.
 1969 *Drugs and society.* 1. Stanford: Jossey-Bass.

CASTANEDA, CARLOS
 1968 *The teachings of Don Juan. A Yaqui way of knowledge.* Berkeley: University of California Press.
 1971 *A separate reality: further conversations with Don Juan.* New York: Simon and Schuster.
 1972 *Journey to Ixtlan.* New York: Simon and Schuster.

CORDOVA-RIOS, MANUEL
 1971 *The wizard of the upper Amazon.* New York: Atheneum.

DOBKIN DE RIOS, MARLENE
 1968a Folk curing with a psychedelic cactus in Northern Peru. *International Journal of Social Psychiatry* 15:23–32.
 1968b *Trichocereus pachanoi* — a mescaline cactus used in folk healing in Peru. *Economic Botany* 22:191–194.
 1970a *Banisteriopsis* used in witchcraft and folk healing in Iquitos, Peru. *Economic Botany* 24:296–300.
 1970b A note on the use of ayahuasca among Mestizo populations in the Peruvian Amazon. *American Anthropologist* 72:1419–1422.
 1972a *Visionary vine: psychedelic healing in the Peruvian Amazon.* San Francisco: Chandler Publishing Company.
 1972b The anthropology of drug-induced altered states of consciousness: some theoretical considerations. *Sociologus* 1:21:147–151.
 1972c "The use of hallucinatory substances in Peruvian Amazonian folk healing." Unpublished Ph.D. dissertation, University of California, Riverside.
 1973a "The non-Western use of hallucinatory agents," in *2nd report of the National Commission on Marihuana and Drug Abuse: Appendix.* Washington, D.C. (in press).
 1973b The influence of psychotropic flora and fauna on Maya religion. *Current Anthropology* (in press).
 1974 "Plant hallucinogens and the religion of the moche — an ancient Peruvian people." Unpublished manuscript.

EBIN, DAVID
 1961 *The drug experience.* New York: Grove Press.

ELIADE, MIRCEA
 1957 *The sacred and the profane: the nature of religion.* New York: Harcourt, Brace and World.

EMBODEN, WILLIAM
 1972 *Narcotic plants.* New York: Macmillan.

FERNANDEZ, JAMES W.
 1972 "Tabernanthe iboga: narcotic ecstasis and the work of the ancestors,"

in *Flesh of the gods: the ritual use of hallucinogens*. Edited by Peter T. Furst. New York: Praeger.

FURST, PETER T., editor
1972   *Flesh of the gods: the ritual use of hallucinogens*. New York: Praeger.

GROF, STANISLAV
1972   Varieties of transpersonal experiences: observations from LSD psychotherapy. *Journal of Transpersonal Psychology* 4:45–80.

HARNER, MICHAEL J.
1968   The sound of rushing water. *Natural History* 78:28–33.
1973   *Hallucinogens and shamanism*. New York: Oxford University Press.

HARRIS, MARVIN
1968   *The rise of anthropological theory*. New York: Thomas Crowell.

HEIM, ROGER, R. G. WASSON
1958   *Les champignons hallucinogènes du Mexiques. Etudes ethnologiques, taxinomiques, biologiques et chimiques*. Archives du Museum National d'Histoire Naturelle, series 7. Paris.

JANIGER, OSCAR, MARLENE DOBKIN DE RIOS
1973   Suggestive hallucinogenic properties of tobacco. *Medical Anthropology Newsletter*. August (in press).

JOHNSTON, THOMAS F.
1973   Datura use in a Tsonga girls' puberty school. *Economic Botany* (in press).

KATZ, FRED, MARLENE DOBKIN DE RIOS
1974   "Music, hallucinogens and the jungle jim of conciousness." Manuscript in preparation.

LONG, JOSEPH K.
1973   *Shamanism: trance, hallucinogens and psychical events*. 9th International Congress of Anthropological and Ethnological Sciences. Chicago (in press).

LUDWIG, ARNOLD M.
1969   "Altered states of consciousness," in *Altered states of consciousness*. Edited by Charles Tart. New York: John Wiley and Sons, Inc.

PITT-RIVERS, JULIAN
1972   "Spiritual power in Central America. The naguals of Chiapas," in *Witchcraft confessions and accusations*. Edited by Mary Douglas. New York: Tavistock Publications.

WALLACE, ANTHONY F. C.
1959   Cultural determinants of response to hallucinatory experience. *AMA Archives of General Psychiatry* 1:58–69.

WASSON, R. G., V. WASSON
1957   *Russia, mushrooms and history*, two volumes. New York: Pantheon.

Peyote and Huichol Worldview: The Structure of a Mystic Vision

BARBARA G. MYERHOFF

ABSTRACT

Huichol worldview, in many respects, constitutes a cultural inflection of what appears to be a highly regular human production: the mystic vision. Among the Huichols, a worldview is elaborated, based on their use of peyote. Cultural expectations for their hallucinogenic experiences combine with a recurrent, possibly pan-cultural mystic vision, which provides the touchstone for their worldview. This worldview emphasizes on overarching a total unity, in human relations, in man's relations to his natural and supernatural world, in his understanding of his history and ultimate destiny. Though distinctively Huichol in flavor, the content and form of the vision is basically familiar from many cultural contexts. The Huichol case offers us a fuller understanding of the mutual influence of culture and hallucinogens, and provides an excellent example of the operation of a hallucinogen in a totally sacred context.

Huichol worldview, in several important features, represents a cultural inflection of what appears to be a highly regular human production: the mystic vision.[1] If dreams and myths are structured, as Freud and Lévi-Strauss have indeed demonstrated, should it come as a surprise to find

[1] Fieldwork on which this article is based was conducted during 1965 and 1966, and was partially funded by a Ford International and Comparative Studies Grant administered through Professor Johannes Wilbert of the University of California, Los Angeles, Latin American Center. My colleague, Professor Peter T. Furst, worked with me in Mexico and collaborated in subsequent interpretations of the data. Many of the Huichol texts were translated by Professors Joseph E. and Barbara Grimes. I acknowledge gratefully this assistance, and especially that of the late Ramón Medina Silva, Huichol *mara'akame*, his wife Guadelupe, and the Huichols who shared so much of their time, their knowledge and their lives. Ramón led the peyote hunt on which Furst and I participated in 1966; to my knowledge this was the first time anthropologists had an opportunity for firsthand observation of this event. Fuller ethnographic description of the Huichols is available in the works of Zingg (1938), Lumholtz (1900, 1902), Myerhoff and Furst (1966), Furst (1967, 1968, 1969, 1971, 1972a, 1972b) and Myerhoff (1970, 1974). Journalist Benítez has written extensive firsthand accounts of the peyote hunt.

that one of the most private, subtle, ineffable, mysterious, and elusive human experiences — the mystic vision — is also structured? Somehow it does, for it is easier by far to deal with cultural regularities in matters of an instrumental nature, pertaining to subsistence and survival, environmental requirements, and similar events where utility and efficiency dictate a fixed number of possible alternatives. In the realms of the imagination of metaphysics, the arts, religion, in areas which are not so clearly rational undertakings, we expect more variation than uniformity. Our explanatory concepts are taxed when we find specific similarities in very different cultural settings where history and diffusion cannot be evoked. We may then fall back on old concepts, such as memory traces, collective-unconscious, instinct, racial memories and the like or on the as-yet incomplete formulations about universal characteristics of the human mind and human nature. Most anthropologists have had to content themselves with descriptions of social processes, short of earlier hopes for the discovery of genuinely lawful regularities. These days, only the intrepid take up problems of psychic unity and common human experience, though these issues, if hazardous, are among the most important and interesting.

From this perspective, recent studies on the relationship between hallucinogenic drugs and religion may be regarded as a significant development in the attempt to enlarge our understanding of universals in human social phenomena. Osmund (1957), Shultes (1963) and Wasson (1969) have demonstrated that the origins and history of religion are inseparable from the use of psychedelic plants. More recently Aaronson and Osmund (1971), Pahnke (1966), Watts (1971), and Dobkin de Rios (1975) have developed typologies which draw our attention to the highly regular factors in psychedelic drug experiences. Watts, Pahnke, and Marsh (1965) have been concerned specifically with isolating the effects of a drug experience which appear to be the same as those associated with the mystical vision, the "Fourth Way," as it is called in the *Mandukya Upanishad*, the way that is not waking dreaming or dreaming sleep; it is "pure unitary consciousness, wherein awareness of the world and of multiplicity is completely obliterated. ... It is One without a second" (*Mandukya Upanished* 1957). In this paper I shall describe the Huichol version of "The Fourth Way."

The Huichols provide a fine example of this experience; more than that, they provide a case in which the mystic vision is extended and elaborated into a worldview, much of which is explicable by reference to their peyote use. That hallucinogenic drugs produce regular experiences is now established: how these Indians use those experiences interests us. It would be an oversimplification to say that peyote directly causes Huichol worldview to be what it is. Peyote use produces the raw material which is built into a system of thought, a *Weltanschauung*. The individual peyote-eater's expectations precede and profoundly influence his perceptions and interpretations of his visions. But these expectations are not random; they are shaped by the regularly recurring results of eating peyote. Thus do culture and individual interlock.

Peyote[2] is the touchstone for the Huichol worldview. In the basic psychedelic experience, we find the source of much of their version of the ideal — in human relations, in man's relations to his natural and supernatural world, in his understanding of his history and ultimate destiny.[3]

THE PEYOTE HUNT[4]

The Huichol Indians realize the climax of their religious life in *Wirikuta*, a high desert plateau several hundred miles from their mountain homeland, conceived of as their sacred land of origin. There is reason to believe that *Wirikuta* represents a historical as well as mythical site of Huichol beginnings.[5] In *Wirikuta*, the First People, quasi-deified ancient ancestors, once dwelled in harmony and freedom as nomadic hunters. According to their traditions, they were driven out, into mortality, into a life of sedentary agriculture in the Sierra Madre Occidental. Yearly, small groups of Huichols, men and women, young and old, are led by a shaman-priest, the *mara'akame*, in a return to *Wirikuta* to hunt peyote.

In order to reenter this sacred land they must be transformed into the deities. The complex cluster of ceremonies and rituals which prepares

---

[2] Peyote, botanically known as *Lophoro Williamsii*, called *hikuri* by the Huichols, is a hallucinogenic cactus which grows in the high central plateau of northern Mexico in the area between the Sierra Madre Oriental and Sierra Madre Occidental.

[3] Huichol worldview may be understood as a combination of several layers of belief: the mystic vision, classical shamanism, and a hunting ideology. Many features typically associated with the latter include the continuity between man and animal; the belief that the animal (deer-peyote) is reborn from its bones; the deer as the *mara'akame*'s familiar spirit; the shamanic flight through dangerous passages to the other world; the shaman's access to direct knowledge of supernatural realism, and so forth. This theme is discussed in more detail in Myerhoff (1974).

[4] The peyote hunt is described here in the ethnographic present. Certainly there are variations between peyote hunts, depending on a great many factors, such as different composition of the party of peyote pilgrims, *mara'akame* leadership, and the like. Nevertheless, there is reason to believe that this is a highly stable event. See for instance, the reports in Lumholtz, Zingg, Furst, and Benítez (1968).

[5] For a detailed treatment of the ethnobotanical, mythical, archeological and cultural historical evidence which supports the interpretation of *Wirikuta* as an historical site of Huichol origins, see Furst and Myerhoff (1966).

them for this return includes a ritual wherein the *mara'akame* dreams their names, the names of the Ancient Ones, and thus determines the pilgrims' godly identities. The peyote hunt pilgrimage is a return to Paradise, for *Wirikuta* is the place where as they say, "All is one, it is a unity, it is ourselves." There, before time began, they "find their lives," and for a while dwell in primordial unity until the *mara'akame* leads them back into ordinary time and life. The climax of the pilgrimage is the hunting of peyote.

For the Huichols, peyote, as a sacred symbol is inseparable from deer and maize.[6] Together, deer, maize and peyote account for the totality of Huichol life and history. The deer is associated with their idealized historical past as nomadic hunters. The maize stands for the life of the present-mundane sedentary, good and beautiful, utilitarian, difficult and demanding. Peyote evokes the timeless, private, purposeless, aesthetic dimension of man's spiritual life, mediating between former and present realities, and providing a sense of being one people despite dramatic changes in their recent history, society and culture. Through the capture of peyote a series of unifications takes place in *Wirikuta*.

The actual pilgrimage lasts several weeks. Each step along the way is highly ritualized and in retracing the steps of the Ancient Ones, the pilgrims or *peyoteros* perform numerous actions attributed to the First People at specific locations, and reenact the feelings and attitudes as well as behaviors of the deities. They rejoice, grieve, celebrate and mourn appropriately as the journey progresses. They do so as a profoundly integrated community. For the hunt to succeed they must pledge their entire loyalty and affection to each other and their *mara'akame*. Unless they are in complete accord, their venture will fail and they will not find the peyote. The journey is very dangerous. One may lose his soul, conceptualized as a fuzzy thread (*kupuri*) which connects each *peyotero* to the deity who gave him life. As the *mara'akame* Ramón Medina Silva stated it, each pilgrim must give his complete heart to him and to the others, for the *mara'akame* to be able to protect them from the danger of soul-loss. Such trust and intensity of affection cannot be sustained in the ordinary social world and when the peyote hunt has ended, it is dissolved. The unity and its dissolution are symbolized by a ritual in which each pilgrim makes a knot in a cord which the *mara'akame* keeps during the journey. When the pilgrimage has been completed, the cord is unknotted and the unity is terminated. In a statement of great sociological acumen, Ramón Medina Silva said,

---

[6] Fuller discussion of the symbolic significance of the deer-maize-peyote complex can be found in Myerhoff (1970).

"It is true that I receive my power from *Tatewarí*, Our Grandfather Fire, but I could not use the power without the complete trust of my peyote comrades."

As the deities, the pilgrims endure many privations, They forego or minimize human physiological needs as much as possible: sleep, sexual relations, excretion, eating and drinking are actually or ritually foresworn during this period, for these are activities of humans not gods.[7] In becoming the gods, the pilgrims are cleansed of their mortality, symbolized by sexual relations. Ritually they confess to all illicit adventures; even children must participate, and even the *mara'akame*. After this confession, they are reborn and renamed and the godly character so received is maintained throughout the pilgrimage.

Sometime before reaching the sacred land, everything is equated with its opposite and reversed. The known world is backwards and upside down[8]: the old man becomes the little child; that which is sad and ugly is spoken of as beautiful and gay; one thanks another by saying "You are welcome," one greets another by turning his back on him and bidding him goodbye. The sun is the moon, the moon the sun. It is said:

When the world ends, it will be like when the names of things are changed, during the peyote hunt. All will be different, the opposite of what it is now. Now there are two eyes in the heavens, *Dios Sol* and *Dios Fuego*. Then, the moon will open his eye and become brighter. The sun will become dimmer. There will be no more difference. No more man and woman. No child and adult. All will change places. Even the *mara'akame* will no longer be separate. That is why there is always a *nunutsi* (Huichol, little baby) when we go to *Wirikuta*. Because the old man the tiny baby, they are the same.

---

[7] Gods are also unmotivated, according to Maslow (1970). In his descriptions of "peak-experiences," that is in states of ecstasy, human beings may become non-striving, non-wishing, asking less for themselves, becoming more unselfish. "We must remember that the gods have been considered generally to have no needs or wants, no deficiencies, no lacks and to be gratified in all things. In this sense, the unmotivated human being becomes more god-like" (1970:176). Such a condition of unselfishness is requisite to the unity among *peyoteros* required for the peyote hunt. The occurrence of a theme of rebirth, as mortals or deities, is reported also in the LSD studies of Grof (1972).

[8] The Huichol theme of opposites fusing in general, and in particular, the old man becoming the child appears in at least one other psychedelically-induced mystic vision: "This theme recurs in a hundred different ways — the inseparable polarity of opposites, or the mutuality and reciprocity of all the possible contents of consciousness ... in this new world the mutuality of things is quite clear at every level. The human face, for example, becomes clear in all of its aspects — the total form together with each single hair and wrinkle. Faces become all ages at once, characteristics that suggest age also suggest youth by implication; the bony structure suggesting the skull evokes instantly the newborn infant" (Watts 1965:40).

These oppositions, like the godly identities, like the hunt of the peyote, are not merely stated, they are enacted. For example, the old man does not gather firewood in *Wirikuta*; it is not fitting work for a baby.

Primeros, those making their first peyote pilgrimage, have their eyes covered on arriving at the periphery of *Wirikuta* so that they will not be blinded by the glory and brilliant light of the sacred land. Only after proper preparation, which involves a kind of baptism with sacred water by the *mara'akame* and a description of what they may expect to see when their eyes are bared to the sight of *Wirikuta*, is it safe for their blindfolds to be removed.

In *Wirikuta*, the party camps and begins to search for the peyote, which is tracked by following his deer tracks. Once sighted, the *mara'akame* stalks the peyote-deer and cautiously, silently drawing near, he slays it with his bow and arrow. Blood gushes upward from it in the form of a rainbow of rays.[9] With his sacred plumes, the *mara'akame* gently strokes the rays back into the body. The *peyoteros* weep with joy at having attained their goal, and with grief at having slain their brother; his "bones," the roots of the peyote plant, will be cut away and saved, to be buried in the brush so that he may be reborn. The peyote is removed from the earth, the resultant cavity surrounded with offerings. Then the cactus is sliced by the *mara'akame* and he gives a segment to each of the peyote companions. Following this, a pilgrim acting as the *mara'akame* assistant, in turn, administers a segment of the peyote to his leader.

This moment marks the fulfilment of the highest goal in Huichol religious life. Unity has been accomplished on every level. The social distinctions among humans have been obliterated: male, female, old, young have been treated and have behaved as if they were the same. The otherwise profound distinctions between *mara'akame* and his followers is deliberately abolished when the former becomes one of them by receiving the peyote from their hands. The separation of the natural and the supernatural order has been overcome, for the *peyoteros* are the deities. The plant and animal realms have likewise merged, as the deer and the peyote are one. And the past and present are fused in the equation of deer-maize with the peyote. All paradoxes, separations and contradictions have been transcended. Opposites are each other. Time itself has been obliterated, for *Wirikuta* is not only the world as it existed before Creation but it is also the world

---

[9] The importance of blinding light, flashing colors, and the general intensification of visual imagery is of course a constant in psychedelic experiences, and indeed the presence of the divine is most commonly signified by dazzling luminosity. Visual imagery is highly stable and fixed sequences occur, according to Kluver (1966) and Marsh (1965), among others.

that will reappear at the end of Time, after this epoch has been completed. Ramón stated this explicitly in saying, "One day all will be as you have seen it there in *Wirikuta*. The First People will come back. The fields will be pure and crystalline... One day the world will end and that beauty will be here again."[10] Thus past and future are the same and the present but a human interlude, atypical and transitory, a mere deviation from the enduring reality represented by *Wirikuta*. This is a foretaste of Paradise and eternity.[11]

Speaking as an outsider, the most encompassing fusion which takes place in *Wirikuta* can be described as what Geertz (1965) has called a merging of "the lived-in order and the dreamed-of order." The attainment of the this dream in reality arouses genuine ecstasy in the *peyoteros*. There are no visions on this occasion, for only a small amount of peyote has been consumed. The rest of the day is spent in gathering more peyote to be eaten later. On the evening following the ritual slaying and token consumption of the first peyote each pilgrim draws into himself, seated with his companions around him before the fire, and eats several segments of his best peyotes. It is generally a quiet affair, and the first release the pilgrims have had from the intense camaraderie and demanding conformity to ritual prescription that have characterized their behavior up to this point. Now each one is alone in his inner world. For it is not the custom, as the Huichols say, to talk of one's visions. Ramón explained it this way:

One eats peyote and sees many things, remembers many things. One remembers everything which one has seen and heard. But one must not talk about it. You keep it in your heart. Only oneself knows it. It is a perfect thing. A personal thing, a very private thing. It is like a secret because others have not heard the

---

[10] The significance of the fields being crystalline may be underscored here. Watts (1970) reminds us that crystal is characteristically used to signify that which is pure, enduring, abstract, and spiritual. Among the Huichols, important ancestors are transformed into rock crystal after life. Crystals stand not only for that which is permanent and lifeless but also signify the enduring unity underlying the multiplicity of shifting forms, again a standard component of mystical and psychedelic visions. Comments Watts, "The cosmos is seen as a multi-dimensional network of crystals, each one containing the reflections of all the others, and the reflections of all the others in those reflections" (1970: 212–213).

[11] Lévi-Strauss (1966) discusses how time and history are altered or abolished in mythology. In myth and ritual, and in what Lévi-Strauss calls "savage thought," man attempts to grasp the world all at once, as a synchronic totality. Savage thought differs from scientific thought in that it does not distinguish the moment of observation from the moment of interpretation. It attempts to integrate synchronic and diachronic events into one system of meaning. This bracketing of the present by the very beginnings and the ultimate end, wherein all is implied, foreshadowed, somehow contained in the present, is exemplified precisely by the Huichol's treatment of time in *Wirikuta*.

same thing, others have not seen the same thing. That is why it is not a good thing to tell it to others.

It is merely said that ordinary people see beautiful lights, lovely vivid shooting colors, little animals and funny creatures. There is no purpose, no message: they are themselves.[12] Each man's experience is his own, and only the vaguest references are made to this part of the ceremony. The visions are always good. The experience can only be happy or even joyous if one has followed the *mara'akame* and done all with a pure heart. There is no nausea, no terror.[13]

Only the *mara'akame* has routinized visions. His are concerned with lessons and messages from *Tatawarí*. He sees *Tatawarí* in the fire and communicates directly with him. Thus the *mara'akame* brings back information from other worlds, information of value and meaning to his people. The Huichol *mara'akame* undertakes a magic flight to help his people understand the regions of the unknown, in classical shamanic fashion. But ordinary folk need not be concerned with such cares; for them peyote brings only extravagant, purposeless beauty and release into the realm of pure aesthetic and spiritual delight.

Peyote visions of ordinary pilgrims are gratuitous. And because peyote produces experiences which are only uniform in being consistently pleasant, it brings to each man who takes it something unpredictable, irregular, spontaneous, and unstructured, though still within safeguards and limits. It permits an experience which is not completely routinized, neither is it dangerous or likely to lead to individual or societal disruption. Peyote constitutes that part of man's life which is private, beautiful, and unique. As such it constitutes that part of religion which has nothing to do with shared sentiments, morals, ethics or dogma. It is within the religious experience but separate from it, and in some philosophical systems, such experiences are considered the most elevated and most intensely spiritual

---

[12] The year before the peyote hunt, in which I participated, before I understood the need for secrecy, Ramón had given me some peyote and watched over me while I had my vision. Afterwards, I attempted to elicit from Ramón an explanation, or interpretation of what I had seen. It took me some time to understand his reluctance as he attempted tactfully to lead me away from questions about meaning or observations about how beautiful it had been. We continued in this fashion for a while until at last he said, "It means itself — no more." I was reminded of this in reading the following from Watts: "The bud has opened and the fresh leaves fan out and curve back with a gesture which is unmistakably communicative but does not say anything except, 'Thus!' And somehow that is quite satisfactory, even startlingly clear. The meaning is transparent..." (1965:33–35).

[13] There is one regular exception to this. When peyote is eaten by one who has not properly prepared himself, truly confessed or gathered "good peyote" under the direction of a *mara'akame*, conventional bad visions are said to occur. This is discussed below.

available to man, providing liberation from structure, within structure, allowing for a voyage into subjectivity, into the unknowable, within a fixed framework. Here one sees peyote as the Huichol provision for that dimension of religious experience which can never be routinized and made altogether public, that sense of awe and wonder, the *mysterium tremendum et fascinans* without which religion is mere ritual and form. It is the ecstatic and enormous moment when the soul departs, flies upward and loses itself in the other reality. The darkness explodes into dancing colors. The Huichol pilgrim knows he has nothing to fear, his flight will not last, he can fling himself into it with immunity. He is safeguarded by the wealth of Huichol tradition, ritual, symbol, and mythology, and the certain knowledge that the *mara'akame* is guarding him, that he is pure in his heart and is one with his comrades. He hears them chatting and singing quietly throughout the night. Gentle laughter and fragments of peyote songs and stories are the ground-base, a cushion on which he can ride, easily wafting upward, then touching down, rising once more. The religious culture of peyote can be thought of as a strong resilient net which allows for greater and greater ascent and freedom.

What does the *peyotero* actually see? Here is the *mara'akame*'s description of an ordinary vision and his contrasting description of his own didactic vision of *Tatawarí*.

And then, when one takes peyote, one looks upward and what does one see? One see darkness. Only darkness. It is very dark, very black. And one feels drunk with the peyote. And when one looks up again it is total darkness except for a little bit of light, a tiny bit of light, brilliant yellow. It comes there, a brilliant yellow. And one looks into the fire. One sits there, looking into the fire which is *Tatewari*. One sees the fire in colors, very many colors, five colors, different colors. The flames divide — it is all brilliant, very brilliant and very beautiful. The beauty is very great, very great. The flames come up, they shoot up, and each flame divides into those colors and each color is multicolored — blue, green, yellow, all those colors. The yellow appears on the tip of the flames as the flame shoots upward, And on the tips you can see little sparks in many colors coming out. And the smoke which rises from the fire, it is also looks more and more yellow, more and more brilliant.

Then one sees the fire, very bright, one sees the offerings there, many arrows with feathers and they are full of color, shimmering, shimmering. That is what one sees.

But the *mara'akame*, what does he see? He sees *Tatewari*, if he is chief of those who go to hunt, the peyote. And he sees the Sun. He sees the *mara'akame* venerating the fire and he hears those prayers. like music. He hears praying and singing.

All this is necessary to understand, to comprehend, to have one's life. This we must do so that we can see what *Tatewarí* lets go from his heart for us. One goes understanding all that which *Tatewarí* has given one. That is when we understand all that, when we find our life over there.

Wirikuta is not less magnificent than the pilgrims had been led to expect in the stories which they had heard throughout their lives. Yet after gathering sufficient peyote to take home and plant in house gardens and use throughout the year, they leave *Wirikuta* precipitously. It is said, "It is dangerous to remain." Not a moment of lingering is permitted and the pilgrims literally run away, following the *mara'akame* beyond the boundaries of the sacred area as speedily as their bundles and baskets of peyote permit. They leave behind their offerings, their deity names, the reversals, their intense companionship and all physical traces and remainders of *Wirikuta*. Spines from cactus, bits of earth, dust, match sticks, cigarette stubs, pieces of food, all that was part of, or was consumed or used in *Wirikuta*, is emptied and scraped and shaken into the fire; the things of the present world and the things of the sacred are kept rigidly apart.[14]

Returning to ordinary reality, the pilgrims are left grief-stricken, exhausted and exhilarated by the experience. An enormous undertaking has been accomplished, they travelled to Paradise, dwelled there as the deities for a moment and returned to mortality. In their lifetimes, they have achieved the most total and complete intention of religion: the experience of entire meaning and coherence in the universe. If, as Bertrand Russell suggested, a minimal definition of religion consists of the relatively modest assertion that God is not mad, the maximum definition of religion might be said to be the insight and knowledge of utter harmony and meaning, the participation in the alleged coherence of the cosmos. It is not merely that the distinction between appearance and reality is blurred; it is that they are the same. It is impossible to find a better way to put it than the Huichol's own description of the peyote hunt and the pilgrimage: "It is one, it is a unity, it is ourselves." Through the *mara'akame* and peyote, the pilgrim has found his place in the divine scheme of things; he is of the divine and the divine is in him.

THE STRUCTURE OF THE MYSTIC VISION AS REVEALED IN *WIRIKUTA*

There is a remarkably large area of agreement among scholars and writers of differing persuasions concerning the nature of the mystical experience. Various terms and interpretations are given of course, but the area of overlap remains relatively stable, whether the phenomenon is called transcen-

---

[14] For a discussion of the significance of observing boundaries between sacred and profane regions, of which this is a clear instance, see Mary Douglas (1966).

dent, peak-experience, poetic vision, ecstatic or mystical; whether it is described in religious or secular terms; whether it is induced by drugs, occurs spontaneously; or is facilitated by techniques which produce biochemical bodily changes (altered respiration, fasting, special diets, flagellation, sensory deprivation, rhythmic behaviors such as drumming, chanting, dancing, physical exercise, and so forth). As previously mentioned, several writers, intrigued by the obvious relationship between religion and psychedelic drugs, have suggested typologies for common constituents of the mystical and the psychedelic experience. I have found several of these to be especially useful: Dobkin de Rios (1975); Pahnke (1966); Watts (1971); Aaronson and Osmund (1971). (Nearly all acknowledge their debt to those giants of religious and mystical phenomenology, William James (1935) and C. G. Jung (1970).) I have drawn upon these schemes selectively in analyzing the Huichol peyote hunt as an excellent example of the mystical experience elaborated into a worldview.

The most significant theme in the peyote hunt is the achievement of total unification, on every level. This sense of unity is the most important characteristic of the mystical experience according to Pahnke (1966). He distinguishes between internal and external unity, the former refers to the loss of the ego or self without a loss of consciousness, and the fading of the sense of the multiplicity of sense impressions. External unity consists of the disappearance of the barriers between self and object.[15] Pahnke puts it as follows:

Another way of expressing this same phenomenon is that the essences of objects are experienced intuitively and felt to be the same at the deepest level. The subject feels a sense of oneness with these objects because he "sees" that at the most basic level all are a part of the same undifferentiated unity. The capsule statement "...all is One" is a good summary of external unity. In the most complete experience, a cosmic dimension is felt, so that the experiencer feels in a deep sense that he is a part of everything that is. (1971: 149).

This most fundamental experience of unity is termed "the panhuman yearning for paradise" by Eliade (1954; 1960). Paradise is the archetype for

---

[15] Watts reminds us that essential to the psychedelic experience is the "vivid realization of the reciprocity of will and world..self and not-self." This puzzles us "from the standpoint of ordinary consciousness: the strange and seemingly unholy conviction that 'I' am God. In Western culture this sensation is seen as the very signature of insanity. But in India it is simply a matter of course that the deepest center of man, *atman*, is the deepest center of the universe, *Brahman*." Watts calls this the mode of inclusive consciousness, in which "the feeling of self is no longer confined to the inside of the skin. Instead, my individual being seems to grow out from the rest of the universe like a hair from a head or a limb from a body, so that my center is also the center of the whole" (1965:63).

the primordial bliss which preceded Creation. The feelings accompanying this condition are characteristically cited as beatitude, peacefulness, bliss, blessedness, a sense of melting and oceanic flowing into the totality.[16] Many explanations have been offered for this yearning toward Paradise. Freudian interpretations conceptualize it as a desire to return to the womb, or as the wish never to have been separated from prenatal dependence. Jungians see it as a form of uroboric incest, a reluctance to individuate and take on the demands of adulthood, for after Creation man must be born, die, suffer, feel pain and confusion. He works, struggles, is vulnerable and ultimately alone, in short, he is mortal. The dangers of attempting to re-enter Eden are couched in many idioms. The Huichol say that one may lose his soul in *Wirikuta*, his *küpuri* may be severed. It may be called the loss of ego, rationality, volition or sanity. The thread of consciousness is felt as fragile in the mystical experience. The awareness of danger and transcience are regularly cited as part of the mystic vision. This is most dramatically portrayed when the *peyoteros* run out of *Wirikuta*, struggling against any temptation to remain or linger inordinately in the sacred realm. This is the explicit recognition that ecstasy cannot be a permanent way of life.

Also regularly mentioned are feelings of brotherly love and camaraderie that are more intense than everyday feelings of friendship and affection. Turner (1969) has suggested that it may be called *communitas;* Buber (1965) referred to it as *Zwischenmenschlichkeit,* the I-Thou intimacy which knows no boundaries, when men stand alongside one another, naked, shorn of the guidelines and expectations of role and persona, a seamless, skinless continuity which is the most intense kind of community conceivable. Watts calls the feelings between those who undertake the mystical voyage together "a love which is distinctly eucharistic, an acceptance of each other's natures from the heights to depths" (1962:51). Among the Huichols this is conceptualized, symbolized and ritualized elaborately and explicitly. The knotted cord binds the *peyoteros* together, the bonds cannot and should not be carried back to regular social life. No mutual expectations are generated among the *peyoteros*, no corporate groups formed on the basis of having shared the journey to *Wirikuta*. Just as the things of the sacred land and the home are separated by leaving behind that which belongs to *Wirikuta*, so are the human connections undone after the peyote hunt. As Durkheim (1915) told us long ago, the sacred by definition is awesome and separate. Pahnke (1966) too says that the drug-induced

---

[16] Images of flowing and blending occur consistently in mystic experiences, as demonstrated by Laski's (1961) content analysis of ecstatic imagery.

mystical experiences he studied were regarded as sacred and not of the everyday realm. The *mara'akame* aids the Huichols in relinquishing ecstasy and shows them that they must leave it behind for another year. *Communitas*, like internal and external unity, is also an experience of wholeness, a form of flowing together, the all is One manifested in social relationships.[17]

Transcendence of time and space is cited by Pahnke (1966) and others as one of the most universal constituents of the mystical experience. Space does not appear to be treated with special significance by the Huichols on the peyote hunt, except that it is clear that the usual spatial categories do not obtain. The entrance to *Wirikuta* is through crashing rocks and is known as the Vagina. Transit through these portals is perilous and shamans must typically pass through such dangerous doorways in the course of their magical flights.[18] Clearly, *Wirikuta* is not in everyday space.

More significant is the notion of time during the peyote hunt. Mythic time prevails. The single moment contains all that was and will yet be, history is obliterated and the present is elongated to imply the beginning and the end of the world. The seamless flow into which the peyote pilgrim slips is eternity and it is a stable feature in mystical visions.

Also significant is the manner in which the individual dwells and behaves and recognizes himself in the sacred realm. Knowledge of this is provided by the ritualization of reversals on the peyote hunt. Several distinct purposes are served by this feature of the pilgrimage. It is not a simple matter to know how to act in Paradise; being named a god is one thing, acting like a god for a while is more difficult. How does one remain in character for an entire day or evening or even for weeks? How does he treat his fellow deities, surely not by following dictates of ordinary norms. The upside-down quality of life in *Wirikuta* serves as a kind of mnemonic, providing a base metaphor by which the pilgrims can coordinate their behaviors and attitudes and understand at every moment exactly what is transpiring. If the sacred realm is just the opposite of the real world, one can picture it in detail, relate to it very concretely and precisely, but not just any metaphor will serve. The utilization of the reversals, as we have seen, is a way of stating that despite appearances, indeed all is One. Not only are differences and multiplicities of form illusory, but things which appear to be the very opposite of each other are shown to be identical, to be completely interdependent, to be part of each other. Subject-object,

---

[17] Turner has considered in detail the matter of *communitas* as part of the religious experience. See especially *The ritual process* (1969).
[18] Furst (1972b) describes the Huichol version of the dangerous passage through the Clashing Clouds. Eliade (1964) elaborates on the significance of the Symplegades theme in shamanic flights.

left-right, male-female, old-young, figure-ground, saint-sinner, police-criminal – all are definable only in terms of each other. Paradoxes are resolved in this experience; formulations which tax the rational mind to its limits are managed comfortably and with lucidity. The deer, peyote, and maize are one. The Holy Trinity in Christian religion is not unfathomable from this perspective. A logic prevails but not the Aristotelian logic which holds that A cannot be B.[19] Eliade has called this the *coincidentia oppositorum* and regards it as the eschatological image *par excellence*. Indeed it occurs in countless societies, in folklore, and in the worlds of dream and imagination, always suggesting the mystery of totality.

The formula *coincidentia oppositorum* is always applied when it is necessary to describe an unimaginable situation either in the Cosmos or in History.... It denotes that Time and History have come to an end — is the lion lying down with the lamb, and the child playing with the snake. Conflicts, that is to say opposites, are abolished; Paradise is regained." (1962:121).

Watts (1971) refers to this feature as awareness of polarity, Pahnke (1966) as paradoxicality; both agree with Eliade that it is essential to the mystical vision.

Ineffability is consistently cited as part of this vision. The experience is essentially non-verbal.[20] In spite of attempts to relate or write about the mystical experience, mystics insist either that words fail to describe it adequately or that the experience is beyond words. "Perhaps," Pahnke suggests, "the reason is an embarrassment with language because of the paradoxical nature of the essential phenomenon" (1971). More than embarrassment, genuine impossibility is the reason for the failure of language according to Jung (1970, first published in 1946). In this discussion of archetypal symbols of wholeness such as the Cross, Jung states:

[The Cross] is given central and supreme importance precisely because it stands for the conjunction of opposites. Naturally the conjunction can only be understood as a paradox, since a union of opposites can be thought of only as their annihilation. Paradox is a characteristic of all transcendental situations because it alone gives adequate expression to their indescribable nature.

Another interpretation for the ineffable nature of the mystic vision may be added to that of paradoxicality. As poets have always known, in order to

[19] Heraclitus rather than Aristotle provides us with the logic in terms of which to conceptualize fusion and unity in his philosophy of universal flow and continuity.
[20] The problem of verbal descriptions of psychedelic experiences, and of all the important events and images of the individual's inner world are treated more fully by Krippner (1971) in his article on "The effects of psychedelic experience on language functioning."

evoke an intense emotional response, effective symbols must be ambiguous to a degree. This has been called the multi-referential feature of symbols by Turner (1967, 1968). The broad spectrum of references embraced by symbols permits one to find in them particulars sufficiently personal to illicit a subjective response. Discussion of ecstatic experiences with full details and specifics would make it clear to those within a mystical community that each person's vision is somewhat distinct. It is more important for each to have his own intense and private experience and at the same time a sense of sharing it with others.[21] Specific language would diminish sense of *communitas* among the Huichol pilgrims, and this is said in so many words by the *mara'akame*. "It is like a secret because others have not heard the same thing, seen the same thing."

Finally one of the recurring explanations of the power of drugs is their ability to loosen social cognitive categories. Conceptualizations are socially provided and given in language. One of the sources of wonder and ecstasy in the mystic experience is the direct perception of the world, without the intervention and precedence of language and interpretation. Huxley (1963) calls this "perceptual innocence"; H. G. Wells spoke of it as providing the Doors in the Wall; for Meister Eckhart it was discovering the *Istigkeit* of objects; Huxley (1954) quotes Goethe on the futile, mediocre and foppish nature of speech. "By contrast, how the gravity of Nature and her silence startle you, when you stand face to face with her, undistracted, before a barren ridge or in the dissolution of ancient hills." We look at the world through a "half opaque medium of concepts, which distorts every given fact into the all too familiar likeness of some generic label or explanatory abstraction." The mystic experience is not verbal precisely because it takes one back behind the word, or more accurately, before the word, to the stunning immediacy of sense data.[22] The Huichol are surely right when they say that it is not good to talk about one's visions.

[21] Krippner (1971) gives an example of the use of language not to describe psychedelic experiences but to signal other users "that one understands." "This language is as much a sign of 'togetherness' and 'belongingness' as it is a device for communicating the content of an experience. Descriptions signify not what the user has 'seen' but that he is a particular kind of person or a fellow member of an important in-group" (1971:230).
[22] In Western tradition, the pre-verbal understanding of the immediacy of sense data is symbolized by the innocence and freshness of the child, whose acquiescence to culturally-provided interpretation is incomplete. The theme appears in the peyote hunt in the form of the presence of the *nunutsi*, and the death of the pilgrims as mortals and rebirth as deities, who like children, are symbols of innocence and non-worldliness. Rites of confession, purification, or atonement usually precede or accompany the shedding of mortality. This ritual among the Huichols has been described in terms of the confession preceding the *peyoteros* and departure of *Wirikuta*.

PEYOTE OUTSIDE OF *WIRIKUTA*

It would be misleading to discuss peyote only in connection with *Wirikuta* for it is a part of ordinary Huichol life as well, and is used on many occasions. One of the most significant features of peyote use among the Huichol is its integration within the society and culture. This is especially relevant from the perspective of contemporary American youth culture in which drug use by comparison is haphazard and promiscuous; with few exceptions, although psychedelic drugs may produce similar visions, these are not integrated into a system of meaning which may be regarded as a worldview.[23]

Among the Huichol, peyote itself is called "very delicate," and generally regarded as sacred. But to be sacred it has to have been gathered in the proper fashion, that is, under the leadership of a *mara'akame* in *Wirikuta*. Peyote purchased in Mexican markets is not sacred, according to Ramón; here are his comments on the matter: "That other peyote, that which one buys, it did not reveal itself in the Huichol manner. One did not hunt it properly, one did not make offerings to it over there [in *Wirikuta*]. That is why it is not good for us." In order to be sure that they always have a supply of peyote from *Wirikuta*, the Huichols plant some which was brought back from the peyote hunt in their gardens. As Ramón says: "When we bring it back we plant it at home, in a little earth. Any amount you bring back you can plant near your house so that it lives. In the dry season one plants it, one waters it a little with care and there it is. Then one has it whenever one wants it."

The references to "that other peyote" which may be purchased, is explained by Huichol ethnobotanical classification which specifies the existence of two kinds of peyote, "good and bad."[24] They are very similar

---

[23] Possible exceptions are found in the philosophical statements about social and psychological implications of psychedelic drugs elaborated by Robert Alpert, Timothy Leary and Ken Kesey. One of the best descriptions of the development of a subculture with at least a nascent worldview based on psychedelic experience is provided in Tom Wolfe's *Electric Kool-Aid acid test* (1969). In Wolfe's interpretation of Kesey and his followers, the number of features which resemble Huichol worldview is striking. The book is a description of an essentially religious pilgrimage inspired by drug-induced visions and the pilgrim's quest for a new way of being. The theme of *communitas* is central, described as "being on the bus." The ineffable nature of the vision is recognized and referred to as "The Unspoken Thing." Imagery of flow and blending abounds. The search for a pattern of totality and unity occurs prominently. Ordinary time is obliterated as "synchronization" replaces the temporal order. The theme of paradoxicality is found here too, in the search for meanings within the meaningless, and patterns within the chaos.

[24] Furst (1972b) has identified bad peyote as *Arioscarpus retusus*, a member of the same cactus subtribe as *Lophoro Williamsii*.

in appearance and only an experienced person, usually a *mara'akame*, can be certain of collecting the good kind. One may accidentally purchase the bad kind, called *tsuwiri*. The results of eating *tsuwiri* are indeed terrible: "If one eats one of those, one goes mad, one goes running into the barrancas, one sees scorpions, serpents, dangerous animals. One is unable to walk, one falls, one often kills oneself in those barrancas, falling off the rocks." (These effects are similar to those attributed to *Datura*.) The hallucinations described due to eating *tsuwiri* are conventional: a common one is the experience of encountering a huge agave in the desert, thinking it is a woman and making love to it.

Eating *tsuwiri* instead of peyote may occur not only as a result of mistaken identity; it may be a supernatural sanction, punishment for going to *Wirikuta* without prior confession. It was said that: "...if one comes there not having spoken of one's life, if one comes not having been cleansed of everything, then this false *hikuri* (peyote) will discover it. It is going to bring out that which is evil in one, that which frightens one. It knows all one's bad thoughts." It is not merely a matter of the *tsuwiri* reading one's thoughts, it is that those who have not confessed honestly or completely will probably behave differently. The pilgrim who knows that he has lied to his companions will eat his peyote in secret "because he does not have good thoughts, he knows he has not spoken honestly with his companions." When such a person hunts for peyote, he will find the *tsuwiri* which "only has the appearance of peyote," and when he returns to his companions after his harrowing visions, the *mara'akame* knows at once what has occurred. The man must then confess and he will be cleansed by the *mara'akame*.

Like maize, peyote can "read one's thoughts" and punish one for being false or evil. The peyote rewards or punishes a man according to his inner state, his moral deserts. The sanction is immediate, just and certain, a most effective regulator of behavior in a small, well-integrated society.

Peyote is eaten or drunk ritually only during dry season ceremonies, but it may be eaten casually at any time of the year. It is also used medicinally for a multitude of problems, eaten to relieve pain, made into a poultice and applied to wounds. It may also be taken for energy, endurance, or courage. In fact it is a panacea.[25] When it is eaten or drunk ritually, it is usually in quantities insufficient to obtain visions, and in this context must be regarded as having the specific symbolic purpose of achieving a kind of communion with the deities.

---

[25] Furst (1972b) reports on recent research which suggests that peyote does indeed exhibit antibiotic activity.

Peyote eating for the purpose of experiencing a vision thus constitutes but one relatively narrow part of a larger set of purposes. It is nonetheless quite an important part, though more for the *mara'akame* than for ordinary folk. When peyote is eaten for visions, non-ritually, it is in a relaxed and convivial atmosphere, much in the manner of the Westerner's use of liquor. In a discussion of this non-ceremonial use of peyote, Ramón said:

Later, during the rest of the year, one eats it when one wants to. If one has planted some peyotes there by one's house, one eats it. One eats it at the ceremonies or one eats it when one wants to. If you want to eat it, you eat it. And if you do not want to eat it, you don't. And if someone asks you for some, if you have it to give, you give it. If you don't, you don't. One eats it like medicine or for whatever purpose one wants to eat it. If one feels weak, if one feels tired, if one feels ill, if one needs strength, then one eats it. That is how it is — if you have it you eat it, if not, then not.

Concerning the first experiences of peyote, which occur early in life, Ramón said the following:

The first time one puts the peyote into one's mouth, one feels it going down into the stomach. It feels very cold, like ice. And the inside of one's mouth becomes dry, very dry. And then it becomes wet, very wet. One has much saliva then. And then, a while later one feels as if one were fainting. The body begins to feel weak, it begins to feel faint. And one begins to yawn, to feel very tired. And after a while one feels very light. One feels sleepy, but he must not go to sleep. He must stay awake to have his visions.

In at least one context peyote may be used prophetically. A very young child may be given a small amount of peyote and if he finds it pleasant tasting this may be a sign that he would make a good *mara'akame*. The interpretation of the taste of peyote is itself an interesting matter; the Huichols insist that peyote is "sweet," "chew it well," they tell each other, "it is sweet, like tortillas." This may be a reversal brought back from *Wirikuta*, for it is clear that though no one vomits from eating peyote, neither is it savored. Huichols eating peyote look like anyone else with a mouth full of peyote: their faces reveal a gamut of grimaces. They suck in their cheeks their eyebrows go up and down in a manner most uncharacteristic of their usual facial composure. The shockingly sour taste of the cactus seems to call forth these reactions despite the official descriptions of peyote as delicious.

Cleansing the peyote is not elaborate; the roots may be cut off and the dust and earth brushed away. The little tufts of hair on the top, called the eyebrows of the peyote (*tsinurawe*) are especially delicate and are eaten always. It is said that different peyotes have different flavors, textures, and colors, and in *Wirikuta*, one of the pleasurable events is comparing peyotes and discussing their aesthetic attributes. Peyotes most valued are those of five segments, five being the Huichol sacred number. In fact, these are often strung together as a necklace and may be used to adorn the deer horns of *Tatawari*. Peyote is often addressed affectionately, called "ti peyote" (our peyote), and even spoken to in baby talk. Often its beauties are likened to states in the growth of maize. "It is new, it is soft like the ripening maize, how fine, how lovely."

The first peyote eaten in *Wirikuta* is touched to the forehead, eyes, breast, voice box, cheeks before being eaten. Other times this is not done. Peyote brought out of *Wirikuta* is carefully packed into baskets in concentric circles from the bottom up, so that it will not be jostled en route, for, as it is said, it is delicate and the trip is long.

Peyote may be eaten fresh, or dried, ground and drunk. It may be taken along on trips and given as a gift to a host, to eat or plant. It is sometimes traded for various items with other Indians, especially the Cora and Tarahumara, who regard Huichol peyote as very desirable. It is always in demand, and its presence is essential throughout the year, since all major religious ceremonies require the presence of peyote, maize and deer meat or blood. The ceremonies constitute an interlocking cycle. The peyote hunt is preceded by the drum and calabash ceremony and followed by the deer hunt; evidently substitutes for deer meat and blood are acceptable, but this is not true for properly gathered peyote.

As an artistic motif, peyote is no less important. As Lumholtz (1900) has shown, peyote is a theme with numerous variations in embroidery and weaving. It provides a key source of inspiration.

CONCLUSIONS

Perhaps in the present context the most significant lesson of the Huichol use of peyote is a fuller understanding of a hallucinogenic drug in a sacred context. Peyote produces certain biochemical changes which are to some degree uniform in their effects. What is done with these effects, what meanings they are given, how they are integrated and eleborated into a context of significance, and coherence and beauty, is what concerns the anthropologist. Simply stated, we see peyote used as a means. Clearly, its effects *per se* are valued but what a relatively small part of the entire picture they are. It would be a profanation to discuss Huichol peyote use in terms of kicks and highs and escape and the other terms which describe the goals of individualistic drug-taking outside of an integrated cultural setting. Peyote is woven into every dimension of Huichol life. It is venerated for its gifts of beauty and pleasure. But this is in reality a Durkheimian kind of projection; it is the Huichol venerating their own customs and traditions, the sense and pattern of a way of life which uses this little plant, this part of its natural environment so wisely and so well.

REFERENCES

AARONSON, BERNARD, HUMPHREY OSMOND, *editors*
    1971 *Psychedelics: The uses and implications of hallucinogenic drugs.* Cambridge: Schenkman.
BENÍTEZ, FERNANDO
    1968 *El la tierra mágica del peyote.* Biblioteca Era. Serie Popular: México.
BUBER, MARTIN
    1965 *Between man and man.* New York: Macmillan Company.
DOBKIN DE RIOS, MARLENE
    1975 "Man, culture and hallucinogens; an overview," in this volume.
DOUGLAS, MARY
    1966 *Purity and danger: an analysis of concepts of pollution and taboo.* London: Penguin.
DURKHEIM, EMILE
    1954 *Elementary forms of religious life.* Translated by J. W. Swain. London: Allen and Unwin. (First published in 1915 as *Les formes élémentaires de la vie religieuse.*)
ELIADE, MIRCEA
    1954 *The myth of the eternal return.* New York: Bollingen (First published in 1949).
    1960 "The yearning for paradise in primitive tradition," in *Myth and mythmaking.* Edited by H. A. Murray. New York: Braziller.
    1962 *The two and the one.* New York: Harper Torchbooks.
    1964 *Shamanism: archaic techniques of ecstasy.* Translated by W. R. Trask. Bollingen Series LXXVI. New York: Pantheon.
FURST, PETER T.
    1967 Huichol conceptions of the soul. *Folklore Americas* 27:39–106.
    1968 The parching of the maize: an essay on the survival of Huichol ritual. *Acta Ethnológica et Linguística* 14. Vienna.
    1969 Ethnographic film: *To Find Our Life: The Peyote Hunt of the Huichols of Mexico.* 16 mm, color and sound, 65 minutes. Distributed by Latin American Center, University of California at Los Angeles.
    1971 *Ariocarpus retusus,* the "false peyote" of Huichol tradition. *Economic Botany* 25 (1):182–187.
    1972a "To find our life: peyote among the Huichol Indians of Mexico," in *Flesh of the gods: the ritual uses of hallucinogens.* New York: Praeger.
FURST, PETER T., *editor*
    1972b *Flesh of the gods: the ritual uses of hallucinogens.* New York: Praeger.
FURST, PETER T., BARBARA G. MYERHOFF
    1966 Myth as history: the jimson weed cycle of the Huichols of Mexico. *Antropologia* 17:3–39.

GEERTZ, CLIFFORD
1965 "Religion as a cultural system," in *Anthropological approaches in the study of religion*. Edited by M. Burton. Association of Social Anthropologists Monographs 3. London: Tavistock.
GROF, STANISLAV
1972 Varieties of transpersonal experience: observations from LSD psychotherapy. *Journal of Transpersonal Psychology* 4:45–80.
HUXLEY, ALDOUS
1963 *The doors of perception and heaven and hell.* New York: Harper-Colophon. (First published in 1954.)
JAMES, WILLIAM
1935 *The varieties of religious experience.* New York: Longmans.
JUNG, CARL G.
1946 *Collected works.* New York: Bollingen.
1970 "Christ, a symbol of the self," in *Personality and religion: the role of religion in personality development*. Edited by William Sadler. New York: Harper and Row. (Abridged from *Collected works*. New York: Bollingen.)
KLUVER, HEINRICH
1966 *Mescal and mechanism of hallucinations.* Chicago: University of Chicago Press.
KRIPPNER, STANLEY
1971 "The effects of psychedelic experience on language functioning," in *Psychedelics: the uses and implications of hallucinogenic drugs*. Edited by Bernard Aaronson and Humphrey Osmond. Cambridge: Schenkman.
LASKI, MARGHANITA
1961 *Ecstasy; a study of some secular and religious experiences.* Bloomington: Indiana University Press.
LÉVI-STRAUSS, CLAUDE
1966 *The savage mind.* Chicago: University of Chicago Press (First published in 1962 as *La pensée sauvage*. Paris: Plon.)
LUMHOLTZ, CARL
1900 *Symbolism of the Huichol Indians.* New York: American Museum of Natural History.
1902 *Unknown Mexico*, volume two. New York: Scribner.
Mandukya Upanishad
1957 New York: Mentor.
MARSH, R. P.
1965 Meaning and the mind-drugs. *ETC* 22:408–430.
MASLOW, ABRAHAM H.
1970 "Religious aspects of peak experiences," in *Personality and religion: the role of religion and personality development*. Edited by William Sadler. New York: Harper and Row. (First published in 1964.)
MYERHOFF, BARBARA G.
1970 The deer-maize-peyote symbol complex among the Huichol Indians of Mexico. *Anthropological Quarterly* 43:64–78.
1974 *Peyote hunt: the religious pilgrimage of the Huichol Indians.* Ithaca: Cornell University Press.

OSMUND, HUMPHREY
   1957   A review of the clinical effects of psychotemimetic agents. *Annals of the New York Academy of Sciences* 66:418–434.
PAHNKE, WALTER N.
   1971   "Drugs in mysticism," in *Psychedelics: the uses and implications of hallucinogenic drugs*. Edited by Bernard Aaronson and Humphrey Osmond. Cambridge: Schenkman. (First published in 1966.)
SCHULTES, R. E.
   1963   Botanical sources of new world narcotics. *Psychedelic Review*.
TURNER, VICTOR
   1967   *The forest of symbols: aspects of Ndembu ritual.* Ithaca: Cornell University Press.
   1968   *The drums of affliction: a study of religious processes among the Ndembu of Zambia.* Oxford: Clarendon and the International African Institute.
   1969   *The ritual process: structure and anti-structure.* Chicago: Aldine.
WASSON, R. G.
   1969   *Soma: divine mushroom of immortality.* New York: Harcourt.
WATTS, ALAN
   1965   *The joyous cosmology: adventures in the chemistry of consciousness.* New York: Vintage. (First published in 1962.)
   1970   *The two hands of God: the myth of polarity.* New York: Collier Books. (First published in 1963.)
   1971   "Psychedelics and religious experience" in *Psychedelics: the uses and implications of hallucinogenic drugs*. Edited by Bernard Aaronson and Humphrey Osmond. Cambridge: Schenkman.
WOLFE, TOM
   1969   *Electric Kool-Aid acid test.* New York: Bantam.
ZINGG, ROBERT M.
   1938   *The Huichols: primitive artists.* New York: Stechert.

Magico-Religious Use of Tobacco among South American Indians

JOHANNES WILBERT

ABSTRACT

Despite the great scholarly attention tobacco has received from a variety of disciplines, no effort has, heretofore, been made to assess its magico-religious significance among South American Indians. The paper examines the prevalence and distribution of techniques of tobacco consumption in indigenous South America (i.e., smoking, drinking, licking, chewing, and snuffing). As a psychotropic agent, tobacco achieved an extensive distribution throughout large parts of the continent. Its use was mainly magico-religious, and only in recent historic times have the manner and ideological foundations of its use shifted increasingly from the magico-religious to the profane.

Few plants have attracted more scholarly attention, or from a greater variety of disciplines, than tobacco. As early as the eighteenth century, Schloezer (1775–1781) suggested that in order to deal adequately with tobacco, its historian had to consider it from religious, therapeutic, medicinal, sociological, economic, commercial and financial points of view. To these Putnam (1938:47–48) added archaeology, philology, linguistics, ethnography, chemistry, and theology. Today, of course, no writer on the subject could afford to ignore the important input of such fields as botany and pharmacology, not to mention geography. Indeed, even this would not exhaust the entire spectrum of professional interest in this most nearly universal of psychodynamic substances employed by man.

The present paper will limit itself to the magico-religious dimension, specifically among South American Indians. Inasmuch as what may appear to the casual observer to be purely medicinal or pharmaceutical use of tobacco more often than not involves a vital magico-religious component (and vice versa), I will also touch occasionally on ethnomedicinal beliefs and practices.

Tobacco (*Nicotiana* spp.) is a native of the New World, derived from a

For Plates, see pp. xxi–xxvii, between pp. 266–267.

variety of different species. Of particular interest to us are the two principal cultivated species — *Nicotiana tabacum* and *N. rustica* — that achieved greater dissemination throughout Indian America as ritual narcostimulants than any of the others. *N. tabacum*, a hybrid formed from *N. tomentosum* and *N. sylvestris*, probably had its origin in the eastern valleys of the Bolivian Andes. It remained closely associated with Arawakan, Cariban, and Tupian tropical forest planters, in the flood plains of the Amazon, in Guayana, and in the West Indies. It may also have spread through portions of coastal Brazil, although like the Brazilian highlands this area of the continent was never typically a part of tobacco dissemination. At the time of European Discovery, the northernmost extension of *Nicotiana tabacum* did not reach beyond the tropical lowlands of Mexico.

By contrast, *Nicotiana rustica*, the hardier of the two cultivated species, diffused far beyond tropical America almost to the very limits of New World agriculture. It was the Indian tobacco of the eastern woodlands of North America, the *piciétl* of the Aztecs, and probably also the *petún* of Brazil. In fact, in its dispersal *Nicotiana rustica* rivalled even maize, and along with such cultigens as cotton and the *Lagenaria* gourd extended farthest into the North American continent. Possibly a hybrid between the progenitors of *Nicotiana paniculata* and *N. undulata*, *Nicotiana rustica* most likely originated on the western slopes of the Andes in the border region between Ecuador and Peru, where the Mochica and Cañari cultures once flourished.

Since man's historic interest in tobacco focused exclusively on the narcotic properties of its principal alkaloid, nicotine, one might conjecture that *Nicotiana rustica* outdistanced *N. tabacum* mainly because of the considerably higher nicotine content of the former. This came to be of special significance in connection with the widespread practice of ritual smoking, especially in South America. Still another consideration may be that after planting, *N. rustica* requires far less attention than *N. tabacum*, a characteristic that surely facilitated its rapid adoption from one tribe to another (Goodspeed 1942; Sauer 1950:522–523; 1969:128–129).

In light of the extensive distribution area of both kinds of tobacco in the Americas, it is safe to say that the Indians made use of the plant thousands of years before Columbus. Likewise, on the basis of its close association with indigenous ideology and ritual at the time of the Conquest and since, it is reasonable to assume that the use of tobacco was always largely confined to magico-religious purposes. Thus the extraordinary geographical distribution of domesticated tobacco in pre-European times and the exclusively ritual use of the plant in Indian America can both be seen as evidence for the great antiquity of the plant as an integral element of American Indian culture.

In the early centuries after Discovery and even more in recent times, tobacco experienced an ever greater tribal and territorial expansion through North and South America, so that today there is virtually no native population, from Canada to Patagonia, that does not know or use tobacco. Especially in northern South America, on the one hand, and the extreme southern area on the other, this phenomenal expansion was increasingly accompanied by the secularization of its once wholly ritual functions. Clearly this profanization was largely due to European influence. The Europeans, to whom tobacco was, of course, completely unknown before the first voyage of Columbus, were slow to recognize the plant as anything more than a new ornamental with certain medicinal properties. Its profound religious significance remained largely concealed to them, and if they referred to it as "divine" or "holy" it was mainly as a euphemism, not because they had somehow assimilated Indian attitudes. Likewise, the miraculous properties that were early ascribed to tobacco by the Europeans were based on its allegedly curative powers as a panacea. Once that had proved to be a fallacy, a purely hedonistic interest in its effects obviously provided sufficient impetus for its swift assimilation into European culture and its wide geographical dissemination throughout the Old World.

Among the Indians, however, secular or hedonistic use continued to be the exception rather than the rule. No doubt there were sporadic instances, for one of the earliest chroniclers, Benzoni (1565:96–98) found the Indians of Haiti smoking cigars "simply because it gave them pleasure." On the other hand, we are told, the priests and doctors among them also smoked ritually to procure dream visions and to consult with their *zemi* deities concerning the sick. As Purchase (1626:57-59), another early writer, put it, they esteemed tobacco not only "for sanetie also for sanctitie" (Plate 1).

Probably there were other indigenous groups that came to use tobacco for pleasure in the early Colonial period. Notwithstanding these exceptions, however, it can be stated as a general rule that "during the period from first Discovery to about 1700, over most of the tobacco area, use was, it seems, exclusively or chiefly magico-religious and/or medicinal" (Cooper 1949:526–527). And indeed, the further we travel away from civilization into the early distribution area of tobacco in the tropical forest, the more we find tobacco still to be closely associated with its ancient ritual meanings. Here at least the native species continue to be employed mainly in a magico-religious context. Smoking for pleasure does occur, but when it does it is commonly restricted to the white man's imported "Virginia tobacco," as it is often called, while the tobacco cultivated by the Indians themselves is reserved for ceremonial occasions.

To summarize, from the combined chronological and spatial evidence bearing on the nearuniversality and cultural functions of tobacco among South American Indians, we conclude the following:

1. In prehistoric and early historic times tobacco achieved a fairly extensive distribution throughout large parts of the tropical forest, the Andes, and the Caribbean, mainly as a psychotropic agent. As such it constituted an integral element of the intellectual culture and ritual practices of tribal South America. Among many Central and North Andean groups tobacco was also or even primarily employed hygienically and therapeutically.

2. During recent historic times, and especially since 1700, tobacco diffused practically throughout the remainder of the continent, down to its extreme southernmost region, the Tierra del Fuego, while at the same time the manner and ideological foundations of its use shifted increasingly from the magico-religious to the profane.

The Indians of South America employ tobacco in many different ways, of which smoking (in cigarettes, cigars, or pipes) is the most common. Of techniques other than smoking, the best known are drinking, licking, chewing, and snuffing. Which of these is the oldest is difficult to say. However, inasmuch as we lack archaeological or historic evidence for smoking in either area of original tobacco domestication, Sauer (1969:48) may well be right when he suggests that "tobacco may have been used first as a ceremonial drink, next in chewing and snuff, and perhaps last, by smoking."

Tobacco is sometimes used in combination or association with true botanical hallucinogens, such as *Coca Datura, Banisteriopsis caapi* (*ayahuasca*) or (especially in Peru) such psychotropic cacti as *Trichocereus pachanoi*. Often it serves its primary sacred function as the supernatural purifying, mortifying, and revitalizing agent during life-crises ceremonies, particularly during the long and arduous initiatory training of neophyte shamans who subsequently begin to use other psychotropic plants as well (e.g. *Banisteriopsis caapi*) (Plate 2).

Finally, tobacco is one of several vehicles for ecstasy in South American shamanism; it may be taken in combination with other plants to induce narcotic trance states or it may, as it does among the Warao of the Orinoco Delta, represent the sole psychoactive agent employed by shamans to transport themselves into the realm of the metaphysical. Unfortunately, largely due to the aforementioned failure to comprehend the profound ideological and ritual significance of tobacco, we lack to this day a systematic study of its magico-religious use in South America. Nevertheless, at least some insight into this complex area of inquiry may be had even from its sketchy treatment in the ethnographic literature.

TOBACCO DRINKING AND LICKING

As Cooper (1949:534) has shown, there exist in South America two major distribution areas of tobacco use in liquid form — the Montaña region and Guyana. In both areas tobacco infusions are of great magico-religious significance. Among the Jivaro of the Montaña ritual tobacco drinking became especially elaborated and formalized. These Indians prepare the liquid by either boiling the leaves in water or by spitting the chewed leaves into their hands or into a container before further macerating them in spittle or water. In Guyana, such Indians as the Barama River Caribs or the Akawaio simply squeeze and steep the leaves in water.

Tobacco juice may be either drunk or taken through the nose. Among the Jivaro the application varies according to sex: women in the main drink it, whereas men inhale it through the nostrils. Some tribes of the tributaries of the Upper Amazon (Jivaro, Witoto, Bora, Campa, and Piro) boil down tobacco leaves in water to a concentrate. An even thicker paste (*ambíl*) is made by adding some thickened casava starch to the soaked and mashed tobacco leaves. In pre-Columbian times this was also the practice among tribes of the Venezuelan Andes and adjacent Colombia. I saw the Ica of the Sierra Nevada still employing small calabashes for this purpose; similarly, the Kogi continue to adhere to this old custom. Interestingly enough, a specially prepared tobacco paste known as *chimó* is also still taken "by a large segment of the modern, non-Indian population" of western Venezuela (Kamen-Kaye 1971:1). In general, however, Indian tobacco concentrates are sufficiently liquid to be drunk in most instances. Licking of liquid tobacco from one or two fingers or from a short stick that is dunked into the syrup is also known. Sometimes *ambíl* and coca are taken together. Whatever the manner of preparation or ingestion, however, the liquid tobacco quickly puts the user into a state of somnolence. The effect of the nicotine is usually felt soon after drinking two or three doses: the face turns pale and the body starts to tremble. Vomiting may occur at this stage, a physiological reaction considered indispensable in initiation and certain life crises rituals, when the body has to be purged of all impurities. Repeated drinking of large doses of tobacco juice or syrup eventually brings on extreme nausea, especially in women, and produces the desired comatose state with its intensive dream-visions.

Among the narcotic plants cultivated by the Jivaro of Ecuador, tobacco occupies first place. The Indians consume most of their tobacco in liquid form, although occasionally it is also smoked in the form of big cigars. As a narcotic beverage tobacco fulfils a very specific magico-religious function in the Jivaro ideational universe, a role that is clearly differentiated from that ascribed to the hallucinogenic *ayahuasca* (*Banisteriopsis*) beverage or to *Datura*.

The Jivaro imbibe tobacco juice on many different occasions and for different purposes. But the common objective they all share is magico-religious. This is true to some degree even when tobacco juice is taken prophylactically against general symptoms of indisposition, colds, or chills. In case of the latter, the shaman holds his sacred rock crystal into the calabash filled with tobacco water and utters a blessing over it before the patient drinks the medicine. Similarly, when used as a remedy for snake bites, the therapeutic value of tobacco juice is mainly magical. When imbibed in large quantities or, for that matter, even when applied externally as body paint, tobacco infusions are believed to fortify a person against evil spirits. Not only does it invigorate his own body but the magical power of tobacco also radiates outward from the drinker and predisposes in his favor the elements of his entire environment.

Finally, as with other psychotropic beverages, the Jivaro consume tobacco water in order to acquire an *arutam* soul (Harner 1973:136) and to be enlightened by a particular spirit concerning their fortune in warfare and life in general. This spirit can appear to them under the influence of the customary ritual hallucinogens. Young men in particular often leave their villages in small bands to retire into the solitude to a special "dreaming-hut" that has been constructed for that purpose away from the village in the immediate vicinity of a water fall. For several days the young men restrict themselves to a diet of tobacco, daily drinking it in considerable quantities. In the mornings they exchange their dream experiences and interpret their visions. Only after several days do they rejoin the community as a whole, physically emaciated but psychically reinvigorated.

The Witoto Indians of Colombia also perform group ceremonies of tobacco licking, when the council of warriors and elders meets to discuss hunting, warfare, and those that have offended the ethical standards of the community. The men are seated on the ground around a vessel filled with tobacco syrup, from time to time dipping their index and middle fingers into the concentrate and licking it off. By their participation in the ceremony the men seal any agreements reached during the session (Koch-Grünberg 1923:329). Padre Gabriel (1944:58) confirms that in 1936 this same population considered the tobacco concentrate to be sacred. Wrongdoers had to lick it standing up and subsequently had to leave the house. During the ceremony "god" would come to provide nourishment for the good and remedies for the sick. In former times gifts of tobacco concentrate and coca were given on the occasion of such life-crises ceremonies as childbirth and marriage (Whiffen 1915).

Tobacco juice that is intended for use during any of the major Jivaro festivals must be especially macerated with saliva. The juice is absolutely indispensable for the nuptial feast for women, the initiation feast for men, and the great victory feast. Preparations for these feasts are invariably elaborate. For instance, only after general preparations and food taboo restrictions that may last for as much as two or three years has the time for the four-day tobacco feast for women finally arrived. The principal purpose of this fertility rite is the initiation of the Jivaro girl into womanhood through the intercession of the tobacco spirit. In the course of a series of elaborate ceremonies of dancing, chanting and the frequent drinking of tobacco water, this spirit enters the woman's body to confer upon her a magic power. Her body impregnated and sometimes externally anointed with the liquid tobacco, the life-giving force radiates out from the young woman, permeating her present and future crops as well as animals. At night she converses with the Great Earth Mother, experiences dream-visions of flourishing gardens and growing flocks, and receives the supernatural promise of fertility and longevity.

An equivalent feast of initiation for boys follows upon an equally prolonged period of preparation, partial fasting, and tobacco drinking. The general purpose of the ceremony — to guarantee an abundant life and fertility — is the same as that for girls. However, there is a difference in the administration of tobacco, in that boys not only take it in liquid form but also swallow it as smoke. The latter is accomplished by the ritual leader, who blows the smoke from a bamboo tube into the mouth of the youngster. Another technique is for the leader to take the lighted end of a cigar into his mouth and blow the smoke through it into the mouth of the initiate, until the entire cigar has been consumed. Immediately after the smoke swallowing, which occurs about six to eight times daily on each of two successive days, the novice has to drink tobacco juice prepared with much saliva by the ritual leader.

Great quantities of tobacco juice are also drunk on the occasion of the Jivaro victory feast, especially during the ceremony of the washing of the trophy head. This ceremony is performed to protect the slayer and his kin from revengeful evil spirits and to endow him with life-giving forces through his *tsansa* (the shrunken trophy head).

Among the tribes of the Peruvian and Ecuadorean Montaña, the shaman drinks tobacco whenever he seeks to communicate with the spirit world. Any shaman may use his power negatively or positively, in that he has the ability not only to cure his kinsmen but cause sickness to enemies by magical means. "Dark" shamans preparing to shoot a magic projectile that will bring sickness or misfortune to the victim must diet for several days on tobacco water. The juice is also efficacious in producing the actual magical pathogen from the practitioner's body and in manipulating the "thorns" that cause illness. However, in his positive or "light" role the shaman also takes large quantities of tobacco water through the nose in order to summon the tobacco spirit and ask him to diagnose and treat sicknesses caused by hostile sorcerers, evil spirits, or other supernatural agencies (e.g. Karsten on the Jivaro 1920, 1935).

Among the Campa, another Montaña tribe, the *sheripiari*, or "tobacco shaman," prepares concentrated tobacco juice of the consistency of syrup. He drinks the syrup (and also beverages of *Banisteriopsis caapi* and *Datura*) to achieve ecstatic trance states, in the course of which he negotiates with the spirit forces to procure health and sustenance for his kinsmen and to retrieve souls that might have strayed or been stolen by demons ("rape of the soul"). The tobacco syrup allows him to alleviate the suffering of those that have been struck by the sickness projectiles of dark shamans, forest spirits, and demonic bees and ants. In his tobacco narcosis the healer is able to diagnose such sicknesses and to treat the patient by anointing him with tobacco concentrate and by blowing on the affected area.

Those who would take on the enormous responsibility of becoming shamans in future years must begin to take tobacco syrup when still tender adolescents. Later, as novices, on the day of their initiation into the company of spirits, future shamans of the Campa are first given an infusion of *Banisteriopsis*, followed by a large quantity of tobacco concentrate. Elick (1969:206–207) quotes the experience of one such neophyte shaman as follows:

Suddenly the room became very brightly lit and after a while Tsori [novice's name] felt that he was slowly withdrawing from his body through the crown of his head. He watched the *sheripiari* [shaman] and his body for a while then found himself walking through the semi-dark forest. He heard a noise and looking in its direction he saw a great jaguar bounding toward him through the trees, but felt no real fear. The jaguar grabbed him tightly with his claws and acted as though it were going to close its mouth over his face and neck. Just at this point the jaguar disappeared and a young woman stood there holding his shoulders with her hands. This was the "Mother of Tobacco," the principal tobacco spirit. He had been told this would happen if he were acceptable as a shaman. Suddenly he was in the hut again, seated on the ground, with the young woman before him. She repeated over and over a new and different song that he realized would thereafter be his own. He sang the song with her until he had it perfectly memorized. This was the only time the new shaman saw the Mother of Tobacco. After this his own tobacco spirit would come to him.

The next night the novice embarked upon a second ecstatic journey to receive the spirit stones of light and/or dark shamanism. The Campa shaman also owns a third sacred stone to which he feeds a daily portion of tobacco syrup. This sacred rock metamorphoses into a jaguar "daughter" when the shaman blows on it. He himself is capable of changing into a jaguar with the assistance of his spirit wife or female spirit helper, who lives in the tubular bamboo tobacco syrup container.

In order to summon their supernatural tobacco wives, daughters and nieces, neophyte shamans must imbibe great quantities of tobacco juice. But as they become more experienced, shamans only need to lick the stopper of their tobacco containers in order to accomplish comparable ends. Female shamans employ the same methods as their male counterparts to summon their tutelary "daughters" and "sons" (Elick 1969).

In Guyana, especially among Cariban tribes, the drinking of tobacco juice is fundamental to shamanic healing practices and the ecstatic trance experience. Here as elsewhere "a man must die before he becomes a shaman" (Wavell, Butt, and Epton 1966:43). For the apprentice preparing to become a so-called tobacco shaman, the initiatory crisis is brought on by prolonged fasting and tobacco drinking. Only thus will he be enabled to gain entrance to the spirit world and use tobacco as do its supernatural denizens. Tobacco belongs to the order of mountain spirits; wild tobacco is searched out and gathered by Akawaio shamans high up in the hills by virtue of their special powers. Since the mountain tobacco was originally received from a spirit only shamans are permitted to use it. This recalls the Jivaro shaman, who also seeks out patches of semi-wild tobacco for ritual purposes.

In order to summon the "old man" tobacco spirit for a healing séance, the shaman first consumes a large quantity of tobacco juice:

The tobacco spirit then comes and can be heard making characteristic whistlings: 'pwee, wee, wee.' He is thought of as an old man. The whistling is shortly followed by the noise of a spirit coming to drink the juice, through the medium of the shaman, who has a cupful by him. A succession of spirits comes during the seance, each in turn seeking to drink the tobacco juice, and everytime when one arrives for this purpose there is a loud and elaborate gurgling, sucking and spitting noise, which denotes the fact that the spirit which is possessing the shaman is sipping its share of tobacco. The tobacco spirit has the power to entice other spirits because no spirit can resist the attraction of tobacco, just as, the Akawaio confess, they themselves are unable to resist it either. Once a spirit has drunk tobacco juice then it is 'glad' and satisfied and can be induced to help the shaman by allowing itself to be interrogated (Wavell, Butt, and Epton 1966:54).

To enter into the ecstatic trance state the shaman takes tobacco through the nostrils. On his supernatural journey he finds himself accompanied by his spirit wife and helper, the clairvoyant bird-woman. Together they join the company of spirits who might assist the shaman in curing the patient. The shaman's flight is made possible through the combined effort of the tobacco spirit and the spirit-bird helper (the swallow-tailed kite), who provide the shaman with magic wings. Upon returning from his cosmic journey, the shaman returns his wings to the bird spirit and once more adopts his everyday human form.

There are also practicing female shamans among Guyana Indians who employ tobacco as a medium of communication with the spirit world. Lacking, however, in this northeastern area of the tobacco drinking complex are the communal tobacco drinking rituals found elsewhere in South America.

TOBACCO CHEWING

The chewing of tobacco has a rather sporadic distribution among South American Indians. It is found mainly in central Guyana and the Caribbean, in the Upper Amazon region, and among several tribes of the Gran Chaco. It was formerly a custom also among the ancient Chibcha and Goajiro of Colombia. As Zerries (1964:99–100) and other writers have pointed out, the scattered distribution of the practice and its occurrence mainly among "marginal" and "submarginal" populations are indications of the great antiquity of this custom.

In tobacco chewing the narcotic juice is swallowed and the nicotine absorbed into the system through the lining of the stomach. Users commonly mix the minced or rolled tobacco leaves with such alkalinic substances as wood ashes, black-niter earth, or pulverized shell. These are either simply added to a pinch of chopped tobacco leaves or sprinkled into a roll made of green or dried tobacco which the chewer holds in his mouth, usually in front of the lower or upper gum:

Before using them [the tobacco leaves], they put them in a cuia [pot] with a little water; then, near the fire, they mix the leaves with ashes until they are dry again. Generally they take three leaves, beat them to remove the ashes and then roll them one over another. If the leaves are very long, they double them over several times, until they make a big long sausage which they put under their lower lip (Biocca 1970:135).

The psychotropic effect of chewing tobacco appears to vary from light to severe. Among the Yanoama of the Upper Orinoco, for example, men and women chew with great frequency and for prolonged periods of time, but I have never noted any acute tobacco intoxication to result from this practice. On the other hand, a Tukano shaman was observed by Nimuendajú (1952:104) falling over backwards with shaking knees after sucking on a wad of cut tobacco that he had placed in each cheek.

In what might be the first recorded observation of tobacco chewing in the New World, Amerigo Vespucci reported in a letter of 1504 to his friend Piero Soderini that the Indians of Margarita Island "each had his cheeks bulging with a certain green herb ... and each carried hanging from his neck two dried gourds, one of which was full of the very herb that he kept in his mouth; the other full of a certain white flour like powdered chalk" (Brooks 1937:189).[1] The mystified explorer was soon to learn that on this island where water is scarce the Indian fishing folk chewed to quench their thirst (Plate 3).

Among the Yanoama of Guyana, where both sexes, adults as well as children, chew (or better, suck) tobacco almost incessantly, the practice appears to be largely hedonistic. However, dying Indians also receive a final roll of tobacco under their lower lip so that Thunder and the spirits of the Other world will recognize them. But even apart from this obviously ritual practice, there is ample evidence that elsewhere magico-religious ideas are closely associated with the chewing of tobacco. Even where masticated tobacco is medicinally applied, it is often intended to ward off the evil spirits that had caused the patient's illness. Patients among the Páez of Colombia also provide their shamans with chewing tobacco and coca which, when taken together, produce dream visions that reveal future events, and especially the patient's likely fate (Bernal Villa 1954:237). These shamans employ chewed tobacco to blow away the rainbow, so that children may not be afflicted with scabies. Among some tribes — the Tukano, for example — tobacco chewing is mainly practiced by the dark shaman who seeks to be possessed by the spirit helpers that supplied him with his magic sickness projectiles (Nimuendajú 1948:723).

TOBACCO SNUFFING

The inhaling of narcotics is a peculiarly New World custom that spread

---

[1] Some scholars suspect, however, that Vespucci's account, published by Waldseemüller in 1507, actually referred to coca chewing rather than tobacco.

to the Old World only in post-Hispanic times, specifically with powdered tobacco. In the Americas, the snuffing of pulverized tobacco was largely restricted to the western regions, especially the humid Amazon Valley. Powdered tobacco as a magic repellent against hostile demons and disease spirits is also employed by the shamans of the Tukano of the Bolivian Andes, who blow the narcotic powder at their supernatural adversaries (Hissink-Hahn 1961). (Rare occurrences of tobacco snuffing have also been reported from Mexico and North America; in Mexico, also, at the time of the Conquest, pulverized *piciétl* [*Nicotiana rustica*] was externally applied to the patient's body rather than inhaled.)

In South America, tobacco snuffing is mainly practiced on the Guaporé, by Arawakan tribes of the Montaña, and by Panoan-speakers of the Jurua-Purús. However, the distribution area also reaches out toward the south, to include Quechua-speakers of central and southern Peru as well as Aymara groups of Bolivia. Outside this main region the snuffing of tobacco seems to have been restricted to only a few tribes of the Orinoco basin and the West Indies (Zerries 1964:96).

Powerful hallucinogenic snuffs were (and still are) prepared in many areas of South America from such species as *Virola* and *Anadenanthera* (Schultes 1972:24-31), but as Schultes noted in an earlier paper (1967: 292), powdered tobacco was certainly a widely used narcotic. There are also several cases on record where tobacco snuff is mixed with coca, *Erythroxylon coca* or *Anadenanthera peregrina*, but generally speaking tobacco was either used by itself or side by side, rather than mixed, with other psychotropic snuffing preparations.

The fairly extensive distribution of tobacco snuffing and its typical association with ecstatic and divinatory shamanistic techniques again suggest considerable antiquity for this custom. In any event, it is likely to antedate the rise of the Andean civilizations rather than to have originated with them and to have subsequently diffused to the less complex populations of the Montaña.

In early contact times Peruvian Indians are reported to have sometimes prepared tobacco snuff from the roots rather than the leaves. Generally, however, the snuff is made by pulverizing the dried leaves. Plant ashes are occasionally mixed with the powdered tobacco, possibly for the same pharmacological reason that ashes are mixed with *Anadenanthera* or *Virola* snuff and lime is taken with coca. Some peoples snuff tobacco without the use of special snuffing instruments, others use single or bifurcated tubes to suck the narcotic powder into their own noses or to blow it into the nostrils of others. These techniques and instruments closely resemble those employed in the use of *Anadenanthera* and other hallucinogenic snuffs (Plate 4).

Like tobacco juice, snuff is sometimes taken prophylactically, for reasons of hygiene, or to forge alliances during peace-making ceremonies. But its main function is in connection with shamanizing, when the practitioner blows it into the patient's nose as a magic remedy, or administers it to participants in ceremonies. Otomac shamans are reported to have taken tobacco snuff (possibly mixed with *Anadenanthera*) in order to experience prophetic dream-visions in the company of the supernaturals. The tobacco snuff of the Tukano included six different ingredients, mainly the bark ashes of several trees but not *paricá* (*Anadenanthera*). It will be recalled that among these Indians the chewing of tobacco is a mark of dark shamans. Snuffing, however, is practiced only in connection with the ceremony of the sacred musical instruments. The sacred trumpet that is sounded during a girl's initiation ceremony to ward off demons and invisible "immortals" can only be blown by men and boys over seven years of age who have been initiated into the use of tobacco snuffing.

The snuff is taken within the compound where the sacred instrument is kept hidden from the girls and the women. It is here also that men enter into ecstatic trance communication with the protective spirits of the sacred instruments, thereby assisting in assuring magical protection for the pubescent girls and the women. The boys are traditionally initiated into this fertility complex when their voices change and when, in the course of formal puberty observances, they are secluded from the community in order to be admitted to the secrets of the sacred trumpet under the influence of the narcotic tobacco snuff (Nimuendajú 1948:718).

Among the tribes of the Guaporé tobacco snuff is commonly used with *Anadenanthera* powder, either in combination or sequentially. Shamans blow it into their patient's nose and take it themselves by means of two to three foot long bamboo tubes. The snuffing tube is sometimes decorated at its mouth with the head of a bird. This avian head may be provided with a pair of eyes which, among the Aikana, for example, facilitate the shaman's vision in the supernatural sphere. Tupari shamans communicate in their trances with ancestral shamans who appear to them "up there" as half-man, half-animal (Caspar 1952:237; 1953:158).

SMOKING

As mentioned earlier, smoking is the most common and most widespread mode of tobacco use. The dried leaves are either smoked as cigars and cigarettes or in a pipe. According to Cooper (1949:527–528), "In earlier times, shortly after and sometime before the period of Discovery — and in large measure at present as well — cigars-cigarettes prevailed over the great northern focal area of the continent and adjacent Antilles and Middle America, pipes over a roughly crescent-shaped belt peripheral thereto on the southeast, south, southwest, and west, a tobaccoless zone peripheral in turn to the pipe zone."

Both cigars and pipe smoking were the first forms of tobacco use witnessed by the Europeans. Two sailors whom Columbus had sent to scout the island of Haiti found the natives there smoking tobacco rolled in dried leaves of maize. Benzoni (1565:81), whose experiences go back to 1541–1555, reports the following:

When these [tobacco] leaves are in season, they pick them, tie them up in bundles and suspend them near their fireplace till they are very dry; and when they wish to use them, they take a leaf of their grain (maize) and putting one of the others into it, they roll them round tight together; then they set fire to one end, and putting the other end into the mouth, they draw their breath up through it, wherefore the smoke goes into the mouth, the throat, the head, and they retain it as long as they can, for they find a pleasure in it, and so much do they fill themselves with this cruel smoke, that they lose their reason. And there are some who take so much of it, that they fall down as if they were dead, and remain the greater part of the day or night stupefied. Some men are found who are content with imbibing only enough of this smoke to make them giddy, and no more.

Other islanders took smoke through the nose. Of this "very pernicious" custom of inhaling smoke from burning tobacco leaves through the nostrils by means of a straight or forked tube, Oviedo (1526) says that the Indians persisted until they became stupefied.

While it was the physical effects of tobacco smoking that struck the Europeans first and foremost, Benzoni (1565:82) did note some of its magico-religious functions:

In La Española and the other islands, when their doctors wanted to cure a sick man, they went to the place where they were to administer the smoke, and when he was thoroughly intoxicated by it, the cure was mostly effected. On returning to his senses, he told a thousand stories of his having been at the council of the gods, and other high visions (Plate 5).

Shamanic healing with tobacco smoke continues to be an almost universal technique through the South American tobacco area and beyond. This is related to the belief that the shaman's breath is charged with magic energy which is reinforced through tobacco smoke. The very "power of the shaman is often linked with his breath or tobacco smoke, both of which possess cleansing and reinvigorating properties which play an important part in healing and in other magic practices" (Zerries 1969:314). "Receive the power of the spirit," exclaims the Tupi shaman when he blows over his people (De Léry 1592:281). The Mbyá-guaraní call the smoke of tobacco "life-giving mist," because they consider it to be the source of vitality, an attribute of the god of spring, the patron of shamans (Cadogan 1958:93).

Generally speaking, the blowing of tobacco smoke by the light shaman, whether over patients and others in different kinds of life-crises situations, or over objects, foodstuffs, gardens, rivers and the forest, invariably has as its principal purpose the purification of what is unclean or contaminated, the reinvigoration of the weak, and the warding off of evil of whatever kind or form.

Thus, the light shaman of the Warao presides over an ancient cult of fertility. In his dream or tobacco-induced ecstatic trance, he travels to the House of Tobacco Smoke in the eastern part of the universe. The celestial bridge of tobacco smoke, which he frequents and maintains between his community and the abode of the Bird-Spirit of the East, is a channel of energy that guarantees health and abundance of life on earth. Protected by a light shaman, no harm can befall the people, even if someone were to be "shot" by the sickness projectile of a hostile shaman. A shaman who feeds his tutelary spirits properly with tobacco smoke can count on their assistance in curing such magically induced disease. When he places his hand on the affected body part of his patient, the spirit helpers diagnose the nature of the arrow of sickness. The healer then sucks it out, inhales great quantities of tobacco smoke, and lets the magic arrow travel through his arm and through an exit hole into his hand, where it is "born" for the patient and all his kin to see.

Dark shamans, on the other hand, reverse the life-conferring energy of the light shaman's blowing of tobacco smoke, for they blow to debilitate and to kill. For example, the dark shaman of the Warao lights a cigar which contains his spirit "sons." While smoking, he chants his destructive song, and with this the ends of a snare of tobacco smoke that he carries wound up in his breast slowly begin to emerge from the corners of his mouth. When these ends arrive at their intended destination, the shaman pulls heavily on his cigar, turns it around and, holding the burning end in his closed mouth, blows into it. Out come ribbons of smoke, and these then transport the magic projectile to the victim. The instant the arrow enters the body, the snare of tobacco smoke closes and the magic projectile travels to the heart to kill (Plate 6, 7).

Not only the shaman but also the ordinary individual can count on the power of the smoke when it comes from his own mouth. I was often told by my Warao friends that I should not smoke on the river or in the forest if I wanted to avoid attracting the spirits. Guyana Caribs, such as the Akawaio, use tobacco in ritual shamanic and personal blowing "because it has an exceptionally strong and powerful spirit"; hence they resort to smoke blowing especially to protect themselves on their way through the forest (Butt 1956). With great piety the Tukano direct private invocations to some animal spirit by uttering a spell and combining it with tobacco smoke. "In all invocations tobacco smoke is the principal medium because the request (or threat, as the case may be) is directly transmitted through the smoke.... Invocation, combined with the use of tobacco is probably the ritual attitude that is most frequently observed by the individual" (Reichel-Dolmatoff 1971: 153, 155).

Within the ideational framework of many indigenous cultures in South America, the concept of life-giving energy associated with tobacco smoke, and with tobacco in general, can be taken quite literally. In the religious symbolism of the Tukano, for example, tobacco has seminal characteristics:

In the act of smoking there is a complex symbolism in which the act of nursing is combined with a phallic symbol, the cigar, and a uterine symbol, burning, and ashes, the latter being the "residue." On the other hand, smoke is *bogá*, an element of fertilizing energy that rises from below in an upward direction to unite the Milky Way with the great universal *bogá*. The tiny seeds of the tobacco plant also have seminal meaning. When the forked cigar holder is used, the sexual symbolism is clear: sticking it into the earth like a world axis, the phallic union between the various planes of above and below is achieved (Reichel-Dolmatoff 1971:152).

Indeed, the most pervasive connotation of tobacco is the concept of fertility in the broadest sense of the word. Fertility is the objective pursued by man through this medium of communication between himself and the supernatural sphere, be it by means of a simple invocation, a curing séance, initiation ceremony, vision quest, or ecstatic trance. The question arises, of course, how tobacco in its various forms came to acquire such a pervasive role. A purely pharmacological explanation would probably be easier than a religious one. However, despite the general paucity of ethnographic data on the metaphysical meaning of tobacco, some general observations are possible.

CONCLUDING REMARKS

It has become obvious that whatever the form in which it is taken, tobacco plays a central role in South American shamanism and religion. Like the sacred mushrooms, peyote, morning glories, *Datura*, *ayahuasca*, the various psychotomimetic snuffs, and a whole series of other New World hallucinogens, tobacco was and is employed by Indians to achieve shamanic trance states, in purification, and in supernatural curing. The chewing of tobacco appears to be the least potent mode of tobacco consumption to achieve these aims, while drinking and snuffing are clearly more effective. Smoking, however, outranks them all, in distribution as well as physiological and metaphysical functions. This may have several reasons. As a vaporous carrier of the nicotine alkaloid, smoke was easily assimilated into pre-existent beliefs about the exhalatory powers of the shaman. Smoke makes his breath visible, and with it the benevolent, or, as the case may be, malevolent, charges that emanate from the shaman. In addition, tobacco smoke, corresponding to the merging of air and fire, acquired the rich antithetical symbolic complex of incense as a medium between earth and heaven through fire.

The non-material smoke is the ideal and most appropriate food of spirits. Taken in liquid form, as, for example, among the Jivaro, Conibo, and Guyana Caribs, tobacco enables one to propitiate and visit the world of spirits and induce it to bestow blessings upon man. Tobacco in smoke form, however, once discovered was quickly recognized as a most immediate and direct way to the spirits and hence became the preferred sacrificial gift to the supernaturals in many parts of the New World. The gods and spirits, it is widely held, crave tobacco smoke so intensely that they are unable to resist it. Since there is no tobacco smoke other than that produced by man through fire, the supernaturals in a very real sense depend on him for their favorite food and sustenance. What seems to have occurred here is the attribution to the gods and other supernaturals of the same near addiction to tobacco that is characteristic of many shamans. Just as the tobacco shaman of the Warao requires tobacco smoke with tremendous physiological and psychological urgency, and is literally sick without it, so the gods await their gift of tobacco smoke with the craving of the addict, and will enter into mutually beneficial relationships with man so long as he is able to provide the drug. Foodstuffs like mead, beer, manioc gruel, moriche flour, etc., are simply not adequate substitutes.

This projection onto the supernaturals of the shaman's tobacco habit in no sense represents a profanization of the gods, however. On the contrary, the essential shamanic quality of the supernaturals (e.g., their craving for tobacco) lies precisely in their origin: the gods and other denizens of the metaphysical sphere are themselves shamans of former times who upon death became transformed into pure spirit.

If tobacco is a life-giving essence for man in the indirect sense by allowing him access to the protective powers of the spirit world, it serves the same life-assuring purpose for the gods themselves in a direct way. Because it is their food and sustenance, they are forced into a dependency relationship with man as their chief provider. In the Mundurucú tobacco myth, even the Mother of Tobacco, who created tobacco smoke *sui generis* and carried it in a calabash from which she periodically sucked her vital sustenance, died as soon as she ran out of the life-giving smoke (Kruse 1951–1952:918).

This relationship of man as provider of nourishment for the spirits has been documented for many tribes in South America, from Brazil to the Caribbean, and from the Atlantic coast to the Montaña. The spirits of the Guyana Indians are said to be "crazy" for smoke, and the shamans control and manipulate them through offerings and regular feedings of tobacco. This is true, above all, of smoke, but it applies as well to its other forms, particularly as a liquid and as snuff, which seem to have preceded the discovery of smoking. The supernatural Tobacco Woman of the Akawaio, for example, is persuaded by a shaman to offer "a drink of tobacco juice ... to *Imawali*, representing the chief order of nature spirits," for the purpose of dissuading other supernaturals of the forest and of vegetation from causing sickness to a fellow tribesman (Butt 1956–1957:170). The Waiwai shaman feeds tobacco smoke to a magic stone as a means of summoning his own helping spirits, whose sustenance is tobacco (Fock 1963:126). And again, much of the Warao Indian's life is spent in propitiating a number of Supreme Spirits, referred to as Grandfathers, and a female spirit called Mother of the Forest, who together inhabit the world mountains at the cardinal and inter-cardinal points of the universe and who require nourishment from the people in the form of tobacco smoke. Like the Balam gods of the four directions in the Maya universe, the Warao gods consume enormous cigars and are well disposed toward mankind so long as men propitiate them with tobacco, moriche flour, honey, fish and crabs. But the spirits keep only the tobacco for themselves, for tobacco is their appropriate food. If neglected in this vital aspect, they spread sickness and death among the people by means of their magic projectiles (i.e., behave like dark shamans of an especially powerful kind).

The shaman-priest of the Warao carries out the feeding of the gods by holding the long cigar vertically and pointing it in the direction of the Supreme Spirits, all the while deeply inhaling with hyperventilation and swallowing the smoke (Plate 8). Smoke offerings are also made to the sacred rattle, as the spirit stones within it require tobacco smoke as well. As in the case of the Tupinambá of Brazil, the Warao rattle is a head-spirit that can be consulted in the fashion of an oracle. However, instead of blowing tobacco smoke into the rattle as do the Warao, the Tupinambá burn tobacco leaves inside the rattle and hold communion with their spirit by inhaling the smoke that emerges through the head-spirit's various orifices (Métraux 1928:67; Wilbert 1972).

A related idea seems to be that of the Mundurucú, whose shaman inhales clouds of tobacco smoke blown on him by fellow practitioners through reversed cigars. In the resulting trance the shaman feeds the Mother of Game Animals with sweet manioc gruel (Murphy 1958:40). In a similar context of hunting magic many other Brazilian tribes propitiate their Master (or "Owner") of Animals (Barbosa Rodrígues 1890:9, 12).

I have previously referred to the Campa of the Peruvian Montaña whose shaman must feed the sacred rock a daily diet of tobacco syrup. Harner (1973:163) reports that among the Jivaro the shaman seeks to reassure himself, by means of periodic tobacco feedings, of the benevolence of his spirit helpers who appear to him under the influence of *Banisteriopsis (ayahuasca)* in "a variety of zoomorphic forms hovering over him, perching on his shoulders, sticking out of his skin, and helping to suck the patient's body." Every four hours he drinks tobacco water in order to keep these spirits fed, so that they may remain his willing helpers and not desert him.

To sum up, on the basis of such widespread evidence we can assume that tobacco was generally considered the proper nourishment of the supernaturals among South American Indians. The supernaturals need man to provide this food for them and hence are anxious to establish and maintain a good reciprocal relationship with him. For his part, man is needful of supernatural protection for his life, his health, and his goods, and only the supernaturals are capable of providing for these needs. Both sides are therefore anxious that, as the Guaraní put it, it "comes to an understanding" (Cadogan 1965:212), and they avail themselves of the services of the shaman to accomplish their respective but interdependent ends. It is in this light that tobacco can clearly be seen in its role as medium between the natural and supernatural worlds. On the one hand, tobacco transports man into the realm of the spirits, where he can learn how "to see" things that are beyond his physical field of vision. He can participate in a life of bliss, devoid of the suffering, starvation, and death of his own world. On the other hand, the spirits and their sphere are attracted through tobacco to the physical earth, where some of the transcendent blessings of their metaphysical world are conferred upon man. No wonder that the Indians considered themselves fortunate, in their humble position as mortals, nevertheless to be able to offer something of value to the immortals! No wonder that in the indigenous world tobacco was considered too sacred for secular or purely hedonistic use.

In South America, then, tobacco served as the bond of communion between the natural and supernatural worlds, functioning, as it were, as the actualizing principle between the two. Without the shaman and his tobacco ceremonies mankind and the spirit world remain separated from each other and may perish. Today, in many tribes, under the varied pressures of acculturation and the disintegration of traditional values, the Indians have increasingly stopped providing tobacco for their supernaturals, and the spirits have indeed faded away. One day, predicted a Cubeo woman, the Indians too will die of hunger and starvation and then "only tobacco would remain" (Goldman 1940:243).

It is this pervasive metaphysical dimension of tobacco that the early European explorers, locked into their own narrow field of vision, were bound to miss and that, sad to say, has largely continued to elude us ever since.

REFERENCES

Listed in these references are only works that have been quoted in the text. However, in preparing to write this paper, the author, together with a group of UCLA students, consulted approximately 600 works on South American Indians and on the subject of tobacco in general. I feel greatly indebted to these men and women for their enthusiastic assistance. The library research was coordinated by Diane Olsen.

BARBOSA RODRÍGUES, JOÃO
   1890   *Poranduba amazonense*. Rio de Janeiro.
BENZONI, GIROLAMO
   1565   *Historia del mundo nuovo*. Venice.
BERNAL VILLA, SEGUNDO
   1954   Medicina y magia entre los Paeces. *Revista Colombiana de Antropología* 2 (2):219–264. Bogotá.
BIOCCA, ETTORE
   1970   *Yanoáma. The narrative of a white girl kidnapped by Amazonian Indians.* New York.
BROOKS, JEROME E.
   1937   *Tobacco: its history illustrated by the books, manuscripts and engravings in the library of George Arents, Jr. (1507–1615)*, volume one. New York.
BUTT, AUDREY
   1956   Ritual blowing. *Taling* as a causation and cure of illness: among the Akawaio. *Timehri* 35:37–52. Georgetown.
   1956–1957   The shaman's legal role. *Revista do Museu Paulista*, 16:151–186. São Paulo.

CADOGAN, LEÓN
1965   A search for the origin of Ojeo, Ye-jharú or Tupichúa. *Anthropos* 60: 207–219.
1958   The eternal pindó palm and other plants in Mbyá-Guaraní myth and legend. *Miscellanea Paul Rivet Octogenario Dicata* 2:87–96. Mexico.

CASPAR, FRANZ
1952   Die Tupari, ihre Chicha-Braumethode und ihre Gemeinschaftsarbeit. *Zeitschrift für Ethnologie* 77 (2):254–260.
1953   "Ein Kulturareal im Hinterland der Flüsse Guaporé und Machado (Westbrazilien)." Dissertation, University of Hamburg.

COOPER, JOHN M.
1949   Stimulants and Narcotics. Smithsonian Institution, Bureau of American Ethnology, *Bulletin 143, Handbook of South American Indians* 5: 525–558. Washington.

DE LÉRY, JEAN
1592   *Americae tertia pars*. Frankfurt.

ELICK, JOHN W.
1969   "An ethnography of the Pichis Valley Campa of eastern Peru." Dissertation, University of California. Los Angeles.

FOCK, NIELS
1963   Waiwai. Religion and society of an Amazonian tribe. *Nationalmuseets Skrifter, Etnografisk Raekke*, 8. Copenhagen.

GABRIEL, PADRE
1944   Los indios Kaimito (Familia Witoto). *Amazonia: Colombiana Americanista* 2 (4–8):56–58.

GOLDMAN, IRVING
1940   Cosmological thoughts of the Cubeo Indians. *Journal of American Folklore* 53 (210):242–247.

GOODSPEED, THOMAS HARPER
1942   The South American genetic groups of the genus Nicotiana and their distribution. *Proceedings Eighth American Scientific Congress* 3.

HARNER, MICHAEL J.
1973   *The Jivaro. People of the sacred waterfalls*. New York.

HISSINK, KARIN, ALBERT HAHN
1961   *Die Tacana; Ergebnisse der Frobenius-Expedition nach Bolivien 1952 bis 1954. 1, Erzählungsgut*. Stuttgart.

KAMEN-KAYE, DOROTHY
1971   Chimó: an unusual form of tobacco in Venezuela. *Botanical Museum Leaflets, Harvard University*. Cambridge, Mass.

KARSTEN, RAFAEL
1920   *Beiträge zur Sittengeschichte der südamerikanischen Indianer*. Drei Abhandlungen. Åbo.
1935   The headhunters of the western Amazonas; the life and culture of the Jivaro Indians of eastern Ecuador and Peru. *Societas Scientiarum Fennica. Commentationes Humanarum Litterarum* 29 (1). Helsinki-Helsingfors.

KOCH-GRÜNBERG, THEODOR
1923   *Zwei Jahre bei den Indianern Nordwest-Brasiliens*. Stuttgart.

KRUSE, ALBERT
- 1951–1952 Karusakaybë, der Vater der Munduruků. *Anthropos* 46:915–932; 47:992–1018.

MÉTRAUX, ALFRED
- 1928 *La civilisation matérielle des Tribus Tupi-Guarani.* Paris.

MURPHY, ROBERT F.
- 1958 Mundurucú religion. *University of California Publications in American Archaeology and Ethnology* 49. Berkeley.

NIMUENDAJÚ, CURT
- 1948 The Tucuna. Smithsonian Institution, Bureau of American Ethnology, *Bulletin 143, Handbook of South American Indians*, 3:713–727. Washington.
- 1952 The Tucuna. *University of California Publications in American Archaeology and Ethnology* 45. Berkeley.

OVIEDO, Y BAÑOS, J. DE
- 1526 *Historia de la conquista y población de la Provincia de Venezuela.* 1940. New York.

PURCHASE, S.
- 1626 *His pilgrimage*, five volumes. London.

PUTNAM, HERBERT
- 1938 *Books, manuscripts, and drawings relating to tobacco from the collection of George Arents, Jr.* Washington.

REICHEL-DOLMATOFF, GERARDO
- 1971 *Amazonian cosmos: the sexual and religious symbolism of the Tukano Indians.* University of Chicago Press: Chicago-London.

SAUER, CARL
- 1950 Cultivated plants of South America and Central America. Smithsonian Institution, Bureau of American Ethnology, *Bulletin 143, Handbook of South American Indians*, 6:487–543. Washington.
- 1969 *Agricultural origins and dispersals: the domestication of animals and foodstuffs.* Cambridge, Mass.

SCHLOEZER, AUGUST L.
- 1775–1781 *Briefwechsel meist statitischen Inhalts.* Göttingen.

SCHULTES, RICHARD EVANS
- 1967 "The botanical origin of South American snuffs," in *Ethnopharmacological search for psychoactive drugs*, 291–306. Edited by D. Efron. U.S. Public Health Service Publication, No. 1645. Washington, D.C.: U.S. Govt. Printing Office.
- 1972 "An overview of hallucinogens in the western hemisphere," in *Flesh of the gods: the ritual use of hallucinogens*, 3–54. Edited by P. T. Furst. New York.

WALDSEEMÜLLER, MARTIN
- 1507 *Cosmographiae introductio.* St. Dié.

WAVELL, STEWARD, AUDREY BUTT, NINA EPTON
- 1966 *Trances.* London.

WHIFFEN, THOMAS W.
- 1915 *The north-west Amazonas: notes on some months spent among cannibal tribes.* London-New York.

WILBERT, JOHANNES
1972 "Tobacco and shamanistic ecstasy among the Warao Indians of Venezuela," in *Flesh of the gods: the ritual use of hallucinogens*, 55–83. Edited by P. T. Furst. New York.

ZERRIES, OTTO
1964 *Waika*. Frankfurt.
1969 "Primitive South America and the West Indies," in *Pre-Columbian American religions*, 230–358. Edited by E. O. James. History of Religion Series. New York.

Coca Chewing: A New Perspective

RODERICK E. BURCHARD

ABSTRACT

Arguments presented by researchers to explain "why" Andean peasants chew coca leaf have traditionally centered around the fact that coca leaf is the source of cocaine alkaloids. Following the presentation of several cocaine-models of coca chewing, this paper argues that we must begin moving toward a new perspective on this complex problem since recent research shows that during the process of chewing, hydrolysis and metabolism, cocaine alkaloids are degraded into ecgonine. Arguing for an ecgonine-model this paper suggests that the chewing of coca leaf may be an important cultural mechanism for the control of the problems of blood glucose homeostasis and carbohydrate utilization which Bolton (1973) has suggested may be widespread in highland Peru.

INTRODUCTION

The genus *Erythroxylon* [family *Erythroxylaceae*] is widely distributed throughout the tropical regions of South America, mainly in Peru and Bolivia, and less extensively in Colombia, Ecuador, Venezuela, and Brazil. The number of different species said to belong to the genus range from as low as 75 (de los Rios 1868) to as high as 250 (Machado 1968). There is general agreement that only a limited number of these species have been cultivated through time. Because of the great plasticity of the plant under varying ecological conditions, Martin (1970:422) argues that several of these might best be considered as cultivated varieties rather than distinct species. In Peru, the two most widely cultivated species (or perhaps varieties) of the

I wish to thank Dr. H. C. Wolfart, Department of Anthropology, University of Manitoba, for the translation of German articles having to do with coca, cocaine, and ecgonine.

genus are *E. coca* lam. and *E. novogranatense* (Machado 1968; Towle 1961). The leaves of these small woody bushes are popularly referred to as "coca."

Coca leaf was probably first cultivated somewhere in the ecological zone referred to as the *montaña* or *yunga* on the eastern slopes of the Andes in Peru or Bolivia sometime in the distant past. Recently, Patterson (1971) has shown that coca was being cultivated in the middle- and upper-river valleys on the western or coastal slopes of the Andes as long ago as 1900–1750 B.C. The antiquity of coca cultivation in Peru therefore is at least 4,000 years and probably longer. Although ethnohistorical data indicate that coca was widely cultivated on the coastal side until the sixteenth century (cf. Rostworowski 1967), today its cultivation is almost totally limited to the eastern slopes of the Andes, or the *montaña*, between altitudes of 1,000 and 6,000 feet (Machado 1968).

The focus of this paper is on the problem of "why" Andean peasants chew coca leaf. Following a background on coca chewing and the general pharmacological and behavioral effects of cocaine hydrochloride, I shall outline several major cocaine-models of coca chewing, or what I refer to as the "food scarcity" hypothesis (Gutierrez-Noriega 1949, Verzar 1955), and a recent argument by Bolton (1973) which he refers to as the "hypoglycemia hypothesis." My major aim in this paper is to move us away from a traditional cocaine-model of coca chewing and toward an ecgonine-model, since ecgonine rather than cocaine is probably the central alkaloid involved in coca chewing.

THE CHEWING OF COCA LEAF

Shortly after the arrival of Europeans in the New World the use of coca leaf as a masticant was reported as far south in South America as the Rio de Plata in Argentina and as far north as the Caribbean. It was even reported in Nicaragua in Central America (Cooper 1946:549). The first description of coca use in northern South America was given in 1499 by Tomas Ortiz, a Dominican missionary (Gagliano 1961:27). Other early descriptions were presented by Alfonso Niño and Cristóbal Guerra who explored the Cumana region of Venezuela in 1500, and Amerigo Vespucci even commented on coca use in a report of 1504 (Bues 1935:2; Gagliano 1961:28).

In the Andean area, the Spanish chronicler, Pedro Cieza de Leon wrote in 1550 that: "All throughout Peru it was and is the custom to have ... coca in the mouth, and they keep it there from morning until they go to sleep without removing it" (Cieza de Leon 1959:259). Several years later, still another Spanish observer, Juan de Matienzo, was writing in 1567 that:

In Peru, from Quito to the ends of the city of La Plata, in all parts, they use and carry [coca] in their mouth. And with it, they put certain powders which they call *llipta* made from certain ground bones and ash from certain grasses... which they call *quinua*, and in certain places with quicklime. And they don't eat it or do anything else with it other than carry it in their mouth (Matienzo 1967 [1557]: 162).

Over four centuries have passed, yet there are probably as many as two million individuals in Peru who can be classified as *coqueros*, or coca chewers. In 1966, Peru produced a total of 9,091,517 kilograms of coca leaf (Banco de la Nación 1967:4). Of this total production, 18,184 kilograms of coca leaf were used within Peru for the government controlled manufacture of cocaine hydrochloride, 261,291 kilograms were exported outside Peru, with 500 kilograms going to France and 260,791 kilograms to the United States, mainly for the extraction of flavorides used in the manufacture of Coca-Cola. The remainder of this official production total, or some 8,812,062 kilograms is said to have been consumed within Peru, principally by the peasant population, for the purpose of "mastication" (*Ibid.*: Anexo II).

The mechanical procedures of chewing coca leaf, or of *chaqchando*, have been described by various researchers (cf. United Nations 1950:20–21; Stein 1961:99–100). I shall only note that it involves little more than a handful of coca leaf and some basic equipment. In the Department of Huanuco, for example, this equipment consists of a *shuti* [coca pouch], an *ishkupuru* [small gourd containing *iskhu*(lime) or *cal*], and a *chupadero* [spatula] which serves to extract the *ishku* from the *puru* as well as a cap for the *ishkupuru* when not in use.

The chewing of coca leaf is both ritualized and stereotyped. The coca leaves are taken from the *shuti*, cupped in both hands and their advice on a certain past or future event or action is requested, generally with the phrase "María Santísima, Mamíta kuquita, avisa me ..." The hands are uncupped and the leaves are examined by the *coquero*. At times the requested information is made public, but more generally it is private knowledge. The leaves are then inserted into the mouth, one or several at a time, and masticated until a *bola* [quid] begins to take shape. The coca *bola* is tucked into the side of the mouth, between the teeth and cheek. The *ishkupuru* is tapped several times against the thumb, knee, chest, or elbow after which the *chupadero* is withdrawn and wet with saliva. It is then reinserted into the *puru*, withdrawn, and tipped with *ishku*, inserted into the *bola* in the mouth. Coca leaf is added throughout the process of mastication until the *bola* has the "correct" size, and *ishku* is added throughout the process until the *bola* is considered to have the "correct" taste and consistency.

"WHY DO YOU CHEW COCA?"

The chewing of coca leaf has long contributed to the visibility of Andean peasants as well as to both curiosity and scientific interest on the part of the non-chewer to know why coca leaf is chewed in the first place. The simplest way to answer this question would appear to be a direct approach to the problem; merely ask. White (1951:242) writes: "Probably the first question asked by the visitor to the sierra and Altiplano is, why do the Indians chew coca?"

The question is not only a logical one, but an old one. Four centuries ago, Cieza de Leon wrote: "When I asked some of the Indians why they always had their mouth full of this plant, which they don't eat, but only keep in their mouth, they said they do not feel hunger, and it gives them great strength and vigor" (Cieza de Leon 1959:259). He added, "I think it probably does something of the sort, though it seems to me a disgusting habit, and what might be expected of people like these Indians" (*ibid.*). In 1567, the Spanish licentiate, Juan de Matienzo wrote: "Asking them why they carry it [coca] in their mouth, they say they feel little hunger or thirst, and they find themselves with more vigor and strength" (Matienzo 1967[1557]:162). The same question was asked by other early observers and they likewise recorded similar responses to their question (cf. Cobo 1890 (I):475; Zarate 1944[1555]:37).

The contemporary researcher who approaches the Andean peasant with questionnaire in hand, and asks: "Why do you chew coca leaf?" will without a doubt receive much the same answers as have individuals who have posed this question over the past four hundred years or more. For example the United Nations Commission of Experts (United Nations 1950:53) noted that "the most prevalent and important belief held by peasants is that coca chewing dispels and relieves hunger, thirst, fatigue, weariness, and even the desire for sleep." Fine (1960:8) writes that his informants claimed that "with coca we are in high spirits, we feel stronger. We want to work." Goddard *et al.* (1969:579) write that according to their study of "attitudes" centering around coca-use, it "reduces sensations of hunger, although apparently not in every case." "In general," they write, "chewers associate coca use primarily with the work situation; it being very common to hear that 'without coca it is impossible to work,' or 'it helps to work,' and 'we always use it because of work.' "

Of the several hundred coca chewers with whom I had contact during the course of fieldwork many dozens of them were asked the same question: "Why do you chew coca?" With few exceptions, I received the same answers as did Cieza de Leon and Juan de Matienzo during the Colonial period, as well as contemporary researchers. On the other hand, many informants simply responded that chewing coca was "customary," and one informant merely stated: "I am an Indian, therefore, I chew coca."

It is relatively easy to document the continuity in peasant responses to their inquisitors over a period of more than four centuries. Since the Spanish conquest to the present day, numerous hypotheses have been presented in an effort to explain these responses. Since the isolation of cocaine alkaloids from coca leaf by Niemann in 1859, the problem of "why" peasants chew coca leaf in the Andes, and elsewhere, has appeared to be rather straightforward. La Barre (1948:67) writes of coca leaf: "These plants contain a certain amount of cocaine, and it is for the purpose of obtaining the stimulation of this drug that coca leaf is chewed."

COCA LEAF ALKALOIDS

At least 14 different alkaloids have been isolated from coca leaf varieties (Martin 1970:422). They belong in the tropane series, together with atropine and scopolamine from the solanaceous genera *Datura*, *Hyoscyamus*, *Atropa*, etc., and are a combination of ecgonines, tropeines, and hygrines. Ecgonine derivatives consist of methyl benzoyl ecgonine [cocaine], methyl ecgonine, and cinnamyl cocaine; tropeines include tropine and pseudotropine, dihydrozypeine, tropacocaine, and benzoyl tropane; and the hygrines include hygrine, hygroline, and cuscohygrine (*Ibid.*:422). The stereoisomers α and β — truxilline have also been isolated, and nicotine has been reported (*Ibid.*).

Since the isolation of cocaine alkaloids, both the pharmacological and behavioral effects of cocaine hydrochloride on humans and non-humans have served as the model for explaining coca-use in Peru and elsewhere.

COCAINE: PHARMACOLOGICAL AND BEHAVIORAL EFFECTS

Classification: Cocaine is generally classified as a CNS [central nervous system] sympathomimetic, or stimulant, since moderate oral doses produce signs of electro-physiological stimulation or arousal of the CNS and peripheral effects indicative of the activation of the sympathetic [adrenalin-like] part of the automatic nervous system (Commission of Inquiry 1973: 312). Cocaine is often grouped together with amphetamines [benzedrine, dexedrine, methedrine, etc.] since, according to Jaffe (1970), their subjec-

tive effects, if not the actual mechanics of these effects, are almost identical.
Subjective Effects: Whereas Lewin (1964[1924]:82) may have been able to comment in 1924 that the "method of its introduction into the body is of no importance," such a statement today would and should be considered as fallacious. Jaffe (1970:293) states that the subjective effects of CNS stimulants are (a) dependent upon the user, (b) the environment [setting], (c) the dose, and (e) the route of administration, i.e. whether taken intravenously or orally since rate and extent of absorption differ with route of administration. Taken intravenously the subjective effects of cocaine are described by Jaffe as follows:

...elevation of mood that often reaches proportions of euphoric excitement. It produces *a marked decrease in hunger*, an indifference to pain, and is *reputed to be the most potent antifatigue agent known. The user enjoys a feeling of great physical strength and increased mental capacity and greatly overestimates his capabilities* [my emphasis]. The euphoria is accompanied by generalized sympathetic stimulation... [resulting in greater epinephrine output — my insertion]. Cocaine is rapidly metabolized and its duration of action is brief, lasting only minutes after intravenous injection. The contrast between the euphoria and the usual affective state, which for many compulsive users is one of chronic depression, motivates the user to repeat the experience. In this way, multiple injections may be taken over a very few hours. When large amounts of cocaine are used, the euphoria becomes mixed with anxiety and suspicion (Jaffe 1965:298–299).

In humans, moderate oral doses [5–30 mg] of cocaine and other CNS stimulants also result in an elevation of mood [euphoria], which may not, however, occur at all times; a sense of increased energy and alertness or decreased fatigue and boredom; and a reduction in appetite (Jaffe 1970:293; Kosman and Unna 1968:21).

Increase in Energy: According to Jaffe (1970:380) there is "no evidence that cocaine increases the strength of muscular contractions" and he therefore concludes that the subjective effect of increased energy or reduction of fatigue, "seems to result from central stimulation which masks the sensation of fatigue."

Anorexogenic Effect [*Reduction of Appetite*]: The reduction of appetite by cocaine and other CNS stimulants probably results from some depressing action on the appetite-regulating centers of the brain (Commission of Inquiry 1973:214). In non-human animals, experimental studies show that cocaine reduces food intake in rats, although chronic doses of cocaine had little effect on the weight-gain curve, except when given in very high doses [200–1200 mg per kg] (Kosman and Unna 1968:243). *In humans the appetite returns to normal following the discontinuance of CNS stimulants* (Commission of Inquiry 1973:23).

Anesthesia: When applied to an abraded area of the skin or mucous membrane, cocaine blocks conduction in the terminal sensory nerve fibers in concentrations as low as 0.02 percent (Ritchie *et al.* 1970:376). Investigations show that the addition of an alkaline substance to local anesthetics will potentiate their activity, and the duration of anesthetic action is proportional to the time it is in direct contact with nerve tissue (*ibid.*).

Body Temperature: Cocaine, according to Jaffe, is "markedly pyrogenic" and a combination of three factors leads to a rise in body temperature: (1) increased muscular activity leads to greater heat production; (2) vasoconstriction leads to decrease in heat loss; and (3) cocaine may have direct effect on the heat-regulating centers, for Jaffe states, the onset of cocaine-fever [sudden rise in temperature following a toxic dose] suggests that the body is adjusting its temperature to a higher level (1970:381).

Respiration: The stimulation of the medulla oblongata by moderate oral doses of cocaine leads to increased respiratory rate, the duration of which is at first unaffected, but later is diminished so that breathing becomes rapid and shallow (Jaffe 1970:380).

Cardiovascular Effects: After moderate oral doses of cocaine, heart rate, pulse rate, and blood pressure increase, and there is widespread vasoconstriction due to stimulation of the vasomotor centers in the medulla oblongata (Grollman and Grollman 1970:405). The rise in blood pressure will later diminish and fall (Jaffe 1970:390). Cocaine intake will also result in a rise of blood glucose levels (Frombach 1967).

Tolerance: Little evidence exists to indicate that cocaine use results in tolerance (Jaffe 1970:294; Commission of Inquiry 1973:23).

Toxicity: Excessive doses [particularly intravenous] may cause seizures and death by respiratory failure (Jaffe 1970:294).

Physiological and Psychological Dependency: Most researchers agree that the chronic use of cocaine does not result in "physiological dependence" and that its abrupt discontinuance will not be characterized by grossly observable withdrawal symptoms or abstinence syndrome (Jaffe 1970; Kosman and Unna 1968). Researchers do argue, however, that chronic cocaine use may result in "psychological dependency" or "habituation" which is defined by Jaffe as follows:

... In the use of drug to alter mood and feeling... some individuals eventually consider the effects produced by the drug, i.e., the condition associated with its use, are necessary to maintain an optimal state of well-being. Such individuals are said to have a psychological dependence on the drugs [habituation] (1970: 276).

He continues:

The intensity of this dependence may vary from a mild desire to a 'craving' or 'compulsion' to use the drug. This need or psychological dependence may give rise to behavior (compulsive drug use) characterized by the preoccupation with the use and procurement of the drug.

The Canadian Commission of Inquiry on the Non-Medical use of Drugs (1973), points out, however, that:

In one sense, psychological dependence may be said to exist with respect to anything which is part of one's preferred way of life. In our society, this kind of dependency occurs regularly in respect to such things as television, music, books, religion, sex, many favorite foods, certain drugs, hobbies, sports or games, and often other persons. Some degree of psychological dependence is, in this sense, a general and normal psychological condition (1973:26).

The Commission of Inquiry continues [citing the Addiction Research Foundation of Ontario]:

It should be recognized, however, that dependency is not necessarily bad in itself, either for the individual or for society. *The question to be evaluated, therefore, is not whether dependence can occur, but whether dependence in a given case results in physical, psychological, or social harm.*

Addiction: The concept of "addiction" has little meaning and is often used interchangeably with physiological or psychological dependence, as well as with "drug abuse" (*Ibid.*). The classical model of the addiction-producing drugs were the opiate narcotics and required the presence of tolerance, as well as psychological and physiological dependency (*Ibid.*). The classical model does not hold up for the non-opiate drugs. In regard to cocaine, its use may produce psychological dependence without tolerance or physical dependence (*Ibid.*: 27). Researchers emphasize that the term "habituated" (Jaffe 1970) or "dependent" be used instead of describing an individual by the term "addict" (Commission of Inquiry 1973:27).

The preceding pharmacological and behavioral effects of cocaine hydrochloride have been incorporated into several cocaine-models of coca chewing in the past few decades.

COCAINE-MODELS OF CHEWING

One of the most active and influential groups of proponents of the cocaine-model of coca chewing in Peru over the past several decades has been the late Carlos Gutierrez-Noriega and his associates, particularly Vicente Zapata Ortiz (cf. Gutierrez-Noriega and Zapata Ortiz 1947). Gutierrez-Noriega (1949:143) states that "the main cause of the coca habit is the deficiency of foodstuffs in the affected areas." Zapata Ortiz (1970:292) likewise writes that "the lack of food is the principal cause of cocaism." I shall refer to the following argument, therefore, as the "food scarcity" hypothesis.

The "Food Scarcity" Hypothesis

"One of the most characteristic actions of coca and cocaine," Gutierrez-Noriega (1949:146) writes, "is the suppression of the sensations of hunger and fatigue." He argues that because of widespread scarcity of food in highland Peru and because coca "suppresses hunger,"

> the coca chewer, as a consequence, takes coca to suppress the disagreeable sensations that result from chronic inanition. But the use of the drug occasions, after some years, the loss of appetite. The habituated chewer prefers the drug to food.... From this, a vicious cycle is established; one begins to chew coca to suppress hunger but later the subject loses his appetite and eats little because he chews coca.
> With such a deficient eating regime, the organism becomes debilitated and as always occurs in poorly fed subjects, they experience chronic tiredness, fatigue at the slightest effort, and apathy. But coca, as well as suppressing the hunger, is a powerful stimulant, perhaps superior to benzedrine and desoxyephedrine. In this way the second condition of the habit of coca chewing establishes itself, the need to counteract the fatigue of the organism with the drug. As a result, those habituated to coca refuse to undertake whatever physical work unless they have previously taken stimulating doses of coca leaf.
> Thirdly, coca is chewed to produce a state of euphoria. The habituated chewers are, in general, depressed and apathetic, which in large part is a result of the bad diet and their chronic intoxication (1952:118).

According to Gutierrez-Noriega, many of the physiological effects of coca chewing also fit within the model of cocaine hydrochloride as well. He writes:

> In general coca addicts do not show, after an ordinary period of coca chewing, strong excitation symptoms as cocaine addicts do. I have found, nevertheless, some physiological changes during the period of chewing, slight mydriasis, moderate increase in respiratory rate, rise in blood pressure, and a definite increase in heart rate.... The metabolic alterations are very constant, even with small doses of coca; there is an increase in body temperature and remarkable increase in basal metabolic rate. *The blood sugar always increases in experimental animals, but only in a very few cases does it increase in man after a period of coca chewing* [my emphasis] (Gutierrez-Noriega and Von Hagen 1950:85).

Moreover, he states that the "symptoms of habituation of the coca chewer are relatively weak" and that "tolerance phenomena are not observed" (Gutierrez-Noriega 1949:148).

A similar position is held by the United Nations Commission of Enquiry on the Coca-Leaf (1950), and I shall also include it under the label of the "food scarcity" hypothesis. This position is best summarized by Verzar (1955), a former member of the above Commission. Verzar writes:

> The alkaloid cocaine which is contained in these leaves in a concentration of 0.5 to 0.6 per cent is the oldest known local anesthetic....
>
> Cocaine has an inhibitory action on peripheral nerves and on sensory nerve endings. It also has a specific action on the central nervous system, even in very low concentrations.... It abolishes the sensation of pain and also of taste and smell. An anesthesia of the stomach with cocaine takes away the sickish feeling in stomach disease. Mucous membranes after cocaine show a vasoconstriction. Stomach secretion is stopped....
>
> *This anesthetic action depends on the presence of the free alkaloid base. At a very acid reaction, as in the gastric juice, a dissociation of the alkaloid takes place and action is destroyed. Only in alkaline solution is the alkaloid stable and active and absorbed in the active state. Obviously, this must be one of the reasons why the coqueo [sic] mixes a strong alkaline substance (lipta) [sic] with the leaves* [my emphasis].
>
> The action on the central nervous system is what is desired by the addicts, the cocainists.... Eichholtz describes the central cocaine action and also the result of coca leaf chewing by saying: 'It satisfies the starving, gives new strength to the tired and exhausted, and makes the unfortunate forget his unhappiness.'
>
> It is... certain that cocaine stops the painful sensation of hunger. The frequently quoted story of Indians who walk for days without food and rest over enormous distances may be true.... The capacity of coca to stop the feeling of hunger is not the result of some nutrient value of the coca leaves.... It is the result of central inhibition of hunger feelings....
>
> *We come to hold the conviction that the chewing of coca leaves is a method for inhibiting the feeling of hunger in a chronically underfed population.... The habit is, however, so much surrounded by mysticism that it is difficult to explain it on a biological basis. No doubt there are many who use this habit without being in the condition for which it was originally used* [my emphasis] (Verzar 1955: 366–367).

This latter point by Verzar of course raises the question of what exactly was the "condition" for which coca chewing was "originally used"? At this point, then, let me turn to still another hypothesis concerning "why" highland peasants chew coca leaf.

The "Hypoglycemia Hypothesis"

In a recent paper "Aggression and hypoglycemia among the Qolla: a study in psychobiological anthropology," Bolton (1973) has presented what surely will become one of the more widely debated arguments for years to come, centering around the "roots of social conflict" in highland peasant communities in Peru. In his paper, Bolton argues that (a) there is a high incidence of "aggressive" behavior in the highland community of Incawatana, (b) that glucose homeostasis problems are widespread among the inhabitants, and (c) that there is a causal relationship between these two phenomena, or what he refers to as the "hypoglycemia hypothesis" (Bolton 1973:241-242). Because it is not possible to outline Bolton's arguments in great detail in this paper, I shall limit my comments only to those aspects of his hypothesis that have to do with the chewing of coca leaf. Although I believe Bolton to be mistaken, I also believe that he has provided us with a starting point from which we can begin moving toward a new perspective on the chewing of coca leaf in Peru. Bolton writes:

If one postulates that the human organism attempts to maintain glucose levels at or above the nominal level, which seems to be the case, then when blood glucose falls below the nominal level, processes occur which will raise the glucose level. In the normal, healthy organism those processes are internal metabolic processes. If, however, these metabolic processes are not operating properly, e.g., because of adrenal exhaustion or liver disease, then behavioral and emotional means might be sought to produce the same effects. The individual may find that by becoming angry or by expressing aggression his glucose level is raised. Anger — the fight-flight reaction — may serve as a stimulus to sluggishly operating glands and organs. Consequently, a person's aggression is reinforced because of the physiological feeling of well-being which accompanies the emotions or aggressive actions. In this way hypoglycemia may lead to aggressiveness because this type of stimulation is extremely effective as a short-run booster of glucose levels....

Consequently, it can be seen that aggressive behavior may become part of the set of mechanisms which are involved in glucose homeostasis. To be sure, this solution to problems of glucose homeostasis, while markedly effective in the short run, is detrimental to the organism if continued for any length of time. While it is probably maladaptive for the individual it has potential eufunctional consequences, too, if, for example, it leads to spacing out or increased access to scarce resources important for an adequate diet (Bolton 1973:249).

Bolton then outlines a number of ecological, biological, and behavioral variables which he feels are interrelated in a systemic way and which account for the etiology of the hypoglycemia present in the community. He presents them in the form of a model of the "Bio-aggression system of the Qolla" (*Ibid.*:251). Included in this discussion are such variables as high population density; low per capita resource base — particularly land; inadequate food production; dietary deficiencies, including hypocaloric intake, low protein intake; vitamin deficiencies, e.g., A,B complex, and C; mineral deficiencies, e.g., calcium; high carbohydrate diet coupled with heavy muscular work; disease, e.g., cirrhosis of the liver; unpredictable weather; anxiety; hypoxia; excessive alcohol intake;

and finally, the chewing of coca leaf (*Ibid.*: 251–253).

Let me briefly illustrate Bolton's argument concerning the systemic interrelationship between these variables and hypoglycemia by focusing on two of them, i.e., hypoxia and coca chewing. Bolton writes:

Hypoxia, too, may serve as a stressor and may be partly responsible for the widespread hypoglycemia in Incawatana residents. But this question is complex. The data (Baker 1969) seem to suggest that permanent residents at high altitude have attained an adaptation which permits equivalent or higher levels of oxygen consumption than is normal for sea-level subjects. However it may be that not all individuals in the Andes are equally adapted to the hypoxic conditions. An individual might in fact be overadapted or underadapted to the hypoxic environment. If a person is overadapted, he would necessarily burn more glucose at a faster rate than is considered normal elsewhere. Thus he might more readily experience glucose deficits, particularly if nutrition is poor and if he encounters other forms of stress. If a person is underadapted, the low oxygen pressure would serve as stressor and possibly lead to the eventual deterioration of the adrenal glands and from there to the development of hypoglycemia. One or both of these situations may exist (cf. Van Liere and Stickney 1963). Picon (1962, 1963, 1966) has been studying the effects of chronic hypoxia on carbohydrate metabolism, comparing groups of subjects at sea level and at high altitudes in Peru. His studies show that there are important differences in metabolic processes between the two groups. Among his findings is the fact that during the intravenous GTT the blood glucose concentration diminishes more rapidly in high-altitude subjects than in sea-level ones, and that the initial hyperglycemic response to glucose is less pronounced in the high-altitude subjects. It was pointed out above that the *highest correlation between aggressiveness and glucose levels occurred when the glucose level in GTT had dropped by the time of the fourth glucose reading, two hours after the beginning of the test. Consequently, the rapidity of the drop seems to be related to both altitude and aggressiveness. Unfortunately, it is not known what causes this rapid drop among high altitude natives* [my emphasis] (*Ibid.*: 252–253).

In regard to the "reciprocal interaction between coca chewing and hypoglycemia," Bolton writes:

The person with hypoglycemia [brought on by such stresses as inadequate food production, dietary deficiencies, hypoxia, etc. — my insertion] becomes hungry and chews coca to dull his hunger pains and to provide himself with energy. The coca has immediate effects in raising the glucose level, probably by stimulating the transformation of glycogen stores, but it probably has long-term detrimental effects which complicate glucose homeostasis problems for the individual who chews (*Ibid.*: 253).

"Hypoglycemia," Bolton writes, "leads to high involvement in aggression" The circle, therefore, becomes complete with aggression becoming, as pointed out earlier, a behavioral means by which the individual attempts to maintain blood glucose homeostasis.

In summary, both the "food scarcity hypothesis" and the "hypoglycemia hypothesis" have a number of points in common. First, both are predicated on a cocaine-model, one explicitly and the other implicitly, of coca chewing. Second, both emphasize food deprivation as playing a major causal role in the chewing of coca leaf to "suppress the sensation of hunger" or to "dull hunger pains," as well as to increase the energy level. Third, both argue that while this may have short-term advantages it probably has long-term disadvantages; in one case, it is argued, the individual eventually "loses his appetite" and "prefers the drugs to food," thereby resulting in a "deficient eating regime" and "debilitation of the organism" (Gutierrez-Noriega 1952:118), and the other argues that it probably "complicates glucose homeostasis problems for the individual who chews" (Bolton 1973:253).

There is, however, one difference between the two models. On the one hand, Gutierrez-Noriega states that "the blood sugar always increases in experimental animals, but only in a very few cases does it increase in man after an ordinary period of coca chewing" (1950:85). On the other hand, Bolton is arguing that "coca has immediate effects in raising the blood glucose level, probably by stimulating the transformation of glycogen stores" (1973:253). The remainder of this paper will be directed at showing that chewing coca leaf does in fact raise blood glucose levels and may in reality be a cultural mechanism for the management of blood glucose homeostasis problems.

TOWARD AN ECGONINE-MODEL OF COCA CHEWING

I believe that Bolton has provided us with an important clue to the problem of "why" Andean peasants chew coca leaf when he showed that there is a widespread problem of hypoglycemia in the community of Incawatana and probably throughout the Andean highlands. Frombach (1967) has clearly demonstrated that the chewing of coca leaf does in fact result in a rise in blood glucose concentration levels (see Figure 1).

What is interesting about the pattern in blood glucose rise during coca chewing that Frombach determines, is that it remains high over an extended period of time, surpassing four hours and still remaining significantly above the initial fasting glucose level of about 72 mg per 100 ml of blood. Using the same criteria as Bolton used for the administration of the oral GTT [glucose tolerance test], i.e., that "a rise in glucose [above fasting level] at the end of four hours or a drop [below fasting level] of 5 mg or less to be normal" (1973:246), then I would say that the chewing of coca

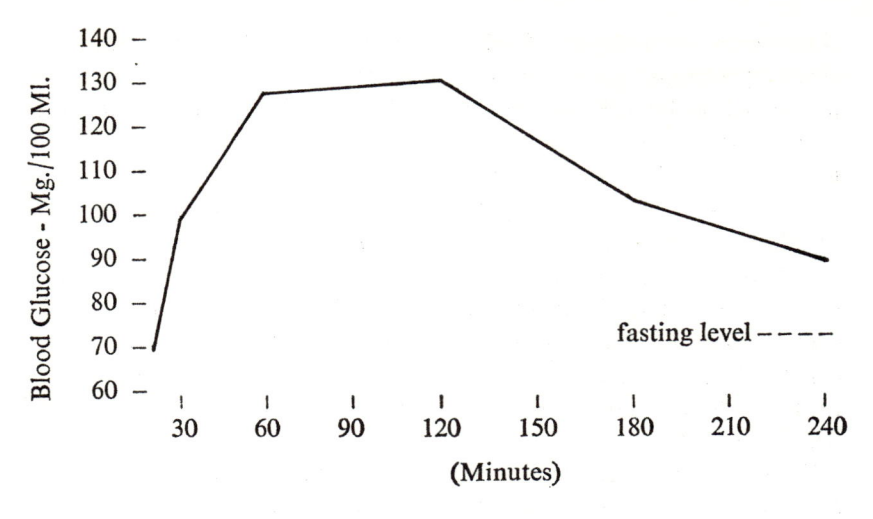

Figure 1. Blood glucose levels in coca chewers after chewing 1–1¹/₂ ounces of coca leaf. Median values of 18 cases, after Frombach (1967:393)

leaf may turn out to be of significance in the management of glucose homeostasis problems, since it may help to "normalize" glucose levels. But this rise in blood glucose is probably not taking place in exactly the way that Bolton would probably argue, i.e., by cocaine stimulation of the sympathetic part of the autonomic nervous system, and the transformation of liver glycogen by increased levels of catecholamines [epinephrine and norepinephrine].

As I pointed out earlier, at least 14 different alkaloids, including methyl benzoyl ecgonine or cocaine, have been isolated from coca leaf varieties (Martin 1970). Several of the most cherished conceptions of the chewing of coca leaf that we may have to put aside are that cocaine is in fact the central alkaloid in coca chewing, and that the *coquero* adds alkaline substances [*cal, llipta, tocra*, etc.] to the coca *bola* during the process of chewing to both facilitate the extraction of cocaine alkaloids and to potentiate their action [refer back to the cocaine-model as outlined by Verzar 1955].

Recently, Montesinos (1965) and Nieschulz and Schmersahl (1969) have demonstrated that the addition of an alkaline substance to coca leaf does in fact facilitate the extraction of the alkaloids from coca leaf, but it does so only by bringing about the degradation of cocaine. Moreover, Montesinos (1965) argues that, beginning in the mouth itself, cocaine alkaloids are further degraded, and ecgonine, not cocaine, is the end product of hydrolysis and metabolism. Montesinos writes:

The amount of cocaine circulating in the addict's [sic] organism is insignificant and the amount of ecgonine very appreciable.

It is quite possible that the addict [sic] may absorb directly through the buccal and gastric mucosa very small amounts of cocaine which are disintegrated by the cocainesterase in the blood, without any appreciable quantities remaining in the circulation or in the tissues (1965:16).

Montesinos outlines the pharmacological effects of ecgonine on mice as follows:

Ecgonine modifies the degree of blood pressure producing slight hypotension, has no influence on the salivary and suderiferous glands, slightly reduces the rate of breathing, produces slight myosis without altering the pupillary reflex, has no effect on the contraction of the striated muscle, and produces moderate relaxation of the muscles of the small intestine in the rat, while maintaining the intensity of its peristaltic movements; the toxic dose of ecgonine is between 100 and 110 mg for a mouse weighing 25 to 30 g (*Ibid.*:15).

More recently, Nieschulz has shown ecgonine to be about 80 times less toxic than cocaine; that it has little or no central stimulating effect on the sympathetic nervous system; no anesthetic or euphoric properties; and that oral doses do increase the exertion capacity of mice, although less so than similar oral doses of cocaine (1971:285). Moreover, Nieschulz demonstrates that the addicting, euphoric, and anesthetic action of cocaine can only occur when the molecule is intact, and because cocaine is degraded into ecgonine, he states that the distinction between the chewing of coca leaf and "cocainism" is "pharmacologically supported" (1971:285).

That cocaine is not the central alkaloid involved in coca leaf mastication should, if nothing else, lead researchers in the future to be very cautious about conducting experiments with pure cocaine hydrochloride on either mice or men and attempting to generalize from this to the mastication of coca leaf, a situation which has been all too common in the past (cf. Gutierrez-Noriega and Zapata Ortiz 1947). Moreover, this should provide us with insights into why, as even the principal opponents of coca cultivation and use agree, and, as one of them states, "the symptoms of addiction to coca leaves... are weak...." (Zapata Ortiz 1970:290).

That cocaine is not the central alkaloid involved in coca-use makes it easier to understand some of the contradictions that appear in the arguments of those researchers who support a cocaine-model of coca-use, especially statements such as those by Gutierrez-Noriega that "the use of the drug occasions after some years the loss of appetite," or "the habituated chewer prefers the drug to food" (1949:143), or the statement by Wolff (1950:147) that "it is evident that the chewing of these leaves for pleasure is incompatible with the regular taking of normal meals."

Close observation by researchers, including myself, who have spent time in the field undertaking participant observation in Andean communities where coca is important indicates that there is no correlation between the chewing of coca and the "loss of appetite" or the preference of the "drug to food." Webster writes: "the conjecture that coca use is actually a cause of inadequate food consumption because it deadens normal hunger drives... is discredited if one appreciates the Indian's nearly obsessive preoccupation with food and food needs as reported by Stein (1961) and Mangin (1954)" (Webster 1970:94). In a comparative study of two brothers from the highland community of Vicos, one of whom chewed coca regularly and the other of whom did not chew coca, Fine (1960) reports that their respective food consumption was equally adequate and their eating patterns almost identical. More recently, Murphy et al. (1969) conducted controlled research on a group of long-term coca chewers and a group of non-chewers. Although their research was not specifically directed at the problem of coca-use and food, nevertheless they write:

Regarding appetite, we had expected that since coca was chewed by the local population to suppress hunger when traveling or working in the fields, the continuing-users might eat less than other experimental subjects. *However, they ate amply, and explained their behavior by saying that coca did not kill their hunger, but merely made it easier to bear and forget* [my emphasis] (Murphy et al. 1969:45).

During the course of my own fieldwork, there were literally dozens of times when, after sitting and chewing coca with peasants for periods of several hours, we were invited to a meal. In these many times, I never once saw a coca chewer refuse to eat because chewing coca resulted in a "loss of appetite," or had suppressed his desire for food. On the contrary, everyone, including myself, ate with great gusto. I have seen both men and women who have spent from 8 to 10 hours in a session [*chaqchupada*] where coca chewing is continuous, end the session with a large meal. When I confronted one of my informants with these contradictions, since he too had told me that he chewed coca to "suppress hunger" ["me quita el hambre"], he turned to me and replied: "Coca is good to chew but you have to eat food to live. All people have to eat food, no matter if they chew coca or not."

I do not mean to imply by the above remarks that when coca chewers say, as they have since and probably even before the Spanish conquest, that they chew coca because it "suppresses hunger" or that it permits them to "work harder," that it may in fact not do just that. What I mean to say is that although these responses, as well as some, but apparently not all, of the physiological responses (cf. Frombach 1967) involved in coca chewing happen to fit within a cocaine-model, perhaps the overemphasis on a cocaine-model of coca chewing and the powerful symbolism of the "cocainist" have been leading us astray in these many years of trying to explain "why" peasants chew coca leaf.

Is it possible, therefore, that in a population where over 70 percent of the diet is based on carbohydrate intake (Mazess and Baker 1964), where hypoxia may impair certain enzymes involved in the transformation of glycogen into glucose and where glucose is used at a much higher rate than at sea level (Picon 1966), and where it has been shown that there are problems of blood glucose homeostasis (Bolton), that since the chewing of coca leaf does result in not only a rise in blood glucose but maintains concentration over an extended period of time, that this may in fact be what the peasant means to imply when he says that it helps to "suppress hunger" and to "work harder"?

I believe that it is, but before I make additional comment, let me turn briefly to the complex problem of coca chewing and peasant health. Although Bolton has argued that chewing coca does result in a rise in blood glucose levels, he also argues that it may have long-term detrimental effects which complicate glucose homeostasis problems for those who chew (1973:253). In fact, the entire problem of coca chewing and peasant health is the center of major debate in Peru and elsewhere today. It is outside the scope of this paper to outline all the arguments that have been brought forth on the subject, but let me present some examples of the complexity of the problem.

Although it is commonly stated that all coca chewers suffer from chronic undernourishment (Gutierrez-Noriega 1949; Zapata Ortiz 1952, 1970; Ricketts 1952, 1954; Buck *et al.* 1970), Baker (1969) has undertaken a nutritional survey of the highland district of Nuñoa, located at an altitude of between 4,000 and 5,000 meters, with a population of some 7,750 inhabitants, most of whom are probably coca chewers. Baker writes:

The results to date indicate that the Nuñoa population has a very delicate, but adequate balance, between nutritional resources and needs... if malnutrition exists, it is probably no more common than in U.S. society (1969:1154).

As an indication of just how delicate the balance is between nutritional needs and resources, Baker points out that the native foods of the area are generally low in calcium, as well as low in certain vitamins, including ascorbic acid [vitamin C] (*Ibid.*). Yet elsewhere, Baker and Mazess (1964) indicate that *cal* and *llipta*, both of which are used in the chewing of coca, are sources of needed calcium. *Cal* contributes between 300 and 1200 mg and *llipta* between 200 and 500 mg of calcium per day to the diet of coca chewers (*Ibid.*:1466). In regard to the deficiency of vitamins in the diet, it should be noted that, the United Nations Commission of Experts states that coca leaf has a relatively high level of vitamin B^1, B^2, and C (United Nations 1950:26). They report that "a quantity of 100 grams of dried leaves could supply a considerable part of the daily human requirements" in the above mentioned vitamins. But they add, because cocaine is involved in coca chewing, that this overshadows any vitamin content that coca leaf might have. But, because cocaine is insignificant, perhaps the vitamin content, as well as the minerals, involved in coca chewing may be significant after all.

In a recent epidemiological study, Buck *et al.* (1968, 1970) point out that they found several indicators which they believe demonstrate the lower nutritional status of coca chewers as opposed to non-chewers. For example, they indicate that coca chewers in the *montaña* community of Cachicoto, Huanuco, Peru, have lower serum protein levels than non-chewers. They write: "Differences in total protein average 0.53 gm% and are on the borderline of statistical significance [$P = .07$]" (Buck *et al.* 1970:26). Yet, in another study, Chahud *et al.* (1969:216) found the total serum proteins of highland coca chewers to be 6.50 gm% and that of non-chewers to be 6.25 gm%, although both groups were lower than coastal "normals" at 6.89 gm%. This indicates that the problem of coca chewing and "poor" health is not as clear cut as we might think on the basis of any one single investigation.

Let me now turn to the topic of coca leaf and blood glucose. Again, I wish to point out that although I am referring to this argument as an "ecgonine-model," that there are other alkaloids in coca leaf, i.e., tropeins and hygrines, and I use the term mainly to try and place emphasis elsewhere than on cocaine. Ecgonine is an amino alcohol base, closely related to tropine, the amino alcohol and active component of atropine (Ritchie 1965:375). Therefore, the combination of ecgonine and the tropeine alkaloids also found in coca leaf may in fact be acting on the parasympathetic nervous system as opposed to the sympathetic, and a parasympathetic response has been reported (Risemberg 1950). Atropine also results in a rise in blood glucose (Berk *et al.* 1970). Moreover, atropine is among the drugs recommended by Miller and Keane (1972:461) "to help control the symptoms of hypoglycemia." Gray (1973:121) points out that malnutrition appears to play a role in the reduced capacity to digest and absorb carbohydrates. He writes: "A study of atropine effect in man... showing an increased absorption of xylose [a sugar] suggests a possible mode of drug therapy that might be of benefit in patients with rapid intestinal transit" of glucose. He notes that atropine increases monosaccharide [of which glucose is the principal one] absorption by increasing the contact-time between carbohydrates and mucosa (*Ibid.*:123).

In short, I believe that the chewing of coca leaf, since tropine is a part of it, may be doing the same thing, and in fact may be important in the control of problems of the malabsorption and too rapid transit of glucose.

CONCLUSION

Bolton (1973:254) writes: "We will need detailed studies on the relationship between coca chewing and hypoglycemia...." This paper, although not as "detailed" as might be needed, is nevertheless, a direct response to the call.

It remains to be seen if the blood glucose rise resulting from coca chewing is due to the transformation of glycogen stores in the liver or merely a result of the concentration of the existing glucose pool and reduced peripheral utilization. Nevertheless, it may very well be that chewing coca leaf is an important cultural mechanism for managing problems of glucose utilization since coca leaf is chewed just as frequently after a high carbohydrate meal as before. After all, Andean peasants classify coca as a medicine and not as a "substitute for food" as many researchers who adhere to a cocaine-model of coca chewing have for too long led us to believe (cf. Gagliano 1961; Hughes 1946; Gutierrez-Noriega 1949; Zapata Ortiz 1952).

REFERENCES

BANCO DE LA NACIÓN
    1967 *Memoria del estanco de la Coca 1966*. Lima, Peru.
BAKER, PAUL T.
    1969 Human adaptation to high altitude. *Science* 163 (3872):1149–1156.
BERK, J. L., J. F. HAGEN, W. H. BEYER
    1970 The hypoglycemic effect of propranolol. *Hormone Metabolism Research* 2:277–281.
BOLTON, RALPH
    1973 Aggression and hypoglycemia among the Qolla: a study in psychobiological anthropology. *Ethnology XII* (3):257–277.
BUCK, ALFRED A., TOM T. SASAKI, J. J. HEWITT, A. MACRAE
    1970 Coca chewing and health: an epidemiological study among residents of a Peruvian village. *Bulletin on Narcotics* 22:23–32.
BUCK, ALFRED A., TOM T. SASAKI, ROBERT I. ANDERSON
    1968 *Health and disease in four Peruvian villages: contrasts in epidemiology*. Baltimore: The Johns Hopkins Press.

BUES, C.
 1935   La coca en el Peru. *Boletín de la Dirección de Agricultura y Ganadería* 18:3–72. Lima.
CHAHUD, A. I., et al.
 1969   Seroproteinas en indígenas coqueros. *Revista Clínica Española* 115: 213–218.
CIEZA DE LEON, PEDRO
 1959   *The Incas of Pedro De Cieza de Leon*. Edited by Victor Wolfgang Von Hagen. Norman, Oklahoma: University of Oklahoma Press.
COBO, BERNABE
 1890–1895   *Historia del Nuevo Mundo*.... Sevilla, four volumes.
COMMISSION OF INQUIRY INTO THE NON-MEDICAL USE OF DRUGS
 1973   *Interim Report*. Information Canada, Ottawa.
COOPER, J. M.
 1946   "Stimulants and narcotics," in *Handbook of South American Indians*, volume two: *The Andean civilizations*. Edited by Julian Steward Smithsonian Institution, Bureau of American Ethnology, Bulletin 143.
DE LOS RIOS, JOSÉ A.
 1868   *Sobre la coca de Peru*. Lima.
FINE, NORMAN LOWY
 1960   "Coca chewing: a social versus a nutritional interpretation." Unpublished paper. New York: Columbia University.
FROMBACH, K. D.
 1967   Beitrag zur Verbreitung und Auswirkung des Koka-Kauens in Peru. *Zeitschrift für Tropenmedizin und Parasitologie*, Stuttgart. 18:387–396.
GAGLIANO, JOSEPH
 1961   "A social history of coca in Peru." Ph.D. dissertation, Georgetown University.
GODDARD, D., S. N. DE GODDARD, P. C. WHITEHEAD
 1969   Social factors associated with coca use in the Andean region. *The International Journal of the Addictions* 4:577–590.
GRAY, G. M.
 1973   Drugs, malnutrition, and carbohydrate absorption. *American Journal of Clinical Nutrition* 26:121–124.
GROLLMAN, A., E. F. GROLLMAN
 1970   *Pharmacology and therapeutics* (seventh edition). Philadelphia: Lea and Febiger.
GUTIERREZ-NORIEGA, CARLOS
 1949   El hábito de la coca en el Peru. *América Indígena* 9 (2):143–182.
 1952   El hábito de la coca en Sud América. *América Indígena* 12 (2):111–120.
GUTIERREZ-NORIEGA, CARLOS, VICENTE ZAPATA ORTIZ
 1947   *Estudios sobre la coca y la cocaína en el Peru*. Lima.
GUTIERREZ-NORIEGA, CARLOS, VICTOR WOLFGANG VON HAGEN
 1950   The strange case of the coca leaf. *The Scientific Monthly* (February): 81–90.
HUGHES, L. W.
 1946   The curse of coca. *Inter-American Monthly* 5:18–22.

JAFFE, JEROME H.
1965, 1970 "Drug addiction and drug abuse," in *The pharmacological basis of therapeutics* (third and fourth edition). Edited by S. Goodman and A. Gilman. New York: Macmillan.

KOSMAN, M. E., K. UNNA
1968 Effects of chronic administration of the amphetamines and other stimulants on behavior. *Journal of Clinical Pharmacology and Therapeutics* 9:240–259.

LA BARRE, WESTON
1948 *The Aymara Indians of the Lake Titicaca Plateau, Bolivia.* American Anthropological Association #68 Memoir Series.

LEWIN, LOUIS
1964 (1924) *Phantastica: narcotic and stimulating drugs their use and abuse.* London: Routledge and Kegan Paul.

MACHADO, FELIX EDGUARDO
1968 "The genus erythroxylon in Peru." Masters Thesis. Department of Botany, North Carolina State University, Raleigh, N.C.

MARTIN, RICHARD T.
1970 The role of coca in the history, religion, and medicine of South American Indians. *Economic Botany* 24:422–437.

MATIENZO, JUAN DE
1967 (1567) *Gobierno del Peru.* Edited and translated by Guillermo Lohmann Villena. Travaux de l'Institut Français D'Etudes Andines, Tome XI. Paris-Lima.

MAZESS, R. B., P. T. BAKER
1964 Diet of Quechua Indians living at high altitude: Nuñoa, Peru. *American Journal of Clinical Nutrition* 15:341–351.

MILLER, BENJAMIN F., CLAIRE B. KEANE
1972 *Encyclopedia and dictionary of medicine and nursing.* Philadelphia: W. B. Saunders Co.

MONTESINOS, F.
1965 Cocaine metabolism. *Bulletin on Narcotics* 17:11–19.

MURPHY, H. B. M., O. RIOS, J. C. NEGRETE
1969 The effects of abstinence and of re-training of the chewer of coca-leaf. *Bulletin on Narcotics* 21:41–47.

NIESCHULZ, OTTO, P. SCHMERSAHL
1969 Untersuchungen über die Bedeutung des Kalkzusatzes beim Kauen von Coca-Blattern. *Pharmakologische und Phytochemische Abteilung der Chemischen Fabrik Promota Gmb. H.*, Hamburg. 178–183.

NIESCHULZ, OTTO
1971 Psychopharmakologische Untersuchungen über Cocain und Ecgonin; ein Beitrag zum Problem Cocaismus und Cocainismus. *Arzneim Forsch* 21:275–285.

PATTERSON, THOMAS C.
1971 Central Peru: its population and economy. *Archaeology* 24:316–321.

PICON-RATEGUI, E.
1966 Effects of insulin, epinephrine, and glucagon on the metabolism of carbohydrates at high altitudes. *Federation Proceedings* 25:iv, 1233–1239.

RICKETTS, CARLOS A.
1952 El cocaismo en el Peru. *América Indígena* XII (4):310–322.
1954 La masticación de las hojas de coca en el Peru. *América Indígena* XIV (2):113–126.

RISEMBERG, M.
1950 Acción de la coca y la cocaína en subjectos habituados. *Revista de Farmacología y Medicina Experimental* 3:317–328.

RITCHIE, J. MURDOCH, P. J. COHEN, R. D. DRIPPS
1965 "Cocaine; procaine and other synthetic local anesthetics," in *The pharmacological basis of therapeutics* (third edition). Edited by L. S. Goodman and A. Gilman. New York: Macmillan.

ROSTWOROWSKI, DE DIEZ CANSECO, MARIA
1967–1968 Etnohistoria de un valle costeño durante el Tehuantinsuyu. *Revista del Museo Nacional, Lima* 25:7–61.

STEIN, WILLIAM
1961 *Hualcan: life in the highlands of Peru.* New York: Cornell University Press.

TOWLE, MARGARET A.
1961 *The ethnobotany of Pre-Columbian Peru.* Chicago: Aldine.

UNITED NATIONS ECONOMIC AND SOCIAL COUNCIL
1950 *Report of the Commisison of Enquiry on the Coca Leaf.* Official Records, Twelfth Session, Special Supplement No. 1. Lake Success, New York.

VERZAR, F.
1955 Nutrition as a factor against addiction. *American Journal of Clinical Nutrition* 3 (5):363–373.

WEBSTER, STEVEN S.
1970 The contemporary Quechua indigenous culture of high-land Peru: an annotated bibliography II. *Behavior Science Notes* 5:213–248.

WHITE, C. LANGDON
1951 Coca chewing in the Andes. *Pacific Spector* 5:242–249.

WOLFF, PABLO OSWALDO
1950 *Annotated bibliography on the effects of chewing the coca leaf.* Annex II. United Nations. Report of the Commission of Enquiry on the Coca Leaf. Lake Success, New York.

ZAPATA ORTIZ, VICENTE
1952 The problem of the chewing of the coca leaf in Peru. *Bulletin on Narcotics* 4:27–36.
1970 The chewing of coca leaves in Peru. *International Journal of Addictions* 5 (2):287–294.

ZARATE, AGUSTIN
1944 (1555) *Historia del descubrimiento y de la conquista del Peru*, volume one. Lima.

Cannabis or Alcohol:
The Jamaican Experience

MICHAEL H. BEAUBRUN

ABSTRACT

Professor Michael Beaubrun of the University of the West Indies was the guest speaker at a joint dinner meeting of the Congress sessions on cannabis and on alcohol. The address provides comparative data from the British West Indies and posits social class and personality factors in the drug of choice — cannabis or alcohol. Beaubrun cites a high correlation between extroversion and heavy drinking; with a preponderance of cyclothymic personalities who are successful in Western cultures, alcohol becomes the "establishment" choice while personality attributes in the "culture of poverty" may lead to cannabis preference.

In giving this address, I feel a little like the eunuch's brother — you know the story of the eunuch who was left behind by the sultan in charge of his harem and when the sultan returned and found three of his wives were pregnant, he asked him for the explanation and the eunuch said, "Well, sir, you see while you were away I was down with flu and I asked my brother to take over. You see, sir, he is not cut out for the job!" I too am not cut out for the job. So if you'll accept my remarks in the light of an after dinner speech rather than a serious contribution to the scientific literature, I will proceed.

The title of my paper is "Cannabis or Alcohol" and it is not as you might think, the choice being offered by the stewardesses on Air Jamaica instead of tea or coffee. It may be that one day it will be, but my guess is that it won't be for quite some time, because the war about cannabis is still being hotly waged and it looks as though it will be for some time. The decision as to which drug is permitted or used in what culture will continue to be made on irrational grounds, or grounds of economic expediency, rationalized afterwards by double-blind controls — you know the blind leading the the blind. But I think that I don't need to stress to an anthropological audience how irrational has been the behavior of mankind through the ages in the sanctioning of psychotropic substances. Yet, I would suggest to you that these choices have not always been quite so capricious as they might seem. A proper study of any given culture usually reveals the reasons why a particular drug has become the drug of choice of a culture or any subgroup within it. In the search for ways of coping with anxiety and depression and ways of making life more meaningful, mankind through the ages has turned to psychoactive substances. The history of drug use is at least as old as agriculture. It would seem that cultures learn to coexist with drugs by adopting rules and by adopting a set of values and attitudes about them and incorporating this into their way of life. Problems with drugs seem related to the attitudes, customs and rules for their use and non-use. Such attitudes and customs are built into the superego of the growing child by the normal processes of socialization, that is to say, by imitation and conditioning. In those cultures where the rules are inconsistent or conflicting, ambivalence, guilt and anxiety arise and problems tend to be created. Where new drugs are introduced into cultures that have no rules for them, there often exists a period of crisis.

McGlothlin pointed out to us that the two drugs most widely used in the world are cannabis and alcohol. He also drew our attention to the fact that cannabis is usually the drug of the have-nots and alcohol the chosen drug of the establishment. It has frequently been suggested that this correlation is no accident, that in fact, there is a causal relationship involved. Two main reasons for this correlation are usually suggested: either (1) that the effect of cannabis is such that it enables the failure to retreat from the world and forget his failures; or (2) that the effect of the drug is such that it actually interferes with his motivation to succeed, or, if not his motivation to succeed, his efficiency and productivity, so that in fact he doesn't get on in the rat-race.

Tonight I'd like to talk to you about our experiences in Jamaica where cannabis has been used for over 100 years, certainly for the whole of this century by the Afro-Jamaicans, and where alcohol has been used for centuries. I'd like to examine the evidence from studies in Jamaica that might help us understand the factors underlying use and non-use of alcohol or cannabis by different socioeconomic and cultural groups, and try and answer two questions: Is the relationship between cannabis use and low socioeconomic status a causal one and, what is the relationship between cannabis and alcohol? Is it possible that in some situations cannabis may be a desirable alternative to alcohol?

Between August 1970 and December 1971, the Research Institute for the Study of Man and the Medical School of the University of the West

Indies carried out a joint collaborative study, a major multidisciplinary study on the long-term chronic use of cannabis in Jamaica, under the aegis of the National Institute of Mental Health, Center for the Studies of Narcotic and Drug Abuse. Detailed anthropological studies were undertaken in seven areas of Jamaica before the clinical studies began. From four of these locations a representative sample of thirty chronic users of cannabis and thirty matched controls was selected and persuaded to remain in the University Hospital for six days and nights undergoing intensive studies — medical, psychological and psychiatric, including EEG findings. The subjects were matched for age, sex, occupation, income, and social class.

The major study has not as yet been published but there were three papers this morning referring to it; the psychiatric findings will appear in the March 11, 1974 edition of the *American Journal of Psychiatry* and there have been other references to it in the literature. I will refer to it as the main background for the points I wish to make tonight, or the guesses I will hazard.

Cannabis has been smoked in Jamaica for nearly 130 years. Though we have evidence that the hemp plant was present in Jamaica as early as the late eighteenth century, the habit of smoking cannabis is thought to have been introduced into Jamaica only in the mid-nineteenth century by East Indian indentured laborers who came to the West Indies after the abolition of slavery. Vera Rubin and Lambros Comitas have documented well the evidence that the Indians introduced cannabis, based on the complex of cultural beliefs about *ganja*, "the *ganja* complex," the methods of preparation and use of the drug and the Hindu names used — like *ganja, kali, chilam* pipe, etc., all in use among working-class Jamaicans today. These are easily identifiable with similar phenomena described by the Indian Hemp Commission Report (1969) in 1894. The working-class Jamaican uses *ganja* as a sovereign remedy for all ills. He uses it to give him energy for work and to relax after work. He believes that giving it to school children makes them brighter and sharpens their understanding. In addition to being a kind of general tonic, he also attributes to it some mystical powers, for example that it wards off evil spirits. This complex of beliefs, attitudes and customs is believed to have been diffused to the Jamaican working class, the descendants of African slaves, and especially to the Rastafarians, a long-haired Afro-Jamaican politico-religious cultural group who preach a back-to-Africa destiny and claim Haile Selassie as their God. The growing child in working-class Jamaica is gradually socialized into the use of *ganja* and has many respectable smoking role models. He is fed it as an infusion even in his infant bottle. He may begin smoking it at the age of seven or eight, but is usually initiated in his early teens by one of his peers or in a group smoking experience which has many of the features described by Dr. Rubin this morning as a *rite de passage*. His response to this initial smoking experience validates his role as a smoker or non-smoker in the *ganja* subculture. An initial unpleasant experience may result in his avoiding *ganja* thereafter and seems to validate his role as a non-smoker.

The anthropological studies of Rubin, Comitas *et al.*, together with the work of Yawney on the Rastafarians, show us clearly how the culture has developed "built in" controls to minimize the ill effects of this drug, for example, the screening mechanism for validating the non-smoking role of those who have "no head for it." The beliefs that you should not smoke when you are angry or on an empty stomach, and above all, the experience of learning to "titrate" so as to achieve the result you need or expect and no more — these are the things that the child learns and I think they are important to the fact that the drug has little ill effect in working-class Jamaica. I can't give you the detailed report of this 500-page manuscript but on the whole, *ganja* comes out remarkably well from the study. The findings show very little long-term damage: in the medical studies only a slight impairment of respiratory function and slight changes in hemaglobin on long-term use (which you would expect) and blood pressure changes.

The psychological tests did not reveal any significant difference between smokers and non-smokers at all. The psychiatric findings, which have been published elsewhere, show no differences between the *ganja* smokers and non-smokers in the incidence of mental illness or of abnormalities of mood or of behavior. Nor did the groups differ significantly with regard to criminal records or the use of other drugs, or in upward or downward social mobility. One finding that was significant relates to the incidence of mental illness in the family. Although there was equal incidence of mental illness among smokers and non-smokers, smokers were found to have more mental illness in the family than non-smokers. This seemed to suggest that in fact *ganja* might be playing a protective role against mental illness, because one would expect a high incidence of psychotic illness in the families of persons with mental illness. It may be that the smoking was protective.

I would like to examine the evidence on the vexed question of the amotivational syndrome. The anthropological findings of the Jamaica cannabis study indicated that chronic use of cannabis, even heavy use, did not seem to result in a loss of motivation or striving toward conventional goals. But one substudy by Dr. Joseph Schaeffer did demonstrate decreased efficiency and productivity immediately after smoking, that is acute smoking, not chronic smoking. The frequency and quantity of use of cannabis also was clearly correlated with socioeconomic status in the villages studied. Heavy smoking was always highly correlated with poverty.

This morning Dr. Schaeffer told us how he and his wife studied the households of cannabis users and made careful recordings with a portable videotape and film, of every movement during periods of agricultural work and kept detailed records of food eaten and energy expended. They also made objective measurements of energy metabolism in special tests. There seems little room for doubt that the subjective descriptions of increased energy output at work are supported in fact by the objective findings. But much of energy may be wasted. Schaeffer reports that in agricultural pursuits, "total space covered, or amount accomplished, or number of plants reaped is usually reduced per unit of time after smoking, and the total number of movements taken to complete the required task is increased after smoking." He also notes, however, that social cohesiveness is enhanced.

Schaeffer was cautious in drawing conclusions from his findings but he does say "intuitively we feel that cannabis use is subtly related to population, land and economic pressures. To oversimplify: land resources in Valley (the name given to this village) are relatively scarce. The topography is not conducive to cultivation. Average farms are small. Common agricultural products in the area do not bring high market profits. A population decrease has ended due to the international pressures against migration and other difficulties of city life. Two results are particularly significant to our concern: (1) the inhabitants of Valley have a vested interest in decreasing total cultivated acreage and consolidating production; (2) social cohesiveness among farmers is now more appropriate than rugged competition."

Note the suggestion that "there may be a vested interest in decreasing total cultivated acreage and reducing competition." I find this thesis may be a little hard to accept in full but it does seem that where social conditions are such that upward social mobility is almost blocked and increased work output results in negligible profits you might expect a lessening of motivation to work. Cannabis seems to be a valuable source of motivation in that it enables the farmers to work hard at repetitive and dull tasks like weeding, which have little reward. Such a situation with rigid economic class lines may be compared to the caste barriers of India where lower caste use of cannabis may serve the short term interests of the middle class as well as it may serve to prevent attempts to overthrow the system or interfere radically with its workings.

Cannabis plays a number of other less obvious roles as it is an unseen subsidy for the economy and a valuable though prohibited small cash crop, as you were told by Lambros Comitas this morning.

How does this compare with alcohol? Now I think that there is little doubt that anyone who attempted to use alcohol regularly for energy, for work in the way that the villagers in Jamaica use cannabis would soon come to a nasty cropper. He would rapidly develop dependency and physical damage. Not only loss of efficiency would result, but other problems. In fact, the closest thing to this perhaps would be the delta alcoholic of wine drinking countries like France. The nearest thing we have to this is the regular consumption of small quantities of wine and we know how damaging that can be.

Alcohol is a major ingredient in our way of life in the Caribbean and Jamaica is no exception. Rum, the by-product of sugar cane, has been central to our way of life since the days of the buccaneers and today social life in the working class revolves around the rum shop. In the upper circles it revolves around the club and the cocktail party and consumption is very high. What is remarkable is that the rates of alcoholism seem to vary tremendously from island to island in the Caribbean.

A number of interacting variables seem to be responsible for this. High rates of alcoholism are found (1) where tourism is highly developed and the country's own national identity is poorly delineated and disparaged; [Examples of this would be the Bahamas and the U.S. Virgin Islands. It is thought there that the tourist provides a role model to emulate — someone who is constantly playing and drinking and never seems to work] (2) where indigenous Indian populations exist, for example Aruba; (3) where East Indians (Hindus and Moslems) are a large part of the population; [Examples of this would be Trinidad and Guyana] and finally, (4) another variable would be where French cultural influences predominate, like Martinique and Guadeloupe.

In all of these places the rates of admission for alcoholism to mental hospitals vary from 20 to 55% of total admissions and the percentage of male admissions is very much higher than that. What is pertinent to my theme tonight is that by far the lowest hospital admission rates for alcoholism for the entire region are found in Jamaica — less than 1% in most years. Compare this with figures of 55% in some of the other places.

Raymond Prince who worked for two years at the 3000-bed mental hospital in Jamaica reported: "Of 600 admissions to one typical ward over a two-year period, less than 2% suffered such problems; not a single case of chronic brain syndrome associated alcoholism was seen and we encountered neither delirium tremens nor alcoholic hallucinosis. The few alcohol-linked disturbances were middle class persons or foreigners." Now note that Jamaica is also the ONLY island where cannabis use is widespread and endemic among the working class — until very recently the only one where there was any smoking of cannabis at all.

The other piece of evidence is a field study of Jamaican drinking practices in four different socioeconomic areas conducted by my students in 1966 which showed that the lowest rates of heavy drinking were found among the Jamaican working class, the very group in which *ganja* smoking was most prevalent. On the basis of this, I hazarded the guess that *ganja* smoking might in fact be an alcohol substitute protecting poor Jamaicans from becoming alcoholics.

Prince, Greenfield, and Marriot followed this up with a study of 106 consecutive male admissions to the Mental Hospital. Of these, 24% used *ganja* regularly once a day or more, 40% had never used it and the rest were occasional users. Using a key informant technique, they estimated that at least as many males in the community from which the sample was drawn used *ganja* once a day or more in the same way. The subsequent anthropological studies have shown that this estimate of *ganja* smoking outside of the hospital is probably an underestimate, indicating that *ganja* smokers are probably underestimated in the *ganja* population in the mental hospitals, again evidence pointing toward the opposite to its being productive of psychosis.

Prince *et al.*, found that *ganja* use was greatest among low income males between 15 and 35 years of age and that they tended to use less as they grew older. Comparing this with our field study of drinking practices which showed that heavy drinking peaked in the mid to late forties, they concluded that as people grow older and a little more affluent they turned to alcohol, adopting middle-class values. This may not be exactly how it happens but certainly there were fewer problems from both alcohol and cannabis.

In view of the fact that few working-class people were hospitalized as a result of either cannabis or alcohol, they concluded that *ganja* was a benevolent alternative effectively protecting poor Jamaicans from the damage due to alcohol.

The subsequent large-scale cannabis study in Jamaica could not prove this but did not disprove it and, in fact, did give it some support. From the data obtained by the psychiatrists and the anthropological field workers, we observed that, although not teetotallers, the cannabis smokers usually drank beer rather than rum, and that in those of the smokers' families where an alcoholic was found, we were usually told that he was the only one who didn't smoke. It did seem as though cannabis smokers were moderate drinkers while their non-smoking peers were more likely to take alcohol to excess.

What then were the factors determining drug choice? Prince suggested only an economic motive, *ganja* being cheaper than alcohol (and it may be that this is significant), but it seems there may be a more complex relationship involving not merely an economic factor but personality factors as well.

Attempts have been made to account for the use of cannabis in terms of the function it serves. But we were repeatedly reminded today that the effect of any drug is a complex interaction of factors including culture. Briefly, the effect of any drug on the individual is the product of (1) the pharmacological action of the drug; (2) the personality of the user; (3) his mental set; and (4) the setting in which he uses it. The last two are considerably colored by cultural factors which determine the expectations of the user.

I would like to consider the factor of personality. In our field survey of drinking practices, we gave each of our 1800 respondents a shortened version of the Eysenck Personality Inventory and found a very positive correlation between high extroversion and heavy drinking. In fact, there was a linear correlation significant at 0.05. Neuroticism did not show any significant correlation. So extroversion is highly correlated with excessive drinking. We used the same tool in the *ganja* study and got no significant correlation with extroversion. I think this is important. As in the classic study by Carstairs on the use of *daru* and *bhang* by the Rajputs and Brahmins, the worldly aggressive extroverts were the ones who chose alcohol. The priestly Brahmins were not poor, because in India they enjoyed high caste for religious reasons, but in most of the Western world the schizothymic personality is less likely to succeed materially than the cyclothymic. It is widely recognized that manic depressive families (i.e. the cyclothymics or people with allied constitutions) are overrepresented at the top of the economic ladder or find their way there, while schizothymics, or the relatives of schizophrenics, tend to drift downwards and to be overrepresented among the poor. Might this be a simple answer to the correlation between cannabis use and poverty? It's too simplistic perhaps to suggest that all the poor are schizothymics and all the rich are cyclothymics, but it could be that there is a significant preponderance of cyclothymic personalities (extroverts) at the top, a sufficient number of them to set the mode and make this the accepted way of life, and this may be why alcohol becomes the establishment drink.

The more introverted — the poet, the academic, the seeker after an inner subjective reality and meaning, and the rugged individualist — may prefer cannabis but they do not really have an unfettered choice.

One of the reasons why the Minnesota Multiphasic Personality Inventory (MMPI) and other personality measures have not given us clear profiles of drinkers versus cannabis smokers is that the profiles are muddied because schizoids, as well as neurotics and other depressives, all abuse alcohol where there is no sanctioned alternative. Is it possible that if a clear choice were available, each equally and comparably priced, that we might find that the extroverts preferred alcohol while the introverts would take cannabis; neurotics might choose either and psychopaths both? This is a simplistic formulation but you know what I mean. I don't mean really cyclothymics and schizothymics but only recognizable profiles. I say simplistic because obviously the relationship between personality and culture is a complex one. Personality is not simply inherited, it is also molded by the culture itself and there is a two-way relationship involved, as well as genetic factors.

Now the pharmacological action of cannabis and alcohol, the other variable. Alcohol after all is a sedative and is needed by those who develop high anxiety levels while striving and competing, those with high levels of aggression, high belligerence. While cannabis is a complex drug, it is a stimulant and a euphoriant, also something of a sedative and something of an hallucinogen. It may be that this is needed more by the less aggressive folk — those unable to communicate, tending to inaction, to dreaming, seekers after meaning.

What answers can we find to the questions that I posed at the start of the talk? First, the causal relationship between cannabis and poverty — is there a causal relationship in this correlation? Well, I think the truth is that from our data so far the answer is still uncertain. Clues suggest rather that it is the personality attributes prevalent in the culture of poverty which leads to cannabis preferences, rather than the self defeating nature of cannabis itself. There is some evidence the other way, so it is rather difficult to give a fair answer to this.

The other question posed was — can cannabis be used as an alcohol substitute? I think in certain situations, in certain places and in certain cultures, it can. There are situations, as we have shown in Jamaica, in which cannabis use may be functional and probably protective against the dangers of alcohol. There is no doubt that alcohol causes more physical damage, dependency and a number of other problems. Going back to the classic study by Carstairs on *daru* and *bhang* among the Rajputs and Brahmins, I think his ideas are still probably right, despite the recent apparent invasion of the Western middle class by cannabis, which I believe is a temporary phenomenon. Cannabis, as Carstairs postulated, is ill-suited to success in the materialist Western world and it is unlikely that it would succed as a drug of choice, in, say, the United States.

What lessons can be learned from the Jamaican experience? If we cannot substitute cannabis for alcohol, we can note that in Jamaica the reason that cannabis works among the poor is because the cultural rules are so well defined; the screening mechanisms, the validation of non-smoking, the other things. We must learn folkways which would enable us to better cope with the drug of choice we already have here — alcohol. We may have to develop the attitudes and practices best calculated to cope with it. This has been advocated in a number of reports, for example, the Cooperative Commission on Alcoholism.

But let us not forget Prince's original finding that the reason that cannabis was being used instead of alcohol in Jamaica in the first instance was probably an economic one. It is really quite simple. *Ganja* is cheaper than alcohol in Jamaica and freely available to the poor. I think we have among us here, people who have also noted the economic factor. Dr. DeLindt of Canada pointed to the importance of beverage price in reducing overall consumption of alcohol and reducing the ill effects. And I think this is part of the lesson that comes out of the Jamaican experience. Perhaps the pricing of whatever is the drug of election or putting it out of reach is one of the ways of dealing with the situation, not forbidding it, because forbidding it only produces the forbidden fruit complex, which makes it all the more desirable. On this note, I think I will end. Thank you.

PART FIVE

The Modern Complex in North America

Cannabis Use in Canada

MELVYN GREEN and RALPH D. MILLER

ABSTRACT

The history of cannabis in Canada extends back to the early 17th century, but non-medical use can be conclusively documented only to the 1930s and popular use to the mid-1960s. Cannabis was first legally prohibited in 1923; criminal penalties for illegal possession, importation, cultivation and trafficking have increased in severity. Convictions of marihuana and hashish doubled annually from the mid-1960s until 1970, and have continued to rise, although at a less dramatic rate of increase, since 1970.

Marihuana and hashish are both routinely available throughout Canada, but the quantity and quality are insufficient to satisfy the demands. Consequently, both marihuana and hashish are smuggled into Canada by sophisticated, criminally-oriented organizations dealing in hundred-pound shipments, and by youthful non-professionals importing small amounts.

The non-medical use of cannabis was primarily restricted to college-aged persons of middle-income families in the mid-1960s, but was quickly diffused to older and younger persons of all class levels. Today, Canada's cannabis-using population appears to increasingly mirror the social characteristics of the general population. Although cannabis users typically take other drugs as well, it is not clear to what extent the use of cannabis adds to, or substitutes for, the use of other drugs such as alcohol.

SOCIAL AND LEGAL HISTORY

The history of cannabis in North America began in 1606 with experimental cultivation in Nova Scotia (then Nova Francia) by Louis Hébert, who was Samuel de Champlain's apothecary. Commercial hemp cultivation was

---

This paper presents the personal opinions of the authors and does not necessarily reflect the official position of the Commission of Inquiry into the Non-Medical Use of Drugs.

The preparation of the manuscript by Lynn Bryan and the editorial assistance of Linda Wright are gratefully acknowledged.

established soon after throughout both French and English New World colonies, encouraged by various systems of legal penalties and incentives. Hemp was considered to be an essential crop for both domestic requirements such as clothing and cordage, and for the colonial powers' naval needs such as sails and rigging (Barash 1971). Commercial hemp production remained a viable industry only until the late 18th or early 19th centuries. Limited cultivation, however, continued in Canada until the early 1930s, when economic developments rendered hemp production an unprofitable enterprise. Unauthorized cannabis cultivation was legally prohibited in 1938, and all hemp fiber used in Canada since has been imported. Untended cannabis, generally of low potency, still grows in several provinces, particularly in parts of Quebec where extensive hemp cultivation occurred a century or more ago. While early Canadian settlers were quick to exploit the agricultural and industrial potential of hemp, it was not until the 20th century that the psychotropic properties of cannabis were generally recognized.

Although cannabis apparently did not play an important role in Canadian medical practice, cannabis preparations were used in conjunction with the treatment of a variety of ailments until relatively recently. Several over-the-counter remedies (primarily cough syrups, sleeping potions and corn removers) were available until 1939, and cannabis-containing medicines were produced for prescription use until 1954. Medical prescribing of cannabis is not prohibited, but there is presently no licit production of cannabinoid medicines. However, old stocks of some cannabis-containing preparations still exist in certain pharmacies.

There are no reliable accounts of the non-medical use of cannabis in Canada which predate the 1930s. The *Canadian Medical Association Journal* first warned of "The Increasing Menace of Marihuana" in 1934 and reported the rising use of the drug in Ottawa, Toronto, Windsor, Montreal, and British Columbia (Canadian Medical Association 1934a). While there may have been small groups of users in these and other areas during the 1930s, cannabis use was not the subject of notable police or media attention until some thirty years later. Dominion Bureau of Statistics calculations, for example, show only twenty-five convictions for marihuana possession in all of Canada between 1930 and 1946, compared to over nineteen hundred convictions for possession of opiates during this period (Josie 1948). According to the Royal Canadian Mounted Police, who are entrusted with enforcing Canada's narcotic legislation: "Prior to 1962, isolated cases of cannabis use were encountered, but generally in connection with entertainers and visitors from the United States. Although marihuana arrests were effected sporadically in the middle 40s, its use on a more frequent basis appeared in Montreal only in 1962, in Toronto in 1963 and in Vancouver in 1965" (Royal Canadian Mounted Police 1969).

Marihuana smoking, however, was supposedly in vogue in the artistic community of Vancouver in the late '50s (Paulus and Williams 1966), and Toronto researchers have estimated that there were about fifteen hundred cannabis users in that city by 1960, and that some middle-class professionals, entertainers and para-criminal persons in Toronto had been smoking marihuana or hashish since the early 1950s (Coleclough and Hanley 1968).

It appears that cannabis use did not develop as quickly or as extensively as in the United States. The virtual explosion of such use in Canada during the mid-'60s was apparently imitative of American developments and a product of the same social forces — such as the evolution of the psychedelic ethos, the mass media's publication of the drug, and the growth of underground newspapers — that can be considered to have contributed to the American situation. In 1962 the Royal Canadian Mounted Police reported only 20 cases connected with cannabis. In 1968 the number of cannabis-related cases had risen to over 2,300, and in 1972 there were nearly 12,000 cannabis convictions in Canada (Royal Canadian Mounted Police 1973).

The supposed dangers of cannabis have been sensationally described by the early Canadian feminist, Emily Murphy (1922), or "Janey Canuck," an Edmonton juvenile court judge and magistrate, in a chapter of her book *The black candle* devoted to "Marijuana — the new menace." This often racially biased monograph presented various flamboyant descriptions of the effects of cannabis which contributed to the prevailing marihuana mythology of that time. Quoting extensively from a letter written by the Chief of the Los Angeles Police, Murphy stated:

Persons using this narcotic smoke the dried leaves of the plant,which has the effect of driving them completely insane. The addict loses all sense of moral responsibility. Addicts to this drug, while under its influence, are immune to pain.... While in this condition they become raving maniacs and are liable to kill or indulge in any form of violence to other persons, using the most savage methods of cruelty without, as said before, any sense of moral responsibility.

When coming from under the influence of this narcotic, these victims present the most horrible condition imaginable. They are dispossessed of their natural and normal will power, and their mentality is that of idiots. If this drug is indulged in to any great extent, it ends in the untimely death of its addict.

Murphy's book had an almost immediate influence on Canadian legislation. One year after its publication — without any scientific evidence or sense of public urgency, and without any explanatory or rationalizing discussion in Parliament — "Indian Hemp" was included in the Schedule of the Opium and Narcotic Drug Act in 1923, and has been legally classified with the opiate narcotics ever since. Thus, cannabis was made illegal in Canada ten years before any empirical evidence of its non-medical use emerged, and fourteen years before federal legislation regarding cannabis was first adopted in the United States, where regional but widespread use had been extensively publicized since 1910 (Cook 1964).

The inclusion of cannabis in the opiate narcotic schedule, and later in the Narcotic Control Act (1961), has meant that occasional increases in the severity of penalties for narcotic offences have been automatically applied to cannabis as well. This situation prevailed until 1970 when the Narcotic Control Act was amended to allow the Crown to proceed by way of "indictment" or "summary conviction" in the case of unauthorized simple possession of cannabis. The indictment procedure was formerly the only option available and provides for a maximum sentence of seven years' imprisonment, while a summary conviction (similar to a misdemeanor in American courts) provides for a maximum sentence of six months' imprisonment and/or a fine of one thousand dollars for the first offense and one year's imprisonment and/or a fine of two thousand dollars for subsequent offences. Since 1972, because of recent revisions in the Canadian Criminal Code, persons convicted of cannabis possession offenses have sometimes been sentenced to "absolute" or "conditional" discharges which involve no fines or imprisonment and allow for the expungement of criminal records related to the offense after a one-year period without further convictions. However, most simple possession convictions result in fines (e.g. $150.00).

The penalties for cannabis-related offenses beyond simple possession have not, as yet, been legislatively altered or separated from the legislation controlling opiate narcotics. Possession for the purpose of trafficking and trafficking itself carry maximum sentences of life imprisonment; unauthorized importation or exportation provides a minimum sentence of seven years' imprisonment and a maximum sentence of life imprisonment; and unauthorized cultivation carries a maximum sentence of seven years' imprisonment. These maximum sentences have never been awarded in the case of cannabis offenders, but unlike the situation with simple possession the majority of persons convicted of trafficking and intent-to-traffic offences are still imprisoned. Importation convictions necessitate a minimum sentence of seven years' imprisonment (which may be reduced by parole), and between a third and a half of those annually convicted of illegal cultivation of cannabis are sentenced to jail or prison terms. Generally speaking, sentencing is far less punitive today than it was during the mid and late 1960s for all cannabis-related offences. However, a consistent, humane and truly realistic legal control model must await the long-promised rewriting of Canadian drug legislation.

In May 1969 the Government of Canada appointed the Commission of Inquiry into the Non-Medical Use of Drugs (the "LeDain Commission"). The Commission has published an *Interim report* (1970), *Treatment report* (1972a), *Cannabis report* (1972b) and *Final report* (1973) in both French and English. The present paper is based primarily on studies conducted while the authors were members of the Commission research staff.

AVAILABILITY AND DISTRIBUTION

Marihuana and hashish are both routinely available throughout Canada, although the former predominates in the West Coast, and the latter is more common in the more Eastern provinces (Commission 1972b). For example, hashish was reported as the "most readily available" drug by three times as many cannabis-using university students as those who named marihuana, British Columbia being the only province where marihuana was claimed to be more easily available than hashish. In most regions of the country high school students reported that the two forms of cannabis were about equally available to them, but in Ontario hashish was reportedly most common, and in British Columbia marihuana was most frequently encountered (Lanphier and Phillips 1971). These data suggest that age, education, and/or social class may be significant factors in determining the relative availability and use of hashish and marihuana. Little research has been directed specifically at this question, but, with this exception, our own social and behavioral studies suggest that the two forms of cannabis are generally used interchangeably in Canada, and that the patterns of use, social characteristics of the users, the general effects of the drugs and the avenues of initiation to use are essentially the same for both. The Canadian experience is significantly different from that of the United States where hashish is relatively less frequently encountered.

In Canada, cannabis is rarely adulterated with other drugs, although various plant materials are sometimes represented as marihuana or are used to dilute or "cut" it. In our national survey of non-forensic "street drug" analysis facilities, and our collection of illicit drug samples, more than three-quarters of those samples presented to the analyst as hashish or marihuana were what they had been alleged to be; almost all of the remainder were inactive substances (Miller *et al.* 1973; Marshman and Gibbins 1970; Commission 1972b, 1973). The drugs submitted to non-forensic facilities for analysis are often those suspected of being in some way unusual; consequently, these studies likely contain a disproportionate number of deviant samples and the data cannot be considered representative of the cannabis generally available in Canada. Tetrahydrocannabinol (THC), the principal active constituent in cannabis, has never been found in isolated form on the illicit market — most of the alleged THC samples analyzed were actually phencyclidine (PCP). Liquid cannabis extract or concentrate ("hash oil") has become intermittently available during the past two years.

The THC content of cannabis in Canada varies over a wide range, with typical values of approximately 5% and 0.6% Δ^9 THC for hashish and marihuana respectively (Miller *et al.* 1973.). With the appropriate seeds, marihuana with high THC content can easily be grown in this country, although much of the domestic material on the illicit market seems to be of rather low potency (Commission 1972b; Small 1971). Sometimes attempts are made to artificially improve the potency of marihuana. Some of these measures include moistening and burying for several days, boiling for several hours, storing with dry ice, or exposing the marihuana to ultraviolet lamp rays.

Royal Canadian Mounted Police (1973) statistics indicate that while the total weight of both marihuana and hashish seized annually has risen considerably since 1968, there has been a relatively greater increase in the hashish figures (See Table 1). The marihuana seizures include some domestically cultivated samples as well as imports, although many plant seizures are not included in the total weight figures. If these quantities are converted to their wholesale Canadian value (assuming a current per-pound selling price of $900 for hashish and $250 for marihuana), the importance of hashish becomes even more apparent (See Table 2).

On the other hand, the Federal Health Protection Branch (HPB) drug laboratories, which conduct most of the forensic drug analysis in Canada, report having analyzed more police seizure exhibits of marihuana than of hashish over the past three years, and that the predominance of marihuana exhibits is increasing (Canada 1973). Unfortunately, these two sets of seizure statistics come from different sources within the government and are not directly comparable. It may be that the R.C.M.P. hashish weight totals (Table 1) contain some very large seizures intercepted in Canada, but which were ultimately bound for the United States market. In contrast, large shipments of marihuana going to the U.S. are much less likely to be routed through Canada and therefore probably would not enter into the Canadian seizure statistics. Most of the individual exhibits analyzed by HPB apparently involve relatively small drug quantities seized in connection with simple possession cases.

If the assumption were made, however, that the bulk of the cannabis

Table 1. Cannabis seizures, in pounds, between April 1968 and September 1972, as reported by the R.C.M. Police

Year[a]	Marihuana	Hashish
1968/69	848	83
1969/70	618	1,171
1970/71	2,692[c]	826
1971/72	4,237[d]	3,957
1972/73 (6 mos.)[b]	3,250[e]	1,045[f]

[a] Fiscal years covering April 1st to March 31st.
[b] First six months only (i.e., April 1st to September 30th, 1972).
[c] Excluding seizures of 26,431 cannabis plants.
[d] Excluding seizures of 93,521 cannabis plants.
[e] Excluding seizures of 12,290 cannabis plants.
[f] Excluding seizures of 37.13 pounds of liquid hashish.

Table 2. Approximate wholesale value of cannabis seizures between April 1968 and September 1972, as reported by the R.C.M. Police

Year[a]	Marihuana[c]	Hashish
1968/69	$ 212,000	$ 74,700
1969/70	154,500	1,053,900
1970/71	673,000[d]	743,400
1971/72	1,059,250[d]	3,561,300
1972/73 (6 mos.)[b]	812,500[d]	1,160,200[e]

[a] Fiscal years covering April 1st to March 31st.
[b] First six months only (i.e., April 1st to September 30th, 1972).
[c] Maximum wholesale value, as these seizures include domestically cultivated marihuana which is less expensive than imported marihuana.
[d] Excluding seizures of cannabis plants.
[e] Including value of 37.13 pounds of seized liquid hashish, assuming a per-kilogram wholesale selling price of $13,000.

seizures were destined for the Canadian market, and that law enforcement authorities are able, at best, to seize approximately ten per cent of the cannabis in Canada, then it would appear that trafficking in marihuana and hashish is at least a forty million dollar a year business at the wholesale level alone. Final Canadian retail sales of marihuana and hashish might, in this case, account for between 75 and 100 million dollars annually.

The Canadian cannabis distribution system is far less tightly organized than some other illicit drug markets (e.g., heroin), is subject to sudden and drastic changes in structure and personnel, and, until recently, was relatively uninfected by professional criminal elements. Traditional criminal organizations have become increasingly involved in the financing and actual importation of large-scale hashish shipments, but most of the foreign cannabis distributed in Canada is smuggled into the country by persons whose criminal ventures are intermittent and generally non-opiate drug-related. The relatively loose structure of both the international and domestic cannabis markets, the wide variety of potential sources, and the absence of any necessary chemical refinement process have made it virtually impossible for any single group or organization to monopolize the distribution network. Generally speaking cannabis trafficking can be viewed as a relatively free market system with nearly infinite opportunities for advancement to higher and more sophisticated levels of distribution.

Although illicit cultivation is becoming increasingly common, in most areas domestically grown cannabis is still considered supplemental to imported supplies of hashish and marihuana. Hashish is ordinarily imported from the Middle East, North Africa or the foothills of the Himalayas. Alternately, hashish importers will purchase the drug in European trans-shipment centers where the cost is much higher but the risks — particularly for the inexperienced smuggler — are considerably reduced.

Much of the marihuana entering Canada is grown in Mexico, purchased in American trans-shipment centers, usually on the west coast, and then smuggled into Canada for domestic distribution. However, American attempts to control Mexican cultivation and exportation of marihuana, coupled with the escalating North American demand for cannabis products, has led to increased marihuana importation from other countries. Colombian and Jamaican marihuana are increasingly prevalent and popular, and it would be of no surprise to discover the existence of long-established supply routes from parts of central Africa and Southeast Asia. The cannabis industry, like all commercial endeavors, is governed by the law of supply and demand and is motivated by the desire to realize a profit. The difficulties recently encountered by importers in some purchasing markets, in combination with a growing number of consumers, has led to an international proliferation of supply avenues and, significantly, the direct transfusion of millions of dollars into the economies of several underdeveloped nations.

Increasing logistics problems related to the importation of cannabis have also led to some manufacturing and importing of liquid or viscous hashish concentrates, generally known as "hash oil." In Afghanistan (which is one of the major Canadian sources of "liquid hashish"), the "oil" is chemically extracted from high quality marihuana pollen which sells *in situ* for between ten and thirty dollars a kilogram. Ten kilograms of pollen are said to produce about one kilogram of potent liquid hashish which, in Canada, sells for between ten and sixteen thousand dollars. The decreased bulk of this substance enables a cannabis courier to transport an amount worth approximately ten times the value of the same volume of hashish smuggled across international borders. At the retail level, this "hash oil" is sold in approximately three gram vials for between fifty and sixty dollars a vial — although prices as high as thirty-five dollars a gram have been reported for particularly potent varieties.

Marihuana and more traditional hashish preparations are much less expensive for the user, but there has been dramatic inflation in price over the past few years as a result of increased international law enforcement efforts, rising world-wide demand, and the decline in value of the Canadian as well as the American dollar. Hashish may still be purchased for under a hundred dollars a pound at some production sources, but its cost in most European trans-shipment centers has risen from about three hundred dollars a few years ago to over five hundred dollars per pound during the past two years. This has had the effect of raising domestic hashish prices by between thirty and seventy per cent. Marihuana prices have escalated along similar lines, and it is not uncommon to find esoteric varieties selling for as much as five hundred dollars a pound in Canada — whereas two hundred and fifty dollars was almost unheard of as recently as 1970.

Most regular cannabis users buy relatively small amounts. In the case of marihuana, an ounce (costing between fifteen and thirty dollars) is the most common measure while hashish purchases may range from" nickel" (five dollar) and "dime" (ten dollar) quantities weighing between one and five grams to "quarter" or "half" ounces (costing between twenty-five and thirty and forty-five and fifty dollars, respectively). Larger purchases may be negotiated (at considerable per-weight savings), but these are usually not for individual consumption and are either divided among friends who provided the money for the purchase, or else some of the surplus may be resold at a profit to subsidize the purchaser's personal cannabis consumption. As noted earlier, in Canada hashish tends to be about five to ten times as potent (in THC) as marihuana — despite the fact that it is only four to five times as expensive throughout most of the country. On a per unit THC basis, then, hashish is by far the better buy,

Excluding "street" sales, very small or hurried purchases, and those involving a highly trusted dealer, most buyers "taste" the cannabis before agreeing to purchase. Except for very low potency cannabis, however, the decision to purchase is usually more of a function of immediate need and the availability of alternate sources than the quality of the tested sample. Individual cultivation of cannabis provides a very inexpensive marihuana supply that may terminate dependency on the commercial cannabis market. Although this practice is increasing, most smokers still find it more convenient and less anxiety-producing to purchase rather than grow their own cannabis. Canadians have only begun to exploit the potential of domestically grown cannabis. We can expect a dramatic impact on the market from local sources in the near future, especially if international controls of illicit importation become more stringent and effective.

Cannabis distribution in Canada can be seen as a complex and growing enterprise in which a few at the top reap healthy profits while many of those involved at the lower levels are fortunate to cover their expenses and escape arrest. Marihuana and hashish, as high-demand commodities, will probably always be available, but the structure of the market, the sources of these drugs, the methods of importation, and the individual participants will continue to change until such a time as distribution is legally sanctioned or professional criminal organizations gain stable monopoly control.

EXTENT AND PATTERNS OF USE

The only national surveys on the extent of cannabis use in Canada were conducted under the auspices of the Commission in the spring of 1970 (Lanphier and Phillips 1971). Three populations — high school students, college and university students, and adult members of randomly selected households — were surveyed, and the results indicated rapid and sharp increases in the use of cannabis by persons in all three categories over the previous five years. The percentage of non-student, adult Canadians who reported ever using marihuana or hashish rose from 0.6% for 1966 to 3.4% in the spring of 1970. The percentage of college and university students who reported ever using cannabis rose from 3.9% to 29.0% for this same period of time, and the percentage of high school students who reported ever having used marihuana or hashish increased from 1.9% to 10.3%. In total, the Commission estimated that at least 850,000 Canadians had used cannabis by the spring of 1970, and that between 1,300,000 and 1,500,000 Canadians had probably done so by the middle of 1971. However, "current" cannabis users appear to account for only about half of those who have "ever used" the drug. In the spring of 1970, for example, only 1.0% of Canadian adults (N = 126,000), 17.4% of college and university students (N = 48,000), and 7.4% of high school students (N = 180,000) reported current use of marihuana or hashish (Commission 1972b).

There has been considerable discussion in Canada as to whether or not the 1971 Commission projections represent a "peaking" of cannabis use rates or are simply indicative of a still-continuing upward trend. While there have been no national surveys conducted since the Commission's 1970 studies, the data collected in more recent local or regional studies including longitudinal surveys of high school populations, suggest that the incidence of cannabis use is still rising, primarily as a result of its diffusion to populations that had remained relatively insulated during the late 1960s.

The Addiction Research Foundation of Ontario conducted a survey of 1,200 randomly selected adults (persons eighteen years of age and over) in Toronto in the spring of 1971 and found that 8.4% had used cannabis at some time during the previous twelve months, and that half of these persons had done so seven or more times during this one year period. Of greater import — as regards future incidence of use figures — was the study's finding that the extent of cannabis use was inversely related to age: approximately 30% of the respondents between 18 and 25 years of age had used cannabis during the previous year, while only about 10% of those between 26 and 35 and only about 1% of those 36 years of age and over had done so (Smart and Fejer 1971). While Toronto survey findings cannot be appropriately generalized to the entire country, the incidence of use in this city is likely typical of that in Canada's larger metropolitan areas and suggests a significant increase over the 3.4% "ever used" rates found by the Commission's national adult survey in 1970. Conclusive evidence regarding contemporary rates of adult cannabis use must await new national survey findings, but, at the moment, there is no good reason to believe that the trend toward increasingly widespread use of marihuana or hashish among Canadian adults has in any way abated.

The Addiction Research Foundation of Ontario has studied the extent of cannabis use among Toronto high school students on several occasions since 1968 (Smart, Fejer and White 1972). In that year 6.7% of the surveyed students reported having used cannabis during the previous six months. Two years later, in 1970, the figure had risen to 18.3%, and by 1972 the percentage of users had further increased to 20.9%.

These longitudinal data indicate a decrease in the rate of cannabis diffusion among urban high school students, but still demonstrate that the incidence of cannabis use is continuing to rise.

Of related interest are the findings of high school surveys conducted in two rural school divisions in southern Alberta in early 1971 (Rootman 1972). Eight percent of the students in one of the school districts and 15.3% of those in the other reported the use of cannabis. While these estimates are not high by comparison with survey findings in Canadian urban communities, they suggest a significant increase in cannabis use since the Commission's national high school survey of one year earlier. If these Alberta findings can be generalized to other rural areas, and if the Toronto high school data is indicative of other urban trends, then the present incidence of cannabis use among Canadian high school students nationally is likely at least twice as high as the 10% "ever used" rates found in the Commission's 1970 study.

It is clear that the use of cannabis is no longer the urban phenomenon almost exclusively indulged in by middle-class young adults and adolescents which it appeared to be in the late 1960s. As use of marihuana and hashish has spread across age and class barriers over the past five years, those social characteristics that were once thought to be related to the use of these drugs have tended to lose significance. In fact, generally speaking, it seems that age and sex (since use tends to be much more common among males than females) are the only remaining social factors related to cannabis use in Canada that have much predictive value.

Apparently, most of the Canadian cannabis-using population is engaged in seemingly very moderate levels of use. According to the Commission's 1970 surveys, about 40% of cannabis- using students and the majority of the adult consumers used marihuana or hashish only once a month or less. Approximately the same proportion of high school students and about one-third of college and university students reported using cannabis between once a month and once a week. Only very small percentages of the three nationally surveyed populations claimed to smoke marihuana or hashish more frequently than once a week (Commission 1972b). While more contemporaneous level-of-use data is not, as yet, available, it is not unreasonable to assume that the regular use of the drug (e.g., between once a month and once a week) will become increasingly common. However, such "stable" patterns of use would likely change with any significant alteration in cannabis availability in Canada.

Certain aspects of cannabis use, common to most consuming occasions involving experienced regular users, are a product of the drug's effects, its illlegal status, and other aspects of the social environment of its use. Although exceptions do occur (particularly in the case of very heavy users), the following discussion describes the social circumstances of regular marihuana or hashish consumption for the majority of Canadian users.

Cannabis users are well aware that they are violating the law and, consequently, often take considerable precautions to avoid discovery of their caches. Some only obtain the drug for special occasions such as parties, while others, who use cannabis more frequently, may retain a minimal quantity in their residence. Larger quantities are frequently stored elsewhere, ideally in a public but secure location, until such time as they are required. Although cannabis may be consumed in a wide variety of circumstances, its use is usually reserved for leisure periods in the evenings or on weekends when it is smoked with a few close friends in a private residence. In increasing numbers of cities the drug may be smoked in the streets, clubs or taverns with relatively little risk of arrest. Smoking in cars, natural outdoor settings and at entertainment activities such as concerts or pop festivals, is also common.

The mode of consumption is very much a function of the drug's form. Marihuana is ordinarily hand-rolled or occasionally machine-rolled into thin cigarettes known as "joints," "J's," or "numbers." Two cigarette papers (often colored, perfumed, or emblazoned with various designs) are sometimes employed so as to retard burning and the "joint" is often thoroughly licked before lighting for same the reason. Marihuana may also be smoked in any one of a large variety of ornate pipes, "hookahs" (water-pipes, which cool the smoke) or "chillums" (Indian-style cylindrical pipes which are held vertically, the smoke being drawn through the narrow bottom of the column), but this style of use is more common with hashish.

In a typical situation, small pieces of hashish are placed in the bowl of a pipe which is relit and refilled as required. Hashish may also be crumbled into small bits or a powder which is then mixed with tobacco and rolled into a joint or "spliff." It may also be smoked by placing a piece on the lit end of a cigarette and inhaling the smoke directly, or through a thin tube (such as a straw or rolled up dollar bill). A similar inhalation procedure is used for smoking burning hashish from the end of a pin or needle.

Typically very little cannabis is wasted during the process of smoking — "joints" or pipes are usually passed quickly from one user to another with relatively little "dead" burning time or lost "side-stream" smoke. Users also typically consume all the material in a "joint," including the butt or "roach." The common inhalation procedure is similarly parsimonious; the smoke is typically taken deep into the lungs and held for a prolonged period before being exhaled, in order to maximize absorption of the active compounds. This style of smoking, common in North America and parts of Europe, results in a much greater proportion of the THC in the cannabis being absorbed, compared to the more casual puffing style with immediate exhalation commonly seen in non-industrial countries with a longer history of cannabis use and easy availability, such as Jamaica or India. These factors, along with likely differences in the efficiency of THC delivery by various forms of pipes and cigarettes, greatly complicate attempts to make quantitative cross-cultural comparisons or estimates.

Both marihuana and hashish can be eaten although this mode of administration is usually restricted to cannabis boiled in tea, or cooked in the proverbial brownies or other dishes that disguise its taste and appearance, as well as often increasing its potency. [Note that high temperatures convert inactive THC-acid to THC]. While eating cannabis produces a "high" of longer duration than smoking, the larger quantities required for ingestion, the inconvenience involved in waiting for the effects to "come on" (usually an hour or more) and the impossibility of controlling the effects by titrating the dose render this method relatively unpopular except for public occasions (attending films or concerts, for example) when it is difficult to smoke in safety. In the past few years virtually an entire new industry has developed to service cannabis users, and in almost every Canadian city one can now purchase specifically manufactured pipes, rolling papers, and assorted other paraphernalia designed to enhance the experience of marihuana or hashish use.

Some persons (mainly long-time or heavy users) occasionally smoke cannabis while alone; the drug may also be consumed at large parties or other public or semi-public gatherings. The most common situation-of-use, however, includes only a few close friends or trusted acquaintances, some of whom may not be smoking. The host typically provides the cannabis (although guests may supplement it with their own supply) and the pipe or "joint" is passed from participant to participant in a circular fashion until the cannabis is consumed or the smokers feel sufficiently "high." Some may stop smoking before others, although they usually remain in the circle, passing the "dope" to the next user. Most smokers, however, continue to smoke even after they are high and, should any one express the desire for more during the session, a fresh "joint" or pipe is usually prepared for circulation. This sharing reinforces the sense of communality that characterizes marihuana or hashish smoking occasions. However, such rituals are increasingly less significant as the use of cannabis becomes more common in Canadian society.

In Canada, marihuana cigarettes rarely contain any tobacco, and may vary in size from a few hundred milligrams up to a several gram "bomber."[1] Our research suggests that a typical "joint" contains about one-third of a gram of marihuana and that, depending on the potency of the material and individual differences in smoking style and reaction, anything from a fraction of a "joint" up to one or two cigarettes might be considered a typical acute dose in this country. We have accumulated a substantial amount of direct and indirect evidence that most cannabis

---

[1] Regular tobacco cigarettes usually weigh about one gram.

users usually smoke less than 6 mg of THC to get "high" or "stoned" (Commission 1972b; Miller *et al.* 1971; Green *et al.* 1971).

While marihuana or hashish smoking sessions involving relatively novice users tend to be deliberate and planned, such use is routinized among more experienced users. Regular users develop increasingly casual attitudes toward cannabis and tend to associate its consumption with social gatherings during which cannabis use is viewed as a means toward an end rather than an end in itself. Smoking-oriented sessions last from under an hour to half a day or longer, the average being several hours. Except for rare occasions when the cannabis is so potent that the users become temporarily immobilized, the duration of a smoking session is more a function of extraneous considerations than the quality of the marihuana or hashish.

The major acute physical and psychological effects of cannabis are generally well known and recognized, but it is worth noting that certain effects are never completely predictable from one occasion to another, even with the same users and identical cannabis samples. The physical and social setting and participants' moods are important variables in determining many aspects of the reaction. Cannabis generally operates as a "social lubricant" and most using occasions are tranquil and relaxed affairs that, for naive observers, are often indistinguishable from many small alcohol-using or non-drug gatherings. Smokers engage in quiet conversation or listen to recorded music in a dimly illuminated room. Arguments appear to occur less frequently than in many other drug-using situations, such as those involving alcohol, although periods of agitated activity are not uncommon. Conversations are often related to drug-associated matters although a diverse range of subjects may be broached — often in a convoluted or seemingly unrelated fashion. While the mood is generally peaceful or jocular, there are occasions when serious discussions involving highly personal matters or existential or spiritual questions occur. Sexual intercourse, reading, eating and watching television are additional activities commonly engaged in by cannabis smokers when they are high. The Commission was unable to find any evidence that cannabis use was a significant factor in aggression, violence or non-drug crime in Canada (Commission 1972b).

Infrequently a user may experience an acute anxiety reaction. Such adverse reactions typically seem to center around fear of legal repercussions of illicit drug use, fear of insanity, fear of death, or basic sexual conflicts, and may be precipitated by a "hassle" or problem of real or imagined significance. Friends usually attempt to assist the individual by assuring him of the ephemeral nature of his condition, trying to distract him, or attempting to uncover the source of his anxiety and convince him that it is insignificant or "not-worth-worrying-about." On rare occasions the disturbed individual may be provided with "downers" (tranquilizers or other sedative-hypnotics, if available), or taken to a street clinic or hospital for professional attention.

During the past few years there have been numerous clinical case reports in Canada of individuals suffering from various acute or chronic psychological problems allegedly associated with cannabis use. However, studies of hospital admissions and resident patients have uncovered an almost insignificant number of hospitalized persons with primary cannabis problems. No cases of so-called "cannabis psychosis" have been identified (Commission 1972b, 1973; Hemmings and Miller 1971; Miller, Brewster and Leathers 1971; Statistics Canada 1972). Although transient phases of anxiety and paranoia, and occasionally more significant panic reactions, occur in some inexperienced and regular cannabis users, it would appear that serious reactions are very infrequent, that only a small proportion of the adverse reactions which do occur come to medical attention, and that such cases rarely require hospitalization or prolonged treatment.

Changes in the extent and patterns of cannabis use in Canada will undoubtedly alter the epidemiological picture of adverse reactions as well: as noted above, long-term or heavy use has up to now been rare. Furthermore, as Becker (1953) suggested, as familiarity with acute effects of cannabis in our culture increases, the frequency of short-term fright or panic reactions will likely decrease. There is some evidence that this process is already occurring in Canada.

For most regular marihuana and hashish smokers, continuous use serves to reinforce favorable interpretation of the cannabis experience and strengthens their defining the laws prohibiting use, rather than use of the drug itself, as immoral or improper. For increasing numbers of persons, then, persistent use of cannabis is evidence of a greater personal commitment to the primarily recreational use. For regular marihuana and hashish users there is no longer any debate: cannabis has been phenomenologically tested and sanctioned; its use is now institutionalized.

The institutionalization of cannabis goes far beyond its incorporation into the lived-in world of its users. Throughout much of urban Canada, cannabis use has been granted *de facto* legitimacy through a combination of more tolerant handling of cannabis-related improprieties by various social control agencies, and by the localization of public use settings to certain bars, clubs and taverns that have come to represent territories generally liberated from the enforcement of cannabis laws (McMullan 1972). These modes of cannabis management may be considered as interim steps on the road to complete institutional normalization of cannabis use in Canada.

CANNABIS IN THE MULTIPLE-DRUG USE CONTEXT

The controversy surrounding the use of cannabis in Canada has resulted in public discussions of non-medical drug use generally — both licit and illicit.

On the basis of the often limited available data, we estimate that at present, Canada has about 15,000 daily heroin and methadone users, between two and three thousand regular users of intravenous amphetamines, several hundred thousand persons who use oral amphetamines and sedatives without benefit of prescription on at least an occasional basis, probably an equivalent number of current hallucinogen users, about one hundred thousand adolescent and pre-adolescent users of volatile solvents, about 12,000,000 alcohol drinkers (including an estimated 300,000 alcoholics), and approximately 7,000,000 daily users of tobacco products. Also, most adult Canadians are regular users of caffeine, in the form of coffee, tea, or cola drinks (Commission 1973).

Despite this extremely high incidence of alcohol and tobacco use — and the indisputable evidence regarding the personal and social potential for harm associated with the use of these substances — it is only since the controversy surrounding the use of cannabis that alcohol and tobacco have begun to be publicly redefined as "drugs." This redefinitional process — which is not yet completed — is likely to have significant legal, educational and treatment consequences. The distinction between legal and illegal drugs — which reflects a moral discrimination at least fifty years old — is now undergoing serious questioning. Ideally, the end result of this process will be a system of drug regulations which discriminates between drugs on the basis of a rational consideration of their potential for physical, psychological and social harm. While such legal developments are not inevitable, one certain result of this public debate will be the legal reclassification of cannabis.

It is clear that in Canadian society the regular use of a single drug is the exception rather than the rule: multiple drug use is the norm. In recent years considerable attention has been turned to the patterns and consequences of the simultaneous and sequential medical or non-medical use of various drugs. The role of cannabis in multiple drug use has been the subject of some controversy. The majority of cannabis users studied in Canada have had regular experience with a variety of other psychoactive drugs

— alcohol, tobacco and caffeine being the most frequently mentioned. Furthermore, the use of amphetamines, LSD and other hallucinogens, barbiturates and other sedative-hypnotics, volatile solvents, cocaine and opiate narcotics is more common among cannabis users than in the general population (Commission 1972b, 1973).

In Canada, cannabis has traditionally been closely tied to tobacco use and there seem to be relatively few regular cannabis smokers who did not initially learn the technique of smoke inhalation from prior experience with tobacco cigarettes. Unlike many non-industrial countries where cannabis is routinely mixed with tobacco for smoking, in Canada, as noted earlier, marihuana is rarely taken with tobacco, although hashish is sometimes smoked in such a combination.

The relationship between cannabis and alcohol use has been the subject of considerable discussion. It has been suggested that cannabis may be a cure for society's alcohol ills. In general, survey studies in Canada indicate that those who use alcohol are much more likely than 'teetotallers' to use cannabis, that most cannabis users still drink alcohol, and that heavy users of cannabis tend to drink more alcohol than light or infrequent users (Bilodeau and Jacob 1971; Campbell 1970; Green and Leathers 1971; Lanphier and Phillips 1971; Russell 1970; Smart and Fejer 1971). On the other hand, in a recent survey in Toronto, heavy users of alcohol reportedly used less cannabis than more moderate drinkers (Smart, Fejer and White 1972).

Many researchers have mistakenly assumed that cross-sectional survey data demonstrating a positive *between subject* correlation of cannabis and alcohol use, at a single point in time, implies a positive relationship between the use of the two drugs *within an individual* over time, which is the relationship of ultimate interest. Such extrapolation is unjustified logically and statistically (Cattell 1952). Evidence of an association (either positive or negative) between the use of two drugs in a population at a given time provides little information as to the relationship (if any) between the levels of use of the drugs within the individuals involved. Changes in behavior within an individual, over time, must be studied directly. Even then, other information in addition to drug-use patterns must be considered in determining causal factors.

The limited retrospective *within-subject* data now available suggest that cannabis use may reduce or interchange with alcohol consumption to some extent in the user population. In several Canadian studies a substantial proportion of cannabis users claimed that they had significantly reduced their consumption of alcohol since using cannabis (Green and Leathers 1971; Green *et al.* 1971; Lanphier and Phillips 1971; Paulus

1969). There is also a reported tendency, with cannabis use, for a greater reduction in the use of hard liquor than of the milder forms of alcohol. However, it is clear that the combined consumption of cannabis with wine or beer is common in some social circles in Canada. None of these reports presents definite objective evidence of a reduction in alcohol use, so conclusions must be guarded.

Apparently, individuals who actually quit alcohol use because of cannabis are uncommon; their choice of drugs may have more to do with their value systems than with the pharmacological properties of the drugs. The hostile attitude towards alcohol expressed in the past by some cannabis-using youth is clearly not reflected in the majority of Canadian users today. Systematic prospective studies have not been conducted, and it is not clear from available data whether, on a large scale, cannabis would tend to replace alcohol as an intoxicant in the user population of this country, or whether the use of these drugs would be additive without significant interaction, or if the use of one might potentiate or increase the consumption of the other. Assessed separately, the incidence of use of alcohol and of cannabis are both increasing in Canada, especially among young people.

In the past two decades, the relationship between the use of cannabis and heroin has been the subject of much dispute. During this period, various reports from the United States suggested that the majority of heroin users had previously used cannabis, although in certain sections of the country this was apparently not the case (Ball, Chambers, and Ball 1968). Before 1950, there has been little evidence or serious discussion of a cannabis-to-heroin progression in North America.

Until recently, there was no evidence of a relationship between the use of cannabis and of heroin in Canada. Heroin users studied had generally been heavy consumers of alcohol, barbiturates, and tobacco, but had little or no cannabis experience (Henderson 1970; Josie 1948; Paulus 1969; Stevenson *et al.* 1956; Williams 1969). The situation has apparently changed, and many young Canadian heroin users also report previous and concomitant use of mariuhana, amphetamines, barbiturate and non-barbiturate sedatives and, less often, LSD (Green and Blackwell 1972; Johnston and Williams 1971).

Older studies of lower-class and/or delinquent populations do not readily generalize to the present phenomenon of middle-class cannabis consumption. It would appear that only a small minority of cannabis users in general have had experience with illicit opiate narcotics. However, an increase in opiate narcotic use in certain younger groups has been reported (Green and Blackwell 1972; Johnston and Williams 1971; Commission 1973).

Almost all of those who have used LSD and similar hallucinogens have also used cannabis, although the majority of cannabis users have not tried LSD. Heavy regular use of LSD is rare in Canada — very intermittent consumption is most common among even confirmed users. The use of "speed" is similarly correlated with cannabis use. Most "speeders" or "speed freaks" have had extensive experience with cannabis, although such individuals make up an almost insignificant proportion of the total cannabis-using population (Commission 1973).

In Canada, peer group values and the establishment of contacts with illicit drug distribution networks have apparently played the major role in concomitant and sequential illegal use of different drugs. Becoming accustomed to "breaking the barrier" of illegal drug use by the consumption of one illicit drug may, in some individuals, reduce inhibitions with respect to other such drugs. It has often been proposed that cannabis frequently provides the initial illicit drug experience in this context. Although previous heavy illicit use of tobacco and alcohol during adolescence is common in adult chronic drug users, their use by young people, even though illegal, is largely condoned and, to some extent, encouraged by our society; it does not have the legal significance of cannabis use. It has been suggested that through the use of cannabis certain individuals may learn to use a drug as a mode of coping or as a simple primary source of reinforcement and satisfaction, and that this lesson might later generalize to other drugs. On the other hand, many investigators contend that persons who ultimately become dependent on opiate narcotics, "speed," alcohol or other "hard" drugs are strongly predisposed in that direction by personal, social and economic factors, and that the use of transitional drugs is of little causal significance. Attempts to empirically identify personal predisposing factors in drug dependence have met with little success, however, and this hypothesis has yet to be scientifically confirmed.

The role of cannabis, if any, in the subsequent use of other drugs is not yet well understood; it is unclear whether cannabis plays a specific predisposing role, or is causally unrelated to other illicit drug use and is often used earlier than certain other drugs simply because of its wider availability and social acceptance. Specific pharmacological properties of marihuana (or any other drug) which might lead to a need or craving for other drugs have not been documented. It would appear that dynamic and changing social, legal, economic and personal factors are the primary determinants of the multi-drug-using patterns seen in Canada, and that the specific pharmacology of the substances involved is often secondary.

It appears that the last few years have marked the beginning of the cultural institutionalization of cannabis in Canada. Cannabis is no longer morally aligned with the opiate narcotics and its legal classification with them must be seen as an historical and moral anachronism. Today cannabis is more frequently equated with the use of alcohol than the use of opiates, and — in the face of common usage and the absence of popularly expected evidence of serious detrimental effects — its *de jure* legitimation for recreational purposes has become simply a matter of time.

REFERENCES

BALL, J. C., C. D. CHAMBERS, M. J. BALL
  1968 The association of marijuana smoking with opiate addiction in the United States. *Journal of Criminal Law, Criminology and Police Science* 59:171–182.
BARASH, L. A.
  1971 "A review of hemp cultivation in Canada." Unpublished research project. Commission of Inquiry into the Non-Medical Use of Drugs. Ottawa.
BECKER, H. S.
  1953 Becoming a marihuana user. *American Journal of Sociology* 59:235–242.
BILODEAU, L., A. JACOB
  1971 *La prévalence de l'usage des drogues de 1969 à 1971, chez les étudiants du secondaire et du collégial de l'ile de Montréal: Quelques résultats généraux.* Quebec: Office de la Prévention et du Traitement de l'Alcoolisme et des Autres Toxicomanies.
CAMPBELL, I. L.
  1970 "Non-medial psychoactive drug use at Bishop's University 1965 to 1970." Unpublished manuscript. Montreal: Sir George Williams University.
CANADA, HEALTH PROTECTION BRANCH, DEPARTMENT OF NATIONAL HEALTH AND WELFARE, COMPUTER SERVICES BUREAU
  1973 "Identity of police drug exhibits." Unpublished reports, Ottawa.
CANADIAN MEDICAL ASSOCIATION
  1934a The increasing menace of marijuana. *Canadian Medical Association Journal* 31:561.
  1934b Marijuana [editorial]. *Canadian Medical Association Journal* 31:544–546.
CATTELL, R. B.
  1952 The three basic factor-analytic research designs — their interrelations and derivatives. *Psychological Bulletin* 49:499–520.
COLECLOUGH, A., L. G. HANLEY
  1968 "Marijuana users in Toronto," in *Deviant behavior in Canada.* Edited by W. E. Mann. Toronto: Social Science.
COMMISSION OF INQUIRY INTO THE NON-MEDICAL USE OF DRUGS
  1970 *Interim report.* Ottawa: Information Canada.
  1972a *Treatment report.* Ottawa: Information Canada.

1972b *Cannabis report.* Ottawa: Information Canada.
1973 in press.
Final report. Ottawa: Information Canada.
COOK, S. J.
1964 "Ideology and Canadian narcotics legislation." M. A. dissertation, Department of Sociology. Toronto: University of Toronto.
GREEN, M., J. C. BLACKWELL
1972 "Continuing survey of sensitive observers in Canada: The final monitoring project." Unpublished research project. Commission of Inquiry into the Non-Medical Use of Drugs. Ottawa.
GREEN, M., B. LEATHERS
1971 "Interviews with 'straight' adult cannabis users." Unpublished research project. Commission of Inquiry into the Non-Medical Use of Drugs, Ottawa.
GREEN, M., *et al.*
1971 "Self-reporting of drug consumption patterns by regular cannabis users: A log book study." Unpublished research project. Commission of Inquiry into the Non-Medical Use of Drugs, Ottawa. (Partial summary in the Commission's *Cannabis report,* p. 40.).
HEMMINGS, B., R. D. MILLER
1971 "Non-medical drug use as a factor in hospitalization: A survey of Canadian psychiatric hospital diagnostic records." Unpublished research project. Commission of Inquiry into the Non-Medical Use of Drugs, Ottawa. (Published in part in the Commission's *Cannabis report,* pp. 88–90; and in the *Final report,* Table A.7 and related text.)
HENDERSON, I.
1970 *An exploration of the natural history of heroin addiction.* Vancouver: Narcotic Addiction Foundation of British Columbia.
JOHNSTON, W. E., H. R. WILLIAMS
1971 *Drug use patterns and related factors of heroin addicts seeking treatment for their addiction.* Vancouver: Narcotic Addiction Foundation of British Columbia.
JOSIE, G. H.
1948 *A report on drug addiction in Canada.* Ottawa: King's Printer and Controller of Stationery.
LANPHIER, C. M., S. B. PHILLIPS
1971 "(a) The non-medical use of drugs and associated studies: a national household survey. (b) Secondary school students and non-medical drug use: a national survey of students enrolled in grades seven through thirteen. (c) University students and non-medical drug use: a national survey." Unpublished Commission research project. Commission of Inquiry into the Non-Medical Use of Drugs." Ottawa. (Published in part in the Commission's *Cannabis report* and *Final report.*)
MARSHMAN, J. A., R. J. GIBBINS
1970 A note of the composition of illicit drugs. *Ontario Medical Review* 37:429–430, 441.
MC MULLAN, J.
1972 "Suburbia in transition: patterns of cannabis use and social control in the suburban community," in *Observations on the normalization of*

cannabis. Co-ordinated by H. T. Buckner. Montreal: Department of Sociology, Sir George Williams University, 1–31.

MILLER, R. D., J. BREWSTER, B. LEATHERS
1971 "Survey of Ottawa-area physicians regarding the non-medical use of drugs." Unpublished research project. Commission of Inquiry into the Non-Medical Use of Drugs, Ottawa. (Published in part in the Comission's *Cannabis report*, 86–88.)

MILLER, R. D. et al.
1971 "A comparison of the effects of Δ^9THC and marijuana in humans." Unpublished research project. Commission of inquiry into the Non-Medical Use of Drugs. Ottawa, (Published in part in the Commission's *Cannabis report*).
1973 "Chemical analysis of illicit drugs in Canada." Unpublished research project. Commission of Inquiry into the Non-Medical Use of Drugs, Ottawa. (Published in part in the Commission's *Cannabis report* [Tables 1 and 2] and *Final report* [Tables A.8 and A.9] and related text.)

MURPHY, EMILY
1922 *The black candle*. Toronto: Thomas Allen.

PAULUS, I.
1969 Psychedelic drug use on the Canadian Pacific coast: notes on the new drug scene. *International Journal of the Addictions* 4:77–88.

PAULUS, I., H. R. WILLIAMS
1966 Marihuana and young adults. *British Columbia Medical Journal* 8 (6): 240–244.

ROOTMAN, I.
1972 Drug use among rural students in Alberta. *Canada's Mental Health* 20:9–14.

ROYAL CANADIAN MOUNTED POLICE
1969 Unpublished brief presented to the Commission of Inquiry into the Non-Medical Use of Drugs, Ottawa.
1973 Unpublished information communicated to the Commission of Inquiry into the Non-Medical Use of Drugs, Ottawa.

RUSSELL, J.
1970 *Survey of drug use in selected British Columbia schools*. Vancouver: Narcotic Addiction Foundation of British Columbia.

SMALL, E.
1971 "Interim report on studies of cannabis undertaken jointly by the Departments of Agriculture and National Health and Welfare." Unpublished report to the Commission of Inquiry into the Non-Medical Use of Drugs, Ottawa.

SMART, R. G., D. FEJER
1971 "Marijuana use among adults in Toronto." Unpublished manuscript, Project J-183, Substudy 6–7 and Jo-71, Addiction Research Foundation, Toronto.

SMART, R. G., D. FEJER, J. WHITE
1972 "Drug use trends among metropolitan Toronto students: a study of changes from 1968 to 1972." Unpublished manuscript. Addiction Research Foundation of Ontario, Toronto.

STATISTICS CANADA
1972 *Mental health statistics*. Vol. 1. *Institutional admissions and separations* (1970). Ottawa: Information Canada.

STEVENSON, G. H., *et al.*
1956 "Drug addiction in British Columbia." Unpublished manuscript, University of British Columbia, Vancouver.

WILLIAMS, H. R.
1969 Treatment of the narcotic addict with some observations on other drug dependencies. *British Columbia Medical Journal* 11:11–13.

cannabis. Co-ordinated by H. T. Buckner. Montreal: Department of Sociology, Sir George Williams University, 1–31.

MILLER, R. D., J. BREWSTER, B. LEATHERS
   1971   "Survey of Ottawa-area physicians regarding the non-medical use of drugs." Unpublished research project. Commission of Inquiry into the Non-Medical Use of Drugs, Ottawa. (Published in part in the Comission's *Cannabis report*, 86–88.)

MILLER, R. D. et al.
   1971   "A comparison of the effects of Δ⁹THC and marijuana in humans." Unpublished research project. Commission of inquiry into the Non-Medical Use of Drugs. Ottawa, (Published in part in the Commission's *Cannabis report*).
   1973   "Chemical analysis of illicit drugs in Canada." Unpublished research project. Commission of Inquiry into the Non-Medical Use of Drugs, Ottawa. (Published in part in the Commission's *Cannabis report* [Tables 1 and 2] and *Final report* [Tables A.8 and A.9] and related text.)

MURPHY, EMILY
   1922   *The black candle*. Toronto: Thomas Allen.

PAULUS, I.
   1969   Psychedelic drug use on the Canadian Pacific coast: notes on the new drug scene. *International Journal of the Addictions* 4:77–88.

PAULUS, I., H. R. WILLIAMS
   1966   Marihuana and young adults. *British Columbia Medical Journal* 8 (6): 240–244.

ROOTMAN, I.
   1972   Drug use among rural students in Alberta. *Canada's Mental Health* 20:9–14.

ROYAL CANADIAN MOUNTED POLICE
   1969   Unpublished brief presented to the Commission of Inquiry into the Non-Medical Use of Drugs, Ottawa.
   1973   Unpublished information communicated to the Commission of Inquiry into the Non-Medical Use of Drugs, Ottawa.

RUSSELL, J.
   1970   *Survey of drug use in selected British Columbia schools*. Vancouver: Narcotic Addiction Foundation of British Columbia.

SMALL, E.
   1971   "Interim report on studies of cannabis undertaken jointly by the Departments of Agriculture and National Health and Welfare." Unpublished report to the Commission of Inquiry into the Non-Medical Use of Drugs, Ottawa.

SMART, R. G., D. FEJER
   1971   "Marijuana use among adults in Toronto." Unpublished manuscript, Project J-183, Substudy 6–7 and Jo-71, Addiction Research Foundation, Toronto.

SMART, R. G., D. FEJER, J. WHITE
   1972   "Drug use trends among metropolitan Toronto students: a study of changes from 1968 to 1972." Unpublished manuscript. Addiction Research Foundation of Ontario, Toronto.

STATISTICS CANADA
　1972　*Mental health statistics.* Vol. 1. *Institutional admissions and separations* (1970). Ottawa: Information Canada.
STEVENSON, G. H., *et al.*
　1956　"Drug addiction in British Columbia." Unpublished manuscript, University of British Columbia, Vancouver.
WILLIAMS, H. R.
　1969　Treatment of the narcotic addict with some observations on other drug dependencies. *British Columbia Medical Journal* 11:11–13.

Memories, Reflections and Myths: The American Marihuana Commission

LOUIS BOZZETTI and JACK BLAINE

ABSTRACT

The National Commission on Marihuana and Drug Abuse was established by the Congress of the United States as a part of the Comprehensive Drug Abuse Prevention and Control Act of 1970. From its inception, the Commission was never given legislative power; rather its function was to study the complex issues involved in marihuana use and related social responses. Given the structures of limited time and budget, the Commission was compelled to limit its activity to separating fact from fiction, reality from myth, and to achieve a balanced judgement on the marihuana issue. The first report was an attempt to clarify the essential issues and concerns of American society regarding marihuana. This knowledge base was then utilized to formulate a reasonable societal response. At the commencement of the Commission's activities it became clear that the marihuana issue was indeed a "signal of misunderstanding." In order to clarify this polarized and politicized phenomenon, a national survey of beliefs, attitudes and experiences with marihuana was undertaken. Compelling findings regarding patterns of use from the survey will be developed in the paper. In order to effectively address the social issues involved the main thrusts of the marihuana investigation were:
1. Use of the drug and its effects;
2. The impact of marihuana use on public health and welfare, on criminal and/or aggressive behavior, and on the dominant social order.

In order to formulate an appropriate social policy regarding the use and control of marihuana in the United States for 1972, the Commission collected and analyzed data on the current societal response to the worldwide use of cannabis.

The incredible short time-frame available to accomplish the above task necessitated an operational strategy which heavily relied upon ongoing research activities, data from cooperating government and private agencies, staff research projects, and contracted research studies and papers by established experts in the field. Further supportive data were collected from public and closed hearings across the country and from international investigative visits by the Commission. The paper will discuss in some detail the processes involved in obtaining and synthesizing these data.

The Commission's real agony began as it attempted to formulate a proposed national policy regarding marihuana use and control. In part, this dealt with the tension existing in American society between individual liberties and the need for reasonable societal restraints. Underlying the Commission's social policy recommendations was the belief that the State is obliged to justify restraints on individual behavior. In its investigations the Commission found that the existing system of controls was not supported by the current concerns of public opinion or scientific fact. In order to express its strong concern for the irresponsible use of cannabis, the Commission chose a social control policy aimed at discouraging use. The processess of choosing and implementing this option of discouragement of use by the partial prohibition model will be explicated in the paper. A hallmark of this policy was the recommendation for decriminalization of possession of marihuana for private use.

The National Commission on Marihuana and Drug Abuse was established by the Congress of the United States as a part of the Comprehensive Drug Abuse Prevention and Control Act of 1970. To assure autonomy, two commissioners were chosen from each of the congressional houses, in addition to nine members who were appointed by the President. From its inception, the Commission was never given legislative power, rather its function was to study the complex issues involved in marihuana use, and related social responses and conduct a study of marihuana including but not limited to the following areas:

a) Epidemiologic studies of the patterns of use, distribution, and law enforcement activities in America;
b) An evaluation of the efficacy of existing marihuana laws;
c) A study of the pharmacology of marihuana;
d) The relationship of the use of marihuana to aggressive behavior and crime;
e) The use of other drugs; and
f) The international control of marihuana.

The study and investigation was to be executed within one year, with recommendations for legislation and administrative action to the President and the Congress.

Given the strictures of limited time and budget, the Commission was compelled to limit its activity to separating fact from fiction, reality from myth, and to achieve a balanced judgement on the marihuana issue. The first report was an attempt to clarify the essential issues and concerns of the American society regarding marihuana. This knowledge base was then utilized to formulate a reasonable societal response.

At the outset of the Commission activities, it became clear that the marihuana issue was indeed a "signal of misunderstanding." Two disparate statements typify this controversy. The President in a news conference at San Clemente in May, 1972, stated that he would never legalize marihuana despite the recommendations of the Commission which was at that time just getting started. On the other hand, Norman E. Zinberg stated at a formal Commission hearing in May, 1973, that the members were biased and had made up their minds from the onset. These positions were exemplar of the public debate regarding marihuana in 1971.

In order to clarify this polarized and politicized phenomenon, a national survey of beliefs, attitudes and experiences with marihuana was undertaken. The survey studied a stratified random sample of U.S. households in which personal interviews with an adult and youth were conducted. Of all adults, 15% reported that they had ever used marihuana, while 5% stated that they were currently using it. Among the youth (12–17 years old), 14% had ever used and 6% reported current use. Interestingly, proportions of users increased during the late adolescent years to 27% (16–17 years old), and peaked during the young adult years to 39% (18–25 years old). There was a steady decline in number of users with advancing age (19%, 26–35 years; 9%, 36–49 years; 6% ,over 50 years). It is noteworthy that both ends of the spectrum report the same percentage of use (6% for 12–13 years old and those over 50 years).

Although trends were noted in the other factors studied (sex, marital status, race, income, etc.), the most striking variation in proportion of marihuana users depended upon age. At the time of the interview, slightly less than half of those who ever used marihuana reported no longer using the substance. The proportions of current adult users followed the same age distribution as those who ever used cannabis.

From the survey data it became apparent that all marihuana users are not the same, i.e., several distinct patterns of use were delineated. Among youth and adults one-half or more of those who had used marihuana either discontinued it or were currently using it episodically at a rate of once a month or less. These were designated experimental users. About 40% of the youth and adults were intermittent users, i.e., they did not use the drug more than once per week. The remaining 10% consisted of moderate and heavy users, i.e., moderate users several times per week to once per day (6% youth, 5% adults); more than once, daily for heavy users (4% youth, 2% adults).

The survey demonstrated that contemporary marihuana use is pervasive, involving all segments of the U.S. population. Indeed, it was extrapolated that 24 million Americans over age 11 have used marihuana at least once.

Additionally, marihuana use does not appear to vary significantly by race. With respect to religious affiliation, Jews and Catholics appeared to be slightly over represented as compared to Protestants. Although males predominate among adult users (2 to 1), the sex differential appears to be diminishing among youthful users. It was also found that users tended to be represented more frequently among clerical and professional workers in the higher socioeconomic categories. Use of marihuana tended to increase with the level of formal education attained. At the same time adult use of the drug is not confined to students. Interestingly, 75% of the 18- to 25-year old users were not students.

Users were found to span social class, income level and occupational classifications. This survey data was confirmed by testimony from individuals in closed hearings before the Commission. During these sessions surgeons, construction workers, policemen, airline pilots, lawyers, stock brokers, air traffic controllers, and bus drivers spoke of their experience with the drug.

As the above description suggests, marihuana use and the marihuana user do not fall into simple and distinct classifications. Although it is possible to sketch profiles of various marihuana-using populations according to frequency, intensity and duration of use, no valid stereotype of "The Marihuana User" can be drawn.

By far the largest group is the experimenters. Experimentation with marihuana is motivated primarily by curiosity and a desire to share a social experience. Usage here is extremely infrequent or non-persistent. This group is rather conventional in life style.

The intermittent users generally continue to use marihuana because of its socializing and recreational properties. They are more inclined to seek and emphasize the social rather than the psychopharmacologic effects of the drug.

In contrast, although the moderate users tend to share many characteristics with intermittent users, they appear to place more emphasis on the psychopharmacologic effects of the drug.

The heavy users seem to need the drug experience more often. Their initial and continued use is motivated not only by curiosity and socialization, but also a desire for "kicks," expansion of awareness, understanding, and relief of anxiety or boredom. Generally these persons use cannabis more than once daily, and exhibit unconventional life styles, values and attitudes.

Hitherto, American research had largely focused on the large majority of individuals categorized as experimental and intermittent users. In order to gain unavailable information about moderate and heavy users, the Commission sponsored the Boston Free Access Study at Harvard University. This study permitted observation of a group of moderate and heavy cannabis smokers and their use of the drug during a 21-day period of free access.

They were superior intellectually; had an average age of 23; had completed on the average of two and a half years of college; had erratic job histories; were itinerant; represented all socioeconomic levels; frequently had family histories of broken homes, alcoholism and drug abuse; and had widespread use of hallucinogens and amphetamines. In contrast to other groups, heavy users almost uniformly reported that marihuana smoking produced relaxation, alteration of perceptions, increased sense of well-being, and decreased hostility.

The heavy users appeared to demonstrate a moderate psychological dependence on the cannabis experience; i.e., it is a pivotal social activity around which conversation, other personal interactions and much of their life style revolve. Indeed, smoking was the focal activity around which activity groups formed. Yet these persons were more inclined to seek the psychopharmacologic effects rather than the socializing effects, in direct contrast to less frequent users. Thus, paradoxically, heavy users tended to be more withdrawn and interact less with each other during their communal drug experience.

During the period of the study, the subjects maintained a high level of interest and participation in a variety of personal, athletic, and aesthetic endeavors. Under the study's confined conditions participants tended to smoke more than they did on the outside. The intermittent users averaged three cigarettes per day ($1/2$–6 a day); the moderate and heavy users averaged $6^1/_2$ cigarettes per day (range $3^1/_2$–8 a day). The marihuana used contained about 20 mgs. $\Delta 9$ THC per cigarette by laboratory assay.

Significantly, several of the heavy users consumed without any significant effects (physiological, psychological or behavioral) a maximum daily dose of cannabis approximately 20 to 30 times that obtained by the average marihuana user in the United States.

The apparent rapid build up of tolerance to the hallucinogenic effects of the drug permitted this combination of atypical heavy use pattern and unusually large daily doses of marihuana. It should be noted that in the non-tolerant individual, i.e., the typical American cannabis user, this pattern of consumption would likely result in toxic psychosis or hallucinations. The results of this study also demonstrated tolerance to the cardiovascular effects (pulse rate), and behavioral effects (time estimation, recent memory, psychomotor coordination). It is important to note that the tendency to increase daily intake by shortening the interval between marihuana cigarettes rather than increasing the number of cigarettes smoked each session suggests tolerance to the desired psychopharmacologic effect of the drug.

One of the most critical tasks facing the Commission concerned the effects of cannabis on the public health and welfare. In order to address itself to the perceived public fears about the effects of cannabis, several items on public beliefs about the drug were included in the first national survey. Marihuana is perceived by the U.S. population as a harmful substance to persons using it, even in small amounts. Heroin and LSD are clearly regarded as the most harmful of all psychoactive substances. Marihuana is listed third with cocaine, morphine, and amphetamines following closely. Barbiturates, tobacco, and alcohol, in that order, follow in perceived harmfulness.

Sixty-five percent of adults and forty-eight percent of youth believed that marihuana was addictive. Interestingly, marihuana was rated as less addictive than alcohol and tobacco by both youth and adults.

The most widely held belief about marihuana by adults and youth is that it, "makes people want to try stronger things, like heroin." Seventy percent of the adults and fifty-six percent of the youth surveyed held this view. Other widely held beliefs are that marihuana is morally offensive, that it makes people lose their desire to work, that many crimes are committed by persons under its influence, that some people have died from using it, and that it is often promoted by persons who are enemies of the United States. The survey revealed that approximately 50% of all adults held these negative perceptions. In contrast, the positive beliefs, e.g., increases enjoyment of art, sex, tension relief, sociability were not widely held by either youth or adults.

Examination of other survey data suggests that these expressions are reflections of a generalized attitude toward marihuana and the user among most adults, and to a lesser extent youth. An example of this was the finding that only one-fourth of the youth and adults surveyed believed that marihuana users lead a normal life. The majority of adults have a mental picture of the marihuana user as someone bored with life, not caring about the world around him, not showing good judgement in selecting friends, poor school performance, emotionally unstable and lazy. Only 10% of adults believed that the marihuana user enjoys life. Interestingly, adults who themselves use marihuana have a much more positive belief system about the user.

In addition to these revealing personal attitudes, it was essential that the Commission also develop an objective knowledge base about the drug and its effects, and its impact upon contemporary American society. A brief historical review of the Commission's earliest operation is needed at this point. This must be done to establish a perspective for understanding the difficulties encountered in commencing a response to the Congressional mandate.

The formal activities of the group began when on March 22, 1971, a $250,000 appropriation was made available from the President's emergency discretionary fund. With this, the legislated time clock began which required that a final report on marihuana, with legislative recommendations, be submitted to the President and the Congress within one year. Compounding budgetary distress the Commission's total appropriation bill was incorporated in the HEW bill[1] which did not clear Congress and the Office of Management and Budget until August, 1971.

The early financial restraint, effectively, (1) delayed early and adequate staff recruitment; (2) precluded the funding of a spectrum of new research projects, particularly in the medical area, and (3) severely limited the time frame to four months for accomplishing, collecting data and reporting on *all* research projects. The above necessitated an operational strategy which heavily relied upon ongoing research activities, and data from cooperating government and private agencies. Further, staff research projects, and contracted studies and papers by established experts in the field were compiled.

The range of studies reviewed included complex endeavors such as the study of chronic *ganja* use in Jamaica by the Research Institute for the Study of Man in New York, and review monographs by accepted authorities. The majority of data in the biomedical areas was graciously supplied by the National Institute of Mental Health and the Food and Drug Administration sponsored investigators. In reality, the focus of commission sponsored projects was in the sociolegal areas.

In order to evaluate the efficacy of existing law, a series of projects was designed to ascertain opinion and behavior within the Criminal Justice System, non-legal institutions, e.g., medical, clerical and business, and the general trend of public opinion. Included were analyses of marihuana arrests (federal and local) and opinion surveys of prosecuting attorneys, judges, probation officers, and court clinicians. From these studies it became evident that the law enforcement community has adopted a policy of containment rather than elimination.

Indeed, the salient feature of the present law was the threat of arrest. The general enforcement pattern is a spontaneous one. Most arrests occur outdoors, in cars, and in the course of other police activity. This leads to heavy concentration of arrests among white males, without prior records, possessing only small amounts of marihuana, for indiscreet use in public. A high percentage of cases (94%) after arrest are disposed of by dismissal or informal diversion from the courts. This attests to the widespread ambivalence among law enforcement personnel about the appropriateness and efficacy of existing law.

[1] The appropriation bill for the United States Department of Health, Education and Welfare.

Other social institutions recognize that the control of marihuana is only partially a law enforcement problem. The majority of legal and non-legal opinion makers are uniformly against incarceration of adults or youth for possession. However, they felt that the drug should not be made available, at least for now.

A substantial amount of confusion underlies public opinion regarding the control of marihuana. There is an awareness of the legal consequences of use. Overshadowing this is a confusion and ambivalence about an appropriate system of control. The public is unenthusiastic about labeling the marihuana user a criminal, but reluctant to relinquish all formal legal controls.

The Commission's real agony began as it attempted to formulate a proposed national policy regarding marihuana use and control. In part, this dealt with the tension existing in American society between individual liberties and the need for reasonable societal restraints. Underlying the Commission's social policy recommendations was the belief that the State is obliged to justify restraints on individual behavior.

The Commission identified four alternative sociolegal policies: approval, elimination, discouragement and neutrality toward use. From the outset, the Commissioners believed that society should not approve or encourage the use of any drug. They concluded that the elimination policy is unachievable and unwarranted. The dissonance between the options of neutrality and discouragement involved the judgement whether society should dissuade persons from using marihuana or benignly defer to individual judgement. The factors which led the Commissioners to opt for the discouragement policy involved beliefs about the dynamics of social change, and the limitation of our current knowledge.

Throughout the Commission's deliberation there was a recurring awareness of the possibility that marihuana use may be a fad which, if not institutionalized, would recede substantially in time. The Commissioners were concerned about the effects of cannabis on the heavy and very heavy users. Although these categories of users are presumably small, the group felt that institutionalization of the drug would greatly increase these numbers. Additionally, it was believed that the general value system of contemporary American society was in a state of flux. In a sense the use of marihuana was seen as a rejection of enduring American values. Further, a substantial majority of the American public (64%) opposes the use of marihuana by themselves or their fellow citizens. For these reasons the Commissioners recommended to the public and its policy makers a social control policy which sought to discourage marihuana use, while concentrating on the prevention of heavy and very heavy use.

From this the partial prohibition approach was recommended which symbolized societal discouragement, while de-emphasizing marihuana as an emotional issue. This approach concentrates on reducing irresponsible use and its consequences. It also removes the criminal stigma and threat from a widespread behavior (possession for personal use), and allows the law enforcement community to focus on drug trafficking and other relevant issues. It also maximizes the flexibility of future public response as new knowledge becomes available.

The hallmark of this policy was the recommendation for decriminalization of possession of small quantities of marihuana for private personal use. In summary, these recommendations fulfill the ultimate objectives of the Commission to demythologize, desymbolize and de-emphasize marihuana as a critical problem in the contemporary United States.

REFERENCES

U.S. NATIONAL COMMISSION ON MARIHUANA AND DRUG ABUSE
  1972 *Marihuana: a signal of misunderstanding*. The official report of the National Commission on Marihuana and Drug Abuse. New York: Signet.
  1972 *Marihuana: a signal of misunderstanding*. Technical Papers of the First Report, Appendix, 2 vols. Washington: United States Government Printing Office.

Sociocultural Factors in Marihuana Use in the United States

WILLIAM H. McGLOTHLIN

ABSTRACT

During the 1960s, the characteristics of the marihuana-using population in the U.S. changed from a predominantly lower socioeconomic minority group to one of middle to upper-upper status. It is argued that this transition resulted from large numbers of middle-class youth participating marginally in the styles set by the hippy or psychedelic movement. This interpretation is supported by the age, social and geographic distributions of current marihuana users, as well as by their attitude, value, personality, and behavior characteristics. The symbolic role of marihuana use also appears to be the most important factor in shaping patterns of use. In comparison with other cannabis-using cultures, the ratio of daily to irregular user appears disproportionately low, and the amounts consumed are definitely much smaller. Most U.S. users can be considered as playing at cannabis use in comparison to patterns in other cultures.

To the extent that symbolic factors play a role in the current marihuana epidemic, as opposed to the pharmacological properties of the drug, usage can be expected to stabilize in the near future and subsequently decline. On the other hand, the extensive introduction of the drug into the culture will undoubtedly result in substantial continued usage. This residual group will likely contain a significant number who consume marihuana or more potent preparations in amounts comparable to heavy users in other cultures, i.e. 200 mg. THC or more.

One of the more interesting sociocultural questions concerning marihuana use can be phrased as follows: How did a drug whose traditional use had been virtually limited to lower socioeconomic groups in the U.S. (and with few exceptions, in other countries as well) suddenly become very widespread among the youth of middle- and upper-class groups? The lower socioeconomic minority group characteristics of early U.S. marihuana use are well documented. There are rare accounts of hashish use in the 19th

This work was supported by Research Scientist Award Number K05-DA-70182 from the National Institute of Mental Health.

century (Brecher 1972), but the first significant non-medical marihuana use was introduced into the southern and western portions of the U.S. by Mexican-Americans around 1910 (Bonnie and Whitebread 1970; Walton 1938). Utah was the first state to prohibit the drug in 1915. The spread was most rapid among the Negro population — four studies of marihuana use in the Army during the 1940's found ninety percent or more of the sample were Negro (Charen and Perelman 1946; Freedman and Rockmore 1946; Gaskill 1945; Marcovitz and Meyers 1944). Most published descriptions characterized the users of this era as rather passive young males, generally unemployed with poor social and psychological adjustment (Goodman and Gilman 1955; Maurer and Vogel 1962; Mayor's Committee 1944). There are two exceptions to the predominantly minority group nature of early marihuana users. First, a high incidence of use existed among jazz musicians (Winick 1960), and pre-1960 usage was generally considerably higher among entertainment and artist personnel than in the general population. The second group is the "Beats" of the late 1940s and 1950s. Marihuana was the drug of choice for this predominantly white protest group, and they also occasionally employed peyote and mescaline along with other drugs (Polsky 1969).

The middle- and upper-class nature of marihuana use in the 1960s is equally well documented. A 1969 Gallup national survey of college students found 30% marihuana usage among students whose parents' income was $15,000 or over in comparison to 12% for those with parental incomes of under $7,000. Surveys of five Houston high schools in 1970 varied from 5% reporting some use in a predominantly black school to 48% in an upper-middle-class white school (Preston 1970). Similarly, Blum (1969) found lower-class high schools in the San Francisco area reported one-third as much marihuana usage as middle-class schools. An interesting footnote to this sharp reversal in socioeconomic status and racial background of marihuana users in the U.S. is the recent adoption of cannabis use by university students in other countries whose traditional use had also been limited to the lower classes, e.g., Greece, Turkey and India. It is clear that this represents the introduction of a Western style rather than an internal diffusion from the lower classes.

THE DEVELOPMENT OF THE MIDDLE-CLASS DRUG SUBCULTURE

To explain the transition from old to new style of marihuana users in the U.S., it is helpful to examine the chronology of the middle-class drug epidemic of the 1960's. The origin actually dates back to the middle 1950s and the emphasis was on LSD – not marihuana. At this time, several small groups began non-medical use of LSD; Blum (1964) describes one such group of mental health professionals in the San Francisco area beginning in 1956. Interest in the hallucinogens had been stimulated by Aldous Huxley's description of his mescaline experiences in "Doors of Perception" (1954). Prior to this time a few students, artists and members of the "Beat" subculture had experimented with peyote, but overall, its use was quite rare outside the American Indian population. Availability of LSD in the 1950s was restricted to licit supplies provided for experimental purposes, and the limited non-medical use was mostly centered around professionals having access to these sources. Such non-medical usage continued on a small scale until the early 1960s. Psilocybin and psilocin were synthesized in 1959, (Hofmann, 1970) and the former was also subjected to limited unauthorized use through diversion from experimental supplies. It should be stressed that most of these early hallucinogen users were well beyond the age of today's typical drug user; that they were to a considerable extent motivated by reports that enhanced self-understanding or other beneficial experiences could result; and that LSD was especially attractive in that it was legal and carried the respectable origin of the laboratory and science rather than the stigma of illicit drugs such as marihuana. Many of these persons had never used marihuana, and those who did regarded it as insignificant in comparison to LSD.

Figure 1 provides a continuing chronology of the significant events leading to the formation of the psychedelic drug subculture, along with the trend in marihuana use as measured by Gallup college and general population surveys. The first LSD to be clandestinely manufactured in the U.S. appeared in California in 1962. Both the source and the market were confined to the small LSD groups described above. By 1964, clandestine LSD manufacture was becoming more common and increasingly sophisticated, however the persons involved in these activities generally continued to be ideologically identified with the emerging drug subculture rather than solely motivated for financial profit. In 1963–1964, a number of leading popular magazines carried feature articles on LSD, particularly in relation to Leary and Alpert and their activities at Harvard University. This national publicity was undoubtedly a major factor in accelerating the spread of LSD use. Also in 1964, the underground press was initiated, providing a means of rapidly disseminating both a psychedelic philosophy and information concerning gatherings and other related activities. Popular music was strongly influenced by the psychedelic

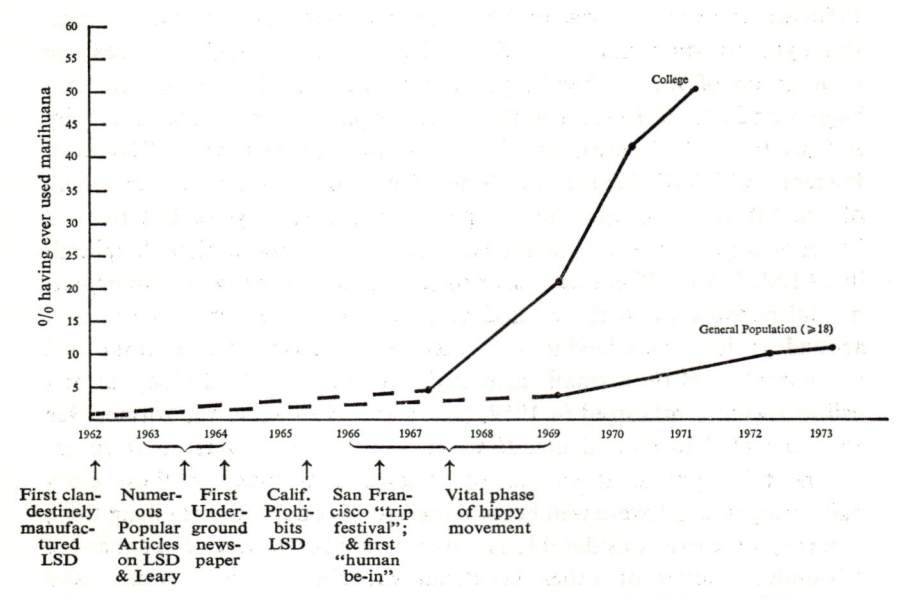

Figure 1. Trend in marihuana use in the U.S.

[Graph showing % having ever used marihuana on y-axis (0-60) vs years 1962-1973 on x-axis. Two lines: "College" rising steeply to ~50% by 1973, and "General Population (≥18)" rising gradually to ~10% by 1973.]

Timeline markers:
- 1962: First clandestinely manufactured LSD
- 1963: Numerous Popular Articles on LSD & Leary
- 1964: First Underground newspaper
- 1965: Calif. Prohibits LSD
- 1966: San Francisco "trip festival"; & first "human be-in"
- 1967: Vital phase of hippy movement

Note: Prevalence of marihuana use is taken from Gallup Public Opinion Index, Feb., 1972 and March, 1973.

movement and, in turn, greatly aided in its growth.

The January 1967 "Human Be-In" in San Francisco was reportedly attended by 20,000 persons, and is generally considered the point at which the mass hippy or psychedelic movement emerged. Similar large-scale gatherings became almost weekly occurrence in various locales in California and spread throughout the country in a matter of months. The LSD trip provided a common ground on an experiential level which served as the unifying principle for hippy communities, and for thousands of otherwise strangers at hippy gatherings. Hippy radio programs sprang up and rock music effectively articulated the flower children's new ethic.

LSD was crucial to the formation of the hippy movement. It produces a very potent drug experience, the major characteristic of which is the temporary suspension of mechanisms which normally provide structure and stability to perceiving, thinking and valuing. This loosening of established associations, beliefs, etc., has been variously described as deactivation of perceptual filters, loosening of constancies, breaking down of ego boundaries, dehabituation and deautomatization. It does not necessarily produce attitude and belief changes, but it can act as a catalyst, permitting rapid changes under favorable conditions, e.g., the use of natural hallucinogens by shamans in primitive tribes.

Once the hippy movement achieved appreciable growth the stage was set for radical modification of beliefs and values on a mass scale — large numbers of impressionable, affluent and uncommitted youth were attracted to take LSD under conditions which strongly encouraged conversion to a radical social philosophy, and sustained these new beliefs and life style through community support, an effective communications system, a creative music industry and various other innovative measures.

Marihuana was also uniformly adopted by the hippy subculture, but for most was little more than a mood modifier utilized in daily social interactions. This was especially true in view of the low potency marihuana generally available. The adoption of marihuana use by the hippies was a natural outgrowth of their general drug orientation. A source of supply was available via the previously existing marihuana traffic, and it produced a mild passive reaction more in accord with their philosophy and life style than that resulting from alcohol. The effects also have some similarities to the more potent hallucinogens. Overall, however, marihuana use cannot be considered as crucial to the hippy movement. On the other hand, it is difficult to envision the movement's full development without the potent LSD experiences which many, if not most, adherents cited as the essential affirmation of their particular belief system.

The argument that interest focused primarily on LSD during this period, and not marihuana, is supported by the citations in the *Readers guide to periodical literature* (1959–1972) shown in Table 1. For the period 1959–1966, there were seventy-six references to LSD compared to only six for marihuana. As seen in Figure 1, the large gains in the per cent of the college and general population using marihuana did not occur until after the vital phase of the hippy movement.

An explanation to the question posed at the beginning of this paper may now be suggested. Marihuana was transformed from a lower-class drug to

Table 1. LSD and marihuana citations in *Readers guide to periodical literature*, 1959–1972

Year	Number of citations	
	LSD	Marihuana
1959–1960	2	0
1961–1962	5	1
1963–1964	13	1
1965–1966	56	4
1967–1968	58	48
1969–1970	17	83
1971–1972	7	73
Total	158	210

a middle- and upper-class drug through the mediating role of the hippy movement. The latter was a highly significant movement in the 1960s and, while it did not fully involve more than a small proportion of the total youth population, it influenced the philosophy, music, dress, attitudes, values, and drug-using behavior of a much larger group. Marihuana was not the essential drug for the hippies, but, along with hair styles, dress and music, it provided a means of marginal participation of the masses in the styles set by the psychedelic or hippy movement.

SOCIOCULTURAL DETERMINANTS

The previous section traced the development of the hippy or psychedelic movement and the subsequent adoption of marihuana usage by the youth of the larger culture. The question remains as to what sociocultural factors contributed to the occurrence at this point in time. As discussed earlier, LSD played a vital role in the hippy movement, but peyote and mescaline had been known for more than one-half century without making headway among the white population. A patent medicine called "Peyotyl" was even advertised as a means to "restore the individual's balance and calm and promote full expansion of his faculties" (Anonymous 1959). As Eric Hoffer (1951) has noted in his study of mass movements, such phenomena require a leader as well as the ripeness of the times. Timothy Leary played a crucial role here by utilizing the mass media to (1) publicize and advocate the use of hallucinogens and (2) simultaneously propound a radical social philosophy. However, it seems likely that if Leary's psychedelic philosophy had been advanced in the depression years of the 1930s, or the war years of the 1940s, it would have gone unnoticed.

Alienation among the younger generation has frequently been suggested as a major contributor to the hippy movement and the middle-class drug epidemic. Weakening of family and community groups, chronic social and technological change, and the lack of historical relatedness have been mentioned in this regard. Others have suggested that the assassinations of the Kennedys added to the disillusionment — undoubtedly the Vietnam war has played a major role.

Another important factor is that social conditions permitted options which did not previously exist. When an adolescent grows up in a structured society which demands he assume adult responsibilities at a relatively early age, the alternative of turning on and dropping out is not available. An affluent society which allows prolonged periods of economic dependence and leisure greatly increases the possible choices as to life styles. Anything which leaves the individual without an established place in the social structure increases the likelihood for radical departures from the existing norms.

WHO WERE INFLUENCED BY THE HIPPY MOVEMENT?

This paper has proposed that the hippy or psychedelic movement was the direct determiner of today's pattern of marihuana use in the larger population. Evidence is provided by the pronounced under-representation of lower socioeconomic and minority groups in the current marihuana-using student population. For obvious reasons, these groups were not responsive to a movement advocating dropping out of an over-materialistic society — hence the hippy population of the 1960's was virtually 100% white, and largely of middle- and upper-class background. Similarly, the subsequent drug-taking spin-out of the hippy movement on the larger youth population continued to have much more impact on middle-class whites than on the lower socioeconomic groups.

When a movement has passed its vital stage it becomes more difficult to trace its impact on the larger culture, but many characteristics of the current marihuana-using population support the interpretation that the behavior developed out of the hippy movement. First, marihuana use continues to be concentrated among youth as shown in the following national surveys (U.S. National Commission 1972:65, 67; Gallup, March 1973:24, 25):

Table 2. Survey of marihuana use among various age groups

Marihuana Commission Survey (1972)		Gallup Poll (1973)	
Age	% ever used	Age	% ever used
12–13	4	18–29	36
14–15	10	30–49	5
16–17	29	50 and over	2
18–21	55		
22–25	40		
26–34	20		
35–49	6		
50 and over	2		

It is generally the same age group that actively participated in the hippy movement, and that most susceptible to the mass adoption of fads and styles. Second, the prevalence of marihuana use is distinctly higher in the West where the hippy movement had its origin and achieved its greatest influence (Table 3).

Table 3. Adult marihuana use by region

Marihuana Commission Survey (1972)		Gallup Poll (1973)	
Region	% ever used	Region	% ever used
Northeast	14	East	13
North Central	15	Midwest	10
South	8	South	9
West	33	West	20

The symbolic role of marihuana use for expressing rebellion and protest has been frequently suggested and is documented in several studies. Smith's longitudinal study of 1800 high school students found self- and peer-ratings of rebelliousness to be one of the best predictors of those who either were, or would subsequently begin, using marihuana (Smith 1973). The adoption of this hippy practice was an especially attractive protest symbol. The establishment had grossly exaggerated the dangers of marihuana and was thus vulnerable to attack. Rebellious youth soon learned that moderate use of marihuana entailed little apparent danger or physical harm. Except for the consequences of the marihuana laws, they could flaunt the establishment's position with little risk. Other more hazardous drugs used by the hippies were less readily adopted.

With more than fifty per cent of the students now having used marihuana in some schools, the behavior is obviously not an indication of statistical deviance. However, studies restricted to the more frequent marihuana users have consistently shown an attitude, value, personality, and behavior pattern which is compatible with that of the hippy or psychedelic movement. One longitudinal study, begun before the marihuana epidemic, found that high school students who subsequently became frequent marihuana users in college exhibited a more non-conformist philosophy, were less disciplined and less decided about future goals than those who used occasionally or not at all (Haagen 1970). Other studies have found frequent users exhibit a more unstable life style with respect to residence, work, school, and goals; receive more traffic violations; are more likely to seek psychiatric counseling; are less religious, belong to few organizations and participate less in athletics; have sexual relations at an earlier age, more frequently and with more partners; exhibit much more liberal and leftish political views, see themselves as outside the larger society, have less respect for authority and are more likely to be activists, especially against the Vietnam war. Personality tests show frequent marihuana users to score lower on dogmatism scales; to be more susceptible to hypnosis and other non-drug regressive states; believe more strongly in para-normal phenomena, such as astrology; demonstrate a strong preference for a casual, spontaneous style of life as opposed to one that is orderly and systematic; and to score high on risk-taking and sociocultural alienation scales. In summary, those individuals who became frequent marihuana users tended to be least accepting of the beliefs, values and behavior of the dominant culture and most responsive to the alternative position advocated by the hippy movement.

PATTERNS OF MARIHUANA USE: OLD AND NEW

If the thesis of this paper is valid, the patterns of current marihuana use would be expected to reflect the symbolic or fad-type motivation for use. In comparison to patterns of cannabis use in other cultures, the ratio of regular to casual users would be expected to be low, the amounts consumed small, the duration of individual use short. In general, it would be expected that the large majority of current marihuana users in the U.S. are essentially playing at cannabis use; that they are participating in a popular style rather than being primarily motivated by the pharmacological effects of the drug.

Frequency of use Recent surveys of U.S. marihuana use have found that, while over twenty million have tried the drug, only a small percentage use it on a daily or more frequent basis. The 1972 national survey conducted for the Marihuana Commission found that, of those having ever used marihuana, the percentages of junior high school, senior high school and college students using daily were 5%, 11% and 17% respectively (U.S. National Commission 1973). A 1971 Gallup survey reported about 10% of college students having tried marihuana were daily users (25 times or more in the past 30 days) (Gallup 1972; No. 80). These percentages of daily users are somewhat larger than those found in the 1971 Marihuana Commission and other 1970–1971 surveys (U.S. National Commission, v. II, 1972).

Since drug-use surveys are a recent innovation associated with the current epidemic, there is little actual data on the relative frequencies of use in other cultures. Some observers have noted that occasional users also far outnumbered those using on a regular basis in the U.S. during the 1930-1940 time period (Bromberg 1934; Mayor's Committee 1944). Much of the older literature on use of cannabis in Eastern countries tends to ignore other than daily users, and the Indian Hemp Commission (1969) specifically concludes that, while *bhang* is often used on an occasional basis, *ganja* and *charas* smoking seldom exists except as a daily habit. A recent study of the extensive use in Jamaica estimated 40 to 50 percent of the male population used on a daily basis (U.S. DHEW 1972).

On the other hand, some Eastern studies have reported considerable less-than-daily usage. Soueif (1967) found an average frequency of 8 to 12 times per month for a sample of Egyptian hashish users, and only one-third of a sample of *kif* smokers in Morocco were daily users (Roland and Teste 1958).

In summary, it appears that for cultures with a long history of cannabis use, the ratio of daily to occasional users is substantially higher than that for the current population of marihuana users in the U.S., however, additional data would be required to verify this conclusion.

Amount consumed   As in the case of alcohol consumption, an adequate description of cannabis-using behavior must include the amount as well as the frequency of use. Here the evidence is quite clear — the typical amount of marihuana consumed per occasion or per day by current U.S. users is quite small in comparison to that for other cultures. The available data on current U.S. use indicates that the average amount consumed by occasional users is around one 1/2-gram marihuana cigarette (McGlothlin 1972). Daily users average around three cigarettes per day with a maximum of about ten. Most marihuana consumed in the U.S. originates in Mexico and averages no more than one percent THC.[1] The casual U.S. marihuana users are estimated to consume about 5 mg. THC per occasion. Daily users average around 15 mg. per day with very heavy users taking 50 mg.

Figure 2 provides a perspective of how this usage compares with experimental data and that reported in other cultures.[2] The maximum amount of smoked THC administered in single-dose experiments in the U.S. is around 20 mg., and the experimental subjects normally report 5 to 10 mg. is sufficient to produce the typical high attained outside the laboratory (Isbell *et al.* 1967; Jones 1971). Thus the experimental data on amount are in agreement with the usage reported in interview studies. In contrast, Miras and Coutselinis (1970: No. 24) report routinely administering smoked-THC doses of 100 mg. to heavy hashish users in Greece.

[1]   Analyses of 40 large seizures (100-2000 pounds each) made by U.S. Customs at the Mexican boundary in 1971 showed only 25 per cent exceeded 1 per cent in THC content (range 0.07 to 2.87 per cent) (U.S. Bureau of Narcotics 1972).
[2]   Except where the actual THC content were cited, the THC estimates in Figure 2 are based on the following assumed THC contents: marihuana or equivalent preparations 1%; Indian *ganja* 3%; hashish 5%.

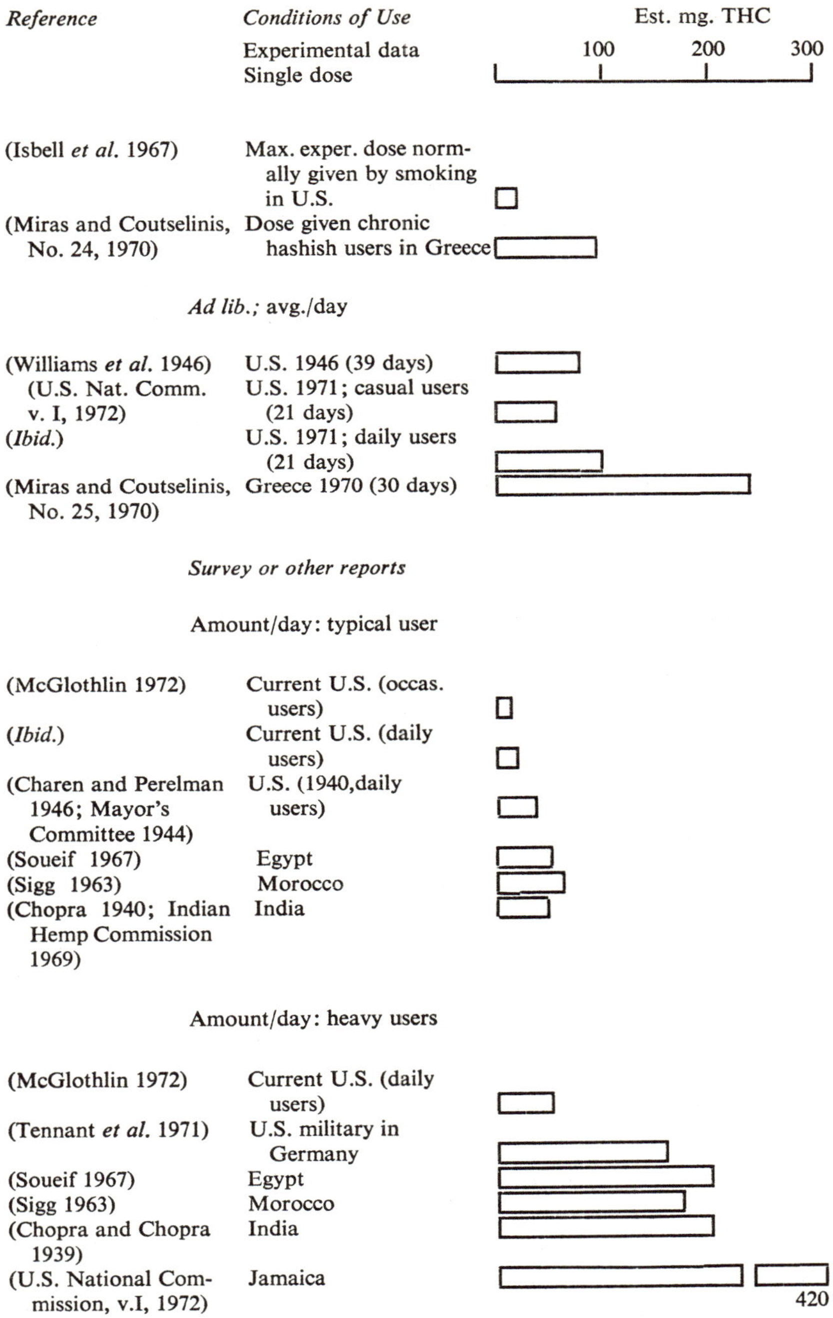

Reference	Conditions of Use	Est. mg. THC
	Experimental data Single dose	100 200 300
(Isbell et al. 1967)	Max. exper. dose normally given by smoking in U.S.	□
(Miras and Coutselinis, No. 24, 1970)	Dose given chronic hashish users in Greece	▭

Ad lib.; avg./day

(Williams et al. 1946)	U.S. 1946 (39 days)	▭
(U.S. Nat. Comm. v. I, 1972)	U.S. 1971; casual users (21 days)	▭
(Ibid.)	U.S. 1971; daily users (21 days)	▭
(Miras and Coutselinis, No. 25, 1970)	Greece 1970 (30 days)	▭

Survey or other reports

Amount/day: typical user

(McGlothlin 1972)	Current U.S. (occas. users)	□
(Ibid.)	Current U.S. (daily users)	□
(Charen and Perelman 1946; Mayor's Committee 1944)	U.S. (1940, daily users)	▭
(Soueif 1967)	Egypt	▭
(Sigg 1963)	Morocco	▭
(Chopra 1940; Indian Hemp Commission 1969)	India	▭

Amount/day: heavy users

(McGlothlin 1972)	Current U.S. (daily users)	▭
(Tennant et al. 1971)	U.S. military in Germany	▭
(Soueif 1967)	Egypt	▭
(Sigg 1963)	Morocco	▭
(Chopra and Chopra 1939)	India	▭
(U.S. National Commission, v.I, 1972)	Jamaica	▭ ▭ 420

Figure 2. Estimated THC content of cannabis used in the U.S. and other countries

A few *ad libitum* studies have been conducted in which subjects smoked cannabis at will over an extended period. Under these conditions subjects tend to use larger amounts than normal because of the unavailability of other activities. An early U.S. study over a period of 39 days reported an average of 17 cigarettes per day (est. 85 mg. THC) (Williams *et al.* 1946). A recent 21-day study found subjects who were casual users averaged about 60 mg THC per day, while subjects who used marihuana daily prior to the study averaged 100 mg THC per day during the experiment (U.S. National Commission, v. I, 1972). These results show that U.S. marihuana users who normally consume 5–15 mg THC per day are capable of taking much larger amounts without apparent ill effects. In a similar *ad libitum* experiment in Greece, chronic hashish users averaged 3 to 7 grams of hashish (est. 150–350 mg. THC) per day for 30 days (Miras and Coutselinis 1970: No. 25).

Figure 2 shows the estimated amount of THC consumed by the current daily marihuana user in the U.S. is about one-fourth that of the typical cannabis smoker in Egypt, Morocco or India. It is also considerably less than the average of 6 to 10 cigarettes reportedly consumed by confirmed U.S. users in the 1940's. The amounts of THC consumed by heavy users in Eastern countries is estimated to be around 200 mg. per day, and even larger amounts are reported in a recent Jamaican study (U.S. National Commission, v. I, 1972). It is of interest to note that some current U.S. military users in Germany report comparable consumption in the form of hashish (Tennant *et al.* 1971).

In summary, the data presented in Figure 2 clearly show that the amount of THC taken by the typical U.S. marihuana user is quite small in comparison to that consumed in cultures where cannabis has been used for many years. Certainly, the estimated 5 mg. of THC per occasion for casual users is almost trivial. This supports the argument that factors other than the pharmacological effects have played an important role in the recent adoption of marihuana use by large numbers of middle-class youth.

Duration of use If participation in a fad or style is a major factor in current marihuana use it would be expected that the period of usage would be relatively short for most individuals. For instance, students primarily responding to peer influence might be expected to terminate usage after leaving school. There is some evidence from recent surveys that the rapid increase in the prevalence of marihuana use has slowed and is perhaps reaching a plateau (Blackford 1972; Gallup, March 1973; U.S. National Commission 1973). Longitudinal studies following individual users are in progress, but the phenomenon is too recent to provide a clear pattern. One 1970 college survey found 77% of those initiated to marihuana 4 to 5 years earlier were still using it to some degree (Lipp 1971). Another 1970 college survey reported 37% of those beginning more than 3 years previously and using more than 10 times had either stopped or were using infrequently (Hochman and Brill 1971). The 1972 Marihuana Commission general population survey found one-half of those 18 years and over having ever used had not stopped (U.S. National Commission 1973).

Studies of cannabis use in other cultures show initiation is also most common in adolescence and may be discontinued in adulthood. However, usage frequently persists for long periods; and, especially in the East, persons using for 20–40 years are not uncommon. At least under conditions of cultural acceptance, cannabis usage appears to have a longevity comparable to that for alcohol and the opiates.

FUTURE USE OF MARIHUANA IN THE U.S.

This paper has depicted the current epidemic of marihuana use as growing out of the hippy or psychedelic movement of the 1960s. The initiation of marihuana use by middle-class youth was interpreted as marginal participation in the styles and protests of the hippy movement, and not related to the earlier use among lower socioeconomic minority groups. This explanation is supported by the chronology of events, the characteristics of the using population and the pattern of marihuana use.

Of course, the symbolic role of marihuana will not sustain its use indefinitely. Either the prevalence of use will decline as the style goes out of fashion, or else the motivation for continued use will shift more to the pharmacological properties of the drug. As the second most popular nrtoxicant in the world, cannabis is clearly a drug which may prove atitactive to large numbers of people on a continuing basis.

Prior to the outbreak of the middle-class drug epidemic, various European observers speculated as to cultural explanations for the choice of alcohol versus cannabis. Bouquet (1950 and 1951) and Porot (1942) both concluded that hashish was suitable for the dreamy, contemplative temperament of the Moslem, where alcohol fitted the aggressive, outward-oriented Westerner. Stringaris (1939) observed that alcohol spreads readily in hashish cultures but not the reverse. The most complete development of this theme is provided by Carstairs (1954) in his explanation of why, in India, the aggressive, action-oriented Rajputs drank alcohol while the passive introspective Brahmins preferred *bhang*.

Some have suggested that the adoption of cannabis use by Western youth heralds a shift away from traditional aggressive, materialistic values. Certainly the tenets of the hippy philosophy would support this view. Whether such a basic shift in values exists in the larger population, whether the West is on its way to becoming a two-drug culture, and whether a relationship exists between the two is still very much open to question. The suggested causal relationship between frequent marihuana use and an amotivational syndrome has given rise to vigorous denials by some authors. Nevertheless, underachievement and the lack of long-term goals do often appear to be associated with, if not causally related to the heavier use patterns. Use of marihuana while working would likely prove more disruptive in the West than among lower-class cannabis users of the East. The effects clearly impair cognitive tasks, whereas cannabis use has occasionally been encouraged among laborers performing repetitive menial work as a remedy for boredom. Also the traditional American cocktail party would have to undergo some rather drastic revisions if alcohol were replaced by marihuana.

In terms of predicting future use of marihuana in the U.S., two conclusions appear to be on relatively safe grounds. First, the introduction of marihuana into the younger age groups has been widespread, and the positive reinforcement resulting from the drug effects *per se* will likely result in substantial continued usage of small amounts on a casual basis for recreational purposes. If marihuana achieves legal status, the number of persons using it in this manner will increase as well as the circumstances of use. The second prediction is that a small proportion of those continuing will consume quantities comparable to the heavy usage observed in other cultures, i.e., 200 mg. or more THC per day. This is substantially above the maximum quantities currently consumed in the U.S. The increasing availability of hashish as well as cannabis extracts will facilitate the intake of such large doses where desired. This pattern of use is comparable to that of the chronic alcoholic and will probably involve considerable overlap with this group.

REFERENCES

ANONYMOUS
   1959 Peyotyl. *Bulletin on Narcotics* 2:16–41.
BLACKFORD, L.
   1972 *San Mateo County, California: surveillance of student drug use; preliminary report*. San Mateo: County Department of Health and Welfare.

BLUM, R. H.
1964 *Utopiates.* New York: Atherton.
BLUM, R. H., et al.
1969 *Drugs II, students and drugs.* San Francisco: Jossey-Bass.
BONNIE, R. J., C. H. WHITEBREAD
1970 The forbidden fruit and the tree of knowledge: an inquiry into the legal history of American marijuana prohibition. *Virginia Law Review* 56 (6): 971–1203.
BOUQUET, R. J.
1950 Cannabis. *UN Bulletin on Narcotics* 2 (4):14–30.
1951 Cannabis. *UN Bulletin on Narcotics* 3 (1):22–45.
BRECHER, EDWARD M., et al.
1972 *Licit and illicit drugs: the Consumers Union report on narcotics, stimulants, depressants, inhalants, hallucinogens, and marijuana — including caffeine, nicotine, and alcohol.* Boston: Little, Brown and Company.
BROMBERG, W.
1934 Marihuana intoxication: a clinical study of cannabis sativa intoxication. *American Journal of Psychiatry* 91 (2):303–330.
CARSTAIRS, G. M.
1954 Daru and bhang: cultural factors in the choice of intoxicant. *Quarterly Journal of Studies on Alcohol* 15:220–237.
CHAREN, SOL, LUIS PERELMAN
1946 Personality studies of marihuana addicts. *American Journal of Psychiatry* 102 (4):674–682.
CHOPRA, R. N.
1940 Use of hemp drugs in India. *Indian Medical Gazette* 75 (6):356–367.
CHOPRA, R. N., G. S. CHOPRA
1939 The present position of hemp-drug addiction in India. *Indian Medical Research Memoirs* 31:1–119.
FREEDMAN, H. L., M. J. ROCKMORE
1946 Marihuana: a factor in personality evaluation and army maladjustment. *Journal of Clinical and Experimental Psychopathology* 7:765–782 (Part I); 8:221–236 (Part II).
GALLUP OPINION INDEX
1969 Public opinion on the controversial issue of legalizing marijuana, No. 53:7–12, November.
1972 No. 80, Princeton, New Jersey, February.
1973 Marijuana use among adults no longer on the increase. Princeton, New Jersey: American Institute of Public Opinion, March.
GASKILL, H. S.
1945 Marihuana, an intoxicant. *American Journal of Psychiatry* 102:202–204.
GOODMAN, L. S., A. GILMAN
1955 *The pharmacological basis of therapeutics.* New York: Macmillan.
HAAGEN, C. H.
1970 *Social and psychological characteristics associated with the use of marijuana by college men.* Middletown, Connecticut: Wesleyan University.

HOCHMAN, J. L., N. Q. BRILL
  1971 "Marijuana use and psychosocial adaption." Paper delivered at American Psychiatric Association meeting in Washington, D.C., May 3rd.
HOFFER, ERIC
  1951 *The true believer.* New York: Harper & Bros.
HOFMANN, A.
  1970 "The discovery of LSD and subsequent investigations on naturally occurring hallucinogens," in F. J. Ayd, Jr., and B. Blackwell (eds.), *Discoveries in biological psychiatry.* Philadelphia: Lippincott.
HUXLEY, ALDOUS
  1954 *Doors of perception.* New York: Harper and Row.
INDIAN HEMP DRUGS COMMISSION
  1969 *Marihuana report, 1893-1894.* Introduction by J. Kaplan, Silver Spring, Maryland: Thomas Jefferson Publishing Co.
ISBELL, H., *et al.*
  1967 Effects of (−)-delta-9-trans-tetrahydrocannabinol in man. *Psychopharmacologia* 11:184–188.
JONES, R. T.
  1971 "Tetrahydrocannabinol and the marijuana induced social 'high' or the effects of the mind on marijuana." Paper presented at the New York Academy of Sciences Conference on Marijuana Chemistry, Pharmacology and Patterns of Social Usage, New York, N. Y., May 21st.
LIPP, M. R.
  1971 Marijuana use by medical students. *American Journal of Psychiatry* 128:207–212.
MC GLOTHLIN, W. H.
  1972 Marijuana: an analysis of use, distribution and control. *Contemporary Drug Problems* 1 (3):467–500.
MARCOVITZ, E., H. J. MEYERS
  1944 The marihuana addict in the army. *War Medicine* 6:382–391.
MAURER, D. W., V. H. VOGEL
  1962 *Narcotics and narcotic addiction.* Springfield: Charles C. Thomas.
MAYOR'S COMMITTEE ON MARIHUANA
  1944 *The marihuana problem in the City of New York.* Lancaster, Pa.: Jaques Cattell Press.
MIRAS, C. J., A. COUTSELINIS
  1970 *The distribution of tetrahydrocannabinol-^{14}C in humans.* Report No. 24, United Nations Secretariat publication ST/SOA/Ser.S/24, November 2nd.
  1970 *The presence of cannabinols in the urine of hashish smokers.* Report No. 25, United Nations Secretariat publication ST/SOA/Ser.S/25, November 4th.
POLSKY, N.
  1969 *Hustlers, beats and others.* Garden City: Doubleday.
POROT, A.
  1942 Le cannabisme. *Annales Medico-Psychologiques* 1 (1):1–24.

PRESTON, J. D.
1970 *A survey of drug use among high school students in Houston, Texas Agricultural Experiment Station, Texas.* Departmental Information Report No. 70–9. Department of Agricultural Economics and Rural Sociology.

Readers guide to periodical literature
1959–1972   S. Robinson and Z. Limerick (eds.) New York: The H. W. Wilson Company.

ROLAND, J. L., M. TESTE
1958   Le cannabisme au Maroc. *Maroc-Medical* 387:694–703. June.

SIGG, B. W.
1963   *Le cannabisme chronique, fruit du sous -dévelopement et du capitalisme: Étude socio-économique et psycho-pathologique.* Alger.

SMITH, G. M.
1973   *Antecedents of teenage drug use.* Presented at the Committee on Problems of Drug Dependence, Chapel Hill, North Carolina, May 21st–23rd.

SOUEIF, M. I.
1967   Hashish consumption in Egypt, with special reference to psychosocial aspects. *UN Bulletin on Narcotics* 19 (2):1–12.

STRINGARIS, M. G.
1939   *Die Haschischsucht.* Berlin: Springer.

TENNANT, F. S., *et al.*
1971   Medical manifestations associated with hashish. *Journal of the American Medical Association* 216 (12):1965–1969.

U.S. BUREAU OF NARCOTICS AND DANGEROUS DRUGS
1972   *Microgram* 5 (10), October.

U.S. DEPARTMENT OF HEALTH, EDUCATION, AND WELFARE. NATIONAL INSTITUTE OF MENTAL HEALTH
1972   *Marihuana and health; second annual report to Congress from the Secretary.* Washington: U.S. Government Printing Office.

U.S. NATIONAL COMMISSION ON MARIHUANA AND DRUG ABUSE
1972   *Marihuana: a signal of misunderstanding.* Technical Papers of the First Report, 2 vols. Washington: U.S. Government Printing Office.
1973   *Drug use in America: problem in perspective.* Washington: U.S. Government Printing Office.

WALTON, R. P.
1938   *Marihuana, America's new drug problem.* Philadelphia: J. B. Lippincott.

WILLIAMS, E. G., *et al.*
1946   Studies on marihuana and pyrahexyl compound. *Public Health Reports* 61 (29):1059–1083.

WINICK, C.
1960   The use of drugs by jazz musicians. *Social Problems* 7 (3):240–253.

Intersections of Anthropology and Law in the Cannabis Area

JOHN KAPLAN

ABSTRACT

The article is concerned with the questions of how knowledge about marihuana is used in the formulation of public policy and how public policy affects the behavior of individuals. Elite opinion tends to be sluggish in changing its views in response to new information and opinions of the elite in turn may exercise important influences on public policy.

Before I move on to the body of my talk let me cover one side point. A number of people have suggested that it is important to determine just how many different species of cannabis there are. To my mind, if it turns out there is more than one species, it will be a matter of interest primarily to textbook publishers, who will have another excuse to put out new editions and to legislative draftsmen, who will have to substitute a more general term wherever *Cannabis sativa* (which we had thought was the only species) appears in the statutes.

Some states, although not all, will have to change their laws so that they comprehend any plant of the genus *Cannabis*. Hopefully, the practical effect of this will be to force many legislatures to rethink the cannabis laws a little earlier than might otherwise be the case. In the meantime, if marihuana offenders have to be released in some states because of the wordings of their statutes, that certainly does not disturb me. On the other hand, we should not exaggerate the importance of such an event. After all, the federal government was without a marihuana possession law for over a year when the Supreme Court, for technical reasons, declared the existing laws unconstitutional. Then, although this state of affairs was not apparently harming the body politic, Congress passed a new law — which avoided the technicality. Similarly, the state of Michigan was without a cannabis law for a while and, though nothing untoward seems to have happened there either, a new law was passed. So, at least from a long term perspective, the botanical issue is not very important.

What I would like to talk to you about is more in the mainstream of anthropology and touches very directly upon my own field of law. There are two questions I want to pose. First, how does information — for instance, knowledge about marihuana — get used in the formulation of public policy? And second, how does public policy, the law, affect the behavior of individuals? You can see that these are two very different questions. Both of them are fascinating and each involves different aspects of the intersection of anthropology and law. I can just hit at the high spots in what I confess will be in an opinionated fashion. There may be people outraged by various things I say, but time does not permit me to be more temperate.

Starting with the problem of transforming knowledge into policy, I find it extremely interesting that when government commissions study marihuana, they study all kinds of facts and theories, but one thing they do *not* study is what has happened to the reports of previous commissions. To me, this oversight suggests a rather curious indifference to whether commission reports will have any effect upon law.

I am not denying that there is some relationship between what the commission recommends and what it thinks can be adopted. Obviously, there is. For instance, I am confident that there are members of both the American and the Canadian commissions who thought to themselves, "Well, what we probably ought to do is just license the sale of the stuff. But if we said that, nobody would pay any attention to anything else we had to say. We'd be too far ahead of the public."

For my own part, though, I can't believe that this amount of reflection on the issue is sufficient. I should know, too, because the very first commission to study marihuana since La Guardia's time was not the *Wooton* Commission in England, nor the *Le Dain* Commission in Canada, nor the Commission on Marihuana and Drug Use in the United States, it was California's Joint Legislative Commission to Revise the Penal Code. It became crystal clear to all the law professors who were the reporters for that commission that the sensible thing for the society to do was to license the sale of marihuana with appropriate controls. We felt that way primarily because of the associated harms that arise from making the traffic illegal: it alienates young people and members of certain ethnic groups by turning them into instant "criminals,"; it creates massive profits for the real criminals; it allows marihuana to be a sort of "loss-leader" for the drug culture, and so on. Although the best solution was clear to us, it was *also* clear that if we recommended licensing, we, the reporters, would be fired, and nobody would pay attention to anything we had said. As a result, we recommended decriminalization — exactly what both the Canadian and American commissions recommended, five years later. And what happened? We were fired and nobody paid any attention to what we said. Not only that but all the other works of the California Joint Legislative Commission, for all practical purposes, disappeared from the face of the earth.

Now somebody should have learned something from that. It's true, of course, that the Le Dain Commission and the Presidential Commission made the same compromise later on and managed not to get fired. On the other hand, they weren't all that effective, either. I would have expected them to at least call in a consultant — a sociologist, maybe — and say to him:

Tell us how we can maximize our effectiveness. Don't tell us what to say. Just tell us, as best you can, what will happen if we recommend X and what will happen if we recommend Y.

That's all. It would have been so simple. But somehow commissions never seem to think that way.

Another interesting thing about marihuana commissions is that the public's outlook influences not only what the commissions recommend once they are appointed, but often also who gets appointed to the commissions in the first place. It has been suggested that most of the members of the Commission in the United States were chosen precisely because they were known quantities, with their minds already made up. That's an extreme position, perhaps, but frankly, if you look at the people the President appointed to the Marihuana Commission, it's clear that he did his very best to stack it. Of the three psychiatrists he appointed, two were known for their outspoken anti-marihuana positions, and the third — although he hadn't really announced either way — was known for a widely quoted article he had written concerning — and exaggerating — the dangers of marihuana. In addition, the pharmacologist on the commission had expressed himself quite strongly against relaxation of the marihuana laws. Where the President made his mistake was in not realizing that these people, although biased, were nonetheless honest and intelligent.

In any event, at least half the people appointed to the United States Commission had to totally reevaluate their positions. They were not coming to the problem with open minds, and it must have been pretty difficult for them to go back on what they had previously said. But to a considerable extent they finally did.

As I hope I have suggested, the problem of translating information into public policy is an extremely interesting and important one, which far transcends the marihuana issue itself. Generally speaking, it doesn't make sense to recommend things that the public is violently against. And in a democracy, at least on issues which tend to polarize people, it may not even make sense to recommend something which a vocal minority is against. Public officials have to get elected. Look what happens to politicians who come out strongly for gun control — even though, so far as we can tell, a majority of Americans are in favor of it.

While we're talking about public attitudes as one of the variables which mediate between information and public policy, I might mention another factor that is at least arguably as important, namely, elite attitudes. I will return to this later, in a different context, but for now I want to disavow any intention to pass judgment on the relative merits of elite attitudes and public attitudes. Indeed, one really striking thing is that *both* public attitudes and elite attitudes in various areas can be, by any standards, incredibly wrong. We have heard that there are psychiatrists in Colombia who are treating marihuana users with shock treatments. What more can I say? I don't doubt that most of them are acting, or shocking, in perfectly good faith. But if they did that in the United States, they would be slapped with suits for malpractice so quickly that they wouldn't even have time to transfer their assets to their wives.

Now it is understandable that elites may initially base their attitudes on incomplete information. The question, however, is how is it that they, who are supposed to have access to all the latest and best knowledge in any area, can often *stay* so wrong for such a long time? And the marihuana issue is only the most obvious example of this.

Obviously, part of the answer is simply human inertia. But a significant part also, I think, has to do with power relationships in the society. Often an elite will have a vested interest — not just a material interest, but perhaps more important, a prestige interest in maintaining positions that they have taken earlier. In some sense, admitting that they were wrong about something, even if reasonably wrong, calls into question their entire capacity to govern. It may be hard to adopt a new position on marihuana when your statements five years ago are on record. And if you do change your position, you may worry that people will question your right to govern a society if you can be that wrong about something.

Now clearly this goes to very sensitive questions about the distribution of power in a society. And I really believe that some of the things members of even the most august commissions do are explicable only in these terms. Their actions are, I think, intimately connected with the problems of both inertia and power. Indeed, a couple of the things both the Le Dain Commission and the United States Commission said are fascinating to me precisely because they are so obviously wrongheaded that they can be explained only on those grounds. For instance, both commissions told us that marihuana might be a fad and just go away, and that therefore we shouldn't do anything too drastic now to make the drug more available through legal channels. Well, I invite you to look at the data showing, for example, that 50% of marihuana users say its use improves sexual enjoyment. If marihuana is as much of a fad as sex is, it's not going to go away. And, basing a public policy on the idea that it may go away seems to me just very wrongheaded.

Or take a second pronouncement by the commissions. They claim — with more hope than conviction, I think — that doing away with the penalty for possession will allow police to focus more on trafficking. If you know anything about law enforcement, you should know that that's just not true. When the legislature does away with the penalties for possession, it de-escalates the whole problem. The police have more time, to be sure, but they don't devote it to trafficking. What they do is to try to cut down on burglaries, armed robberies, rapes — in short, to deal with the problem of violent crime. To my mind, that is a much more sensible use of police time. There is not a shred of evidence to prove that if we do away with penalties for possession, the police will pay more attention to marihuana trafficking. Indeed, there is strong reason to believe quite the contrary.

In short, we may conclude that a major problem with bringing information to bear on the formulation of public policy is that elite opinion seems to be relatively sluggish in changing its views in response to information. This is, of course, a double problem since not only are opinions important in themselves as a shaper of public policy but typically the elite acts as a transducer of information to the rest of the citizenry whose opinions may also exercise important influences on public policy.

If I had the time, I could go on at some length discussing the relationship between information and public policy. Some of the things that I have said are obviously biased, almost designed to elicit a response. Others, I think, are very sensible things that just have to be understood by anyone trying to figure out the relation between the two variables.

But let's go on to the next area: how public policy influences behavior. This is, to my mind, even more interesting. One thing I have been struck by again and again in the papers presented here is the irrelevance of public policy to so much of behavior. Anyone just reading through the statute books of countries like Colombia, Costa Rica, India and Jamaica would immediately conclude that marihuana use is severely punished there and hence rarely used. But neither of these things is true. If one goes out in the field, one finds that the drug is widely and almost openly used. What does the legal system do about it? Well, it manages to inflict a certain toll. It's almost as if you mined the oceans and every 150th freighter went down. You're not going to stop people shipping things. You're just going to raise insurance rates a little.

Basically, all that strict marihuana laws in these countries accomplish is to ruin a certain number of lives. Otherwise, they have no real effect. I might say, as a first approximation, that in this area the law is by and large irrelevant. And that leads to the rather intriguing question: in what kind of societies does this occur? For convenience, I'd like to talk of a tripartite division of legal systems. The first type — perhaps China and the Soviet Union are examples — is a legal system where one has the feeling (and let's assume it's true) that the government is in essentially complete control. In terms of the behavior of the citizens within very wide limits, what it wants done gets done, and what it doesn't want done doesn't get done. In a legal system like that, one would not expect that the government would have any serious problems enforcing laws against marihuana. People just wouldn't smoke the drug, at least in those areas in which the government cared about enforcing the law — though the government might well allow it in, say, backward rural areas. But where the government cared at all about it, people wouldn't dare violate the law. And therefore there would be relatively few associated costs (police, prison upkeep, etc.). Laws are not enforced there with great expense and effort because they don't have to be.

The second kind of legal system is one like that of the U.S. or Canada, one which has a formal structure of authority but also many rights for individuals. Marihuana is forbidden, but the government is not able to enforce the prohibition. And from this situation there is considerable resulting harm: police corruption, marihuana marketing by organized crime, a whole subculture based on drugs, large numbers of people arrested with consequent damage to their lives. Because the law is incapable of enforcment it causes serious social harm.

The third type of legal system is one for the most part like that attributed here to Costa Rica. In such a system, although the law, on paper, prohibits something, nobody really pays a great deal of attention to that law. As a result, in gross terms, it doesn't really do much harm. Now this is not a response to a problem which is easy in most industrialized societies. The law in developed societies tends to be a fairly fine instrument. It's only when the authorities attempt to enforce laws which illegalize actions they would like to prevent, but can't, that they do real damage to the legal fabric. This seems not to be the case in underdeveloped countries. There, while it may be that the laws are wrongheaded, they don't do a great deal of harm because nobody — public *or* authorities — pays attention to them.

To move on, because time is running out, let me point out what appears to happen in a Western developed country's legal system (say, the U.S. system) when in response to their perceived inappropriateness the laws begin to relax. The relaxation occurs in basically four steps, although they run together somewhat. First, the actual inflicted penalty starts dropping, in practice, if not in law. This has already, for the most part, happened in dramatic fashion, in both the United States and Canada. There's a wonderful case in Canada, where, although the law hasn't been changed very much partially because of the Le Dain Commission's work, attitudes have greatly changed. In Toronto, somebody has just been convicted for a fourth time on marihuana possession charges. For his first offense, with no other previous convictions of any kind, he was given six months in jail. For his second offense, he was given a month in jail. And for his fourth offense, he was given three months in jail. For his third offense, he was fined and put on probation.

Now what happened there is interesting. The generally accepted practice as to punishments for subsequent offenses puts the cases on the up-escalator, as it were. On the other hand, the whole law as to marihuana, because of the society's increasing appreciation of the problem, has been on a down-escalator, moving even faster in the direction of lessened sentences.

The same thing has taken place in the United States. At present, over 90% of Americans convicted of marihuana possession don't go to jail. This certainly wasn't true ten years ago. The seriousness of punishments given have gone down very sharply, but not primarily as a function of statute law. Although that, of course, has been happening, too. The main reason is that the judicial enforcement policy has been changing — in response to a whole range of social pressures.

After the judges start dropping the penalties actually given, the behavior of the police begins to change. More and more, police in the United States are beginning to just forget about the whole business. If the people they catch with marihuana haven't done anything else, they often give them a warning and throw away the stuff. Sometimes they won't even take it away from those they catch. A sizable percentage of officers simply ignore the matter, so that potential offenders don't come into the criminal system at all.

The third step occurs when the statutory penalties themselves start dropping. We're pretty close to the end point of that, so far as possession is concerned, in parts of the United States, such as Oregon. Both Denmark and the Netherlands have already reached it. In those countries, there is essentially no penalty for possession.

As for the final step, licensing the sale of marihuana that will be a big one. I have no doubt we'll do it in the United States — in maybe five years. Once people realize that there is in fact no penalty for possession, then they're going to begin to think,

Well, as long as so many people are using it, who should make the profit on selling the drug? The government can have it through taxes, or the drug culture can get it and use it to support other activities (including, I might point out, the feeding of large amounts of more dangerous drugs to people who still will have to buy their marihuana covertly).

So the issue becomes then, given that marihuana is going to be sold, is it going to be sold by government licensed, taxed dealers or by dope peddlers? Once we have come to that, people will conclude, as they must, that it is better to have the sales made legal.

The one thing that could retard statutory change — at least, in the licensing area — is an international agreement. International agreements are, by their very nature, the most sluggish type of law to reform. They are also the variety least based on public policy considerations, and the most heavily bureaucratic in their operation. These could be serious problems, but there are legal means around them.

There is one other thing I'd like to mention. I was very impressed with the discussion of Colombia, where we talked about the other social control agents than the courts and police. Something we tend to forget is that the criminal law is by no means the only agency of social control. The psychiatrist who gives shock treatments to marihuana users is punishing people just as much as are the prisons. Indeed, he is probably more of a threat to the people than is the actual legal system. And the psychiatrists aren't the only social control mechanism. There are also the newspapers and the governing elites or opinion-leaders.

I wish I could go on at greater length about the various means of social control, but the most significant thing I want to point out is that we come full circle. The social control agents including, of course, the police and the courts are also the elites who mould attitudes in this area and, in a very real sense, make the law. They are the governing class in our society but theirs is an acutely uncomfortable position. They are required by their institutional roles to help enforce a societal proscription on the use of marihuana. Simultaneously, because the laws in this area have come increasingly to be seen as simply ridiculous, more and more people are coming to them and demanding that they change things. They are unsympathetic to changes in the laws they are enforcing in part, due to cognitive dissonance — the basic principle that says we are unwilling to credit people who describe a job as unnecessary, in direct proportion to the amount we are investing in doing the job.

In other words, the involvement of the elites in social control prevents their acting as appropriate transducers and interpreters of unbiased information to the general population on the laws they are helping to enforce. In the absence of such mediators of information the general population does not press for change — or at least accepts change at a reduced rate. Moreover, insofar as these governing elites have independent power to mould the law — either as law-makers or as tranducers of information to the law-makers — the same processes of reluctance to accept new information will occur.

It is for this reason primarily, I postulate, that the incorporation into public policy of information on cannabis moves at such a sluggish pace. I would hope that someone would undertake to verify that the more involved elites are in the task of social control on an issue the greater their inertia, and the less is their willingness to accept new information at odds with that upon which the law is based, and the more sluggishly they will react to information challenging the purposes of the control.

Cannabis Conference Participant-Observers

Dr. Michael Agar
Division of Research
New York State Narcotic Addiction Control Commission
New York, New York

Dr. Khem Bahadur Bista
Center for Economic Development and Administration
Tribhuvan University
Kathmandu, Nepal

Dr. Monique Braude
Acting Chief
Pre-Clinical Studies Section
Biomedical Research Branch, Division of Research
National Institute of Drug Abuse
Rockville, Maryland

Mr. Miguel Carranza
Department of Sociology and Anthropology
University of Notre Dame
Notre Dame, Indiana

Mr. Louis Cavanaugh, Jr.
Agency for Health and Drug Control
Bureau of International Organization Affairs
Washington, D.C.

Mr. Jon Cowan
Department of Pharmacology
University of California
San Francisco, California

Dr. José de la Isla
Director
Fellows Program, Drug Abuse Council
Washington, D.C.

Mr. James Helsing
Liaison Officer
Division of Research
National Institute of Drug Abuse
Rockville, Maryland

Mr. Matthew Huxley
Special Advisor on Standards
Office of Director
National Institute of Mental Health
Rockville, Maryland

Dr. Denise Kandel
Biometrics Research
College of Physicians and Surgeons
Columbia University
New York, New York

Mr. Alberto G. Mata
Department of Sociology and Anthropology
University of Notre Dame
Notre Dame, Indiana

Dr. Helen Nowlis
Director
Bureau of Drug Education
Office of Education
Washington, D.C.

Dr. Vincent Nowlis
Drug Abuse Council
Washington, D.C.

Dr. Robert Petersen
(Formerly Chief, Center for Studies of Narcotic and Drug Abuse)
Special Assistant to the Director
Division of Research
National Institute of Drug Abuse
Rockville, Maryland

Dr. Maynard Quimby
Department of Pharmacognosy
University of Mississippi
University, Mississippi

Dr. Arthur Rubel
Center for the Study of Man
Notre Dame, Indiana

Dr. Moshe Shokeid
Head
Department of Sociology and Anthropology
Tel Aviv University
Tel Aviv, Israel

Dr. Jean Paul Smith
Chief
International Activities
National Institute of Drug Abuse
Rockville, Maryland

Mr. Willian Stablein
Department of Anthropology
Columbia University
New York, New York

Mr. James Taccoh
Department of Sociology and Anthropology
University of Notre Dame
Notre Dame, Indiana

Dr. Coy W. Waller
Research Institute of Pharmaceutical Sciences
University of Mississippi
University, Mississippi

Biographical Notes

ASSAD ABBAS (M.D.) is Chief Psychologist at Queen Mary's Childrens Hospital in London, England.

MICHAEL H. BEAUBRUN (M.B., Ch.B., D.P.M.) resides in Jamaica where he is Professor and Head of the Department of Psychiatry of the University of the West Indies and Senior Consultant of the University Hospital. His major research interests include alcoholism and drug abuse, psychiatric education, and community psychiatry. In 1968 he was named a Distinguished Fellow of the American Psychiatric Association and is a member or consultant of numerous medical and psychiatric organizations, including the World Psychiatric Association and the World Health Organization. Dr. Beaubrun is currently serving as President of the World Federation for Mental Health.

SULA BENET (Ph.D.) is a Professor of Anthropology at Hunter College of the City University of New York. She has authored numerous publications on archaeology, folklore, social organization of Eastern Europe and the USSR, Soviet gerontology, and hashish. Her principal interests include social aspects of gerontology, the diffusion of hashish, and Eastern European Slavic cultures.

JEAN BENOIST (M.D., D.Sc.) is a Professor of Anthropology and Director of the Center for Caribbean Studies at the University of Montreal. He has conducted fieldwork in the West Indies, Israel, India and islands of the Indian Ocean, and has published extensively on population structure in the West Indies, and on social structure and change in plantation societies of the Caribbean and Indian Ocean areas. At present Dr. Benoist is working principally in the field of medical anthropology.

JACK D. BLAINE (M.D.) is currently Psychiatry Resident at the University of California, San Diego. His major fields of interest include adolescent and adult psychiatry and research on psychopharmacology and drug abuse. He has served as a consultant for the National Institute of Mental Health at their Center for the Studies of Narcotic and Drug Abuse, as Assistant Director for Medical Science of the National Commission on Marihuana and Drug Abuse, and since 1972 has been a member of the Drug Abuse Research Advisory Committee of the Food and Drug Administration's National Institute of Drug Abuse.

LOUIS P. BOZZETTI (M.D.) is currently affiliated with the University of California at San Diego, where he holds the positions of Associate Clinical Professor of Psychiatry, Head of the Community Psychiatry Program of the Department of Psychiatry, and Medical Director of the University Psychiatric Clinic. His major research interests include drug addiction and cross-cultural studies of drug use.

RODERICK E. BURCHARD (Ph.D.) is presently an Assistant Professor of Anthropology at the University of Manitoba, Canada. His major research interests include medical and nutritional anthropology and he is a specialist on the use of coca in the Andean regions of South America.

WILLIAM E. CARTER (Ph.D.) has served as Director and Professor of the Center for Latin American Studies at the University of Florida, Gainesville, since 1968. He has conducted extensive research in Central and South America and is the author of numerous articles and books. Dr. Carter is currently engaged in a study on the chronic use of cannabis in San Jose, Costa Rica. He has been the recipient of various grants and fellowships, including a Fulbright-Hays research award and grants from the National Science Foundation and the National Institute of Mental Health.

HELEN CODERE (Ph.D.) is currently Professor of Anthropology at Brandeis University. Among her interests are method and theory in anthropology, economic anthropology, historical anthropology and primitive art. She has conducted extensive research among North American Indian populations and in Africa. She is the author of numerous scholarly books and articles.

LAMBROS COMITAS (Ph.D.) is currently affiliated with Teachers

College, Columbia University, where he is Professor of Anthropology and Education, and Director of the Center for Education in Latin America. He is also a consultant for the Department of Health, Education, and Welfare in their Center for Studies of Narcotic and Drug Abuse; co-principal investigator on a cannabis project in Jamaica; an Associate Director of the Research Institute for the Study of Man, in New York. Dr. Comitas has authored numerous publications on the Caribbean, among them *The ganja complex: marihuana in Jamaica*, co-authored with Vera Rubin.

ALVARO RUBIM DE PINHO (M.D.) is currently Head of the Department of Neuropsychiatry and Professor of Psychiatry of the Faculty of Medicine at the Federal University of Bahia, Brazil. He is a former President of the Brazilian Psychiatric Association and has numerous publications in his field. His main current research interest is cultural influence in the treatment of mental disease.

MARLENE DOBKIN DE RIOS (Ph.D.) is currently an Associate Professor of Anthropology at California State University at Fullerton. From 1967 to 1969 she worked as Research Associate at the Institute of Social Psychiatry of the National University of San Marcos in Lima, Peru. Her many research papers include reports on folk healing and ritual, non-Western use of hallucinogens, and altered states of consciousness. In addition to her teaching duties, Dr. Dobkin de Rios serves as a consultant for the National Commission on Marihuana and Drug Abuse.

BRIAN M. DU TOIT (Ph.D.) is an Associate Professor of Anthropology and African Studies at the University of Florida. He did postgraduate work in the United States and South Africa, and conducted his first formal research among the Zulu. Other field projects include community studies among rural and urban Africans, research in the central highlands of Papua, New Guinea, and a current study concerning cannabis in Africa. Various publications reflect Dr. du Toit's interests in the fields of culture change, the anthropology of religion and new religious movements, and migration and urbanization.

B. R. ELEJALDE (M.D.) is an Assistant Professor of the Faculty of Medicine and Head of the Genetics Laboratory of the Department of Pathology at the University of Antioquia in Medellín, Colombia. He has served as Research Fellow of the British Council in the Cytogenetics Laboratory, Paterson Laboratories, Christie Hospital, and Holt Radium

Institute in Manchester, England. He is on the editorial board of *Antioquia Médica*, Consultant to the Fondo Colombiano de Investigaciones Científicas (*Colciencias*), and a member of various scientific and medical organizations. Dr. Elejalde is the author of numerous cytogenetic and chromosomal studies.

JAMES F. FISHER (Ph.D.) is an Assistant Professor in the Department of Anthropology at Carleton College. He taught English at the elementary, secondary, and college levels while he was a Peace Corps Volunteer from 1962–1964 in Nepal. Since then, he has served as consultant and coordinator of various language, education, and Peace Corps Training programs in Nepal and India. Among his special interests are central and south Asia, economic anthropology, and cultural change. In 1973, Dr. Fisher was Director of the Associated Colleges of the Midwest Indian Studies Program held at Kathmandu.

MELVYN GREEN, presently completing his doctoral dissertation, is a co-organizer of a Drug Abuse Council sponsored survival manual for "free clinics" and other alternative health care agencies. He has served in various positions, as a sociological lecturer on deviant behavior, drug research associate, and recently worked as Assistant Director of a videotape production on treatment for acute adverse drug reactions.

K. A. HASAN (Ph.D.) is an Associate Professor of Anthropology in the Indiana State University, Terre Haute. He is the author of numerous papers published in medical and anthropological journals in India, Europe, and the United States, as well as a book, *The cultural frontier of health in village India*. Dr. Hasan is particularly interested in medical anthropology and holds a Masters degree in Public Health from the University of California, Berkeley.

H. W. HUTCHINSON (Ph.D.) is currently Professor and Chairman of the Department of Anthropology at the University of Miami, Florida. He has published extensively on plantation communities and social organization in Brazil. From 1954 through 1959 he taught anthropology in Brazilian universities, first in the Escola de Sociologia e Politica de São Paulo, and later in the Faculdade de Filosofia of the Universidade da Bahia. Concurrent with Dr. Hutchinson's interest in Brazil, are his interests in sociocultural factors in health behavior and services, and the epidemiology of mental illness.

KNUD JENSEN (M.D.) is currently Consultant Psychiatrist and Neurologist at Odense University Hospital and a Lecturer at Odense University in Denmark. His major fields of research are psychopharmacology and clinical and social psychiatry.

ROGER JOSEPH (Ph.D.) is the Research Director of the Institute of Science, Technology, Arts, and Culture, in Fullerton, California. He has conducted fieldwork in Mexico, the Caribbean, Lebanon, and Morocco, and for the academic year 1973–1974, served as a Visiting Associate Professor at the American University of Beirut. Dr. Joseph, in addition to a number of papers and articles, has produced two documentary films.

JOHN KAPLAN (LL.B.) is currently affiliated with Stanford University, where he is a Professor of Law. He is the author of numerous articles and books, including *Marijuana — the new prohibition* (1970).

AHMAD M. KHALIFA (Ph.D.) is currently President of the National Center for Social Research in Cairo. He has taught in the Universities of Cairo, Ein-Shams, and Baghdad, and is the author of numerous publications on narcotic drugs, the sociology of deviant behavior, and the penal system of the United Arab Republic. Dr. Khalifa is Chairman of the United Nations Committees on Crime Prevention and Control, and on the Prevention of Discrimination and the Protection of Minorities.

MUNIR A. KHAN (M.D.) is a Research Fellow at the Institute of Psychiatry, Odense University Hospital, Denmark. He has worked in Switzerland and England, and is currently engaged in research in the field of psychopharmacology, with emphasis on the interaction of alcohol and other psychopharmacological drugs.

HUI-LIN LI (Ph.D.) is currently affiliated with the University of Pennsylvania where he is a Professor of Botany and Director of the Morris Arboretum. He received his education in China and the United States, and has taught biology and botany at Soochow and Taiwan Universities. Dr. Li has carried out extensive research in biology, plant taxonomy, economic botany, and biosystematics, as a Fulbright, Guggenheim, and National Academy of Science Research Fellow.

MARIE ALEXANDRINE MARTIN (Ph.D.) is Head of Research at the National Center of Scientific Research, Paris. She has conducted and published studies of botanical research in Cambodia and eastern Thailand

and is currently engaged in ethnoscientific and linguistic research in those two countries.

WILLIAM H. McGLOTHIN (Ph.D.) has held the position of Professor in Residence in the Department of Psychology at the University of California, Los Angeles, since 1971. He is a member of the Scientific Advisory Boards for the National Council on Drug Abuse and the National Commission on Marihuana and Drug Abuse and also serves as a consultant to the World Health Organization and as a Research Scientist of the National Institute of Mental Health. Dr. McGlothin's major research interest is the psychological effects of psychotropic drugs and their social implications. He has published extensively on hallucinogens, cannabis, and other drugs.

RALPH D. MILLER (Ph.D.) presently is residing in Vancouver, British Columbia, where he is engaged in consultation and research in the field of drug usage. He has served on the faculty of McMaster University in Hamilton, Ontario, and from 1969 to 1973 was Research Director and principal scientific writer for the Commission of Inquiry into the Non-Medical Use of Drugs, in Ottawa.

BARBARA G. MYERHOFF (Ph.D.) is an Associate Professor in the Department of Sociology and Anthropology at the University of Southern California. She is the recipient of numerous awards and grants, and a member of several anthropological and sociological organizations. Dr. Meyerhoff has also published extensively, including articles and a book on the symbolism and use of peyote among the Huichol Indians of Mexico.

PHYLLIS PALGI is Chief Anthropologist of the Mental Health Division of Israel's Ministry of Health, and also teaches Anthropology in the Behavioral Science Department of the Medical School. She has authored a number of publications in the field of anthropology and mental health, with special reference to immigrant adjustment problems. Her other areas of studies include death, bereavement, and mourning rites, and family types in Israel.

WILLIAM L. PARTRIDGE, who will receive his Ph.D. in Anthropology in August, 1974, is currently a predoctoral Research Fellow of the National Institute of Mental Health. He is the author of a number of publications, including a book *The hippie ghetto: the natural history of a subculture.* His principal interests include community studies and applied anthropology in the United States and South America; he has done field work in the Caribbean and on the north coast of Colombia.

VERA D. RUBIN (Ph.D.) is Director of the Research Institute for the Study of Man in New York. She was previously affiliated with Brandeis University, where she taught in the Department of Anthropology. She is an Honorary Fellow of A.A.A.S., New York Academy of Sciences, and a Fellow of a number of other anthropological organizations. She is also an Associate of the Joint Program in Applied Anthropology, Center for Education in Latin America, Teachers College, Columbia University. Her major research interests include applied anthropology, anthropology and medicine, and population dynamics. A recent book, *The ganja complex: marihuana in Jamaica*, co-authored with Lambros Comitas, is one of Dr. Rubin's numerous publications.

JOSEPH H. SCHAEFFER (Ph.D.) is a Professor of Anthropology and Communication at Marlboro College in Vermont. Some of his major interests include communication in complex urban settings, general systems theory as it relates to communication, human ecology, and the development of audiovisual techniques related to the acquisition of permanent anthropological records. He has done fieldwork in the Caribbean and urban New York. In 1970–1971 he participated, with his wife, in a multidisciplinary study of the effects of cannabis upon behavior in a defined socioeconomic setting in Jamaica, West Indies.

RICHARD EVANS SCHULTES (Ph.D) is currently affiliated with Harvard University where he is the Paul C. Mangelsdorf Professor of Natural Sciences, Director of the Botanical Museum, and Curator of Economic Botany. He has published extensively in taxonomic botany, ethnobotany, and plant chemistry, and is present Editor of *Economic Botany* and the *Harvard Botanical Museum Leaflets*. His specialty is the taxonomy of useful plants, particularly narcotics and poisons, of the New World Tropics, and Dr. Schultes has engaged in plant exploration in these areas.

ALVIN BURTON SEGELMAN (Ph.D.) is an Assistant Professor in the College of Pharmacy, Rutgers University. He is the author of numerous publications, Contributing Editor for *Pharmacognosy Titles*, and Scientific Reviewer for the *Journal of Pharmaceutical Sciences* and *Lloydia, The Journal of Natural Products*. Dr. Segelman is currently engaged in a number of research projects, including work to isolate and identify previously unknown biologically active components of cannabis.

WILLIAM THOMAS STEARN (D.Sc., Sc.D., Ph.D.) is the Senior Principal Scientific Officer in the Department of Botany of the British

Museum (Natural History). His major research and interests include plant collection in Australia, Europe, Jamaica, and the United States; the history of botany and botanical exploration; bibliography of natural history; and the life and work of Carl Linnaeus. Dr. Stearn is a member of numerous scientific and academic societies and organizations, and has an extensive list of publications to his name.

COSTAS N. STEFANIS (M.D.) is currently Professor and Chairman of the Department of Psychiatry of Athens University Medical School, and Director of Eginition University Psychiatric Hospital. He is also President of the Hellenic Association of Neurology and Psychiatry. Dr. Stefanis has served in academic and clinical positions in neurology and psychiatry in Greece, Canada, and the United States. His major research interests include clinical psychiatry, psychopharmacology, psychosocial aspects of schizophrenia, and physical and sociocultural aspects of drug abuse.

NIKOLAAS J. VAN DER MERWE (Ph.D.) recently assumed the post of Professor of Archaeology at the University of Capetown, South Africa. He received his education in the United States, has conducted fieldwork in Africa, Italy, and the U.S., and previously taught anthropology in the State University of New York, Binghamton. He has a number of publications in archaeology and soil chemistry to his name. Dr. van der Merwe's major fields of research are African prehistory and archaeometry (physical and chemical analysis in archaeology.)

JOHANNES WILBERT (Ph.D.) currently holds the positions of Professor of Anthropology and Director of the Latin American Center at the University of California at Los Angeles. He also holds the position of Guest Professor at the University of Vienna. From 1956 through 1966 he served in Caracas variously as Director of Anthropology for the Society of Natural Sciences, Director for the Caribbean Institute of Anthropology and Sociology, and Chairman of Anthropology for the same organization. In addition to his teaching responsibilities Dr. Wilbert is editor of the Venezuelan journal *Antropológica* and of the "Latin American Studies" monograph series.

ROBERTO WILLIAMS-GARCIA (M.A.) is currently Investigator for the Instituto de Antropología, Universidad Veracruzana, in Xalapa, Veracruz. His major fields of interest include Mexican myth and ritual, and documentary film-making.

Index of Names

Aaronson, Bernard, 402, 418, 427
Abbas, Assad, 345–354
Achenbach, K., 395
Afendoulis, Th.: *Pharmacology*, 311
Agustín, Pedre, 134, 135, 137, 138, 141
Alarcón, José C., 150
Albany, J.: *Zamal*, 231
Albers, Patricia, 263
Alberti, Ludwig, 95
Allauddin Khilji (king of India), 236
Allen, M., 335
Al-Magraby, S., 199
Alpert, Robert, 432, 533
An Chih-min, 53
Anderson, Charles John, 93
Anderson, E., 23
Anderson, Loran C., 32
Anderson, J. G., 53
Antonio (Mexican priest), 134, 135
Antzyferov, L. V., 46
Aranújo, Alcen Maynard, 148
Arbousset, T., 93
Ardila Rodríguez, Franciso, 149, 168
Arensberg, Conrad M., 167
Argota, G., 341
Aristotle, 430
Ashcroft, Michael, 369
Asuni, T., 101
Ataide, Luis, 175
Athenaeus, 304
Atherton, J., 78
Atkinson, Edwin T., 253
Aurangzeb (Moghal kind), 236
Ausubel, David P., 169

Baard, E., 103, 105
Bagshawe, F. J., 100
Baines, Thomas, 96, 106
Baker, Paul T., 474, 479
Bal, Mary, 369
Balfour, Henry, 104
Ball, J. C., 515
Ball, M. J., 515
Ballas, C., 303–326
Barash, Lucille, 7, 498
Barber, Theodore X., 409, 411
Barbosa Rodrígues, João, 457
Barbour, R. G., 281
Barrow, John, 93
Barry, H., III, 274, 278, 279, 280
Baudelaire, P. C., 231, 264
Bauhin, C., 15, 27
Beaubrun, Michael, 6, 485–494
Becker, H. S., 512
Beckstead, H. D., 270
Benet, Sula, 2, 10, 39–49
Benetowa, Sula, 258
Benítez, Fernando, 417, 419
Benoist, Jean, 227–234
Bensusan, A. D., 83
Benton, A. L., 395
Benzoni, Girolamo, 441, 452
Berk, J. L., 480
Bernal Villa, Segundo, 449
Bharati, A., 250
Biegeleisen, H., 46
Bilodeau, L., 514
Biocca, Ettore, 448
Bird, John, 96

Bista, Khem Bahadur, 247
Blackford, L., 542
Blackwell, J. C., 515
Blaine, Jack, 8, 521–529
Blum, Richard, 403, 532, 533
Blumenfield, M., 332, 339
Bolton, Ralph, 463, 464, 472–476, 479, 481
Bonnie, R. J., 532
Borgen, L. A., 275, 334, 335, 337
Boroffka, A., 101
Bouquet, R. J., 270, 277, 543
Bozzetti, Louis, 8, 521–529
Braadtvedt, H. P., 97
Bradbury, J. B., 274
Braenden, O., 33
Braude, Monique C., 269, 270, 272
Brawley, P., 270, 272
Brecher, Edward M., 532
Bretschneider, E. V., 45, 56
Brewster, J., 512
Breyer-Brandwijk, M. G., 89, 106
Brill, Leon, 196
Brill, N. Q., 543
Bromberg, W., 539
Brooks, Jerome E., 449
Brunel, R., 309
Bryan, Lynn, 497
Bryant, A. T., 97
Buber, Martin, 428
Buck, Alfred A., 479, 480
Buess, C., 464
Bukinich, D. D., 23, 25, 33
Burchard, Roderick E., 463–484
Burchell, William, 94, 95
Burkill, Isaac Henry, 68
Butt, Audrey, 447, 448, 454, 456

Cadogan, León, 453, 457
Camp, W. H., 22, 23
Campbell, I. L., 514
Campbell, J., 104
Campbell, J. Gabriel, 247
Carlini, E. A., 275
Carlota Joaquina (queen of Portugal), 175, 179
Carstairs, G. Morris, 238, 149, 493, 543
Carter, W. E., 9, 389–398
Casalis, E., 96
Casper, Franz, 451
Castaneda, Carlos, 403, 407, 412
Cattell, Raymond B., 394, 514
Chahud, A. I., 480
Chambers, C. D., 515

Charen, Sol, 532, 541
Chaudenson, R., 227
Chittick, Neville, 84
Chopra, G. S., 244, 258, 541
Chopra, I. C., 244, 248
Chopra, R. N., 244, 248, 541
Cintra, Assis, 175
Clark, Edith, 360
Cobo, Bernabe, 466
Codere, Helen, 217–226
Coelho, Pedro, 175
Coggins, W. J., 9, 389–398
Coleclough, A., 499
Columbus, C., 78
Comitas, Lambros, 6, 119–132, 162, 361, 488, 490
Conder, C. R., 96
Conklin, H. C., 362
Cook, S. J., 500
Cooper, John M., 441, 443, 451–452, 464
Copland, Samuel, 83
Cordeiro de Farias, R., 178
Cordova-Ríos, Manuel, 406
Cotton, M. de V., 270, 272
Coutselinis, A., 540, 541, 542
Crawford, D. M., 395
Crawford, J. E., 395
Crévost, C., 31, 73
Cruickshank, Mrs. Eric, 369
Cureau, A. L., 99
Curry, S. H., 270 271, 272; *Botany and chemistry of Cannabis*, 18

Dale, Andrew M., 98
D'Aléchamps, 15, 27
Dandy, J. E., 19
Dapper, O., 92
Darwin, Charles, 23, 82
Daumas, F., 93
Davidian, G. G., 22, 23
Davis, W., 334, 335, 337
De Candolle, A. L. P. P., 22, 25, 47
De Champlain, Samuel, 497
De Cieza León, Pedro, 464, 466, 467
Decle, L., 97
De Grevenbroek, J. G., 92
De Laeger, L., 217
De Léry, Jean, 452
De Pinho, Alvaro Rubim, 8, 178, 179, 182, 293–302
De Renzi, E., 397
Dewey, L. H., 39
De Zeeuw, R. A., 278

Index of Names

D'Hertefelt, Marcel, 217
Diocletian, 45
Dioscorides, 45, 305, 306
Dix, Robert, 153
Dobkin de Ríos, Marlene, 9, 185, 401–416, 418, 427
Doke, Clement, 86
Dombrowski, J. C., 78
Doorenbos, N. J., 33
Doria, Rodrígues, 295
Dorman, M. R. P., 99
Dornan, S. S., 85, 94
Douglas, Mary, 426
Dragendorff, Georg, 45
Dreher, Melanie C., 119, 385
Drury, R.: *Vocabulaire de la langue de Madagascar*, 228
Durkheim, Émile, 428
DuToit, Brian, 5, 80, 81–116

Eberhard, W.: *Guilt and sin*, 61
Ebin, David, 402
Eckler, C. R., 274
Edery, H., 272
Efendi, Eulogio, 309
Elejalde, B. R., 9, 327, 343
Eliade, Mircea, 408, 427, 429, 430
Elick, John W., 446, 447
Ellenberger, D. F., 96
Ellington, A. C., 275, 334
Ellis, William, 83
Emboden, William A., Jr., 42, 82, 181, 258, 403
Epton, Nina, 447, 448
Evans, W. C., 274

Fabrega, Horacio, Jr., 162
Faga, Brian M., 84–85
Faglioni, P., 397
Fals Borda, Orlando, 153, 155
Farias, Roberval C., 296
Farrington, B., 93
Fejer, D., 507, 514
Fennell, E., 395
Fentiman, A. F., Jr., 272
Fernández, James W., 403, 407
Fetterman, P. S., 270
Fine, Norman Lowy, 466, 478
Fisher, James, 247–255
Fluharty, Vernon Lee, 152, 153
Fock, Niels, 456
Fort, Joel, 265
Freedman, H. L., 532
Freud, Sigmund, 417

Freyre, Gilberto, 294; *O nordeste*, 175
Fritsch, Gustav, 95
Frombach, K. D., 469, 475, 476, 478
Furst, Peter T., 403, 417, 419, 429, 432, 433

Gagliano, Joseph, 464, 481
Gagneux, Pierre Marie, 63
Galanter, M., 275
Gamal Ad-Din Fath Moussa Ibn Aghmour (prince of Egypt), 198
Galvão, Eduardo, 148, 174
Gandhi, Mahatma, 237
Gaoni, R., 270, 271
García Márquez, Gabriel: *Cien ãnos de soledad*, 152
Gardiner, Allen F., 96
Garriott, J. C., 279
Gaskill, H. S., 532
Gauteir, Théophile, 231, 264
Geber, W. F., 275, 334
Geertz, Clifford, 423
Gelpke, R., 309
Gershon, S., 270, 272
Ghosh, J. J., 275
Gibbins, R. J., 501
Gill, E. W., 276
Gilman, A., 244, 532
Goddard, D., 466
Godwin, H., 13, 22
Goldman, Irving, 458
Goode, E., 355, 356
Goodman, L. S., 244, 532
Goodspeed, Thomas Harper, 440
Gopal, R., 235
Gourves, J., 286
Gray, G. M., 480
Green, Melvyn, 8, 497–520
Greenway, P. J., 84
Grimes, Barbara, 417
Grimes, Joseph E., 417
Grinspoon, Lester, 82, 258, 355, 356
Grof, Stanislav, 407, 410, 421
Grollman, A., 469
Grollman, E. F., 469
Grunfeld, Y., 272
Guerra, A., 341
Guerra, Cristóbal, 464
Gunn, J. W., 280
Gutiérrez de Pineda, Virginia, 164
Gutiérrez-Noriega, Carlos, 464, 470, 471, 475, 477, 479, 481
Gutsche, Thelma, 95

Haagen, C. H., 538
Hadley, K., 33
Hager, K., 44
Hahn, Albert, 450
Hahn, Hugo, 94
Haile Selassie (emperor of Ethiopia), 487
Hamberger, E., 197
Hamilton, H. C., 31, 274
Hanley, L. G., 499
Harner, Michael., 403, 410, 444, 457
Harris, M., 369, 412; *The nature of cultural things*, 371
Hartwich, Carl, 305
Hasan, Khwaja, 2, 235–246, 248
Hays, D., 286
Hébert, Louis, 497
Heim, Roger, 403
Heinz, H. J., 95
Hemmings, B., 512
Henderson, I, 515
Heraclitus, 430
Herodotus, 2, 40, 41, 77, 209, 258, 304, 305
Heyndrickx, A., 281
Hilton-Simpson, M. W., 99
Hissink, Karin, 450
Hively, R. L., 272
Hochman, J. L., 543
Hoffer, Eric, 536
Hofmann, A., 533
Hollister, L. E., 270, 272, 355, 356
Hooper, D., 274
Houghton, E. M., 31
Hsieh, Ping: *Hsin-chiang yu-chi (Account of travel in Sinkiang)*, 62
Hsü, F. L. K.: *Under the ancestors' shadow: Chinese culture and personality*, 60
Hua T'o, 56
Hughes, J. E., 98
Hughes, L. W., 481
Hussein, M. K., 199
Hutchinson, W. H., 5, 173–183
Huxley, Aldous, 259, 431; *Doors of perception*, 533

Idanpaan-Heikkila, J., 334
Inskeep, R. R., 91
Isbell, H., 271, 272, 356, 540, 541

Jacob, A., 514
Jaffe, Jerome H., 467, 468, 469, 470
James, S., 78
James, Theodore, 83, 105, 108
James, William, 427
Janiger, Oscar, 403
Jenny, Hans, 94
Jensen, Knud, 345–354
João III (king of Portugal), 174, 293
João VI (king of Portugal and Brazil), 175
Johnson, D. W., 280
Johnston, Harry H., 98, 99
Johnston, Thomas F., 404–405
Johnston, W. E., 515
Jones, R. T., 356, 540
Joseph, Roger, 185–195
Josie, G. H., 498, 515
Joyce, C. R. B., 270, 271, 272, 286; *Botany and chemistry of Cannabis*, 18
Jung, C. G., 427, 430
Junod, Henri A., 85

Kabelik, Jan, 7, 258
Kamalaprija, V., 150, 152, 153
Kamen-Kaye, Dorothy, 443
Kaplan, John, 549–557
Karniol, I. G., 275
Karsten, Rafael, 446
Katz, Fred, 408, 409
Keane, A., 99
Keane, Claire B., 480
Kesey, Ken, 432
Kerim, F., 309
Khalifa, Ahmad, 5, 195–205
Khan, Munir A., 9, 345–354
Kimball, Solon T., 147
Kiplinger, G. F., 272
Klein, F. K., 276
Klein, Siegfried, 41
Klein, William M., 21–38
Kluckhohn, Clyde, 167
Kluver, Heinrich, 422
Knight, J., 270
Koch-Grünberg, Theodor, 444
Kolb, Peter, 93
Kolberg, O., 43
Kollmann, Paul, 86
Komarov, V. L., 25; *Flora of the U.S.S.R.*, 34
Kosman, M. E., 468, 469
Kostis, N., 310–311
Koukou, E., 308
Kouretas, D., 311, 313
Krause, E. H. L., 31
Krim, Abdel, 186
Krippner, Stanley, 430, 431
Kroeber, A., 207, 212

Index of Names

Kruse, Albert, 456
Kubena, R. K., 273, 274, 278, 280

La Barre, Weston, 467
Lamarck, Jean, 3, 16, 21, 24, 29, 30, 32, 33
Lambo, T. A., 101
Langner, Jeanette, 81
Lanphier, C. M., 501, 506, 514
Laski, Marghanita, 428
Latrobe, C. I., 93, 96
Laufer, B., 27, 84; *Sino-Iranica*, 53
Leary, Timothy, 432, 533, 534, 536
Leblond, M. A.: *Sortilèges*, 231
Leech, Kenneth: *A practical guide to the drug scene*, 334
Lefranc, A., 14
Lemarié, C., 73
Leathers, B., 512, 514
Le Vaillant, M., 93
Levin, Aubrey, 108
Levin, D. A., 15
Lévi-Strauss, Claude, 417, 423
Levy, R., 208
Lewin, Louis, 468
Li, Hui-Lin, 2, 51–62, 248
Lichtenstein, Henry, 89, 93
Linnaeus, Carolus, 3, 13, 15, 16, 17, 18, 19, 21, 24, 27, 28, 29, 30, 35, 40
Lipp, M. R., 543
Li Shih-chên, 56
Livingstone, David, 84, 98, 99
Lockwood, Tom E., 21–38
Long, Joseph K., 407, 410
Lucena, José, 175, 299
Ludlow, Fitzhugh, 259
Ludwig, Arnold M., 408
Lumholtz, Carl, 417, 419, 435
Lunardi, Federico, 328
Luther, Martin, 41

McGlothlin, William H., 8, 259, 486, 531–547
Macgregor, J. C., 96
Machado, Felix Edguardo, 463, 464
Mackenzie, D. L., 236
McMullan, J., 512
Madianou, D., 303–326
Magre, Maurice, 231
Manning, Peter K., 162
Manno, J. E., 272, 277, 355
Maquet, J. J., 217
Marcovitz, E., 532
Marsh, R. P., 418, 422

Marshman, J. A., 501
Martin, Marie Alexandrine, 63–75
Martin, Richard T., 463, 467, 476
Marwick, Brian, 97
Maslow, Abraham H., 421
Matienzo, Juan de, 465, 466, 467
Maugh, Thomas H., II, 181
Maurer, D. W., 532
Mazess, R. B., 479
Mechoulam, R., 270, 271, 272, 277, 286
Medina Silva, Ramón, 417, 420–421, 423, 424, 432, 434
Meerlsman, R. P., 228
Meissner, B., 40
Mentzel, O. F., 93
Merlin, M. D., 22, 77
Métraux, Alfred, 457
Meyers, H. J., 532
Mikesell, Marvin W., 185, 186
Mikuriya, Tod H., 185, 187, 188, 192
Miller, Benjamin F., 480
Miller, F. A., 274
Miller, George, 370
Miller, N. G., 25
Miller, Philip: *Gardeners dictionary*, 15
Miller, Ralph D., 8, 497–520
Millman, D. H., 339
Mills, L. A., 270, 272
Minns, Ellis H., 41
Miras, C. J., 334, 540, 541, 542
Mitra, S. K., 236
Mohammed II (conqueror of Constantinople), 307–308
Moldenke, A., 39
Moldenke, H., 39
Montaña Cuellar, Diego, 152
Monteiro, Joachim, 99
Montesinos, F., 476–477
Moorhead, P. S., 335
Moreau, Jacques-Joseph, 273, 355
Moreno, García, 175, 179
Murphy, Emily (Janey Canuck): *The black candle*, 499
Murphy, H. B. M., 478
Murphy, Robert F., 457
Musinga (ruler of Rwanda), 218
Myerhoff, Barbara, 9, 417–438

Nadel, S. F., 120
Nahas, G. G., 270, 272, 273, 281, 286
Nassonov, V. A., 32
Neumeyer, J. L., 270, 272
Nienaber, G. S., 89, 96
Nieschulz, Otto, 476, 477

Index of Names

Nigm Ad-Din Ayoub (sultan of Egypt), 198–199
Nimuendajú, Curt, 449, 451
Niño, Alfonso, 464
Nordal, A., 33
Nowliss, H. H., 21

O'Flaherty, W. D., 240
Ogilby, John, 92
Olsen, Diane, 458
O'Neil, Owen Rowe, 97
Ortíz, Tomas, 464
O'Schaughnessy, W. B., 259, 272
Osmond, Humphrey, 402, 418, 427
Oviedo y Baños, J. de, 452

Pace, H. B., 334, 335, 337
Pages, A., 217
Pahnke, Walter N., 418, 427, 428, 429, 430
Palgi, Phyllis, 207–216
Pan Chi-hsin, 54
Papadopoulos, D. N., 304, 306, 311, 314
Paparigopoulos, C., 308
Parker, Seymour, 263
Parreiras, Décio, 181
Partridge, William, 6, 9, 147–172
Patai, R., 44
Pate, Jame B., 160
Patiño, Victor Manuel, 148, 149, 162
Patterson, Thomas C., 464
Paulus, I,. 499, 514, 515
Pentzopoulos, D., 308
Pereira, Jayme R., 179
Perelman, Luis, 532, 541
Pérez de Barradas, José, 328
Persaud, T. V. N., 275, 334
Petropoulos, E., 313, 314
Phillips, Ray E., 109
Phillips, S. B., 501, 506, 514
Picón-Rategui, E., 474, 479
Pires da Veiga, E., 296, 297
Pitt-Rivers, Julian, 409
Pliny the Elder, 304
Plowman, Timothy, 21–38
Plutarch, 305
Poddar, M. K., 275
Polo, Marco, 77, 208
Polsky, N., 532
Polunin, Nicholas, 82
Porot, A., 543
Postma, W. P., 26
Preston, J. D., 532
Preuss, K., 328

Prince, Raymond, 490, 491, 492, 494
Purchase, S., 441
Purvis, J. P.. 100
Putnam, Herbert, 439
Pye, Orrea, 369
Pyrros, Dinoysos: *Doctors' textbook*, 310

Quimby, M. W., 22, 270
Quiñones, A., 330, 333, 339

Rabelais, Antoine, 14
Rabelais, François, 13, 14, 15, 19, 258
Rana, Prakrita S., 252
Raven, J. C., 396
Raven-Hart, R., 89, 92, 95
Ray, J., 15, 17, 19
Raymond, W. D., 99
Reichel-Dolmatoff, Gerardo, 148, 263, 454
Reiniger, W., 304, 306
Reitan, R. M., 395
Ricketts, Carlos A., 479
Ríos, José A. de los, 463
Risemberg, M., 480
Ritchie, J. Murdoch, 469, 480
Ritter, M., 207
Rockmore, M. J., 532
Rogers, Claudia, 126
Roland, J. L., 540
Rootman, I., 507
Rosado, Pedro, 174
Roscoe, John, 100
Rosenthal, Franz, 82, 84, 86
Rostovtzeff, M., 42
Rostworowski de Diez Canseco, Mariá, 464
Rubin, Vera, 1–10, 65, 131, 162, 257–266, 488
Rudenko, S. I., 2, 42, 258
Russell, J., 514

Sagoe, E. C., 102
Saint-Lager, J. B., 15
Salzberger, G., 42
Samuelson, L. H., 97
Sandis, E. E., 310, 320–321
Satz, P., 395, 396
Sauer, Carl, 440, 442
Sauer, Monica, 81
Savage, M. Spencer, 27
Schachtzabel, Alfred, 99, 103
Schaeffer, Jane, 360, 369
Schaeffer, Joseph, 6, 163, 355–388, 488–489

Index of Names

Schapera, I., 93, 103, 105
Schebesta, Paul, 100–101, 103
Schloezer, August, 439
Schmersahl, P., 476
Schneider, Kurt, 300
Schramm, L. C., 275, 334
Schreyer, Johan, 92
Schrijver, Isaq., 92, 94
Schultes, Richard Evans, 1, 3, 21–38, 47, 77, 82, 160, 173, 182, 270, 273, 341, 418, 450
Schwanitz, F., 21
Scigliano, J. A., 272
Seale, C. C., 148
Segelman, Alvin B., 269–291
Segelman, Florence H., 269–291
Shagoury, R. A., 270, 272
Shapiro, H. A., 108
Shaw, George, 83
Shaw, M., 102, 103, 104, 105–106
Shên-hung (emperor of China), 56, 77
Sibree, James, 83
Siegel, Ron, 408
Sigg, B. W., 541
Silberbauer, George B., 95
Simoons, Frederick J., 84
Simopoulos, K., 309
Singer, A. J., 270, 272
Sloane, Hans, 19
Small, E., 25, 26, 270, 502
Smart, R. G., 507, 514
Smith, Andrew, 96
Smith, D. E., 129
Smith, Edwin, 98
Smith, G. M., 538
Sofia, R. D., 279
Sofia, R. Duane, 269–291
Soják, J., 34
Solomon, David, 264
Sonnerat, M. Pierre, 29
Soueif, M. I., 196, 200, 540, 541
Speight, W. L., 106
Stayt, Hugh A., 97
Stearn, Wiliiam, 3, 13, 19
Stefanis, C., 303–326
Stein, William, 465, 478
Stenchever, M., 335
Stern, Michael, 247
Stevenson, G. H., 515
Steyn, Douw G., 106
Stokes, J.: *A botanical Materia Medica*, 30–31
Stott, H. H., 106
Stow, George, 93, 94

Stringaris, M. G., 309, 311, 313, 314, 543
Suramarinth (king of Cambodia), 66
Sutherland-Harris, Nicola, 85
Syrenius, S. Z., 45–46

Taillard, C., 67
T'ang Shên-wei, 56
T'ao Hung-ching, 56
Tart, C. T., 355
Teich, J., 207
Tella, A., 101
Tennant, F. S., 541, 542
Ten Rhyne, Wilhelm, 92
Terry, C. E., 236
Teste, M., 540
Theal, George, 95
Theophrastus, 305
Tobias, Phillip V., 95
Torday, E., 99, 100
Torres Ortega, Jorge, 149, 166
Towle, Margaret A., 464
Trease, G. E., 274
Truitt, E. B., Jr., 272
Ts'ai Lun, 54
Tsaousis, D. G., 310
Tschirch, A., 46
Turk, R. F., 78
Turner, C. E., 33
Turner, Victor, 428, 431; *The ritual process*, 429
Tutin, T. G.: *Flora Europaea*, 13, 25, 34

Underhill, M. M., 240
Unna, K., 468, 469
Urquhart, Thomas, 14

Vamvakaris, N., 312, 313
Van der Merwe, Nikolaas, 5, 77–80
Van Riebeeck, Jan, 88, 90, 92, 94
Vansina, J., 85
Varasarin, Uraisi, 63
Vavilov, N. I., 22, 23, 25, 33, 47, 77
Veda, Atharva, 258
Vedder, Heinrich, 94
Vergara y Velasca, F. J., 148, 150
Verzar, F., 464, 472, 476
Vespucci, Amerigo, 449, 464
Victoria (queen of England), 98
Vogel, V. H., 532
Von Hagen, Victor Wolfgang, 471
Vougoucas, C. N., 315

Wagley, Charles, 148, 174
Waldseemüller, Martin, 449

Wallace, A. F. C., 402
Waller, C. W., 272
Wallis, T. E., 274
Walton, James, 82, 83, 102, 103, 104, 105
Walton, R. P., 532
Warren, E., 286
Wasson, R. G., 404, 418; *Russia, mushrooms and history*, 403; *Soma: divine mushroom of immortality*, 240
Wasson, V., 403, 404
Watt, J. M., 83, 89, 106
Watts, Alan, 418, 421, 423, 424, 427, 430
Wavell, Steward, 447, 448
Webster, Steven S., 478
Wechsler, J., 397
Weil, A., 209, 355, 356
Wells, H. G., 431
Wen Huey, M. A., 339
Werner, A., 100
Westphal, E. O. J., 90, 100
Whiffen, Thomas W., 445
White, C. Langdon, 466
White, J., 507, 514
Whitebread, C. H., 532
Wilbert, Johannes, 9, 264, 417, 439–461

Wille, L., 286
Williams, E. G., 541, 542
Williams, H. R., 499, 515
Williams García, Roberto, 133–145
Wilson, Monica, 91
Winick, C., 532
Wissman, H., 45, 99
Wo (emperor of China), 54
Wolfart. H. C., 463
Wolfe, Tom: *Electric Kool-Aid acid test*, 432
Wolstenholme, E. W., 270
Wood, H. C., Jr., 274
Wright, Linda, 497
Wylie, Judith, 369

Zabathas, E., 315
Zapata Ortíz, Vicente, 470, 477, 479, 481
Zarate, Agustín, 466
Zerries, Otto, 448, 450, 452
Zhukovsky, P. M., 13, 22, 25; *Cultivated plants and their wild relatives*, 34
Zinberg, Norman E., 522
Zingg, Robert M., 417, 419

Index of Subjects

Acculturation, 207–216, 458
Activity patterns, 335 356–357, 368–387
Adaptive radiation, 22–23, 32
Addiction, 9, 39, 43, 69, 106–107, 108, 195–196, 197, 198, 203–204, 235, 293, 297, 298, 299, 300, 301, 315, 341, 349–350, 455, 469–470, 471, 477, 516, 526
Addiction Research Foundation of Ontario, 470, 507
Adulteration of drugs, 269, 280–281, 297, 501–502
Aegean, 311, 318–320
Aenos peninsula, 304–305
Aesculapian shrines, 305
Afghanistan, 24, 32, 33–34, 286, 504
Africa, 5, 6–7, 44–45, 48, 77–80, 81–110, 120, 148, 174, 177, 185–193, 195–204, 207–208, 209–214, 217–225, 293–294, 363, 404, 487, 504. *See also* Names of individual countries
African herders, 86–87, 90–94, 95, 100
Afro-Brazil cultism, 178, 179, 294
Afro-Cuan ritual, 338
Age differences in cannibis use, 106, 109, 126–128, 130, 190, 197, 233, 247, 249, 251, 253, 298, 300–301, 321–324, 331, 491, 497, 501, 506–508, 523, 537, 543
Age of initiation into cannabis smoking, 68, 126–127, 164, 201–202, 260, 297, 316, 323–324, 331, 332, 348, 363, 375, 377, 379, 487–488, 543
"Aggression and hypoglycemia among the Qolla: a study in psychobiological anthropology" (Bolton), 472–475
Ahir (Hindu caste), 239, 243

Aikana, 451
Akawaio, 443, 447–448, 453–454, 456
Alagoas (Brazilian state), 174, 295
Alberta (Canadian province), 507–508
Alcohol, 1, 6, 46, 57–59, 70–71, 105, 107, 108, 109, 124–125, 126, 152, 154–155, 161, 162, 164, 165–166, 170, 181, 185, 189, 190, 198, 199, 201, 203, 204, 208, 209, 223, 224–225, 233, 235–240, 243–244, 249, 251, 252, 254, 274, 281–286, 294, 298, 301, 307, 309, 327, 333, 338–339, 340, 341, 342, 345, 346, 348, 349–350, 391, 403, 434, 473, 485–494, 497, 511, 513–515, 516, 517, 526, 535, 540, 543–544
Alcoholism, 6, 46, 234, 296–297, 298, 350, 392, 490–494, 513, 525, 544
Alcohol or cannabis, choice between. *See* Cannabis or alcohol, choice between
Alexandria, 306
Alhucemas (Moroccan province), 186–189
Alhucemas, Morocco, 186, 189
Alienation, 7, 197–198, 215–219, 312, 536, 538–539, 550
Altai region (Siberia), 42, 258
Amahara, 84
Amahuaca, 402, 406
Amanita muscaria (fly-agaric), 240, 403–404
Amasili/Masarwa, 85
Amazonas (Brazilian state), 174
Amazon region, 263, 294, 341, 402, 405–406, 440, 443, 448, 450
American Journal of Psychiatry, 487

580 Index of Subjects

Amerindian, 2, 45, 48, 257, 262–263, 264, 273, 440, 450, 490, 533. *See also* South American Indians
Amotivational syndrome, 7, 129, 391, 488–489, 544
Amphetemines, 108, 197, 298, 317, 337, 467–468, 513–514, 515, 516, 525, 526
Analgesic, 7, 63, 70, 72, 175, 258, 280
Anadenanthera, 450, 451
Anglo-Saxon (language), 27
Angola, 86, 98–99, 102, 103, 174, 177, 293–294, 295
Animal familiars, 405, 406, 409–410, 419
Animals, use of hallucinogens by, 408
Animation of plant spirits, 403–404, 409
Ano Hora (village on Syros), 311
Anomie, 196
Antecedent variables, 402, 406, 411–414
Antibiotic, 7, 285, 433
Antilles, 149, 452
Antioquia group (Colombia), 337–339
Antisocial behavior, 8, 332, 341. *See also* Effects of cannabis, criminal
Antitoxican Law (Brazil), 300
Aphrodisiac, 46, 47, 98, 161, 164, 167, 196, 202, 210–211, 212, 213, 251, 265
Arabia, 42, 77, 84, 95
Arabic, 40, 89, 101, 193, 208
Arabs, 5, 64, 67, 80, 82–84, 86–87, 96, 98, 100, 154, 157, 191, 210, 211, 213, 214, 236, 306–307, 309, 311, 312
Aralian region, 47
Aramaic, 2, 40
Arambi (Africa), 101
Ararat, 41
Arawakans, 440, 450
Archaeological studies, 2, 5, 47, 51, 53, 77–80, 82, 83, 91, 104–105, 258, 304, 327–328, 402–403, 419, 439, 442
Argentina, 464
Argolis, Greece, 311
Armenia, 41, 306
Aruba, 490
Aryans, 235, 248
Ashkenaz, 41–42. *See also* Sythian (people)
Asia, 2, 4, 6–7, 16, 21, 22, 25, 27, 28, 29, 30, 31, 40, 42, 45, 46, 47, 48, 51–62, 63–75, 77, 81, 82, 101, 192, 253, 257–258, 270, 304–305, 504. *See also* Names of individual countries
Asia, Southeast. *See* Southeast Asia
Asia Minor, 2–3, 42, 309, 310, 311, 313, 315, 318, 320–321

Associability, 300, 301
Assassins' cult, 77, 208
Assyria, 2, 40, 41
Assyrian (language), 40, 305
Atropa, 467
Atharvaveda, 45, 258
Athens, Greece, 303, 309, 310, 312–313 314, 316–321
Athens Metropolitan Police, 316
Athens Suburban Constabulary, 316
Atlantic Coast group (Colombia), 337–339
Atlas Mountains, 210
Atoli (Africa), 101
Attika (Greek department), 317, 318–321
Attitudes, elite, 549, 552–553, 556–557
Attitudes of cannabis users toward other drug users, 203
Attitudes toward cannabis use, 6, 7–8, 9, 74–75, 119, 130–131, 163, 166–167, 189–190, 191, 199, 211, 215–216, 220, 221–225, 229, 231, 245, 247, 249, 251, 253–254, 259, 298, 300, 301, 327, 328, 329, 330–338, 339–341, 345–346, 350, 366–367, 372, 391, 499, 511, 512, 516–517, 521–523, 525–526, 527–529, 538, 543, 549, 551–553, 555–557
Audiovisual records, 6, 163, 355, 368–371, 372, 376, 381, 385, 489
Auditory hallucinations, 404–405
Austria, 311
Ayahuasca (Peruvian hallucinogen). *See Banisteriopsis*
Aymara, 450
Ayurvedic practices, 247, 251
Ayyubid dynasty (Egypt), 199
Aztecs, 440

Babylon, 2, 40
Babylonia, 41, 42
Babylonian (people), 41
Baden, Germany, 43
Badjok, 99
Baganda, 100
Bagishu, 100
Bahamas, 490
Bahia (Brazilian state), 8–9, 174, 177–178, 179, 293, 294, 296, 297, 299
Bambuti, 101, 103
Bangi complex, 81, 82, 84–87, 97–99, 101
Bangongo, 100
Ban Het Kansa, Vietnam, 67
Banisteriopsis (Ayahuasca), 149, 402,

405–406, 408, 442, 444, 446, 454–455, 457
Bantu, 83, 84, 86, 88, 91, 95, 99, 105, 109
Bara (district of Nepal), 248
Baralong, 96
Barbiturates, 108, 317, 329, 514, 515, 526
Barranquilla, Colombia, 149, 332
Bashi, 221
Bashilenge, 45, 99
Basoga, 100
Batapin, 104
Batetela, 99
Bathlapin, 96
Bechuana, 96
Bedouins, 214
Beersheba, Israel, 214
Begemeder (Ethiopian province), 77–80
Behavior stream, 356, 368–369, 386–387
Beizan (Palestine), 41
Bengal, India, 82
Beni Seddath, Morocco, 186
"*Benk u Bôde*" (Mohammed Ebn Soleiman Foruli), 309
Berbers, 185–193, 210, 211
Bergdama. *See* Damara
Bhagats, 235, 238–239, 242–243
Bhujwa (Hindu caste), 239, 243
Bible, 2–3, 39, 40–41, 42, 44, 120, 123, 209, 258, 304, 367
Biochemical studies of cannabis, 1, 7, 21, 33, 35, 77–80, 106, 261, 265, 269–287
Biological activity, 269, 272, 273, 275–276, 281, 287
Birth defects. *See* Teratogenic effect
Black candle, The (Murphy), 499
Black Sea region, 47
Bloemfontein, South Africa, 105
Blood glucose, effect of coca chewing on, 463, 469, 471, 472–477, 479, 480–481
Boers, 88
Bogotá, Colombia, 148, 150, 332
Bolívar (Colombian department), 163–164
Bolivia, 450, 463, 464
Bora, 443
Boston Free Access Study, 524–525
Botanical aspects of coca, 463–464
Botanical materia medica, A (Stokes), 30
Botanical studies of cannabis, 1, 2, 3, 7, 13–19, 21–36, 52, 106, 173, 176, 270, 341, 549–557
Botany and chemistry of cannabis, The (Joyce and Curry), 18
Botswana (Africa), 104
Brahman, 6, 235–236, 238–239, 242, 243,
249, 250, 492, 493, 543
Brahmanism, 235–236, 427
Brazil, 5, 8–9, 148, 173–182, 293–301, 440, 456, 457, 463
Brazilian Indians, 173–174, 294
British, 5, 150, 178, 236–237, 258, 311, 497–498
British Columbia, 498, 501
British Museum of Natural History, 13, 17, 19, 28
Buddhism, 60, 236, 248
Bugakwe, 95
Bureau of Narcotics (Cambodia), 66
Bushmen, 83, 88, 90, 93, 94–95
Byzantium, 303, 306–207

Cachacos (Colombia), 153–155, 157, 159, 160, 166
Cachicoto, Peru, 480
Caffeine, 513–514
Caffer, 96
Cairo, Egypt, 82, 195, 196, 200
Caja Agraria (Colombia), 151
Calcutta, India, 231, 273
Cali, Colombia, 332
California, 533, 534, 550–551
Cambodia, 63–75
Campa, 443, 446–447, 457
Canada, 4, 8, 494, 497–517, 554, 555
Canadian Commission of Inquiry into the Non-Medical Use of Drugs, 7, 356, 467, 468, 469, 470, 497, 501, 506–508, 510–511, 512, 513–514, 515, 516, 550–551, 552–553, 555
Canadian Criminal Code, 500
Canadian Federal Health Protection Branch (HPB), 502
Canadian Medical Association, 498
Canadian Medical Association Journal, 498
Cañari culture, 440
Candomblé (Brazilian sect), 179, 294
Cannabidiol (CBD), 78–79, 271, 274, 277, 282–285, 334, 372
Cannabinol (CBN), 67, 78–79, 271, 274, 277, 282–285, 334, 372
Cannabinolic agents, 9, 21, 30, 33, 35, 67, 77–80, 98, 269–287, 334–335, 356, 372, 374, 378, 502, 505, 509, 510–511, 525, 540–542, 544
Cannabis as symbol of rebellion, 8, 190, 197–198, 215, 231, 340, 531, 538–539, 543–544
Cannabis oil, 5, 13, 22, 40, 44–45, 55–56, 82, 173, 251–252. *See also* "Hash oil"

Cannabis or alcohol, choice between, 6, 170, 185, 189–190, 198, 199, 203–204, 208, 209, 224–225, 234, 235–245, 249, 254, 298, 301, 307–310, 327, 333, 338–340, 342, 345–346, 485–494, 497, 514–515, 553, 543–544
Cannabis Report (Canadian Commission on Inquiry into the Non-Medical Use of Drugs), 501
Cannabis smoking places, 126, 160, 163–164, 179, 309, 314, 315, 348
Cape Town, South Africa, 105
Caribans, 440, 443, 447–448, 453–454, 455, 456
Caribbean area, 149, 162, 442, 448, 456, 464, 490
Cartagena, Colombia, 148, 149, 163–164
Casablanca, Morocco, 212, 213, 214
Cash cropping of cannabis, 6, 62, 66–67, 122, 123–124, 154–155, 157–160, 185, 186–189, 192–193, 250, 252–253, 254, 295, 327, 328, 329, 333, 363, 365–366, 375, 489–490, 504
Caste, 217–225, 235–245, 249, 250–251, 252, 410, 489, 492, 543
Catholic Church, 43, 133, 135, 338, 339–340
Catholics, 311, 312, 339–340, 523
Catimbó (Brazilian sect), 179
Cauca valley (Colombia), 149
Caucasus, 41, 42–43
Ceará (Brazilian state), 174
Center for Studies of Narcotics and Drug Abuse (National Institute of Mental Health), 81, 119, 486–487
Central America, 389–398, 409, 464, 553–550. *See also* Names of individual countries
Ceylon, 29
Chainouqua, 94
Chaldean (language), 40
Chamar (Hindu caste), 239, 243, 244
Chaudec (Vietnam), 67
Chelsea Physic Garden, 19
Chemical Abstracts, 271
Chêng-lei pên-ts'ao (T'ang), 56
Chhatris (Hindu caste), 249, 250
Chibcha, 448
Chieng Mai, Thailand, 68
Children, use of cannabis by, 47, 100, 121, 124–125, 126, 128, 161, 162, 230, 251, 252, 265, 487–488
Chile, 148
China, 2, 4, 28, 29, 31, 48, 51–62, 72, 73, 77, 192, 212, 236, 248, 252, 257–258, 554
Chinaura, India, 238–239, 242–244, 245
Chinese (language), 51, 54–55, 57, 58, 61, 64
Chinese (people), 51–62, 72, 73, 105, 227, 228–229
Chinese Turkistan, 62
Chios (Greek island), 311
Christian religion, 306, 307, 430
Christians, 127, 129, 212, 308–309
Chromatographic technique, 77, 78–79, 274, 277, 282–285
Chromosomes, 8, 9, 327, 335–337, 342
Chuckchee, 403
Churchville, Jamaica, 362
Cinais, France, 14
Class. *See* Social class
Classification of drugs, 107, 197, 204, 254, 259, 264, 311, 467–468, 499–500, 513, 516–517
Class markers, 119, 130
Clifford Herbarium, 17
Clinical studies of cannabis use, 1, 6, 7, 8–9, 106–107, 108–109, 124, 173, 176, 180, 182, 233, 244–245, 260–261, 293, 295–297, 298–300, 301, 303–304, 314, 316, 317, 323–324, 327, 334–337, 341–342, 345–354, 355–357, 369–371, 381–382, 383, 387, 389–398, 487, 491–492, 512, 524–525, 527
Clinical studies of hallucinatory phenomena, 402, 406–407, 412, 421, 488
Club de Diambistas, 179
Club des Hachichins, 4, 258–259
Coca, 3, 149, 181, 196, 327–328, 442, 443, 445, 449, 450, 463–481
Cocaine, 108, 181, 197, 203, 274, 314, 463, 464, 465, 467–479, 480, 481, 514, 526
Cocaine models of coca chewing, 463, 464, 467, 470–476, 477–479, 481
Codeine, 337
Coincidentia oppositorum, 430
"Collection of Brazilian writings on Maconha, A" 176
Colombia, 6–7, 8–9, 147–170, 327–342, 443, 444–445, 448, 449, 463, 504, 552, 553–554, 556
Colombian Institute for Family Welfare, 340
Coloureds (in South Africa), 105, 107–108
Columbia University, 369

Comisión de Planificación (Colombia), 150, 153
Communitas, 428–429, 431, 432
Community Mental Health Center (Jaffa, Israel), 207
Comores, 228, 232, 233
Comprehensive Drug Abuse Prevention and Control Act (United States), 521, 522
Conformity, 130, 201, 202
Confucianism, 59–61
Congo basin, 85, 99, 101
Congolese, 221
Conibo, 455
Consequent variables, 411–414
Constantinople, 307–308, 309, 311
Consumption level of cannabis, individual, 124, 163, 164, 200–202, 260–261, 347–348, 363, 364. 372, 375, 377–378, 379, 489, 491, 508, 523, 524–525, 531, 539–542, 544
Consumption of cannabis as food. *See* Uses of cannabis, food
Consumption of cannabis as incense, 40, 42
Consumption of cannabis as tea, 121, 124, 126, 128, 142, 180, 269, 270, 276–286, 295, 363, 366, 372, 510
Consumption of cannabis by simultaneous smoking and drinking, 269, 276–280
Consumption of cannabis by smoking, 5, 6–7, 8, 45, 46, 48, 62, 63, 65, 66, 67–69, 70, 71, 72, 74–75, 77–80, 81, 83, 84, 86–87, 89, 91, 93, 94–107, 109, 120–121, 124, 126–131, 142, 148–149, 156, 157, 159, 160, 162–165, 166, 175, 178, 179, 185, 187–192, 200, 202–203, 207–208, 209, 210, 211, 212, 213, 214, 216, 217, 219, 221–225, 229, 230, 231, 232–233, 235, 240, 241–242, 243, 244, 249, 250–251, 252, 257, 260, 261–265, 269, 270, 272, 275, 276–286, 293, 294, 295, 297, 309, 313, 314–324, 327, 335, 336–337, 342, 345–350, 352, 355–356, 363–386, 487–489, 491–492, 499, 509, 510–511, 525
Continuous Choice Reaction, 397
Cooperative Commission on Alcoholism, 494
Cora, 435
Corinth Canal, 313
Costa Rica, 9, 149, 389–398, 553–555
Costa Rican Ministry of Health, 389, 390

Costa Rican Social Security Hospital of San José (Hospital Méjico), 389, 394
Cough syrup, 108, 498
Crete, 306–307, 311, 318–320
Crimea, 47
Cross-cultural approach, 1–2, 10, 195, 403, 509
Crossing Ridge, Jamaica, 362
Crusaders, 208, 258
Cubeo, 458
Cultivated plants and their wild relatives (Zhukovsky), 34
Cultivation of cannabis, 3–4, 6, 13–15, 21–23, 25, 26, 35, 43–44, 45, 51, 52, 54–55, 62, 63, 66, 67, 73, 81–82, 93–94, 95, 97–98, 107, 109, 119, 120, 121–123, 125, 127, 141, 147, 154–155, 157–160, 166, 169, 185, 186–188, 190, 191, 192–193, 199, 221–222, 227, 237, 247–248, 250, 252–253, 254, 258, 293, 295, 300, 304, 305, 306, 313–314, 315, 327, 328, 329, 330, 331, 333, 340, 342, 363, 365–366, 367, 372, 375, 390, 398, 489–490, 497–498, 502, 504, 505–506
Cultivation of cannabis, large-scale, 4, 45, 62, 73, 157–160, 295, 327, 329, 340, 366
Cultivation of cannabis, rituals concerning, 43–44, 221–222, 295
Cultivation of cannabis, small-scale, 3–4, 6, 63, 66, 121–123, 154, 157–159, 185, 186–188, 190, 295, 327, 328, 329, 363, 365–366, 372, 375, 489–490, 505–506
Cultural evolution, 35, 401, 410
Cultural expectations, 6, 259, 260–265, 401, 402, 404, 414, 417, 419, 492
Cultural materialism, 412
Culture Fair Intelligence Test, 394–395
Culture free investigations, 109, 394
Cundiboya (Cundinamarca-Bohacá) group (Colombia), 337–339
Cundinamarca (Colombian department), 153, 337–339
Curanderos, 161–162
Cyclades (Aegean islands), 311
Cyclothymic personality, 485, 492–493
Cyprus, 306–307, 313
Czechoslovakia, 7, 46

Dagga complex, 81–110
Damara (also, Dama, Bergdama), 90, 93–94
Datura, 92, 108, 149, 305, 404–405, 442, 444, 446, 454–455, 467

584 *Index of Subjects*

Decriminalization, 8, 286, 522, 528–529, 551
Delaware, 277
Delhi, India, 236, 237
Denmark, 556
Departamento Administrativo Nacional de Estadística (Colombia), 153
Dependence on cannabis, 9, 43, 69, 106–107, 108, 144, 245, 298–300, 301, 345, 349–350, 364–365, 524, 525
Dependence on drugs. *See* Addiction
Dependency, prolonged childhood, 536–537
Dervishes, 309
Description of Greece (Pausanias), 306
Deviance, 7, 129–130, 157, 196, 213, 261–262, 300, 538
Dhanusa (district of Nepal), 248
Dharamsutras (Indian text), 235–236
Dhobi (Hindu caste), 239, 243, 244
Diamba complex, 81, 86, 99–101
Diario del Caribe (Colombia), 160
Diet. *See* Nutrition
Dietary taboos and use of hallucinogens, 411, 413–414, 421, 445, 446, 447
Diffusion of cannabis, 2–3, 4–5, 7, 8, 16, 21, 22–23, 26, 27, 39–48, 51, 52, 57, 63, 64, 65, 77, 80, 81–88, 91, 95, 97–101, 119, 120, 148–149, 174–176, 191, 199, 207–216, 217, 227–229, 233, 248–249, 257–259, 260, 293–294, 297, 301, 304–315, 363, 390, 398, 487, 497–498, 507, 531–532, 543
Diffusion of cannabis to the New World, 5, 119, 120, 148–149, 174–176, 257, 260, 293–294, 301, 363, 487, 497–498
Discouragement of cannabis use, national policy of, 522, 528–529
Dispensatory of the United States of America, The, (Wood, et al.), 274
Distribution of cannabis, 6, 63, 66–67, 94, 107–108, 119, 120, 121, 123–124, 125–126, 127, 147–148, 154–155, 156–157, 158, 159, 160–161, 166, 169, 170, 187–189, 191, 192–193, 199, 203, 204, 229, 232, 236–237, 241, 247, 252, 253, 261, 296, 297–298, 300, 313–314, 327, 328, 329–330, 331–332, 339, 340, 342, 363, 365–366, 367, 375, 390, 391, 398, 497, 500–506, 516, 522, 535, 550, 553, 554, 556
Divination, 44, 56, 60, 97, 293, 294, 305, 402, 405–406, 408, 410–411, 444, 446, 449, 450, 456

Doctors' textbook (Pyrros), 310
Dodecanesus, 310
Dolpa (district of Nepal), 251–252
Dom (Hindu caste), 239, 243, 244
Domestication of cannabis, 21–23, 25–26, 35, 52, 77, 81–82
Dominion Bureau of Statistics (Canada), 498
Doors of perception (Huxley), 533
"Downers," 512
Dravidian religion, 229
Dromokaiteion Mental Hospital, 314
Durban, South Africa, 106
Dutch (language), 89
Dutch (people), 88, 90–91, 92–93, 95
Dutch East India Company, 92
Dutch Settlement at the Cape of Good Hope, 88, 90–91, 92

Eastern Woodlands Indians, 440
East India Company, 236
East Indies, 29, 88, 119, 120
Ecogonine, 463, 464, 467, 475, 476–477, 480
Ecogonine model of coca chewing, 463–481
Economic botany, 185
Ecuador, 440, 444, 446, 463
Efe, 100–101
Effects of cannabis, 2, 6–9, 59, 61, 69, 98, 100, 106–107, 108–109, 128–129, 130–131, 137–140, 142, 163, 164–165, 168, 169, 180, 181, 199, 215–216, 217, 221, 222, 223–224, 225, 228, 229–230, 231, 244–245, 250, 251, 260, 269–287, 293, 296–301, 303, 306, 314, 327, 328, 330, 332, 334–337, 339–342, 345–354, 355–387, 389–398, 486, 488–489, 491–492, 493, 501, 508, 510–512, 516, 521, 522, 524, 525, 526, 527, 528, 531, 535, 539, 542, 543, 544
Effects of cannabis, criminal, 7, 59, 61, 69, 130–131, 168, 181, 208, 215, 222, 223–224, 225, 228, 229, 231, 244–245, 296–297, 301, 314, 340–341, 350, 367, 368, 488, 499, 511, 521, 522, 526
Effects of cannabis, pathological brain damage, 9, 108–109, 199, 392, 394–397
Effects of cannabis, pharmacological, 269–287, 293, 299, 492, 493, 516, 522, 524, 525, 531, 539, 542, 543
Effects of cannabis, physiological, 4, 6, 8–9, 69, 100, 108–109, 199, 244, 250, 293, 298, 303, 306, 327, 330, 334–337,

339, 340–342, 345–354, 355–358, 364–365, 367–368, 369–387, 389, 391–398, 488, 492, 493, 499, 511, 525, 526
Effects of cannabis, productivity and, 6, 9, 98, 128-129, 163, 222, 223-224, 300, 355-387, 391, 486, 488-489, 526
Effects of cannabis, psychological, 6, 8–9, 69, 106–107, 108–109, 164, 199, 215, 222, 244, 251, 293, 296–297, 299–300, 301, 303, 341, 350, 355–358, 364–365, 367–368, 381, 383, 385, 387, 389, 391–398, 486, 488, 491–492, 493, 499, 511–512, 524, 525
Effects of cannabis, speaking, 137–139, 142
Effects of cannabis, subjective, 355, 356–358, 364–365, 367–368, 370, 372, 374–375, 376, 378, 379, 384–385, 386–387, 391, 489, 524, 525
Effects of chronic smoking of Cannabis in Jamaica (Rubin and Comitas), 119
"Effects of psychedelic experience on language functioning, The" (Krippner), 430
Egypt, 5, 8, 39, 41, 42, 48, 82, 84, 101, 195–204, 208, 209–210, 258, 304, 311, 312, 313, 540, 541, 542
Egyptian (people), 92, 195–204, 209–210, 311, 313, 540, 541, 542
Egyptian Islam Mufti, 203
Egyptian National Center for Social and Criminological Research, 195, 196, 200
Electric Kool-Aid acid test (Wolfe), 432
Elis (Peloponnesus), 306
Elites. *See* Attitudes, elite; Upper class
Encyclopédie méthodique (Lamarck), 29
Energy expenditure, 368–386, 489
Energy measurement, 6, 368, 369–370, 373, 376, 378, 379, 380, 381–382, 385, 468, 489
England, 5, 15
English (language), 37, 192, 501
Epirus, 310, 318–320
Erythroxylon. *See* Coca
Escalation from cannabis to other drugs, 7, 108, 298, 301, 341, 479, 513–514, 515, 516, 526
Espectador (Colombia), 160
Estonia, 43
Ethiopia, 5, 77–80, 84
Ethnic group, 211–216, 217, 225, 227–234, 306, 307–310, 550. *See also* Minority group
Ethnic group identity, 211–216, 217, 225

Ethnobotany, 2, 3, 5, 8, 63–75, 240, 419, 432
Ethnohistory, 2, 3, 5–6, 8, 81–110, 147–149, 235–237, 240, 257, 464
Ethnomedicine. *See* Folk medicine
Eurasia, 26, 403
Europa, 2–3, 4, 13–14, 16, 19, 23, 25, 28, 31, 40, 42–44, 45, 46–47, 48, 82, 88, 93, 150, 192, 212, 214–215, 227, 228, 258, 303–324, 441, 504, 505, 509. *See also* Names of individual countries
European (people), 5. 39, 43, 46, 48, 88, 89, 107, 159, 214–215, 227, 228–229, 312, 441, 452, 464, 543
Excerpt of the 1890 report of the health council (Greece), 314
Exertcitia Phytologica (Gilibert), 30
Excise taxes, 236–237, 247, 248, 252–253
Exodus (Bible), 40, 41, 44
Expressive behavior, 407
Eysenck Personality Inventory, 492

Facial Recognition Memory Test (University of Florida modified version), 396
Fad, cannabis consumption as, 8, 528, 531–544
Females, 43–44, 46–47, 68–69, 70–71, 95–96, 100, 101, 106, 121, 133–134, 141, 163–164, 179, 210–211, 213, 215, 221, 223–224, 241–243, 244, 249, 251, 265, 295, 317, 336, 363–364, 365, 369, 383, 443, 445, 447, 448, 449, 451, 478, 508
Fertility, 335–337. *See also* Sterility
Fertility rites, 404–405, 445, 451, 453, 454
Fez, Morocco, 210
Final Report (Canadian Commission of Inquiry into the Non-Medical Use of Drugs), 501
Finger Localization Test, 395–396
Finger Oscillation Test, 395
Fingo, 91, 95–96, 106
Finno-Ugrian (language), 27
Flora Europaea (Tutin, *et al.*), 13, 25, 34
Flora of the U.S.S.R. (Komarov), 34
Flora von Deutschland (Sturm), 31
Folk medicine, 3–4, 6, 7, 9–10, 39, 40, 43, 44–48, 51, 56–57, 63, 64, 67, 68, 69–73, 88, 92, 121, 124–125, 128–129, 161–162, 164, 167, 173, 174, 177–178, 180, 181, 198, 208, 210, 221, 223, 227, 230–231, 240, 247, 251, 257–258, 259, 260–261, 265, 293, 294, 295, 305–306, 310, 327, 341, 372, 401, 402, 403–404, 405–406,

408, 409–410, 412, 433, 434, 439, 441, 442, 444–457, 481, 487, 498
Folk use of cannabis, 1, 2, 3–4, 5–7, 39–48, 51–57, 63, 64, 66–75, 77, 90, 81–82, 83, 88–110, 119–131, 133–145, 148, 161–170, 173–182, 185–193, 197, 198, 207–216, 217–225, 227–234, 235–245, 247–255, 257–265, 293–296, 302–315, 327–334, 345–350, 352, 355–387, 485–494, 509, 513, 514, 532, 539–543, 544
Folk use of hallucinogens, 1, 2, 9–10, 48, 56–59, 133–145, 148–149, 174, 181, 195–196, 235–236, 257–265, 273, 294, 327–328, 333–334, 401–414, 417–436, 439–458, 534
Food scarcity hypothesis of coca, 464, 470–472, 475
Ford Foundation, 417
France, 30, 179, 186, 227, 228, 232, 233, 465, 490
French (language), 193, 501
French (people), 150, 178, 179, 211, 212–213, 227, 228, 231, 232, 233, 258–259, 490, 497–498
French Congo, 99
French Protectorate (in Indochina), 66, 73
Funeral practices and cannabis, 2, 40, 41, 42–43, 54, 258, 304

Gallup Public Opinion Index, 532, 533, 534, 537, 538, 539, 542
Ganaqua, 94
Gangs, 101, 109
"Ganja complex," 4, 5–7, 119–131, 257–265, 485–494
Ganumqua, 94
Gardener's dictionary (Miller), 15
Gene pool, 26
Genera Plantarum (Linnaeus), 16–17
Genesis (Bible), 41
Germany, 31, 43, 46, 191, 304, 541, 542
Ghana, 101–102
Glue sniffing, 108 .*See also* Volatile solvents
Goajiro, 448
Goldman Weekers adaptometer, 393
Gonaqua, 93, 104
Graeco-Latin (language), 27
Gran Chaco Indians, 448
Great Lakes region of Africa, 84–85, 86, 87
Greece, 303–324, 532, 540, 541, 542
Greek (language), 27, 40, 306, 307
Greek (people), 41, 303–324

Greek Department of the Interior, 314
Greek Orthodox Church, 311, 312
Greek Pharmacopoeia, 310
Grihya (Indian text), 235
Griqua, 105
Grower-vendor relationships, 154–155, 157
Guadeloupe, 490
Guaporé, 450, 451
Guaraní, 452–453, 457
Guyana, 440, 443, 447–448, 449, 453, 455, 456, 490

Hadza, 100
Haiti, 441, 452
Haitian ritual, 338
Hallucinatory experience, idiosyncratic, 257, 264–265, 402, 406–407, 423–425, 431, 432
Hallucinogenic themes, 401–402, 407–411, 421, 427–431, 432
Halstead Tactual Performance Test, 395
Hancumqua, 94
Handbook of pharmacology (Kostis), 310–311
Handbook of South American Indians (Steward), 174
Han dynasty, 54, 60, 62
Harmine, 405
Harvard University, 160, 524, 533
Harvesting cannabis, 15, 42, 43–44, 68, 159, 187, 295, 300
Hasan-ibn-al-Sabbah (assassins' cult), 77
Hashishin, 208
"Hash oil" (also, liquid hashish), 286, 502, 503, 504–505
Hebrew (language), 2, 40–41, 42
Hebrew (people), 41, 44
Heichware, 104
Heikum, 102
"Herb camp," 126
"Herb yard," 126
Herero, 103
Hermoupolis (capital of Syros), 310, 311–313
Heroin, 7, 181, 197, 204, 253, 254, 317, 503, 513, 515, 526. *See also* Opiates
Heusequa, 92
Himalayas, 81, 248, 249–250, 253, 504
Hindi, 4, 65, 83, 85–86, 248, 250, 487
Hindu religion, 229, 236, 237–245, 249–250, 252, 254–255
Hindus, 223, 235–245, 247–255, 490
Hippies, 197, 214, 247, 252, 253, 297,

Index of Subjects

533–539, 543–544
Holy scriptures The (Jewish Publication Society of America), 42
Honan (Chinese province), 53
Horticulturalists, 406–407
Hortus cliffortianus (Linnaeus), 16–17, 19, 27, 28
Hortus malabaricus (Rheede), 16
Hottentot, 83, 86, 87, 88–90, 92, 93, 94, 96
Hou-Han shu (history of Han dynasty), 54, 56
Houston, Texas, 532
Huantla (Mexico), 144
Huanuco (Peruvian department), 465, 480
Huichol, 9, 417–436
Human Relations Area Files, 174, 403
Hunter-gatherers, 90–91, 94–95, 100, 408, 410
Hutu, 217–225
Hybridization, 26, 32, 34, 88
Hygienic Institute of the Palacky University (Czechoslovakia), 7
Hyoscyamus, 305, 467
Hypoglycemia, 464, 472–476, 480–481

Iberian Peninsula, 175
Ica, 443
Idealistic approach, 412
Illustrated London News, 105
Incan empire, 328
Incawatana, Peru, 472–475
INCORA, 151
"Increasing menace of marijuana, The" (Canadian Medical Association), 498
India, 2, 4, 5, 6, 13, 16, 19, 24, 28, 29, 30, 48, 51, 53, 57, 60, 62, 65, 77, 82–83, 84, 85, 86, 93, 119, 120, 175, 176, 198, 227, 229, 231, 235–245, 247–249, 252, 257–258, 259, 260, 270, 273, 274, 311, 352, 487, 489, 492, 493, 509, 532, 539–540, 541, 542, 543, 553–554
Indian Hemp Commission, 4, 236, 248, 260, 487, 539–540, 541
Indians (people of India), 64, 65, 81, 92, 93, 120, 227, 228–231, 235–245, 247, 248–250, 252, 257, 260, 274, 311, 363, 487, 490, 492, 493, 541, 542, 543
Indians, American. *See* Amerindian; Mexican Indians; South American Indians
Indochina, 31, 66
Indochina, French, 66
Indo-Chinese nations, 53

Indo-European (language), 27, 39, 40
Indonesia, 29, 30
Ineffability, 430–431, 432
Institutionalization of cannabis use in Canada, 8, 512–513, 516–517
Instrumental behavior, 407, 418
Interim Report (Canadian Commission of Inquiry into the Non-Medical Use of Drugs), 501
International Association for Psychiatric Research, 303–304
International code of botanical nomenclature, 16–17
International Archiv für Ethnographie, 104
International drug control, 107, 192–193, 197, 236–237, 247, 253–254. 502–506, 522, 529, 556. *See also* Legal status of cannabis
Interpol, 197
Intoxicants Act (Nepal), 252–253
Intoxicants Rules (Nepal), 252–253
Ionian Islands, 307, 310, 318–320
Iquitos, Peru, 402, 405–406
Iran, 214
Iron Age, 84–85, 91
Ishihara plates, 392
Islam, 62, 199, 203, 208, 209, 212, 236, 308
Israel, 44, 207–216
Italy, 310

Jamaica, 5, 6–7, 119–131, 257–265, 355–387, 390, 398, 485–494, 504, 509, 527, 540, 541, 542, 553–554
Japan, 212
Jeremiah (Bible), 41
Jerusalem, 214, 306
Jewish law, 209
Jewish Publication Society of America, 42
Jews, 42, 207–216, 532
Jívaro, 443, 444, 445, 447, 455, 457
Joint Legislative Commission to Revise the Penal Code (California), 550–551
Ju-Chia. *See* Confucianism
Jumla area (Nepal), 252
Juruá-Purús area, 450

Kaffir, 91
Kalahari, 85, 94, 102
Kalamata, Greece, 319
Kali, cult of, 229
Kansas State University, 32
Kasai (province in Zaire), 99
Kashmir, 62

Index of Subjects

Kastro area (Syros), 312
Kathmandu, Nepal, 248, 249, 250, 252–253, 254
Kayastha (Hindu caste), 238, 239
Ketama, Morocco, 186–188, 192
Khanpur region, Pakistan, 246–248
Khmer (language), 65
Khmer (people), 63–75
Khoikhoi, 90–91, 92–95, 100, 101, 103, 104
Khoikoin, 90
Khoisan, 90, 93
Killie Campbell Africana Library, 81
Kilwa, 84, 85, 87
Kingarawanda, 219
Kingston, Jamaica, 123, 124
Kofrani-Michaelis respirometer, 369–371, 373, 376, 379, 380, 381
Kogi, 443
Koran, 208, 210, 212, 309
Korea, 212
Korsakoff syndrome, 299
Koryak, 403
Kshatriya (Hindu castes), 238, 241
!Kung Bushmen, 102

La Española, 452
La Estrella, Colombia, 328
Lahore, Pakistan, 346–348
Lalibela Cave (Ethiopia), 77–80
Lamba, 86
Laos, 63–68, 72–73, 74
Latin America, 8, 328, 390. *See also* Central America; Mexico; South America
Latins (Romans), 306
Latvia, 43
League of Nations, 107, 217. *See also* United Nations
League of Nations Advisory Committee on Traffic in Opium and Dangerous Drugs, 107
Lebanon, 210, 286
Lectotype, 17–18, 19, 28. *See also* Type specimen
Le Dain Commission. *See* Canadian Commission of Inquiry into the Non-Medical Use of Drugs
Legal status of cannabis, 2, 3, 6, 8, 24, 27, 46, 66, 67, 70, 82, 83, 93, 99, 101–102, 105, 106, 107–108, 119, 120, 121, 122–123, 125, 129, 130–131, 149, 155, 156, 160–161, 166–167, 175, 178, 181–182, 185, 188, 189, 190, 191–193, 199, 203–204, 208, 209–210, 215, 232–234, 236–237, 247, 252–255, 257, 260, 261, 286, 294–295, 297, 300, 314, 315, 328, 363, 365, 366–367, 390, 398, 485–486, 497–501, 505, 506, 508, 512–513, 516–517, 521–529, 532, 533, 544, 549–557
Legal status of cannabis in Africa, 93, 99, 101–102, 105, 106, 107–108
Legal status of cannabis in Brazil, 175, 178, 194–295, 297, 300
Legal status of cannabis in Canada, 497–501, 506, 508, 512–513, 516–517, 554, 555
Legal status of cannabis in Colombia, 149, 155, 156, 166–167, 328, 553–554, 556
Legal status of cannabis in Costa Rica, 149, 390, 398, 553–555
Legal status of cannabis in Denmark, 556
Legal status of cannabis in Egypt, 199, 203–204, 210
Legal status of cannabis in Greece, 314, 315
Legal status of cannabis in India, 236–237, 553–554
Legal status of cannabis in Israel, 215
Legal status of cannabis in Jamaica, 119, 120, 121, 122–123, 125, 129, 130–131, 257, 260, 261, 363, 365, 366–367, 553–554
Legal status of cannabis in Morocco, 185, 188, 189, 190, 191–193
Legal status of cannabis in Muslim society, 82, 189, 190, 208, 209–210
Legal status of cannabis in Nepal, 247, 252–255
Legal status of cannabis in Réunion, 232–234
Legal status of cannabis in Southeast Asia, 66, 67, 70, 75
Legal status of cannabis in Spain, 191
Legal status of cannabis in the Netherlands, 556
Legal status of cannabis in the United States, 500, 512–529, 532, 533, 544, 549–557
Legal systems, typology of, 554–555
Leopard-men Society (secret society of Nigeria), 101
Lesotho, 96
Le Tiers Livre des Faictz et Dictz Héroiques du Noble Pantagruel (Rabelais), 14
Liberia, 79, 87
Li Chi (Book of Rites), 54, 55

Index of Subjects

Linguistic studies, 2, 27, 39–41, 47, 51, 54, 55, 57, 58, 61, 63, 64–66, 83–84, 85–90, 100, 120, 148, 176–177. 227–228, 293–294, 305, 439, 487
Linnaeus's classification of cannabis, 13, 16–19, 27–29, 35
Linnean Herbarium, 27, 28
Linnean Society of London, 18, 27, 28
"Liquid hash." *See* "Hash oil"
Lisbon, Portugal, 5, 175
Literature, ancient, 2–3, 39–41, 51, 52, 53–56, 61, 77, 208–209, 235–236, 340, 257–258, 304, 305–307, 308
Lithuania, 30, 43, 46
Lloyd-Haldane gas analysis apparatus, 369–371, 373, 381
Lone user. *See* Solitary use of psychogenic agents
Lophoro williamsii. See Peyote
Los Angeles Police Department, 499
Lower class. *See* Working class
LSD, 7, 108, 197, 259, 264, 274, 280–281, 335, 339, 341, 407, 409, 410, 421, 514, 515, 516, 526, 533–536
Luba, 87–88, 99
Lung-shan, 53

Macedonia, 310, 318–320
Macropsia, 403, 409
Macumba (Brazilian sect), 179, 294
Madagascar, 29, 83–84, 227–228
Magars, 251–252
Magdalena (Colombian department), 164
Magdalena River valley, 149
Mahatari (district of Nepal), 248
Makololo, 98
Malagasy, 227–228, 229, 231
Malawi, 98, 104
Malaysia, 68
Males, 6–7, 44, 47, 68, 74, 95–96, 100, 101, 106, 108, 120–121, 126–128, 129–130, 133–134, 141, 155, 162–163, 164, 190, 191–192, 210, 213, 215, 221, 223–224, 232, 242–243, 244, 247, 249, 250–251, 257, 261–265, 317–324, 327, 333, 339, 345–350, 363–364, 368–369, 371–386, 391, 443, 444, 445, 446–448, 449, 451, 478, 480, 491, 508, 527, 532
Mandragora, 305
Mandukya Upanishad, 418
Man-plant relationship, 21–23, 25–26, 35, 51, 52, 54, 182, 227, 233
Mantinea, Greece, 313–314

Manual laborers, 4, 6
Maranhão (Brazilian state), 174
Margarita Island Indians, 449
Marginality, 101, 130, 157, 168, 169, 188, 203–204, 214–216, 232, 259, 296–297, 301, 327, 391, 448
"Marihuana complex," 4, 7, 259, 265
Marihuana Tax Act (United States), 259, 260
Marital status and cannabis use, 167–168, 200, 321, 523
Markets, sale of cannabis in, 63, 66, 187–189. *See also* Distribution of cannabis
Martinique, 490
Masaba (Africa), 100
Masara (Indian intoxicant), 235–236
Mashonaland, 98
Massachusetts, 277
Matabele, 85, 97, 103, 104
Materia medica (Dioscorides), 305
Mauritius, 228, 323, 233
Maya, 410, 456
Mayor's Committee on Marihuana (New York), 355, 356, 532, 539, 541
Mbyá, 452–453
Mecca, 191
Medeans (Medes), 41
Medellín, Colombia, 332, 335, 336, 339
Medical, Dental, and Pharmacy Act (South Africa), 107–108
Medicinal uses of cannabis. *See* Uses of cannabis, medicinal
Mediterranean region, 53, 304–305
Men. *See* Males
Mescaline, 259, 264, 273, 274, 339, 504, 532, 533, 536. *See also Trichocereus pachanoi*
Mesopotamia, 306
Methadone, 513
Mexican (people), 7, 133–145, 412, 417–436
Mexican-Americans, 259, 532
Mexican Indians, 133–142, 417–436, 440, 450
Mexico, 133–145, 148, 153, 417–436, 440, 450, 504, 540
Mexico City, 142
Michigan, 549–550
Micropsia, 403, 409
Middle America, 452
Middle classes, 4, 7–8, 150–152, 197, 198, 199–200, 215, 232, 247, 253, 259, 261, 265, 297–298, 300–301, 311–312, 315, 320, 329–330, 332, 336, 341, 390, 402,

489, 490–491, 493–494, 497, 508, 515, 531–544
Middle East, 82, 101, 124, 151, 207–216, 270, 304–305, 312, 504,
Migration, 2–3, 4, 5, 41–43, 51, 57, 81, 82–88, 90–91, 93, 95, 97–98, 101, 148–149, 153, 158, 167–168, 169, 191, 199, 207–216, 227–229, 232, 248–249, 257, 258, 260, 293–294, 296, 306–307, 310, 311, 312, 313, 315, 317–321, 333, 384, 386, 489
Ming-i pieh-lu (T'ao), 56
Minnesota Multiphasic Personality Inventory (MMPI), 439
Minni (Medea), 41
Minority group, 8, 62, 107–108, 120, 209, 211–216, 217–225, 228, 315, 531–532, 537, 543. See also Ethnic group
Mishna, 41
Mississippi, 24, 32
Mochica culture, 440
Moghal dynasty (India), 236
Monark ergometer, 370
Monastiraki, Greece, 309
Mongoloid people, 248
Monotypic species, 3, 13, 16, 21, 23–27, 35, 52, 77, 270, 549
Montagnard Tribes, 73
Montaña region of South America, 443, 446, 450, 456, 457, 464, 480
Montpellier Botanical Garden (France), 31
Montreal, 498–499
Moors, 258
Moraceae, 34
Moravia, 46
Morning glories, 454–455
Moroccan Jews, 207–216
Morocco, 6–7, 185–193, 198, 207–208, 209–214, 540, 541, 542
Morphine, 74, 204, 214, 274, 314, 526. See also Opiates
Motivational syndrome, 119, 129
Motives for beginning cannabis use, expressed, 201, 202, 348
Movement, organization of, 371–382, 385–386
Mozambique, 83, 96
Mubanbi (Africa), 99
Multidisciplinary approach, 1–2, 6, 9, 260, 355, 387, 486–487
Multiple drug use, 108, 109, 298, 299, 301, 335, 336, 339, 488, 497, 513–517, 522, 553

Mundurucú, 456, 457
Mushrooms, 144–145, 240, 333, 403–404, 409, 454–455
Music and use of hallucinogens, 408–409, 414
Muslims, 82, 84, 92, 189, 190, 208–214, 215, 216, 228, 236, 239, 306, 307–310, 490, 543
Mwami, 224
Mysiri, 313

Nama, 89, 90, 94
Namaqua, 94
Namkunqua, 94
Narcotic Control Act (Canada), 500
Narcotics subculture, 197
Nariño group (Colombia), 337
Natal, 96, 109
National commissions on drug use, 1, 2, 7, 497, 501, 506–508, 521–529, 550–557. See also Canadian Commission of Inquiry into the Non-Medical Use of Drugs; Indian Hemp Commission; United States National Commission on Marihuana and Drug Abuse
National Institute of Mental Health (United States), 81, 109, 119, 147, 260, 269, 303–304, 357, 389, 486–487, 527, 531
National Institute of Personnel Research (South Africa), 108–109
National Institute on Drug Abuse (United States), 269
National Institutes of Health (United States), 24, 173
National Museum of Natural History (France), 73
National Panchayat of Nepal, 253
National Press (Portugal), 175
Nature of cultural things, The (Harris), 371
Navpaktos, Greece, 311
Near East, 2, 6, 39, 40–42, 44–45, 48
Necromancy, 51, 56. See also Divination; Shaman; Witchcraft
Neolithic, 2, 3, 51, 52, 53–54, 57
Nepal, 6–7, 237, 247–255
Nepali (language), 250
Netherlands, 556
Network, 6–7, 109, 123–124, 125–128, 129–130, 164, 211, 329, 368, 370, 387, 391, 503–504, 516
Neuropsychological tests, 392–393, 394–397

Newari (language), 250
New Jersey, 277
New Orleans, 259
New World, 5, 48, 78, 120, 149, 174, 258, 409, 439, 440, 449–450, 454–455, 464, 497–498
Ngoni, 104
Nguni, 91, 95–96, 103
Nicaragua, 464
Nigeria, 101
Nile Delta (Egypt), 82
Nomothetic theory, 412
Norte de Santander (Colombian department, 153, 159
North America, 4, 5, 8, 23, 121, 148, 262–263, 270, 440, 441, 450, 497–517, 521–529, 532–544, 549–557
North Americans, 150, 151, 152, 159, 178, 197, 242, 253, 259, 296, 333–334, 432, 497–517, 521–529, 531–544, 549–557
Nova Scotia, 497
Nuñoa (Peruvian district), 479
Nutrition, 241, 293, 297, 298, 327, 334, 368, 369–370, 373, 374, 383, 391, 463, 464, 470–481, 489
Nyamwezi, 99
Nzega, Rwanda, 223

Odozi-Obodo (secret society in Nigeria), 101
Old Testament. *See* Bible
Old World, 4, 9–10, 48, 53, 441, 449–450
On hashish: a report by the Mayor of Orchomenus in Montinea, 313–314
O nordeste (Freyre), 175
On rivers' and mountains' names (Plutarch), 305
Ontaria (Canadian province), 501
Opiates, 70, 72, 197, 470, 498, 499–500, 514, 515, 516–517, 543. *See also* Heroin; Morphine; Opium
Opium, 3, 52, 59, 61–62, 66, 67, 68, 70, 72, 74, 92, 107, 108, 197, 201, 203, 208, 210, 214, 215, 236–237, 251, 280–281, 307, 309, 348, 499–500. *See also* Opiates
Opium and Narcotic Drug Act (Canada), 499–500
Oracles, ancient Greek, 305
Oral tradition, 2–3, 51, 56
Orange Free State, 91, 93
Orchomenus, Greece, 313–314
Oregon, 555, 556

Organized crime, 181, 497, 503–504, 506, 554
Origin of cannabis, 2–3, 13, 16, 19, 21, 22, 23, 25, 27, 39, 47–48, 51–62, 63, 64, 77, 80, 81–82, 84, 110, 191, 248, 257, 270, 304–305
Orinoco region, 442, 449, 450
Otis Group Intelligence Test, 394–395
Otomac, 451
Ottawa, Canada, 498
Ottoman Empire, 303, 307–310
Ova herero, 94
Ovambo, 94
Overseas Hindustan Times, 237

Pacific Coast group (Colombia), 337
Páez, 449
Pakistan, 6–7, 8–9, 345–354
Palestine, 2, 39, 41–42
Panama, 149
Panama Canal, 149
"Panhuman yearning for paradise," 427–428
Panaons, 450
Pantagruelion, 13, 14, 19, 258
Paper, invention of, 54
Pará (Brazilian state), 174
Paradigm, shared, 412
Paradigm of reality, scientific, 407, 410
Paranormal phenomena, 407, 410–411, 538–539
Paricá. *See Anadenanthera*
Paris, 4, 259
Parsa (district of Nepal), 248
Partial prohibition model, 522, 528–529
Pasi (Hindu caste), 239, 243, 244
Pastoralists, 403–405. *See also* African herders
Patras, Greece, 310, 316
Pazaryk (Siberia), 42
Peasants, 4, 6, 39, 40, 42–44, 46–47, 48, 63–75, 151, 152, 153, 154–155, 157–159, 160, 161, 162–170, 185–193, 264, 295, 317, 320, 333, 401, 405, 410, 463–481. *See also* Rural sector
Peer group, 6–7, 126–128, 129–130, 167, 192, 198, 261–264, 487–488, 516, 542
Peloponnesus, 306, 310, 311, 312, 313–314, 318–320
Pemba, 84, 87
Pennsylvania, 277
Pentecostal Church in Jamaica, 123
Pen-ts'ao Ching (earliest Chinese pharmacopoeia), 51, 56

Pen-ts'ao kang-mu (li), 56
Pergamum, 306
Peripatetic School, 305
Pernambuco (Brazilian state), 174
Persia, 28, 82-83, 84, 85, 86, 95, 102, 208, 214, 311
Persian (language), 40
Personality as factor in reaction to cannabis, 293, 297, 299-300, 301, 492, 511-512
Personality factors in choice between cannabis and alcohol, 485, 492-493
Peru, 148, 402, 405-406, 440, 442, 446, 450, 457, 463-481
Peruvian Indians, 402, 405-406, 440, 442, 446, 450, 457, 463-481
Peruvian Mestizos, 402, 405-406
Peyote, 2, 9, 10, 259, 273, 339, 417-436, 454-455, 532, 533, 536
Pharmacology (Afendoulis), 311
Philippines, 29
Phoenician (people), 42, 211
Phnom Penh, Cambodia, 66
Physiological factors in hallucinatory patterns, 407, 409, 427, 435
Pipes, 5, 45, 48, 65, 68, 69, 71, 77-80, 81, 82, 83, 84-85, 86, 95-97, 98-99, 100-106, 107, 124, 178, 179, 187, 200, 202, 203, 210, 214, 219, 221-223, 224, 235, 240, 241-242, 243, 244, 250-251, 253, 260, 261, 295, 451-452, 487, 509, 510
Piraeus, Greece, 312-313, 314, 316-320
Piraeus Metrolpolitan Police, 316
Piro, 443
Plains Indians, 257, 262-263
Poland, 43, 44, 46
Polytypic, 3, 13, 21, 24-36, 52, 77, 549
Ponducherry (India), 29
Pontos (Greece), 312
Population Registration Act (South Africa), 105
Port, Réunion, 232
Portland State College (Oregon), 78
Portugal, 5, 174-176
Portuguese (people), 5, 64, 65, 83, 90, 96, 99, 174-176, 293
Portuguese royal court, 5, 174-176, 178
Potency of cannabis, effects of preparation on, 269-278, 502, 510
Power broker, 123
Power structure, use of psychogenic agents as threat to, 311, 181, 203, 410, 521, 528, 552-555, 556-557
Practical guide to the drug scene, A

(Leech), 334
Preadaptation, 23
Pretoria Mental Hospital, 106-107
Priests, 4, 6, 133-141, 198, 229-230. *See also* Ritual specialists
Prison populations, studies of, 173, 176, 180, 195-204, 244-245, 296-297, 298
Productivity. *See* Effects of cannabis, productivity and
Prostitution, 179, 199, 113, 214, 232, 296-297
Protestantism, 212, 523
Prusa, 309, 313
Psara (Greek island), 311
Psilocin 533
Psilocybin, 259, 264, 533
Psychedelic ethos, 499, 533, 536, 537, 544
Psychedelic subculture, 197, 531, 532-539, 543-544
Psychic unity, 418
Psychological set, 356, 386, 423-414, 492
Psychosis, 8-9, 106, 293, 299-300, 301, 314, 488, 491, 512, 525
Publicity as a factor in use of psychoactive agents, 329-333, 339, 499, 533-534, 535, 536
Pygmies, 100-101

Qolla, 472-475
Quebec, 498
Quechuans, 450

Race and cannabis use, 523, 532
Racism, 7, 131, 499
Rajasthan, India, 249
Rajput (Hindu caste), 249, 492, 493, 543
Ras Tafarians (Jamaica), 363, 487, 488
Rate of incidence of cannabis, 8, 120-121, 127-128, 130, 315, 327, 328-334, 338-341, 342, 363, 491, 497, 498-499, 506-508, 512, 515, 522, 523, 528, 531-532, 534, 535, 537-538, 539-540, 542-544
Raven's Progressive Matrices, 396
Readers' guide to periodical literature, 535
Rebetiko music (Greek), 312-313, 314
Religious affiliation and cannabis use in the United States, 523
"*Remarques historiques sur les mots 'plantes males' et 'plantes femelles'*" (Saint-Lager), 15
Report of the Indian Hemp Drugs Commission 1893-1894, 4
Reproductive isolation, 25, 26
Research Institute for the Study of Man

Index of Subjects 593

(United States), 119, 120, 124, 126, 260, 383, 385, 486–487, 527
Resources, pressure on, 383–386, 489
Rhytmic movement. *See* Movement, organization of Réunion, 8, 227–234
Rg Veda, 240
Rhapta (Africa), 84
Rhodes (Greek island), 311
Rhodesia, 91, 97–98, 104
Rhône basin (France), 15, 304
Rif Mountains (Morocco), 185–193
Río de Janeiro, 5, 175, 294–295, 296
Río Grande del Norte (Brazilian state), 174
Rites of passage, 45, 129, 257, 260, 261, 264, 327, 488
Ritual, 2–4, 6, 9–10, 39, 40–45, 48, 57, 60, 73, 123, 130, 154, 155, 163, 164, 165, 170, 174, 178, 179, 181, 190, 196, 198, 203, 208, 209, 221–222, 227, 229–230, 231, 233, 235–236, 239–240, 242, 247, 249–251, 263, 264, 293, 294, 295, 304, 305, 307, 309, 327, 338, 390, 401, 402–406, 408–411, 412, 413–414, 417–436, 439–458, 465, 534
Ritual process, The (Turner), 429
Ritual specialists, 2, 9, 51, 57, 62, 73, 74, 123, 243, 258, 402, 403–406, 408, 409–411, 412, 413–414, 419–436, 442, 444, 446–458, 534. *See also* Priests
Role model, 126, 201–202, 487, 490
Role validation, 6, 257, 261–264, 488, 494
Roman Empire, 304
Royal Canadian Mounted Police, 498–499, 502, 503
Royal Society of London, 19
Rumania, 311
Rural sector, 4, 5, 6, 109, 120–131, 147–170, 187–188, 200–202, 232, 260–261, 264, 293–296, 301, 312, 317–320, 327–342, 345–354, 355–387, 507–508, 545 *See also* Peasants
Russia, 4, 5, 24, 31, 32, 42–43, 46, 47, 258, 304–305, 311, 403
Russia, mushrooms and history (Wasson and Wasson), 403
Russian botanical studies, 3, 21, 24–25, 31–32, 33–34, 47
Rwabda, 217–225

Sahara, 45, 101
Saint-Denis, Réunion, 232
Salonika, 214
San, 90, 93, 94–95, 100, 102, 103, 104

San Agustín culture, 328
Sanctions, 6, 8, 24, 66, 82, 99, 105, 107–108, 120, 122–123, 130–131, 149, 155, 160–161, 166–167, 175, 178, 185, 189, 190, 192, 198–199, 202, 203, 204, 208, 209–210, 232–233, 235, 238–239, 243–244, 247, 252–255, 261, 294–295, 297, 300 309, 315, 316, 327, 328, 329, 330–332, 339, 340, 342, 362, 365, 366–367, 368, 390, 398, 410, 485–486, 494, 497–501, 506, 511, 512, 516, 521–522, 527–529, 532, 533, 549–557
Sanctions, legal, 6, 8, 24, 66, 82, 93, 99, 105, 107–108, 120, 122, 123, 125, 130–131, 149, 155, 160–161, 166–167, 175, 178, 189, 190, 192, 198–199, 203, 204, 232–233, 247, 252–255, 294–295, 297, 300, 315, 316, 328, 329, 330–332, 340, 324, 363, 365–367, 390, 398, 410, 485–486, 494, 497–501, 506, 511, 512, 516, 521–522, 527–529, 532, 533, 549–557
Sanctions, religious, 185, 198, 190, 198–199, 203, 208, 209–210, 236, 238–239, 309, 327, 329, 339
Santions, social, 8, 166–167, 209, 235, 238–239, 243–244, 261, 329, 512, 516, 528–529, 533, 556
Sandawe, 100
San Francisco, 532, 533, 534
San José, Costa Rica, 389, 397, 398
Sanskrit, 40, 63, 64, 65
Santa Marta, Colombia, 148, 149, 152
Santander (Colombian department), 153
Santos, Brazil, 296
São Paulo, Brazil, 296
Satapatha brahmana, 240
Satz Block Rotation Test, 396
Satz Neuropsychology Laboratory (University of Florida), 395, 397
Saudi Arabia, 82, 85
"Savage thought," 423
Schizophrenia, 299–300, 301, 492
Schizothymic personality, 492–493
Screening mechanism, 7, 261, 488, 494
Scythian (language), 40–41
Scythian (people), 2, 39, 40–43, 77, 209, 258, 304, 305, 307
Secret society, 99, 101
Selection, 21, 22, 25, 26, 35
Selection, natural, 22
Semite, 2–3, 41
Semitic languages, 39, 40–41
Sena (Africa), 84
Senusi, 45

Index of Subjects

Septuagint, 40
Serbia, 46
Seres (Peloponnesians), 306
Sergipe (Brazilian state), 174
Sex differences in cannabis use, 68–69, 74, 100, 101, 121, 141, 164, 179, 221, 249, 251, 317, 345, 363–364, 508, 523, 532
Sex differences in tobacco use, 166, 443, 445, 451
Sexual abstinence and use of hallucinogens, 411, 413–414, 421
Sexual dimorphism of cannabis, 14–19, 51, 54, 55, 64–65, 67–68, 70, 270, 366
Shagana-Tsonga, 402, 404–405
Shaman, 2, 9, 51, 57, 62, 258, 402, 403–406, 409–411, 412, 419–436, 442, 444, 446–458, 534. *See also* Priests; Ritual specialists
Shangaan (language), 83
Shi Ching (Book of Odes), 55
Shivites, 229, 249–250
Shona, 83, 85
Short account of the Cape of Good Hope and of the Hottentots who inhabit that region, A (Ten Rhyne), 92
Shudre (Hindu castes), 238, 241, 243
Siam, 68
Siberia, 30, 31, 42, 52, 258, 402, 403–404
Siberian (people), 42, 402, 403–404
Sierra Nevada (South America), 153, 154, 157, 160, 443
Sinai desert, 214
Singha Durbar (Nepal secretariat), 255
Sinkiang (Chinese province), 62
Sino-Iranica (Laufer), 53
Siraha (district of Nepal), 248
Six Day War, 214
Slavs, 43
Small Parts Manual Dexterity Test, 395
Smyrna, 309, 313
Social apathy, 203–204. *See also* A-motivational syndrome
Social caste and cannabis use, 217–225, 237–245, 249, 250–251, 252, 489, 543
Social class, 2, 4, 5–6, 7–8, 9, 51, 57–59, 108, 109, 119–131, 161, 178–179, 197–198, 199–200, 202–203, 210, 214–215, 231, 232–233, 257–265, 293–301, 309, 311–315, 317, 319–321, 327, 328, 329–330, 332, 336, 338–339, 340, 341, 346–347, 390–391, 398, 410, 485–494, 497, 501, 508, 515, 524–525, 531–544
Social class and cannabis use, 2, 4, 5–6, 7–8, 9, 108, 109, 119–131, 161–165, 166–170, 178–179, 191–192, 197–198, 199–200, 202–203, 210, 214–215, 231, 232–233, 257–265, 293–301, 309, 313–315, 319–321, 327, 328, 329–330, 332, 338–339, 340, 390–391, 398, 485–494, 497, 501, 508, 515, 523–525, 531–544
Social class and *Wu-Shih san* use, 51, 57–59
Social group cohesion and cannabis, 4, 6–7, 43–44, 45, 48, 63, 74, 109, 126–128, 129–130, 161, 198, 202–203, 214–216, 241, 247, 250–251, 261–264, 366, 374–375, 376, 380, 386, 489, 510, 511, 524, 525
Social mobility, 119, 128, 130, 169, 232, 261, 488, 489
Social setting, 6–7, 43–44, 48, 74, 109, 126–128, 129–130, 191–192, 201–210, 241–242, 261–265, 295, 297, 348, 366, 372, 374–375, 386, 413, 414, 487–488, 490, 492, 508–509, 510, 511, 512, 524, 525
Sociocultural factors in reaction to cannabis, 2, 6, 10, 143, 180–181, 257–265, 492
Sociocultural factors in reaction to psychogenic agents, 2, 6, 10, 143, 180–181, 196, 257–265, 300, 301, 401–414, 417–419, 432
Sociocultural factors in use or nonuse of cannabis, 2, 51–52, 57–62, 109, 189–192, 195, 196–204, 207–216, 217–225, 227–234, 235–245, 249–255, 257–265, 293–301, 303–324, 327, 328–334, 337–341, 342, 355, 382–387, 485–494, 508, 516, 523–525, 531–544, 549–557
Sofala (Africa), 84, 91
Solanoids, 305, 467
Solitary use of psychogenic agents, 7, 43–44, 48, 163, 170, 201, 297, 366, 372, 377, 379, 510
Soma, 235, 240, 305
Soma: divine mushroom of immortality (Wasson), 240
Sortilèges (Leblond), 231
Sotho, 86–87, 96, 98, 103
South Africa, 6–7, 89, 100, 105–109
South African Institute of Medical Research, 106
South African Medical Congress, 106
South African Medical Journal, 108
South African Minister of the Interior, 106
South African Museum, 102

Index of Subjects

South African Secretary of Social Welfare and Pensions, 109
South America, 23, 88, 147–170, 173–182, 293–301, 327–342, 439–458, 463–481. *See also* Names of individual countries
South American Indians, 9, 173–174, 264, 294, 402, 405–406, 439–458, 463–481, 490
Southeast Asia, 6–7, 63–75, 77, 504
Spain, 5, 48, 85, 148, 186, 191, 258
Spanish (language), 193, 397
Spanish (people), 5, 9, 64, 148–150, 186, 191–192, 258
Spanish Civil War, 191
Spanish Protectorate (in Morocco), 186, 191–192
Spanish Republican Army, 191
Spatial distortion, 59, 355, 356
Species plantarum (Linnaeus), 13, 16–18, 27–28, 29
"Speed." *See* Amphatemines
Spontaneous abortion, 8, 327, 335–337, 342
Srautasutras (Indian text), 235–236
Stability of cannabis preparations, 273–276, 277–278
Stanford-Binet Intelligence Test, 394–395
State Hospital at Tashkent (U.S.S.R.), 46
Statistics Canada, 512
Sterility, 9, 306. *See also* Fertility
Strandloopers, 90–91
Stream of consciousness, 355, 356, 364, 368, 370, 386–387
Stress, 169, 170, 176, 181–182, 300, 337, 473–474
Stress, physiological, 473–474
Stress, psychological, 169, 300, 337
Stress, social, 169, 170, 176, 181–182, 300
Stress and cannabis use, 169, 170, 176, 181–182, 300
Subcultural groups, 147–170, 303, 486, 488, 531–539, 554. *See also* Middle class; Minority group; Peasants; Upper class; Working class
Subjective reality, 356, 492–493
Sudanese, 294
Sura (Indian intoxicant), 235–236
Surat, India, 228
Swahili, 85, 86, 87, 99, 101, 223
Swazi, 86, 91, 96, 97, 102
Sweden, 28
Swiss, 44
Switzerland, 46
Syracuse (Greek city-state), 304

Syria, 5, 42, 199, 309
Syrians, 306
Syros (Greece), 303, 310, 311–313

Tamil-Nadu traditions, 229, 231
T'ang dynasty, 57
Tantric ritual, 250
Tanzania, 99, 100
Taoism, 60
Tarahumara, 435
Targuist, Morocco, 186
Taxonomy, 3, 13–19, 21–36, 52, 77, 88, 89, 270, 549–550
Tembu, 91
Temporal distortion, 56, 59, 142, 355, 356, 368
Tenetehara, 174
Teratogenic effect, 275, 327, 334, 335–337, 342
Terai (Nepal), 248, 251
Tetuan (Moroccan province), 187
Teutonic (language), 27
Thailand, 63–75
THC (tetrahydrocannabinol), 9, 78–79, 98, 261, 265, 269–287, 334–335, 356, 372, 378, 502, 505, 509, 510–511, 525, 531–542, 544
Theory of drug-induced hallucinations, 401, 411–414
Thessaloniki, Greece, 318, 319, 320
Thonga, 83, 85, 103
Thought content, 377, 378
Thrace, 304, 305, 307, 310, 318–320
Tibet, 212, 248
Tibetan (people), 53, 248
Tibet autonomous Region of the People's Republic of China, 248
Tibeto-Burman language, 250
Tiempo (Colombia), 160
Tierra del Fuego, 442
Times of India, 237
Tobacco, 1, 2, 3, 9–10, 47, 48, 51–52, 59, 63, 65, 67, 68, 71, 72, 78, 79, 80, 84, 86, 87, 89, 92, 93, 94, 95–96, 97, 99, 100, 103, 104, 105, 124, 149, 159, 162, 163, 165, 166, 170, 174, 175, 178, 179, 181, 187–188, 189, 210, 221, 230, 235, 240, 241, 242, 243, 264, 280, 294, 327, 328, 363, 373, 391, 403, 439–458, 510, 513–514, 515, 516, 526
Tobacco, ritual use of, 2, 9–10, 48, 174, 181, 230, 264, 327, 439–458
Tobacco, secular use of, 9–10, 181, 441–442, 457

Index of Subjects

Tobacco chewing, 9, 439, 442, 448–449, 455
Tobacco drinking, 439, 442, 443–448, 455, 456, 457
Tobacco smoking, 48, 63, 65, 67, 68, 71, 72, 78, 79, 80, 86, 87, 89, 92, 94–96, 97, 99, 103, 104, 124, 149, 163, 166, 175, 178, 179, 187, 189, 210, 221, 230, 235, 240, 241, 242, 243, 294, 363, 373, 439, 440, 441–442, 445, 451–454, 455–457, 510, 514
Tobacco snuffing, 48, 87, 96, 97, 149, 439, 442, 449–451, 455, 456
Tonkin (Vietnam), 73
Toronto, 498, 499, 507, 508, 514, 555
Trade, 3, 4, 5, 41, 42, 45, 48, 82, 83–85, 93–95, 99, 101, 107–108, 121, 148, 156, 157, 228, 258, 296, 297, 300, 304–305, 311–313, 329, 435
Trancaucasia, 47
Transcedence of time and space, 429, 432
Transvaal, 91, 104, 402, 404–405
Treatment report (Canadian Commission of Inquiry into the Non-Medical Use of Drugs), 501
Trichocereus pachanoi (mescaline cactus), 405, 442. See also Mescaline
Trinidad, 490
Tswana, 96, 103, 104
Tukano, 449, 450, 451, 454
Tupari, 451
Tupi, 452
Tupians, 440
Tupinambá, 456–457
Turkey, 84, 192, 214, 315, 532
Turkish (language), 27
Turks, 84, 306, 307–310, 311
Tutsi, 217–225
Twa, 217–225
Type specimen, 28–32, 33. See also Lectotype
Tyre, 42

Uigur, 62
Ukraine, 43, 44, 46
Umbanda (Brazilian sect), 179, 294
Underground cookbooks, 281
Union of Soviet Socialist Republics, 46, 554. See also Russia
United Fruit Company, 150–153, 155, 156, 169
United Kingdom, 121, 236
United Nations, 196, 217, 247, 254, 465, 466, 471–472, 480. See also League of Nations
United Nations Bulletin on Narcotics, 196
United Nations Commission of Enquiry on the Coca-Leaf, 465, 466, 471–472, 480
United Nations International Narcotics Control Board, 254
United Provinces Excise Act IV (India), 236–237
United States, 4, 7–8, 32, 107, 150, 151, 152, 155, 160, 165, 166, 169, 177, 197, 199–200, 214–215, 247, 253, 259, 260, 269, 270, 272, 273–274, 276–277, 303, 329, 332–333, 339, 377, 398, 432, 465, 479, 490, 493–494, 498, 499, 500, 501, 502, 504, 505, 514, 521–529, 531–544, 549–553, 554, 555–557. See also Names of individual states
United States Bureau of Narcotics, 540
United States Congress, 521, 522, 526–527, 549
United States Department of Agriculture, 160, 369
United States Department of Agriculture Handbook No. 8, 369
United States Department of Health, Education, and Welfare, 163, 165, 270, 272, 356, 527, 540
United States Food and Drug Administration, 269, 527
United States National Commission on Marihuana and Drug Abuse, 165, 401–402, 521–529, 537, 538, 539, 541, 542, 543, 550–551, 552–553
United States Pharmacopoeia, 259, 273–274
United States Public Health Service, 269
United States Virgin Islands, 490
Unity against Marihuana (Colombia), 340–341
Universidad del Valle (Colombia), 341
University of Athens, 303, 310
University of California, Los Angeles, 408, 417, 458
University of Florida, 389, 395, 396, 397
University of Ghana, 78
University of Manitoba, 463
University of Massachusetts, 119
University of Miami, 126
University of the West Indies, 119, 260, 369, 370, 383, 485, 486–487
Untouchable castes, 238, 241, 243
Upper class, 4, 6, 7, 51, 57–59, 108, 130–131, 150–152, 156–157, 159, 160, 165–

Index of Subjects 597

166, 169, 170, 178–179, 190, 199, 210, 231, 297–298, 300–301, 309, 312, 315, 317, 320, 327, 329–330, 332, 336, 338–339, 390, 410, 531, 532, 535–536, 537
Urals, 47
Urbanization process, 317–318
Urban sector, 4, 5, 106, 109, 120, 156–157, 158, 159, 163–164, 167, 187–189, 190, 200–202, 212–213, 214, 215, 228, 232, 233, 247, 260, 264, 294–301, 311–324, 327–342, 345–354, 507–508, 509
Urticaceae (Nettle family), 34
Uses of cannabis, 1, 2–4, 5, 6, 7–8, 13–14, 22, 30, 35, 39–48, 51–62, 63, 64, 66–75, 81–82, 83, 88–89, 97, 98, 99, 100, 106–108, 109, 119, 121, 124–125, 128–129, 133–145, 148–149, 161–163, 167, 170, 173, 175, 177–178, 179–180, 181, 185, 186, 187, 190, 196–199, 201, 202, 208, 209, 210–211, 215–216, 221, 223, 227, 229–231, 233, 235, 239–241, 247–252, 253, 259–261, 264–265, 293–296, 304, 305–306, 307, 309, 310–311, 314, 327, 338, 341, 372, 398, 487, 489, 497–517, 521–529, 531–532, 535, 544
Uses of cannabis, food, 1, 3–4, 22, 43, 46, 47–48, 51, 52, 54–56, 63, 66, 68, 73, 74, 121, 124, 125, 173, 210, 240–241, 251–252, 257–258, 259–261, 311
Uses of cannabis, manufacturing, 4, 5, 13, 22, 73, 148, 187, 257–258, 304, 305–306, 497–498
Uses of cannabis, medicinal, 1, 2, 3–4, 6, 7, 22, 35, 39, 40, 43, 44–48, 51, 52, 56–57, 63, 64, 67–68, 69–73, 82, 88–89, 121, 124–125, 128–129, 161, 167, 170, 173, 177–178, 179, 180, 181, 198, 202, 208, 210, 221, 223, 227, 230–231, 247, 251, 257–258, 259–261, 265, 293, 294, 295, 305–306, 307, 310–311, 327, 341, 372, 487, 498
Uses of cannabis, mind-altering, 1, 3–4, 6, 7–8, 13–14, 22, 30, 35, 40, 42, 43–44, 45–48, 51–52, 56–57, 63, 67–69, 74–75, 83, 89, 97, 98, 99, 100, 106–108, 109, 148–149, 161–163, 167, 170, 173, 175, 177–178, 179, 180, 181, 185, 186, 190, 196–199, 201, 202, 208, 209, 210–211, 215–216, 223, 227, 231, 233, 247, 249–252, 257–261, 264–265, 294–296, 304, 305, 307, 314, 327, 487, 489, 497–517, 521–529, 531–532, 535, 544
Uses of cannabis, ritual, 2–4, 6, 39, 40–45, 48, 57, 73, 97, 133–145, 178, 179, 181,
190, 198, 208, 209, 227, 229–230, 231, 233, 235, 239–240, 247–251, 257–258, 260, 293, 294, 304, 305, 307, 309, 338
Use of cannabis, textile, 1, 2, 3–4, 5, 13, 22, 41, 42, 51, 52–54, 55, 73, 81–82, 83, 148, 173, 187, 209, 249, 257–258, 304, 305–306, 498
Uses of cannabis, work-aiding, 6, 63, 74, 98, 119, 128–129, 161, 163, 167, 170, 223, 264–265, 398, 487, 489, 544
Utah, 532

Vaisya (Hindu caste), 243
Vancouver, 498–499
Variability of cannabis, 21–36, 52
Vedic texts, 45, 77, 240, 258
Veeder-Root counter, 395
Venda, 86, 97, 103
Vendor-client networks, 123–124, 125–126, 127, 232
Venezuela, 156, 264, 443, 463, 464
Venitions, 311
Verbal Memory Task, 397
Veterinary practices, 4, 46, 230–231, 247, 251
Vicos, Peru, 478
Videotape, 6, 163, 355, 368–371, 372, 376, 381, 385, 489
Vietnam, 63–67, 72, 73, 536, 538
Virgin Islands. *See* United States Virgin Islands
Virola, 450
Visions, 6, 9, 134, 137, 138–140, 142, 143–145, 165, 180–181, 208, 257–265, 273, 356, 401–414, 417–436, 443–444, 445–447, 449, 451, 452–453, 454–456, 457
Visual distortion, 165, 356, 392–393
Visual Reaction Times, 397
Vocabulaire de la langue de Madagascar (Drury), 227–228
Volatile solvents, 513–514. *See also* Glue sniffing
Volga region (Russia), 31
Voortrekkerhoogte (South African military academy), 108

Wad Ghis (Morocco), 186
Wad Nkqur (Morocco), 186
Waiwai, 456
Warao Indians, 264, 442, 453, 455, 456–457
Wechsler-Bellevue Intelligence Test, 394–395

Wechsler Memory Scale, 397
Wenner-Gren Foundation for Anthropological Research, 185
Western influence in secularization of tobacco use, 441–442
Western influence on use of psychoactive agents, 4, 7, 8, 52, 59, 65–66, 75, 107, 159, 178, 190, 191–193, 214–216, 227, 231–233, 247, 252–254, 296, 333–334, 350, 532
West Indies, 5, 6–7, 119–131, 151, 257–265, 355–387, 390, 398, 440, 450, 485–494, 504, 509, 527, 540, 541, 542, 553–554
Wild populations of cannabis, study of, 3, 21–26, 31, 34, 47, 52, 64
Wilmersdorf, Germany, 304
Wilson Memorial Hospital (Johnson City, New York), 78
Windsor, Canada, 498
Wirikuta, 419–436
Witchcraft, 44, 402, 405–406, 409, 410, 411, 446, 449, 453, 456
Witoto, 443, 444–445
Women. *See* Females
Wooton Commission (England), 550
Work groups, 6–7, 125, 127, 130, 155, 156, 162–163, 164, 167–168, 170, 374–375, 376, 380, 390
Working class, 4, 5, 6, 7, 8, 119–131, 150–152, 155–156, 157, 160, 161, 162–170, 179, 198, 199, 210, 214–215, 228, 231, 232, 233, 257–265, 293, 296–298, 300, 301, 312–315, 317–324, 327, 329–330, 332, 338, 340, 341, 346–347, 390, 398, 487–494, 515, 531, 535–536, 537, 543, 544
World Health Organization (WHO), 192, 356
Worldview, 417–436
Wu-shih san (Chinese drug), 51, 57–59

Xango, 179
Xhosa, 91, 95–96, 105

Yang-shao, 53
Yanoama, 449
Yin-Shang, 57
Youth "drug culture," 1, 4, 7–8, 106, 108, 181, 197–198, 199–200, 203–204, 214–215, 227, 232–233, 247, 252–253, 259, 269, 280–281, 293, 297–298, 300–301, 315, 327, 328–334, 338–340, 350, 390, 432, 497–517, 521–529, 531–544
Yurak Samoyed, 404

Zaire, 86, 99, 100
Zamal (Albany), 231
Zambezi River region, 84–85, 86, 102, 104
Zambia, 86, 98
Zanzibar (Africa), 83, 84, 85, 86, 87, 99
Zend-Avesta, 45
Zulu, 85, 86, 91, 96–97, 103, 104, 105, 109

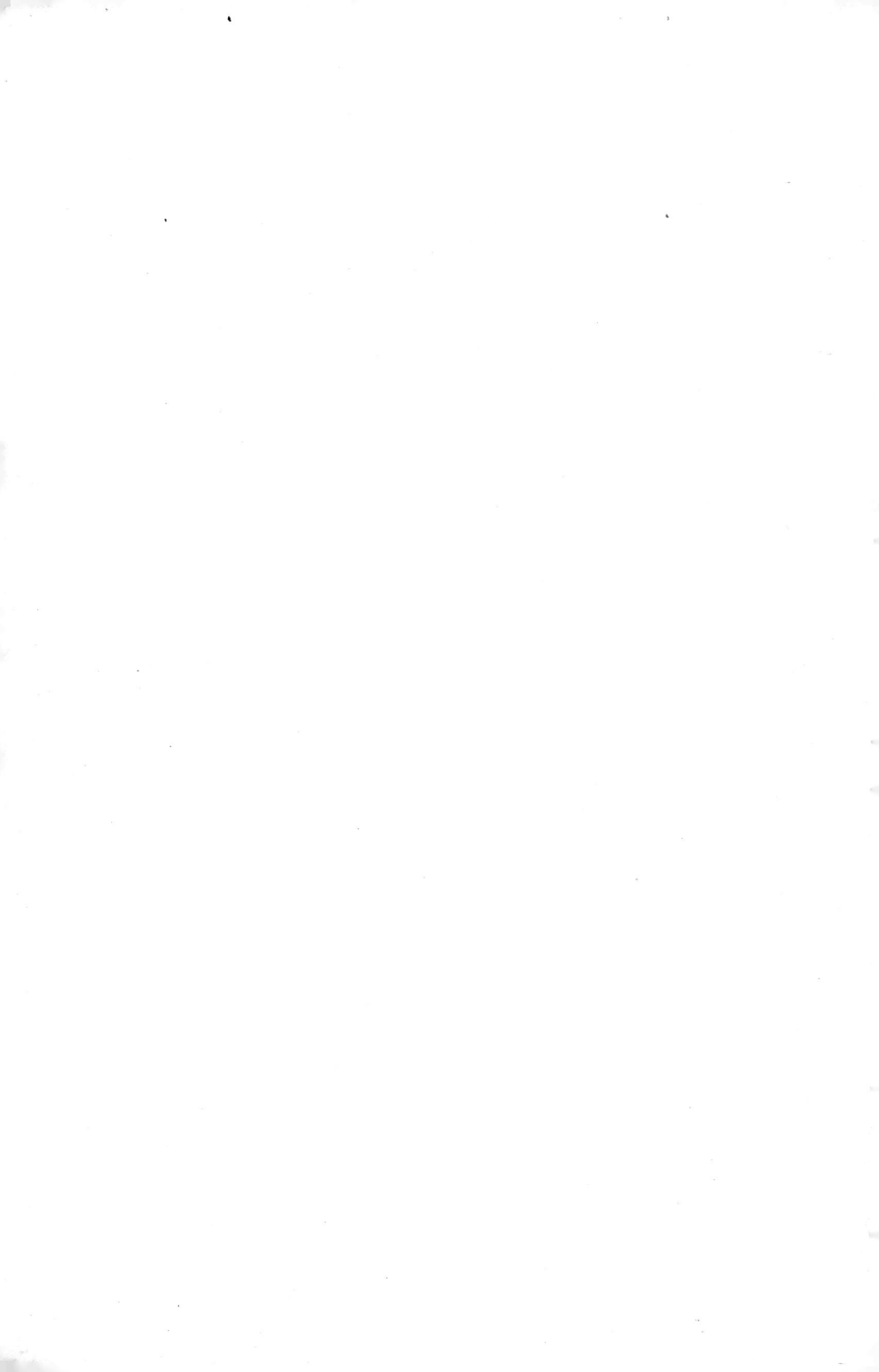